Essentials of Surgical Pediatric Pathology

D1388614

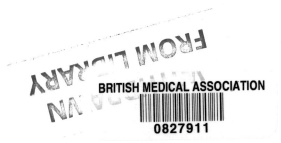

Essentials of Surgical Pediatric Pathology

Edited by

Marta C. Cohen
Consultant Paediatric and Perinatal Histopathologist at Sheffield Children's Hospital; Honorary Senior Lecturer, University of Sheffield, UK

Irene Scheimberg
Consultant Paediatric and Perinatal Pathologist, Royal London Hospital, Barts Health NHS Trust;
Honorary Senior Lecturer, Barts Medical School, Queen Mary University, London, UK

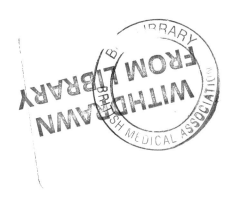

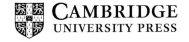

CAMBRIDGE
UNIVERSITY PRESS

CAMBRIDGE
UNIVERSITY PRESS

University Printing House, Cambridge CB2 8BS, United Kingdom

Cambridge University Press is part of the University of Cambridge.

It furthers the University's mission by disseminating knowledge in the pursuit of education, learning and research at the highest international levels of excellence.

www.cambridge.org
Information on this title: www.cambridge.org/9781107430808

© Cambridge University Press 2014

First published 2014

Printed in Spain by Grafos SA, Arte sobre papel

A catalog record for this publication is available from the British Library

Library of Congress Cataloging in Publication data
Essentials of pediatric surgical pathology / edited by Marta C. Cohen, Irene Scheimberg.
    p.   ;   cm.
Includes bibliographical references and index.
ISBN 978-1-107-43080-8 (mixed media)
I. Cohen, Marta C., 1961– editor.   II. Scheimberg, Irene, editor.
[DNLM: 1. Pathology, Surgical – methods.   2. Pediatrics. WO 925]
RD57
617.1'07–dc23

2014010863

ISBN 978-1-107-43080-8 Mixed Media
ISBN 978-1-107-66752-5 Paperback
ISBN 978-1-107-43077-8 (DVD)

Contents

Contributors

Rita Alaggio
Anatomia Patologica,
University of Padova,
Padova, Italy

Paula Borralho
Professor of Anatomical Pathology,
Lisbon University & Lisbon School of Health
Technology and Department of Anatomical
Pathology, Hospital and Descobertas, Lisbon, Portugal

Marie-Anne Brundler
Professor,
Departments of Pathology and Laboratory
Medicine, and Paediatrics,
Alberta Children's Hospital,
Calgary, Alberta, Canada

Mariana M. Cajaiba
Assistant Professor of Pathology and
Laboratory Medicine, Ann and Robert
Lurie Children's Hospital of Chicago,
Northwestern University Feinberg School of
Medicine, Chicago, IL, USA

Eumenia Castro
Assistant Professor,
Texas Children's Hospital,
Baylor College of Medicine,
Houston, TX, USA

Justin M. M. Cates
Associate Professor,
Department of Pathology,
Microbiology and Immunology,
Vanderbilt University Medical Center,
Nashville, TN, USA

Allison Cavallo
Department of Pathology,
University of Chicago Medical Center,
Chicago, IL, USA

Cheryl M. Coffin
Retired Clinical Professor of Pathology,
(volunteer)
Microbiology and Immunology,
Vanderbilt University,
Nashville, TN, USA

Marta C. Cohen
Consultant Paediatric and Perinatal
Histopathologist,
Sheffield Children's Hospital NHS FT;
Honorary Senior Lecturer,
University of Sheffield,
Sheffield, UK

Isabel Colmenero
Consultant Paediatric Pathologist,
Birmingham Children's Hospital,
Birmingham, UK

Aurore Coulomb
Department of Histopathology,
Hospital Armand Trosseau,
Paris, France

Jane E. Dahlstrom
Professor of Anatomical Pathology,
Australian National University Medical
School,
Canberra, ACT, Australia

María T. G. de Dávila
Patóloga Pediátrica,
Hospital Nacional de Pediatría
"Dr Prof J. P. Garrahan",
Buenos Aires, Argentina

Derek de Sa
Professor Emeritus of Pathology,
University of British Columbia
Children's and Women's Health Centre,
Vancouver, BC, Canada

Gail Deutsch
Associate Professor,
University of Washington,
Department of Laboratories,
Seattle Children's Hospital,
Seattle, WA, USA

Paul S. Dickman
Professor,
Department of Child Health,
University of Arizona College of Medicine,
Phoenix;
Clinical Professor,
Departments of Pathology and Pediatrics,
University of Arizona College of Medicine,
Tucson;
Professor,
Department of Pathology,
Mayo Clinic College of Medicine;
Department of Pathology and Laboratory Medicine,
Phoenix Children's Hospital,
Phoenix, AZ, USA

Paola Domizio
Professor of Pathology Education,
Barts and the London Hospital and Queen
Mary's School of Medicine and
Dentistry,
London, UK

Julie C. Fanburg-Smith
Professor of Pathology GUH, HUH, USUHS,
Department of Anatomic and Clinical Pathology,
Sibley Memorial Hospital of Johns Hopkins
Medicine,
Surgical Pathology Consultation Services,
Orthopedic, Soft Tissue and Surgical
Pathology Consultant,
Washington, DC, USA

Laura Galluzzo
Patóloga Pediátrica,
Hospital Nacional de Pediatría "Dr Prof J. P.
Garrahan",
Buenos Aires, Argentina

Katja Gwin
Assistant Professor of Pathology,
University of Texas Southwestern Medical
Center at Dallas,
Dallas, TX, USA

Riitta Karikoski
Head of Department
Department of Pathology,
of Kanta - Häme Central Hospital,
Hämeenlinna, Finland

Roman Kodet
Head,
Department of Pathology and Molecular
Medicine,
Charles University Prague,
Prague, Czech Republic

Megan S. Lim
Professor,
Department of Pathology,
University of Michigan Medical School,
Ann Arbor, MI, USA

Dolores López-Terrada
Professor of Pathology and Pediatrics,
Baylor College of Medicine, and
Director, Molecular Oncology and Cancer
Cytogenetics,
Texas Children's Hospital Department of Medicine,
Houston, TX, USA

Fabiana Lubieniecki
Patóloga Pediátrica- Neuropatología,
Hospital Nacional de Pediatría "Dr. Prof. J. P.
Garrahan",
Buenos Aires, Argentina

Pamela Lyle
Bay Pines VA Healthcare System,
St. Petersburg, FL, USA

Jo McPartland
Consultant Paediatric Pathologist,
Alder Hey Children's Hospital NHS Foundation
Trust,
Liverpool, UK

Bo-Yee Ngan
Assistant Professor,
Department of Laboratory Medicine and
Pathobiology,
University of Toronto;
Division of Pathology,
Department of Pediatric Laboratory Medicine,
Hospital for Sick Children,
Toronto, Ontario, Canada

Luc Laurier Oligny
Associate Director, and Associate Professor,
Department of Pathology and Cellular Biology,
University of Montreal;
Head,
Department of Pathology, CHU Sainte-Justine,
Montreal, Quebec, Canada

David A. Ramsay
Neuropathologist,
Department of Pathology,
University Hospital,
London Health Sciences Centre,
London, Ontario, Canada

Miguel Reyes-Múgica
Marjory K. Harmer Endowed Chair in Pediatric Pathology,
Chief of Pathology and Head of Laboratories,
Children's Hospital of Pittsburgh of UPMC;
Professor of Pathology,
University of Pittsburgh School of Medicine,
Pittsburgh, PA, USA

Erin R. Rudzinski
Assistant Professor,
Department of Laboratories,
Seattle Children's Hospital,
Seattle, WA, USA

Melinda E. Sanders
Associate Professor,
Department of Pathology, Microbiology and
Immunology,
Vanderbilt University Medical Center,
Nashville, TN, USA

Irene Scheimberg
Consultant Paediatric and Perinatal Pathologist,
Royal London Hospital,
Barts Health NHS Trust;
Honorary Senior Lecturer,
Barts Medical School,
Queen Mary University,
London, UK

Rajeev Shukla
Consultant Paediatric Pathologist,
Alder Hey Children's Hospital NHS
Foundation Trust,
Liverpool, UK

Naveena Singh
Consultant Pathologist,
Department of Cellular Pathology,
Barts Health NHS Trust,
London, UK

Alena Skálová
Professor,
Department of Pathology,
Charles University Prague,
Faculty of Medicine in Plzen,
Plzen, Czech Republic

Jens Stahlschmidt
Consultant Pediatric
Histopathologist,
Leeds Teaching Hospital NHS
Foundation Trust,
Leeds, UK

Antonio Torrelo
Pediatric Dermatologist and Head of
the Department of Pediatric
Dermatology,
Hospital Niño Jesús,
Madrid, Spain

Jo-Anne Vergilio
Assistant Professor,
Department of Pathology,
University of Michigan Health System,
Ann Arbor, MI, USA

Gordan Vujanic
Professor of Pediatric Pathology,
Institute of Cancer and Genetics,
Cardiff University School of Medicine,
Cardiff, UK

Foreword

Essentials of Surgical Pathology has been written for general pathologists who occasionally encounter pediatric cases in the course of their mainly "adult" work, and for pediatric pathologists in training.

Babies and children are not "small" adults. The incidence, rarity, and peculiarity of many diseases and conditions are such that they justify the need for a different subspecialty. However, the practice of pediatric pathology is not always carried out in specialist centers where experts in this discipline are available. This is true in many countries around the world where there are few exclusively pediatric hospitals. Referral centers may be far away and it is not always possible to send these cases for second opinion.

Essentials in Surgical Pathology is designed and written as a practical bench-book, where experts in the relevant field write each chapter.

The book is organized by systems, except for individual chapters dedicated to typical pediatric tumors. Children's tumors are rare. They are of different types and have different morphological features from adults. The book includes a chapter those in dedicated to small round blue cell tumors, which are almost always found in children and only occasionally in adults. Soft tissue tumors, another difficult area in pediatric pathology, has its own chapter. The chapter dealing with skin pathology, a subject deserving a whole book, prioritizes skin diseases found in children, many of which have a genetic component. This is true of all the systemic chapters where the authors concentrate on predominantly pediatric diseases.

The authors aim to describe the most common and important conditions found in pediatric patients. The book does not pretend to have in-depth understanding of each condition. A very complete list of references may guide interested pathologists.

We are grateful to our colleagues and friends who agreed to co-author the chapters that constitute *Essentials in Surgical Pathology*. We are indebted to them for their skillful contribution, thoughtful advice and enduring patience, which helped us shape the book that we initially envisioned two-and-a-half years ago. Pediatric and fetal autopsies have been covered in the companion book *The Pediatric and Perinatal Autopsy Manual*.

Marta Cohen dedicates this book to her parents, Elsa and Ramon Cohen, who as pediatricians nurtured and encouraged her love for pediatric medicine. She also dedicates the book to Roc Kaschula, her mentor during her time as a young trainee in Cape Town, South Africa, whose inspiration, careful guidance, and continuous friendship have influenced all her accomplishments.

Irene Scheimberg dedicates this book to her wonderful parents Rosa and Augusto, excellent clinicians in their own fields, and to Fernando Paradinas, whose knowledge and love of pathology inspired her to pursue this exciting career path.

Sincere thanks are due to our families: our spouses and children, who provided the necessary emotional support while being deprived of invaluable family-time during week-ends and holidays.

Preface

Of all the subspecialties into which the discipline of pathology has been segmented, some with better justification than others, one of the most distinct is that of pediatric and developmental pathology (PDP), especially the latter. To begin with, a perinatal autopsy in this field requires knowledge of two "specimens" (the placenta and the fetus/neonate), plus the connector that joins them. In the case of surgical specimens, one needs to always be mindful of the ever-changing features of the growing tissues as they undergo development. Secondly, it calls for expertise in matters which are usually of generally less import in adult pathology, such as embryology, physiology, cytogenetics, and special branches of bacteriology.

Most importantly, an autopsy in PDP has, more often than not, a greater clinical relevance than its adult counterpart, as attested by the genuine interest of pediatricians and obstetricians in the autopsy findings and the high percentage of such autopsies that are carried out in general hospitals. Whereas the number of adult autopsies keeps decreasing despite the constant pleas of pathologists, no such solicitation is needed from their PDP counterparts.

The special standing that PDP has in the wide field of pathology is also borne out by disorders exclusive of this specialty, such as rare cancers, early pregnancy loss, intrauterine growth restriction, *hydrops fetalis*, and twin pregnancies.

Equally unique is the area of placental pathology, which in expert hands can provide a wealth of clinico-pathologic correlations and morphologic clues to specific inflammatory condition in the infant.

Another area in which PDP reigns supreme is that of the congenital anomalies and metabolic disorders. Yet another, perhaps the most difficult to master, is that of congenital heart defects and associated syndromes. I will never forget watching, as a first-year resident, a perinatal autopsy demonstration by an expert in congenital heart disease, and how the intricated physiopathology of that particular cardiopathy came alive by the master rotating the specimen, inserting fingers, and pointing to bundles of hypertrophic muscle, holes that should not be there, and missing components of the organ. Which reminds me of the comment made by a famous pathologist to the effect that the expert in pathology is not necessarily the one who finds extraneous tissues, but the one who notices the absence of an important piece of the anatomy.

And what about the enigmatic infant sudden death syndrome? Isn't PDP the best team equipped to elucidate once and for all the pathogenesis of this disastrous event?

This wealth of opportunities is skillfully covered in this attractive book by Dr. Marta Cohen and Irene Scheimberg, two UK-based PDP of Argentinian background, a fact worth mentioning because of the great tradition of excellence in PDP in that country, exemplified by representatives of the caliber of Luis Becù, Roberto Gallo, and Ricardo Drut. The editors have garnered a cadre of experts in pediatric surgical pathology, covering the most salient points of the wide spectrum of pediatric and developmental surgical pathology. This volume is complementary to the book dedicated to *Pediatric and Developmental Postmortem Pathology*, also edited by Drs. Cohen and Scheimberg.

Overall, this clearly written and well-organized book should be an ideal introduction to the field of pediatric and developmental surgical pathology for general pathologists, and perhaps induce some of them to consider becoming members of this outstanding league of specialists. If they do, they will not be disappointed.

Juan Rosai, MD
Milano, Italy

Skin

Isabel Colmenero, Antonio Torrelo, and Miguel Reyes-Múgica

Skin diseases are very frequent in children. Most of them, including the most common disorders, such as atopic dermatitis, hemangiomas, nevi, acne, or bacterial and viral infections, are readily diagnosed through an adequate anamnesis and clinical examination. However, some skin tumors and inflammatory disorders may require a biopsy. The patient's age and relevant clinical history, in addition to the site from which the skin biopsy was obtained, should be known by the pathologist.

A sound basis of pediatric dermatological epidemiology is necessary, since the entities most frequently observed in children differ significantly from those seen in adults.

The specimens and biopsies most frequently sent for histopathological analysis in children are melanocytic nevi, inflammatory dermatoses such as Henoch–Schönlein purpura, psoriasis, pityriasis lichenoides, pityriasis rosea, lichen planus, pityriasis rubra pilaris, erythema multiforme, atopic dermatitis, granuloma annulare, and pigmented purpuric dermatosis, as well as infections, vascular anomalies and benign tumors/hamartomas/cysts. Genodermatosis and malignancies are rarely seen.

In this chapter, we will be dealing with the histopathology features of the most commonly biopsied skin diseases in children.

Inflammatory skin disorders

We will follow the pattern analysis approach and discuss an important example in each pattern.

Spongiotic dermatitis

Spongiotic dermatitis (SD) is defined by the presence of intraepidermal intercellular edema. Pronounced spongiosis results in the formation of intraepithelial spongiotic vesicles. When large enough, these vesicles can be grossly appreciated. These vesicles contain lymphocytes and/or Langerhans cells in most cases, but sometimes eosinophils or neutrophils can be the dominant element. spongiotic dermatitis is further subclassified into acute, subacute, and chronic. As the lesions progress, the spongiosis decreases and parakeratosis appears. In the late stage the spongiosis is mild to absent, but there is pronounced irregular acanthosis, hyperkeratosis, and parakeratosis.

The pattern of SD is caused by a variety of clinical conditions. These include atopic dermatitis, allergic/contact dermatitis, nummular dermatitis, dyshidrotic dermatitis, seborrheic dermatitis, drug reactions, Id reaction, dermatophytosis, miliaria, Gianotti–Crosti syndrome, and pityriasis rosea (1). The differential diagnosis of spongiotic dermatitis is shown in Table 1.1.

Atopic dermatitis is the most prevalent cause of spongiotic dermatitis, and is generally diagnosed clinically; however, some atypical cases can occasionally undergo biopsy.

Atopic dermatitis (AD)

Atopic dermatitis is a chronic, eczematous condition of the skin, often related to atopic states (including asthma, hay fever, and other allergic diseases).

Clinical presentation: Atopic dermatitis affects 5–15% of children in the industrialized world. Its prevalence has increased steadily in recent years, to become the most prevalent skin disease in children. The main clinical features include a combination of eczema, prurigo, and lichenification. It usually runs a chronic course with exacerbations. Most cases of AD begin in infancy with head and face eczema that can spread to the extensor areas of the limbs and trunk. By the age of two, the typical flexural involvement

Table 1.1 Spongiotic dermatitis

Usual type spongiotic dermatitis (spongiosis distributed randomly through the epidermis with no specific localization)
- Contact dermatitis
- Pompholyx
- Juvenile plantar dermatosis
- Autoeczematization ("id" reaction)
- Papular acrodermatitis of childhood (Gianotti–Crosti)
- Spongiotic drug reactions

Miliarial spongiosis (intraepidermal edema centered on the acrosyringium)
- Miliaria rubra

Follicular spongiosis (intercellular edema in the follicular infundibulum)
- Infundibulofolliculitis
- Atopic dermatitis
- Apocrine miliaria
- Eosinophilic folliculitis

Pityriasiform spongiosis (microvesicles within areas of spongiosis that contain lymphocytes, histiocytes, and Langerhans cells)
- Pityriasis rosea
- Pityriasiform drug reaction
- Erythema annulare centrifugum
- Nummular dermatitis
- Lichen striatus

Neutrophilic spongiosis
- Pustular psoriasis
- Pemphigus foliaceus
- IgA pemphigus
- Infantile acropustulosis
- Acute generalized exanthematous pustulosis
- Palmoplantar pustulosis
- Staphylococcal toxic shock syndrome
- Dermatophytoses and candidiasis
- Pustular contact dermatitis
- Periodic fever syndromes

Eosinophilic spongiosis
- Pemphigus
- Bullous pemphigoid
- Allergic contact dermatitis
- Atopic dermatitis
- Arthropod bites
- Eosinophilic folliculitis
- Incontinentia pigmenti (first stage)
- Drug reactions
- Autoeczematization ("id" reaction)
- Still's disease
- Wells' syndrome

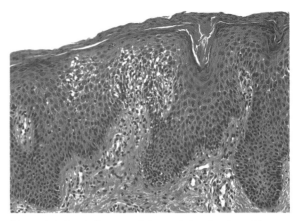

Figure 1.1 Atopic dermatitis. Subacute lesion showing mild spongiosis, exocytosis of lymphocytes, and parakeratosis, in a perifollicular distribution.

Genetics: Atopic dermatitis is due to a genetic defect in the skin barrier. In about 40% of patients, a semi-dominant genetic defect in the FLG gene, encoding the epidermal protein filaggrin, is responsible. Deficient filaggrin function leads to weaker corneocytes and skin barrier derangement, thus leading to an increased passage of irritants and allergens throughout the epidermis, and to a higher adherence of bacteria due to impaired natural immunity (3,4).

Classification: Atopic dermatitis is a heterogeneous disease; different types of genetic defects are supposed to result in an epidermal barrier defect. Most types of eczema in infants are regarded as "atopic," although there may be clinical differences that might reflect different genetic backgrounds.

Histology: Atopic dermatitis cannot be reliably or consistently distinguished from other forms of eczematous dermatitis based on assessment of histopathological features alone. Biopsies of atopic dermatitis are usually taken from subacute or chronic lesions, so parakeratosis, epidermal hyperplasia, and superimposed features of lichen simplex chronicus are typical, rather than prominent spongiosis (Figure 1.1). Secondary impetiginization with Staphylococcus aureus or secondary herpes simplex virus infection (eczema herpeticum) may occur.

Psoriasiform dermatitis

Psoriasiform dermatitis is characterized by the presence of regular epidermal hyperplasia, elongation of the rete ridges, hyperkeratosis, and parakeratosis. Thinning of the suprapapillary plates, a superficial

affecting mainly the elbow and knee folds is patent. Chronic disease and a vicious circle of itch and scratch lead to a typical thickening of the skin named lichenification. Prurigo lesions, consisting of papules and papulo-vesicles scattered throughout the skin surface are also common in older children and adolescents (2).

Table 1.2 Psoriasiform dermatitis

- Psoriasis
- Psoriasiform drug eruption
- Pityriasis rubra pilaris
- Lichen simplex chronicus
- Chronic spongiotic dermatitides
- Erythroderma
- Pityriasis lichenoides chronica
- Inflammatory linear verrucous epidermal nevus
- Chronic fungal infections
- Lamellar ichthyosis
- Secondary syphilis
- Pellagra and other nutritional deficiencies

Table 1.3 Interface dermatitis

Interface dermatitis, vacuolar-type
- Erythema multiforme
- Erythema multiforme-like drug eruption
- Fixed drug eruption
- Lichen sclerosis et atrophicus
- Erythema dyschromicum perstans
- Lupus erythematosus
- Dermatomyositis
- Viral exanthemas
- Phototoxic dermatitis
- Acute radiation dermatitis
- Acute graft vs. host disease

Interface dermatitis, lichenoid-type
- Lichen planus
- Lichenoid drug eruption
- Lupus erythematosus
- Chronic graft vs. host disease
- Lichen nitidus
- Pigmented purpuric dermatosis
- Pityriasis lichenoides chronica
- HIV dermatitis
- Syphilis
- Mycosis fungoides
- Urticaria pigmentosa

perivascular inflammatory cell infiltrate, and dilated, tortuous blood vessels within these papillae are also present. Numerous conditions can result in psoriasiform dermatitis (Table 1.2).

Psoriasis

Psoriasis is a common, chronic, relapsing, papulosquamous disorder of the skin with highly variable presentation.

Clinical presentation: Psoriasis is very common, and around 20% of cases begin in childhood or adolescence. The main clinical feature is the psoriatic plaque. It appears as an erythematous, flat-topped plaque, with thick, adherent scales, generally on the extensor surfaces of the elbows and knees, but areas such as the scalp, trunk, arms, legs, and virtually any part of the skin surface can be affected. The extension of the disease may range from a very few plaques to whole skin involvement (5).

Genetics: Psoriasis' heterogeneity and multiple gene involvement make it difficult to establish a clear genetic base of the disease. Certain genes are known to predispose to psoriasis, and there is a strong relationship with genes involved in the immune response.

Classification: Plaque-type psoriasis is the most common variant. Other variants include pustular psoriasis, with a predominance of pustules usually arranged in arcs and annuli; erythrodermic psoriasis, with erythema and scales covering more than 95% of the body surface; palmo-plantar psoriasis, with variable presentations including plaques and pustules; and psoriatic arthritis, among many others.

Histology: Fully developed lesions exhibit parakeratosis with neutrophils, hypogranulosis, psoriasiform hyperplasia, thinning of suprapapillary plates, tortuous blood vessels within papillary dermal tips, and

superficial perivascular predominantly lymphocytic dermal infiltrates. Neutrophilic spongiosis, intraepidermal spongiform pustules (of Kogoj), and neutrophil aggregates in the stratum corneum (Munro microabscesses) can also be present.

Interface dermatitis

Interface dermatitis is characterized by epidermal basal cell damage, which may be manifested by cell death, basal vacuolar change, or both. The basal cell death usually presents in the form of Civatte bodies (shrunken eosinophilic cells with pyknotic nuclear remnants) scattered along the epidermal basal layer. Based on the pattern of inflammation, interface dermatitis can be divided in two groups: vacuolar and lichenoid. Vacuolar interface dermatitis (such as erythema multiforme) is characterized by sparse inflammation along the dermo-epidermal junction. Lichenoid interface reactions (such as pityriasis lichenoides) are characterized by a denser band-like infiltrate (6). Differential diagnosis of interface dermatitis in pediatric patients is displayed in Table 1.3.

Erythema multiforme (EM)

Erythema multiforme (minor) is an acute, self-limited, and sometimes recurring reactive condition of the skin due to direct infection by herpes simplex virus (HSV).

Clinical presentation: Target lesions, consisting of a central papule or vesicle, a surrounding pale elevation and peripheral erythema, are the hallmark of the disease. They appear in attacks of cropped lesions, affecting mainly the cheeks, forearms, hands, and palms, but they may also involve the elbows, knees, and feet. The lesions usually disappear in 2–3 weeks without scarring. They may be preceded or coincide with a typical HSV on the lips, but may appear without any visible HSV infection or recurrence; polymerase chain reaction (PCR) has revealed HSV viral DNA in erythema multiforme lesions.

Classification: There has been considerable confusion and overlapping with two other conditions, erythema multiforme major and Stevens–Johnson syndrome (SJS). In erythema multiforme major, mucosal involvement of at least three different mucosae is seen, mainly the oral, eye, and genital mucosae. Some cases of erythema multiforme major in children are related to HSV infection, but also to mycoplasma and drugs. Stevens–Johnson syndrome shows preferential mucosal involvement with purpuric target-like lesions that resemble toxic epidermal necrolysis (TEN); in fact, SJS and TEN are part of the same disease spectrum. Toxic epidermal necrolysis is the most severe reaction, defined as widespread sloughing of the epidermal surface on greater than 10% of the total body surface area. The cause of TEN and SJS is drug intake, but there may be cases of SJS related to HSV (7,8).

Histology: Erythema multiforme is the prototypical vacuolar interface dermatitis showing a lymphocytic infiltrate along the dermo-epidermal junction associated with vacuolar degeneration and apoptotic basal keratinocytes. Because most cases present acutely, there is usually "basket weave" orthokeratosis. Occasionally, severe papillary edema is present. A mild-to-moderate lymphocytic infiltrate around the superficial vascular plexuses is also seen. As the lesions progress, partial-to-full-thickness epidermal necrosis or subepidermal blisters may appear (Figure 1.2). In TEN there is always progression to full-thickness epidermal necrosis and subepidermal blistering.

Differential diagnosis: Erythema multiforme, SJS, and TEN cannot be reliably distinguished from one another on histopathological grounds alone; distinction requires clinical context. Prodromal upper respiratory tract syndrome, mucous membrane involvement, extensive exfoliation, and association with medication use are features of SJS/TEN. The most important clinical differential diagnosis of TEN

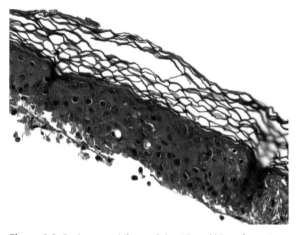

Figure 1.2 Erythema multiforme. Subepidermal blister formation.

is staphylococcal scalded skin syndrome (SSSS), the latter exhibiting a superficial intraepidermal cleavage plane, akin to that observed in pemphigus foliaceus.

Pityriasis lichenoides (PL)

A papulo-squamous disease of the skin of unknown origin, PL can range from a relatively mild chronic form to a more severe acute eruption.

Clinical presentation: Pityriasis lichenoides appears as a generalized exanthema of discrete, red-brown papules, affecting mainly the trunk and flexor surface of the arms and forearms, although a widespread distribution can occur. Shortly after, the papules develop a round, pale-brown scale that can be easily shed. Finally, when the lesions eventually disappear, hypopigmented areas appear (9,10).

Classification: There is an acute and a chronic form. In the acute form, also known as PLEVA (pityriasis lichenoides et varioliforme acuta), there is an acute onset of lesions, usually developing a hemorrhagic and vesicular component leading to small dark crusts. In chronic PL (CPL), there are recurrent attacks of less severe lesions leading to a long-lasting eruption that can even span through many months. The possible relation of PL with cutaneous lymphoma is virtually absent in children.

Histology: Pityriasis lichenoides et varioliforme acuta lesions are characterized by a wedge-shaped superficial and deep dermal lymphocytic infiltrate, interface dermatitis with lymphocyte exocytosis, papillary dermal hemorrhage, parakeratotic neutrophilic crust, and variable death of epidermal keratinocytes (Figure 1.3). Epidermal necrosis may involve

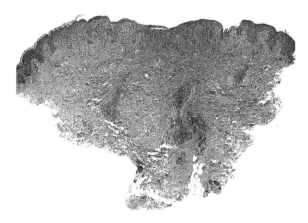

Figure 1.3 Pytiriasis lichenoides. An interface dermatitis with lymphocyte exocytosis and a wedge-shaped superficial and deep dermal lymphocytic infiltrate.

Table 1.4 Bullous dermatitis, differential diagnosis according to blister location

Subcorneal/intracorneal blister
- Miliaria crystallina
- Bullous impetigo
- Staphylococcal scalded skin syndrome
- Subepidermal pustular dermatosis
- Pustular psoriasis
- Acropustulosis of infancy
- Transient neonatal pustular melanosis
- Erythema toxicum neonatorum
- Acute generalized exanthematous pustulosis
- Pemphigus foliaceus

Intraspinous blister
- Pemphigus variants
- Hailey–Hailey disease
- Darier's disease
- Grover's disease
- Spongiotic vesicles
- Herpetic dermatitis
- Friction
- Edema

Suprabasilar blister
- Pemphigus vulgaris
- Darier's disease

Subepidermal blisters
- Linear IgA bullous dermatosis
- Epidermolysis bullosa
- Dermatitis herpetiformis
- Bullous pemphigoid
- Burns and cryotherapy
- Toxic epidermal necrolysis
- Bullous urticaria
- Bullous acute vasculitis
- Bullous lupus erythematosus
- Sweet's syndrome
- Epidermolysis bullosa acquisita
- Suction blisters
- Blisters overlying scars
- Drug reactions
- Kindler's syndrome
- Wells' syndrome
- Arthropod bites

scattered single cells or sheets of cells, resulting in confluent necrosis. Fully developed lesions have a lichenoid infiltrate. Dense infiltrates of lymphocytes in and around blood vessels is often noted, but a true vasculitis, with fibrin within vessel walls, is only occasionally present. In CPL, neutrophilic crust, necrosis of keratinocytes, and erythrocyte extravasation may be minimal or absent, and the perivascular lymphocytes are usually sparser and superficial.

Bullous dermatitis

This pattern is characterized by intraepidermal or subepidermal blister formation, resulting from a defect, congenital or acquired, in the adhesion of keratinocytes. A blister is a fluid-filled space within or beneath the epidermis that can be primary or appear as a secondary event caused by different factors (infections, burns, ischemia, etc.). Assessment of the associated inflammatory infiltrate, identification of the mechanism of tissue split, and determination of the histologic plane of the blister are the first steps in the histopathological diagnosis of a vesiculo-bullous disorder.

The blister may be subcorneal/intracorneal, intraspinous, suprabasilar, or subepidermal. See Table 1.4 for differential diagnosis.

Bullous pemphigoid (BP) and linear IgA disease of childhood (LAD)

Bullous pemphigoid and LAD are bullous diseases due to the development of autoantigens directed to certain structures of the basal membrane. In BP, the autoantigens are usually IgG, IgM, and sometimes IgA type, whereas in LAD, antigens are IgA type. There is considerable overlap between these two entities, and thus they are discussed together (11,12).

Clinical presentation: Both are infrequent. Bullous pemphigoid usually presents as an annular, urticarial eruption; later, a few vesicles develop within the urticarial plaques, and finally, a striking bullous eruption appears. The perioral region, neck, trunk, limbs, and especially hands and feet may be involved. In LAD there is predominant perineal involvement. Bullae

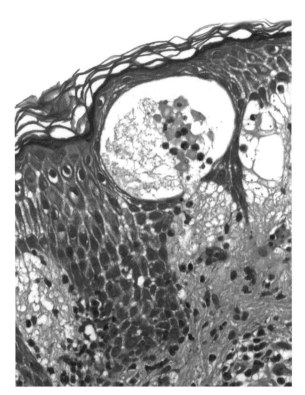

Figure 1.4 Bullous penphigoid. Eosinophilic spongiosis is frequently seen in the erythematous non-bullous skin.

often show a typical peripheral beading, with blisters surrounding a central area of erythema. Both BP and LAD run a chronic course, but eventually the disease disappears in most cases.

Classification: In BP and LAD, certain basal membrane antigens are targeted by autoantibodies. Antibodies against the BP230 antigen are typically present in BP patients' serum, and in both BP and LAD, different epitopes of the BP180 antigen (corresponding to collagen XVII) are targeted.

Histology: In LAD, also known as chronic bullous dermatosis of childhood, the blister is subepidermal and neutrophils are usually the predominant cells in the infiltrate. Papillary microabscesses are seen in some cases, making the lesion indistinguishable from dermatitis herpetiformis on light microscopy. Direct immunofluorescence reveals a homogeneous linear pattern of IgA deposition along the basement membrane of non-lesional skin. IgG, IgM, and/or C3 may also be present.

In BP there is also a subepidermal blister, but eosinophils are the predominant cell in the dermis and blister cavity. Eosinophilic spongiosis may be

seen in the clinically erythematous skin surrounding the blister (Figure 1.4). Direct immunofluorescence shows a linear deposition of IgG and/or C3 along the basement membrane. IgM and IgA can sometimes be positive. In early stages of the disease only C3 may be present.

Vasculitis

Vascular diseases can be classified as non-inflammatory purpuras, vascular occlusive diseases, urticarias, neutrophilic dermatoses, and vasculitis. Schönlein–Henoch purpura (SHP) is the most commonly biopsied condition in this heterogeneous group of disorders (13,14).

Schönlein–Henoch purpura

Schönlein–Henoch purpura is a peculiar type of leukocytoclastic vasculitis, mediated by IgA immune complexes that can affect the skin and internal organs.

Clinical presentation: Usually an infectious episode precedes the skin eruption. Palpable purpura is the hallmark of SHP, and appears as small purpuric papules surrounded by a halo of flat purpuric erythema. These lesions usually appear on the ankles, feet, and legs, but can also affect the thighs, buttocks, arms, and, rarely, the face. IgA immune complexes deposit in the vessel walls leading to necrotizing vasculitis and blood extravasation, visible as purpura. Vasculitis can affect other organs such as joints, gastrointestinal tube, kidneys, and, more rarely, central nervous system (CNS), lungs, and virtually any other organ. Accompanying symptoms include fever, malaise, joint swelling, gastrointestinal hemorrhage, and proteinuria. Schönlein–Henoch purpura usually affects children and adolescents. In infants, a similar vasculitic condition called acute hemorrhagic edema of infancy is recognized. It shows large purpuric macules with acral distribution and edema of ankles, wrists and ears, but usually there is no systemic involvement.

Histology: Recent lesions are characterized by small-vessel neutrophilic vasculitis affecting the superficial dermal plexus. Fragmented nuclei (leukocytoclasia) around small vessels are typical (Figure 1.5). Focal intravascular fibrin and thrombosis can be present. The dermis shows variable edema and extravasation of red blood cells. In some cases, the subepidermal edema is pronounced, resulting in vesiculo-bullous lesions. In resolving lesions, there is usually a mild perivascular infiltrate of lymphocytes and some

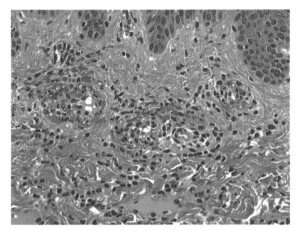

Figure 1.5 Schönlein–Henoch purpura. Neutrophilic vasculitis with leukocytoclasia and fibrinoid necrosis involving dermal postcapillary venules.

eosinophils. In most cases biopsied early in the course of the disease IgA can be demonstrated in vascular walls of involved and uninvolved skin. In infantile acute hemorrhagic edema the histopathology is the same, but IgA deposition is negative (15).

Granulomatous dermatitis

Granulomas are discrete collections of histiocytes or epithelioid histiocytes with variable numbers of admixed multinucleate giant cells and other inflammatory cells. Different histological patterns of granulomas are recognized: sarcoid ("naked" granulomas), epithelioid, or tuberculoid, necrobiotic (collagenolytic), suppurative and foreign-body granulomas. Some granulomas do not fit neatly into one of the above categories. Differential diagnosis is shown in Table 1.5.

Granuloma annulare (GA)

Granuloma annulare is a fairly common benign inflammatory skin condition of unknown etiology, which most often affects children and young adults (16).

Clinical presentation: There are four main clinical variants: localized, subcutaneous, disseminated, and perforating. Localized lesions usually appear on the distal extremities of children and young adults as smooth, flesh-colored to erythematous, firm papules that may coalesce into an annular papule or plaque. Subcutaneous GA is characterized by firm or hard asymptomatic nodules in the deep dermis or subcutaneous tissues; they are prevalent on the anterotibial zone, ankles, dorsal feet, buttocks, hands, scalp, and eyelids (17). Disseminated GA occurs predominantly

Table 1.5 Granulomatous dermatitis

Sarcoidal granulomas (epithelioid histiocytes and giant cells with a paucity of surrounding lymphocytes)
- Sarcoidosis and Blau's syndrome
- Foreign body reactions
- Secondary syphilis
- Crohn's disease
- Orofacial granulomatosis
- Granuloma annulare (sarcoidal type)
- Immunodeficiencies

Tuberculoid granulomas (epithelioid histiocytes and Langhans giant cells with a rim of lymphocytes and a central "caseation" necrosis).
- Tuberculosis
- Tuberculids
- Leprosy
- Late syphilis
- Leishmaniasis
- Rosacea
- Lupus miliaris disseminatus faciei
- Perioral dermatitis
- Crohn's disease
- Idiopathic facial aseptic granuloma

Necrobiotic granulomas (usually poorly formed and composed of histiocytes, lymphocytes and giant cells with associated 'necrobiosis'. The inflammatory component may form a palisade around the necrobiosis)
- Granuloma annulare
- Necrobiosis lipoidica
- Rheumatoid nodules
- Rheumatic fever nodules
- Crohn's disease
- Immunodeficiencies
- Reactions to foreign materials and vaccines

Suppurative granulomas (epithelioid histiocytes and multinucleate giant cells with central collections of neutrophils).
- Non-tuberculous mycobacterial infections
- Fungal infections (chromomycosis and pheohyphomycosis, sporotrichosis, blastomycosis, paracoccidioidomycosis, coccidioidomycosis,
- Nocardiosis and actinomicosis
- Ruptured cysts and follicles
- Cat-scratch disease
- Lymphogranuloma venereum
- Pyoderma gangrenosum

Foreign body granulomas (epithelioid histiocytes, foreign body-type giant cells, and variable numbers of other inflammatory cells with identifiable foreign material)
- Endogenous materials (calcium deposits, keratin, hair)
- Exogenous materials (tattoo material, cactus bristles, wood splinters, suture material, injected hyaluronic acid, bovine collagen, insect mouth parts, pencil lead, etc.)

in adults. In the rarer variant called perforating GA, there is a variety of superficial umbilicated papules with or without discharge, that heal with scarring. Localized disease is generally self-limited and resolves within one to two years, whereas disseminated disease

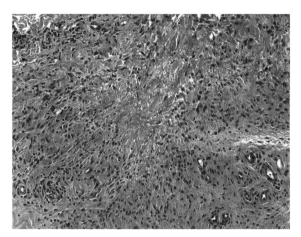

Figure 1.6 Granuloma annulare. Necrobiotic dermis surrounded by palisading granulomatous inflammation.

lasts longer. Granuloma annulare may be associated with diabetes, but association with other systemic disease is rare.

Histology: The fully developed GA lesions reveal foci of degenerative collagen with palisading granulomatous inflammation (Figure 1.6). Necrobiotic areas frequently show a pale, homogeneous, light-blue appearance due to the presence of mucin. There are associated perivascular and interstitial lymphocytes, occasionally neutrophils and nuclear dust. In the incomplete or interstitial variant, there is only an interstitial histiocytic infiltrate with minimal or absent palisading or increased mucin. In subcutaneous GA the palisading granulomas are located in the subcutaneous fat. In the perforating variant of GA there is transepidermal elimination of abnormal collagen fibers.

Panniculitis

The panniculitides include a group of disorders of varied etiology that manifest as inflamed nodules in the subcutaneous tissue. They are rarely seen in infants and children (18,19). Panniculitides can be classified into three distinct categories: septal panniculitis, lobular panniculitis, and panniculitis associated with large-vessel vasculitis. Septal panniculitides with no vasculitis include erythema nodosum, necrobiosis lipoidica, deep morphea, subcutaneous granuloma annulare, and rheumatoid nodule. Lobular panniculitides without vasculitis comprise a large series of disparate disorders, including sclerema neonatorum, subcutaneous fat necrosis of the newborn, post-steroid panniculitis, lupus erythematosus profundus, pancreatic panniculitis, α-1 antitrypsin deficiency

panniculitis, subcutaneous Sweet syndrome, infective panniculitis, factitial panniculitis, traumatic panniculitis, etc.(20). Lobular panniculitis with vasculitis is represented by erythema induratum of Bazin (21). Finally, polyarteritis nodosa can mimic a primary panniculitis, and many serial sections are needed in some cases to definitely rule out vascular involvement.

Specific panniculitides of children include subcutaneous fat necrosis of the newborn, post-steroid panniculitis, sclerema neonatorum, and cold panniculitis. The panniculitides of the newborn represent a unique response of the infant's fat to different injuries, and are a specific type of panniculitis that is only seen in neonates and very young infants (18).

Subcutaneous fat necrosis of the newborn (SFNN)

SFNN is a self-limited panniculitis, present at birth or appearing in the first few days of life.

Clinical presentation: Subcutaneous fat necrosis of the newborn is an uncommon disorder, usually affecting healthy, full-term children that undergo some form of obstetric trauma such as meconium aspiration, asphyxia, hypothermia, or peripheral hypoxemia. In most cases, hypothermia is the common factor that leads to SFNN and extensive subcutaneous fat necrosis of the newborn has been described associated with therapeutic hypothermia (22). A not uncommon and life-threatening complication of SFNN is hypercalcemia (23).

Newborn fat has a lower fusion point than children's fat, and thus lower body temperatures lead to fat solidification, crystallization, and adipose tissue necrosis and inflammation. Clinically, erythematous or violaceous subcutaneous nodules appear on the back, shoulders, arms, or buttocks in newborns. Most cases resolve spontaneously, but in some patients the nodules melt and break, leading to external extrusion of the necrotized tissue. Prognosis is generally good, except for the development of hypercalcemia in severe cases (24).

Classification: There is considerable overlap with a condition called sclerema neonatorum, which is also a type of newborn panniculitis usually appearing in severely sick preterm newborns in which a diffuse induration of the back is the main symptom.

Histology: Subcutaneous fat necrosis of the newborn is characterized by necrosis of the subcutaneous fat with needle-shaped crystal formations within the adipose cells. This initiates a localized inflammatory process with foreign-body giant cell formation. There

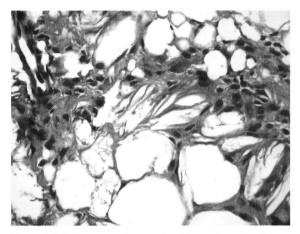

Figure 1.7 Subcutaneous fat necrosis of the newborn. Needle-shaped crystals and necrotic adipocytes.

is mostly lobular panniculitis, with a dense inflammatory infiltrate composed of lymphocytes, histiocytes, lipophages, and multinucleated giant cells. At a higher magnification, narrow needle-shaped clefts radially arranged are seen within the cytoplasm of the adipocytes and multinucleated giant cells (Figure 1.7).

Infectious disorders and bites

Bacterial skin infections are rarely biopsied; a clinical and microbiological diagnosis is usually made. Common viral infections, such as warts or molluscum contagiosum may require a skin biopsy for a correct diagnosis. Certain mycobacterial, parasitic, and fungal disorders are diagnosed on histopathological grounds, and thus a skin biopsy is required.

Warts

A wart (*verruca vulgaris*) is an epidermal proliferation induced by human papilloma virus (HPV) infection of the skin (25,26).

Clinical presentation: Warts are very common, especially in school-age children. They usually present as discrete verrucous papules that may appear in virtually every area of the skin surface. Palmar and plantar warts often take the form of translucent papules. Facial lesions may have a filiform shape. Mucosal lesions appear as moist masses, and are called condylomata. Different types of HPV cause different variants; both skin and mucosal types are recognized. Types 1, 2, and 4 are the most common in palms and soles, whereas types 6 and 11 are the most common mucosal types in children.

Histology: Warts show a papillomatous hyperplasia of the epidermis with hyperkeratosis and a prominent granular cell layer with enlarged keratohyaline granules and, sometimes, intracytoplasmic eosinophilic viral inclusions. Columns of parakeratosis overlie the tips of the papillomatous peaks. Koilocytes are frequent in the upper epidermis; they have a small, dark, hyperchromatic nucleus with irregular contours, surrounded by clear cytoplasm. Mild variation of the architecture and cytological features is seen in flat warts, myrmecial warts, and filiform warts. *In situ* hybridization or PCR studies can be used to detect HPV in paraffin-embedded tissue. In cases of warts involving genital or perianal skin, the possibility of sexual abuse may require investigation.

Molluscum contagiosum (MC)

This is a viral infection of the skin due to a poxvirus (27).

Clinical presentation: Molluscum contagiosum is very common in children, especially those attending swimming pools, atopic patients, and children affected by immunodeficiency. Individual lesions consist of small, discrete, pearly papules, sometimes with an umbilicated center. Their size ranges from 1 mm to 1 cm diameter nodules. There may be a single lesion to hundreds. The trunk, limbs, face, groin, and face are the most common sites. They are virtually never seen on mucosae, palms, or soles. In adolescents and adults, MC may be acquired throughout sexual contact (28,29).

Histology: Lesions appear as cup-shaped invaginations of the epidermis into the dermis. Eosinophilic inclusion bodies (Henderson–Patterson bodies) form in the cytoplasm of keratinocytes just above the basal layer. They accumulate and progressively enlarge, replacing the entire cell. These molluscum bodies are eventually extruded with keratinous debris into dilated ostia, which lead to the surface. Some lesions show a florid dense lymphocytic inflammatory infiltrate.

Leishmaniasis

Cutaneous leishmaniasis is due to infestation of the skin by protozoa of the genus Leishmania.

Leishmaniasis is present worldwide, with great species and clinical variation according to geographical distribution. It is endemic in the Middle East, North Africa, and in parts of Asia. Most cases in Europe are restricted to the Mediterranean basin, in relation with the vector mosquito population. Dogs are the most

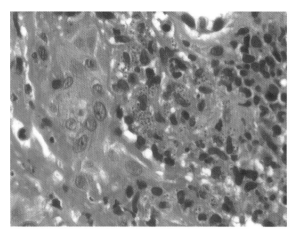

Figure 1.8 Leishmaniasis. Amastigotes within the cytoplasm of hystiocytes.

common reservoirs; mosquitoes act as vectors, and inoculate Leishmania on the human skin (30).

Clinical presentation: Leishmania growth within macrophages leads to an erythematous papule topped by a grayish, adherent crust that usually lasts for many months and is resistant to topical corticosteroids and antibiotics. There is usually a single lesion, most commonly on the cheeks. Rarely, multiple lesions can develop on the face.

Histology: Depending in the clinical type and stage, the epidermis may be either ulcerated with marked secondary changes and epidermal reaction, or it may be quite unremarkable or even atrophic. In *acute* lesions there is a massive dermal infiltrate of parasitized macrophages intermixed with lymphocytes, epithelioid cells and plasma cells. There may be a few eosinophils and variable numbers of neutrophils. The infiltrate may surround neurovascular bundles akin to lepromatous leprosy. Although Leishmanias can be seen in H-E stained sections (Figure 1.8), the morphological details are better seen on Giemsa stain. The parasites are 2–4 μm round to oval basophilic structures, with an eccentrically located kinetoplast. Leishmania organisms are difficult to find late in the disease, when there is a resolving granulomatous and sclerotic inflammatory reaction. Polymerase chain reaction is the most sensitive method for diagnosis and can be used to demonstrate the presence of amastigotes in tissue sections or lesional scrapings (31,32).

Differential diagnosis: Cutaneous leishmaniasis is frequently misdiagnosed in areas where it is not endemic, particularly if organisms are not seen. It may be misinterpreted as sarcoidosis, foreign-body reaction, granulomatous rosacea, and even granuloma annulare. When organisms are present, the lack of a capsule in Leishmanias is helpful in distinguishing them from *Histoplasma capsulatum.*

Melanocytic lesions

Melanocytic nevi (MN) are benign proliferations of nevocytes 3. that are present virtually in every person. Recognizing the many variants of MN avoids confusion with malignant melanoma (MM), which is very uncommon in children.

Dermal melanocytosis (DM)

DMs are cutaneous hyperpigmented lesions characterized by scattered pigmented dendritic melanocytes in the reticular dermis.

Clinical presentation: At least three different types are recognized: Mongolian spot, nevus of Ito, and nevus of Ota. Mongolian spots appear as one or multiple hyperpigmented patches on the lower posterior trunk with predilection for the sacro-gluteal region. Nevus of Ito typically involves the supraclavicular, deltoid, or scapular area. Nevus of Ota usually involves the sclera, conjunctiva, and skin around the eye, and zygomatic and temporal areas.

Histology: All types of DM are histologically similar. The epidermis appears unremarkable, but may show increased melanin in basal cells and a mild increased number of basal melanocytes. Scattered dendritic or spindle-shaped, often deeply pigmented melanocytes are recognized in the superficial and mid-dermis. Melanophages in the papillary dermis may be seen.

Simple lentigo (SL)

Simple lentigo is a common, benign lesion showing basal melanocyte proliferation.

Clinical presentation: Simple lentigo may appear anywhere on the skin surface as small, sharply demarcated macules about 3–5 mm in diameter, with a uniform light to dark-brown color. Sun-exposed skin of the trunk and extremities in individuals with white complexion is most frequently involved.

Histology: Simple lentigo is characterized by basal hyperpigmentation and increased melanocytes in the basal layer. The melanocytes are usually single and cytologically normal. Small junctional nests are sometimes seen. Epidermal acanthosis and melanophages in the papillary dermis are additional histological features.

Differential diagnosis: SL needs to be distinguished from small lentiginous junctional melanocytic nevi, which may have only very few junctional nests. Melanotic macules show hyperpigmentation of basilar keratinocytes, but lack increased cellular density of melanocytes, or show just a slight increment. Several syndromes are associated with multiple melanotic macules/lentigines (Peutz–Jeghers, Carney complex, etc.).

Congenital melanocytic nevi (CMN)

Congenital melanocytic nevi represent benign proliferations of nevocytes (cells derived from melanocytic precursors that have most commonly undergone *NRAS* mutations) usually present at birth or within the first few months of life (33,34).

Clinical presentation and classification: Several classification systems, based on size, exist. A recently proposed system (35) offers a more objective and reproducible classification:

LARGE/GIANT CMNS (L/GCMN) are larger than 20 cm, in neonates, larger than the palm of the patient at birth (36). L/GCMN occur in approximately one in 20 000 births (37), most commonly involve the posterior trunk ("bathing trunk" or "garment-like nevus"), and feature a verrucous surface, significant hyperpigmentation, color variation within the dominant background color and irregular margins; often, smaller so-called "satellite" nevi are associated.

MEDIUM-SIZE CMNS are those >1.5 cm but <20 cm in diameter.

SMALL CMNS are those <1.5 cm in diameter and usually present as solitary, well demarcated, light tan to dark-brown uniformly colored macules or slightly raised papules. They can occur in any location and be clinically indistinguishable from the so-called common acquired nevi (38).

There is a higher risk of developing MM in patients with CMN, proportional to lesional diameter (39). Other, non-melanocytic malignancies, most frequently, rhabdomyosarcoma may also arise (10).

Histology: Congenital melanocytic nevi may have a papillomatous epidermis. Their superficial portion is similar to acquired nevi with a junctional component. However, CMN, and specially L/GCMN, show a thick, multilayered pattern of skin involvement, with nevocytes present from the reticular dermis all the way up to the papillary dermis, and some may even have an intraepidermal ("pagetoid") component. Not infrequently, subcutaneous tissue, and even

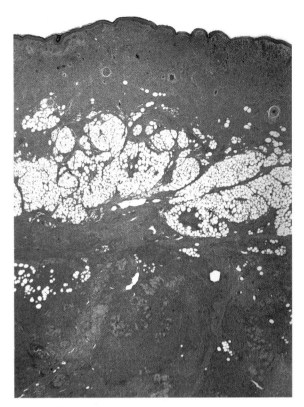

Figure 1.9 Congenital melanocytic nevus.

deep fascial planes show proliferating nevocytes (Figure 1.9). They frequently feature significant "neurotization," represented by formations that reveal the neural crest origin of these cells, with Masson or Wegner–Meissner bodies. Heterologous elements may also be found.

Differential diagnosis: Histological features that help in distinguishing CMN from common acquired melanocytic nevi are not very specific or reliable, but they are used to suspect their congenital nature when no documentation of the nevus at birth exists. These histological features are shared by small and L/GCMN, and include the presence of nevocytes within the lower two-thirds of the dermis and within the subcutaneous tissue; nevocytes splaying or extending between the collagen bundles of the reticular dermis as single cells, or cords of cells; extension of nevocytes around and within hair follicles, sebaceous glands, eccrine apparatus, vessel walls, and nerves; a perivascular and perifollicular distribution of nevocytes simulating an inflammatory reaction such as figurate erythema; and arrector pili that may be enlarged, distorted, and infiltrated by nevocytes (38,40–42).

Proliferative nodules (PN) in CMN must be differentiated from MM arising in the deep dermal component of CMN. Proliferative nodules are defined as atypical nevocytic proliferations which manifest predominantly in the neonatal period within a pre-existing L/GCMN (43). The vast majority of atypical nodular proliferations developing in CMN are benign. Features that favor a benign nature include blending of these cellular aggregates with the surrounding nevocytes, low mitotic rate, absence of diffuse high-grade cytologic atypia, and absence of inflammatory infiltrate or necrosis (38). A subgroup of PN is represented by atypical PN, which appear sharply demarcated; show an expansile pattern of growth and epidermal effacement, pleomorphism and higher mitotic activity. They feature an increased Ki67 and PHH3 staining compared to those seen in non-atypical PN and the adjacent nevus cells surrounding the nodule. However, they show the same pattern of *BRAF* and *NRAS* mutations seen in non-atypical PN and surrounding nevus cells (44).

Common acquired melanocytic nevus (CAMN)

Melanocytic nevi are a heterogeneous group of lesions generally manifesting as melanin-producing cellular proliferations, although sometimes these are non-pigmented cutaneous lesions. The prototypical example is the common acquired nevus.

Clinical presentation: Common acquired melanocytic nevus are often <6 mm in diameter, with smooth, regular borders and evenly distributed pigmentation. Depending on the size and elevation, CAMN may present as macules, papules, or nodules.

Histology: In general, CAMN are symmetrical and well circumscribed. The microscopic appearance depends on its subtype and the type/location of skin it involves. Histologically, they are composed of nevocytes organized in nests, leading to the following designations according to the location of these nests: junctional, with nests located only at the dermal–epidermal junction; compound, with nests at the dermal–epidermal junction and dermis; and intradermal, when nests involve only the dermis. In junctional nevi, the nests are discrete and situated at the tips of the rete ridges. The architecture of the rete is regular and without bridging or fusion, lentiginous proliferation of single cells, with no pagetoid migration. Nevus cytology is bland, with nuclear sizes typically smaller than in adjacent keratinocytes. In compound nevi, nests at

the dermal–epidermal junction are discrete, accompanied by an underlying collection of dermal nevocytes. Classically, the dermal component of compound and intradermal nevi have been said to undergo a phenomenon called "maturation" (a rather erroneous concept in light of modern theories regarding nevogenesis). Mitoses in superficial nevocytes are not worrisome, but deeper mitoses are and should raise the possibility of a more aggressive lesion. Peculiar histological findings are sometimes seen in intradermal nevi or the dermal portion of compound nevi, including neurotization, adipocyte or ossifying metaplasia, amyloid deposition, multinucleation, etc. Epidermal hyperplasia overlying a CAMN is frequently seen.

Differential diagnosis: This includes all the benign and malignant melanocytic lesions discussed in this chapter.

Spitz nevus (SN)

Described originally as "juvenile melanoma" (45), SN is a benign proliferation of large, spindled, oval or round (epithelioid) nevocytes that begins in the epidermis, and evolves into compound or intradermal stages (43).

Clinical presentation: Spitz nevus usually presents as a single, dome-shaped papule or nodule with a diameter of 6 mm or less, but larger lesions are not uncommon. Most SN occurs on the face and head in children, or the lower extremities in young adults, particularly women. They may vary from non-pigmented to pink, red-brown and even black in color. Spitz nevus commonly appears suddenly, and after a period of rapid growth reaches a plateau and remains stable. However, color changes, bleeding, and pruritus may occur. Unusual variants include grouped or agminated (46–49), disseminated (50), and eruptive (51).

Histology: The classic SN is dome-shaped and symmetric, with abrupt attenuation of the junctional nests at the lateral borders of the lesion. The epidermis is acanthotic, hyperplastic, with hypergranulosis and hyperkeratosis. The nevus is composed of variable proportions of spindly and epithelioid nevocytes, plump and with abundant cytoplasm, featuring a centrally located vesicular nucleus, often with prominent nucleolus (Figure 1.10). The proliferating cells sometimes show bizarre shapes, and multinucleated cells may be present. The cytoplasm may have a ground glass appearance, and melanin is usually absent.

A common feature in SN is the presence of Kamino bodies (52), which are eosinophilic and

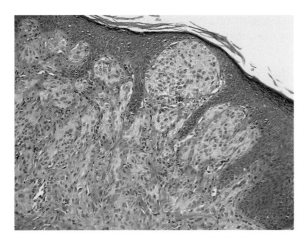

Figure 1.10 Spitz nevus. Large nests composed of epithelioid nevocytes with abundant cytoplasm.

globular deposits of basement membrane material found within the epidermis, usually above dermal papillae. Kamino bodies are present in variable numbers from case to case (53). Spitz nevus usually features a compound histological pattern, although junctional and intradermal lesions are not uncommon. Compound SN is symmetric, well circumscribed, and often wedge-shaped, with large nests of nevomelanocytes in the epidermis and in the underlying dermis. The proliferating cells are of relatively uniform in size and shape, typically orientated perpendicular to the epidermis. Artefactual clefts around the nests are usually seen. Pagetoid spread of nevomelanocytes can be present, mainly in the lower half of the epidermis. This process is usually confined to the center of the lesion; however, it can be quite marked in developing junctional SN in young children (54). There is progressive reduction of melanocytic nests and cellular size from the top to the bottom (55). Nevocytes in the dermis are mostly nested or arranged in fascicles and do not form sheets. There are often single cells infiltrating in between collagen bundles in the reticular dermis at the base of the lesion. Non-atypical mitoses may be seen, but they are usually not numerous, seen in the mid-to- upper portion of the lesion, and are more prevalent in the compound type of SN compared with the junctional and intradermal SN (55).

Lymphocytic inflammatory infiltrate is often seen around vessels and at the base of the lesion. Blood vessels might be dilated and prominent. Histological variants of SN include desmoplastic, angiomatoid, myxoid, plexiform, and rosette-like SN (56).

Differential diagnosis: Although distinction between SN and spitzoid MM cannot be reliably made on immunohistochemical basis, some stains may be useful in distinguishing spitzoid melanocytic neoplasms from non-melanocytic tumors. HMB-45 and tyrosinase diminish toward the base of SN, in contrast with the diffuse pattern seen in spitzoid MM. The percentage of MIB-1-positive cells is higher in MM than in SN (29.7% vs. 4.0%, respectively). S100 and Melan A are diffusely expressed in both SN and spitzoid MM, therefore, they are useful only to discriminate SN from non-melanocytic tumors (57–61).

Comparative genomic hybridization and fresh tissue fluorescence *in-situ* hybridization (FISH) are increasingly promising ancillary tests (62); the sensitivity and specificity of these techniques is improving fast, although there are still some pitfalls, including false-positive and false-negative results, and the fact that some histologically "borderline" lesions show "borderline" cytogenetic features as well. Among the newer and most useful approaches is the use of a FISH probe set, including 9p21, 6p25, 11q13, and 8q24, which has recently been demonstrated to reach a sensitivity of 94% and a specificity of 98% (63).

Atypical spitzoid neoplasms (ASN)

This is a poorly defined and likely heterogeneous group with morphological overlap between melanoma and Spitz nevus. In contrast to classic SN, ASN exhibit more worrisome features such as larger size (>1 cm in diameter), ulceration, increased cellularity or prominent confluence of nevomelanocytes in the dermis, extension into dermis or subcutaneous fat, dermal mitoses, cytological atypia, and lack of "maturation" at the base (64).

Although ASN have generally been reported to have a good prognosis, well-documented cases of metastasis and death exist (65–67). Because the malignant potential of these lesions is uncertain, many clinicians and patients make decisions to treat them as if they were melanomas with excision and, often, a sentinel lymph node biopsy if the thickness is >1 mm (68).

Nevus of Reed (NR)

Nevus of Reed is characterized by non-atypical, uniform, heavily pigmented and spindled nevocytes (69,70). Nevus of Reed can be histologically or clinically misinterpreted as melanoma (70). There is significant controversy as to whether the NR represents a separate clinical entity or a variant of the classical Spitz nevus.

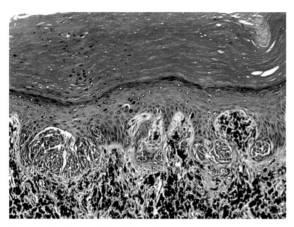

Figure 1.11 Nevus of Reed. Vertical nests of spindle melanocytes at the dermoepidermal junction. Numerous melanophages are seen within the dermis.

Clinical presentation: Nevus of Reed presents as a well-circumscribed, uniformly dark-brown or black lesion, averaging 3–5 mm in diameter.

Histology: Nevus of Reed is symmetrical and shows a sharp lateral circumscription. The nevocytes are arranged in vertical nests at the dermal–epidermal junction and sometimes may involve the papillary dermis. Occasional mitoses may be found. Epithelioid nevocytes are seen in a minority of cases. Commonly, the epidermis is slightly hyperplastic and shows marked hyperpigmentation of the basal keratinocytes. Kamino bodies may be observed in about half of the cases. An inflammatory infiltrate composed of lymphocytes and histiocytes with many melanophages is found within the papillary dermis (Figure 1.11; 41,70,71).

Halo nevus

Halo nevus of Sutton is the name given to a pre-existing melanocytic nevus surrounded by a depigmented halo. The immunological reaction to the proliferating nevocytes leads to the formation of the halo.

Clinical presentation: Many halo nevi show depigmentation of the pre-existing nevi; these may even later disappear. The halo can affect just one or multiple nevi in the patient, and this benign reaction should not be confused with melanoma regression. In 5% of patients with halo nevi there is a personal or familial history of vitiligo.

Histology: Halo phenomena can affect any type of melanocytic nevus. Residual nevocytes may show heavy infiltration by lymphocytes and histiocytes.

Differential diagnosis: Halo phenomena can also affect malignant melanomas. Features that help to distinguish between halo nevus and halo melanoma are the same as in lesions without the halo phenomena.

Blue nevus (BN)

Blue nevus is a subset of melanocytic proliferations containing cells reminiscent of the embryonal neural-crest-derived dendritic melanocytic precursors (72). The blue color is due to the deeper location of the pigment.

Clinical presentation: Blue nevi appear usually as small blue or blue-black macules or papules, mostly on the dorsum of hands and feet, scalp and buttocks. They are usually acquired, but congenital lesions are also recognized. Multiple blue nevi may be associated with LAMB (lentigines, atrial myxomas, mucocutaneous myxomas, and blue nevi) syndrome.

Histology: Symmetrical mid- and/or upper-dermal proliferation of heavily pigmented dermal nevocytes adopting an inverted wedge-shaped configuration, with the base of the lesion parallel to the surface of the epidermis (classic BN). Blue nevi frequently involve deep reticular dermis and infiltrate along adnexal structures. Most cases are associated with some degree of stromal fibroplasia. The overlying epidermis lacks a junctional component, except when a blue nevus is part of a combined nevus. Nevocytes are variably pigmented, spindly, dendritic cells revealing a slender, branching network of processes without significant cytologic atypia or mitoses. Dendritic cells – the diagnostic cells of blue nevi – are usually intermixed with non-dendritic elongated, oval to spindle nevocytes. Melanophages are variably present.

The cellular variant of blue nevus is a pigmented biphasic tumor with a component of classic blue nevus and distinct cellular areas composed of spindly to oval nevocytes with clear or finely pigmented cytoplasm. In most cases, the cellular areas involve the deep portion of blue nevus with vertical projections joining superficial portions with the deep reticular dermis and subcutaneous tissue, forming a dumbbell-shaped outline. In many cases, the cellular areas are sharply demarcated from the common blue nevus component and form distinct nests or nodules (Figure 1.12). Other histological variants include sclerosing (desmoplastic), amelanotic/hypomelanotic, and epithelioid (pigmented epithelioid melanocytoma).

Differential diagnosis: Rare variants may be confused with other entities. Non-neoplastic and inflammatory conditions resulting in cellular or extracellular pigment accumulation can also be mistaken for blue nevus. Hemosiderin deposition can sometimes mimic

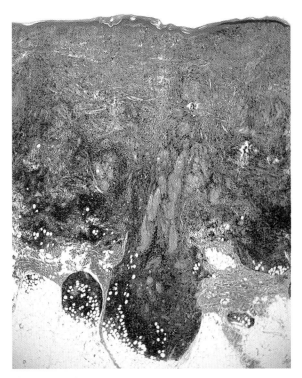

Figure 1.12 Blue nevus.

dendritic cells of blue nevus and may require iron staining to distinguish it from Fontana–Masson-positive melanin pigment. Another condition that can mimic blue nevi is postinflammatory hyperpigmentation.

Malignant blue nevi are recognized by the presence of atypical cytologic features such as pleomorphic nuclei, large eosinophilic nucleoli, brisk mitotic activity, or atypical mitoses. Other features, especially tumor necrosis and frank invasion with destruction of anatomic structures, can also be helpful.

Malignant melanoma

Pediatric MM is generally defined as melanoma occurring in patients <21 years and includes fetal cases. Pediatric melanoma can be subdivided into several groups, including congenital (*in utero* to birth), neonatal or infantile (birth to 1 year), childhood (1 year to puberty), and adolescent melanoma (puberty to 21) (73). In children and adults, most melanomas develop *de novo*. However, atypical, amelanotic, and nodular melanomas are more common in children (74).

Clinical presentation: Malignant melanoma in prepubertal children is so rare that it is usually unsuspected. Clinical findings of MM in children, and particularly in adolescents, are similar to those seen in adults. Atypical morphological features are more frequently seen in young patients. Congenital MM is also very rarely seen and can present *de novo* (75) in neonates with giant CMN (76) or may be secondary to transplacental migration of malignant melanocytes from an affected mother (77).

In an early series of 125 patients with pediatric melanoma, the most common clinical presentations included a nevus increasing in size, bleeding, color change, itching, palpable lymphadenopathy, and palpable subcutaneous mass (78). Compared with adult melanoma, a significant proportion of pediatric MM is amelanotic (50%) or has a nodular configuration (30%), and presents with greater median thickness (3.5 mm) (79).

The "ABCDE clinical rule" (Asymmetry, Border irregularity, Color variability, Diameter >6 mm, and Evolving) often used in identifying suspicious skin lesions in adults may be difficult to apply to pediatric cases because common lesions in children, such as Spitz nevi or benign nevi that grow as the child grows, may show these features, and, as mentioned before, pediatric patients are more likely to present with amelanotic lesions, not a common feature in adult melanoma (79).

Most patients (>80%) present with localized disease at diagnosis; the remainder have either regional lymph node disease (10–15%) or distant metastasis (1– 3%). Any organ may be involved in metastasis, including lung, liver, lymph nodes, subcutaneous tissue, and brain (80).

Malignant melanoma is the most common skin cancer during childhood, followed by basal cell carcinoma (BCC) and squamous cell carcinoma (SCC). Malignant melanoma accounts for <3% of all cancers seen in children. The incidence is higher in older children (81–83).

Melanoma can present at any site; however, the extremities are the most common primary sites in patients under 20 years of age, followed by trunk, head, and neck (80).

Most predisposing factors leading to melanoma in adults may have been present since childhood (84). In addition to the inherited syndromes that confer increased risk of melanoma in children, such as xeroderma pigmentosum (XP) and familial atypical multiple mole melanoma syndrome (FAMMMS), other significant predisposing factors are listed in Table 1.6 (81,82,85,86).

15

Table 1.6 Predisposing factors for malignant melanocytic skin tumors

- Impaired DNA repair, especially xeroderma pigmentosum
- Familial atypical mole syndrome
- Immunosuppression
- Previous malignant disease
- Congenital melanocytic nevus, especially giant nevus
- Melanoma in the family
- Large number of common melanocytic nevi
- Several atypical melanocytic nevi
- Light skin, red or blond hair, and/or light eyes
- Freckles and/or actinic lentigines (sun spots)
- Tendency to sunburn when exposed to UV light
- Intermittent intensive exposure to UV light

Pediatric melanoma appears to have a better prognosis compared to adult melanoma, even when matched for stage (82,87). Clinical characteristics associated with poor prognosis include male gender, earlier age at diagnosis, and head-and-neck location of primary tumor.

Pathogenesis and genetics: The exact etiology of MM in children remains unclear. Interplay of inherited and environmental factors is likely. Malignant melanoma development has been linked to germline mutations in genes encoding *CDKN2A*, *CDK4*, and *MCIR*, as well as to somatic mutations in the proto-oncogenes *B-RAF, N-RAS,* and *KIT,* and tumor suppressor genes *CDKN2A*, p53, and PTEN. Somatic mutations in *B-RAF* are the most common genetic alterations, occurring in up to 66% of cases. There are at least 30 documented mutations of B-RAF that activate the MAPK pathway, the most common being V600E (88). Targeting these mutations with specific inhibitors offers a new therapeutic approach.

Higher levels of microsatellite instability (MSI) and loss of heterozygosity (LOH) were found in pediatric melanoma compared with adult melanoma (96).

Histology: The criteria used for adult patients should also be used for pediatric melanomas (Table 1.7).

The most useful features distinguishing MM from nevi are: large size (>7 mm), ulceration, high mitotic rate (>4 mitosis/mm^2), mitosis in the lower third of the lesion, asymmetry, poorly demarcated lateral borders, lack of so-called "maturation," finely-divided melanin, and marked nuclear pleomorphism (89,90).

Melanoma in children is classified into three groups (43):

Table 1.7 Histological features of malignant melanoma

Histopathology
- Asymmetry
- Ill-defined borders
- Lack of "maturation"
- Atypia of melanocytes (variable)
- Mitoses
- Irregular pagetoid spread
- Lentiginous junctional proliferation
- Ulceration and/or "consumption of the epidermis"
- Predominance of solitary units of melanocytes
- Marked confluence of melanocytes along the dermal-epidermal junction
- Marked dyscohesion of melanocytes
- Lichenoid inflammatory reaction may be present
- Fibrosis and dermal regression may be present

Immunophenotype
- Positive for S100, Melan-A, HMB-45, tyrosinase

Variants
- Common MM (superficial spreading, nodular, acral lentiginous)
- Small-cell melanoma
- Spitzoid melanoma

Differential diagnosis
- Spitz nevi
- Atypical spitzoid neoplasm
- Reed nevi
- Proliferative nodule in CMN
- Acquired or congenital nevi with pagetoid melanocytosis and lentiginous melanocytic proliferation

Conventional melanoma: Most melanomas in children are in this group. Of the four classical histologic subtypes (superficial spreading, nodular, acral-lentiginous, and lentigo maligna), superficial spreading melanoma is the most common type in both pediatric and adult patients (Figure 1.13; 86). Young patients appear to have a greater frequency of nodular melanoma. Melanomas of glabrous skin are exceedingly rare in childhood. Lentigo malignant melanoma does not occur in childhood (91).

Small-cell melanoma: These tumors may appear *de novo* or develop in a congenital nevus, are frequently localized in the scalp, show striking Breslow thickness, and are associated with a fatal outcome in most patients. Small-cell MM is composed of monomorphous cells arranged in sheets or in organoid configurations. The high cellular density, lack of "maturation," and high mitotic rate are the clues to recognize this lesion (89,90).

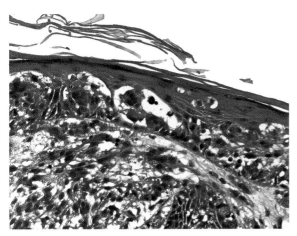

Figure 1.13 Malignant melanoma. Marked nuclear atypia and epidermotropism in a superficial spreading melanoma.

Spitzoid melanoma: Some melanomas may exhibit features like those seen in a Spitz nevus, such as large epithelioid cells and spindle cells arranged in fascicles, epidermal hyperplasia, wedge-shaped configuration, epidermal clefts surrounding intraepidermal nests, etc. Although most of these lesions also show unequivocal features of a malignant melanocytic neoplasm, some may be extremely difficult to differentiate under the microscope, and require additional molecular analyses for definitive discrimination.

Vascular anomalies

Vascular anomalies are the most common lesions of soft tissues in children and adolescents (92). They are very frequent in neonates and infants. One in three newborns has a vascular birthmark, which may either fade away or remain asymptomatic. However, some patients are born with deforming or life-threatening vascular anomalies.

The classification system from the International Society for the Study of Vascular Anomalies (ISSVA), separates them into vascular tumors and vascular malformations (93).

Vascular tumors

Infantile hemangioma (IH)

Infantile hemangioma is the most common pediatric benign vascular tumor, affecting approximately 40% of infants.

Clinical presentation: Infantile hemangioma is more common in Caucasian girls, especially with fair hair. Approximately 80–85% of patients have a solitary cutaneous lesion. The remaining 15–20% show multiple cutaneous lesions and are at higher risk for visceral hemangiomas involving the liver, lungs, and gastrointestinal tract, in that order. IH classically appears as a soft strawberry-like appearance, though deep lesions may have a bluish hue.

The natural history is characterized by a marked proliferative phase from the first few months of life until the end of the first year, rarely persisting beyond that time. After the first year of age, the hemangiomas begin a slow involuting phase, which may extend up to 10 years of age. Once they reach the involuted phase, they remain unchanged. Even a large, protruding hemangioma can regress completely, leaving near-normal skin.

Histology: The proliferative phase lesions are richly cellular, composed of plump endothelial cells and pericytes forming capillaries with small, sometimes almost undetectable lumina, arranged in delicately defined lobules. The basement membrane is multilaminated; brisk mitotic activity is common, but no abnormal mitoses are present. Mast cells are numerous (94) and supportive arteries and veins are prominent. During involution, lesional capillaries progressively "drop out" and are replaced by loose fibroadipose tissue. Endothelial cells and pericytes flatten, lumina enlarge, and the number of mitoses decreases (Figure 1.14a). Residual lesions may mimic vascular malformations.

Infantile hemangioma endothelial cells express GLUT1 (Figure 1.14b). This is highly specific for IH and persists even during involution. Panendothelial markers and WT1 are also expressed by the endothelial cells (95,96).

Congenital hemangiomas: RICH and NICH

Rarely, hemangiomas start to grow *in utero* and are fully developed at birth, i.e. they are truly congenital hemangiomas (CHs), representing a lesion with clinical and histopathological features different from those of IH.

Clinical presentation: The diagnosis is usually reached on clinical grounds. Congenital hemangiomas appear as large, reddish or bluish plaques, generally with a paler rim and prominent telangiectasia. They do not grow after birth, but may show two possible outcomes. Some will experience a very rapid resolution (within 1–4 months), and are called rapidly involuting

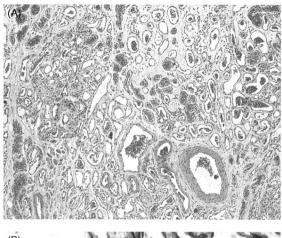

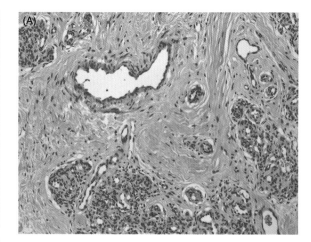

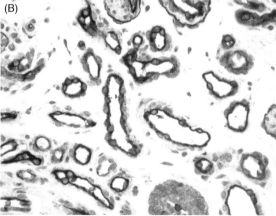

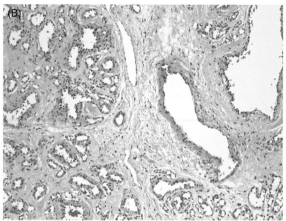

Figure 1.14 Infantile hemangioma. (A) Involuting lesion showing lobules of dilated capillaries with thickened walls, lined by flattened endothelial cells. (B) Intense endothelial positivity for GLUT-1.

Figure 1.15 Congenital hemangiomas. (A) RICH. (B) NICH.

congenital hemangioma (RICH). Other cases will persist unchanged throughout life, and are called non-involuting congenital hemangioma (NICH).

There is, however, some overlap between RICH and NICH: the involution process of RICH can stop at any time, transforming them into a NICH (97).

Histology: Rapidly involuting congenital hemangioma and NICH can be separated histologically from infantile hemangioma, and sometimes also from each other. Rapidly involuting congenital hemangioma have small to large lobules of capillaries with moderately plump endothelial cells and pericytes. The lobules are surrounded by fibrous tissue with large, abnormal draining channels and may contain hemosiderin, thrombosis, cyst formation, focal calcification, and extramedullary hematopoiesis (Figure 1.15a). Zonation with advanced involution in the lesional center is sometimes observed (97). Non-involuting congenital hemangioma show

generally large fibrotic lobules of vessels with curved lumina, hobnailed endothelial cells, endothelial cytoplasmic eosinophilic inclusions, prominent lobular draining channels, arteriolobular and arteriovenous fistulae, and a prominent interlobular vascular network (Figure 1.15b). Some lesions also have lobules of capillaries with multi-laminated basement membrane, as observed in the involuting and involuted phase of IH (97,98). Rapidly involuting congenital hemangioma and NICH are negative for GLUT1 and exhibit positive cytoplasmic endothelial staining for WT1. GLUT1 staining is the easiest method to separate these lesions from IH (97,99).

Verrucous hemangioma

The term verrucous hemangioma (VH) is used for dermal and subcutaneous vascular lesions with an overlying verrucous surface.

These lesions are considered variants of vascular malformations with secondary reactive epidermal acanthosis, hyperkeratosis, and parakeratosis (100). Despite its clinical features, similar to those seen in vascular malformations, VH exhibits some histological characteristics and an immunophenotype similar to vascular neoplasms, expressing WT1 (101) and GLUT1 (101,102).

Clinical presentation: VHs are congenital or identified in early infancy, exhibit proportional growth without regression, and are located mainly on the limbs. Fully developed VHs are composed of well-circumscribed hyperkeratotic linear vascular plaques ranging in size from 2.5–20 cm in diameter (101). In the early stages, these lesions are non-keratotic, soft, and bluish-red, but with time they become increasingly hyperkeratotic.

Histology: The epidermis generally shows compact hyperkeratosis, papillomatosis, and irregular acanthosis overlying dilated capillaries, which involve the papillary dermis, the deep dermis, and the subcutaneous tissue (Figure 1.16). The vessels are organized in a diffuse or lobular pattern. Thick-walled round capillaries with a multilayered basement membrane, closely resembling those of infantile hemangioma in its involuting phase, are frequently observed. Verrucous hemangioma show cytoplasmic immunoreactivity for WT1 and GLUT1 within endothelial cells lining the lesional vascular structures, but the lymphatic endothelial marker D2–40 is negative (101,102).

Differential diagnosis: Verrucous hemangioma can be clinically confused with "angiokeratomas," but this lacks a deep vascular component making the diagnosis easier. Combined vascular malformations composed of capillary, lymphatic, and venous components can also show varying degrees of hyperkeratosis and acanthosis; however, they are always negative for GLUT1 and WT1, and the vessels show features reminiscent of veins and lymphatic channels (101,102).

Pyogenic granuloma

Pyogenic granuloma (PG), also termed "lobular capillary hemangioma," is one of the most common benign vascular proliferations in childhood, with an estimated prevalence of 0.5–1%.

Clinical presentation: About 12% of all cases present during infancy beyond the age of 4 months (103); it is very rare in infants of <3 months of age (104). Pyogenic granuloma is characterized by friable vascular papules that erupt preferentially on the head and neck. They can also be located on the oral mucosa (105) and conjunctiva (106). Disseminated (104) as well as agminated PG (107) have been reported.

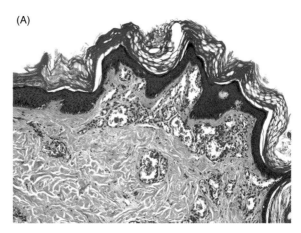

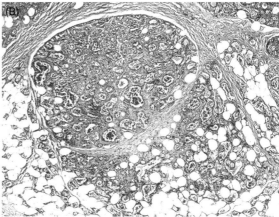

Figure 1.16 Verrucous hemangioma. (A) Superficial part of the lesion showing a verrucous epidermis and dilated capillaries in the papillaru dermis. (B) Lobular arrangement of the vessels in the deeper part of the lesion.

Their size ranges from 1–100 mm (103). PG is a benign, reactive lesion adequately treated by local excision. Neither recurrent nor disseminated forms are associated with bad prognosis (92).

Histology: Exophytic, often ulcerated lesions characterized by lobulated proliferation of capillary sized vessels in a loose and edematous stroma (108). The superficial epithelium is attenuated and characteristically forms an epidermal collarette around the lesion. Ulceration and associated neutrophilic inflammation are frequently seen. Normal mitoses may be present.

Spindle-cell hemangioma

Spindle-cell hemangioma (SCH) is an uncommon benign vascular lesion commonly occurring in children or young adults. Spindle-cell hemangioma development correlates with histological and/or clinical evidence of a malformed vasculature at the affected site (109,110). A small percentage of patients with SCH also have Maffucci syndrome (111), congenital lymphedema, or Klippel–Trenaunay syndrome (109).

Clinical presentation: Spindle-cell hemangioma is seen equally in both Sexes; it most frequently occurs distally on the extremities, and less commonly proximally on the limbs, trunk, head, and neck. The tumor usually presents as a superficial, slow-growing, painless, solitary purplish mass, or with multiple nodules within an anatomical region. Most nodules are <2 cm (112).

Histology: Spindle-cell hemangiomas are mostly found in the dermis and subcutis, and occasionally in the deep soft tissues. They are well-circumscribed but non-encapsulated lesions characterized by intricate blending of cavernous and solid spindle-cell zones. Cavernous areas are composed of thin-walled blood vessels lined by flattened endothelial cells containing red blood cells and thrombi. In the solid regions, short fascicles of spindle cells are interspersed with ramifying narrow vascular spaces. The spindle cells possess uniform, elongated, dark nuclei, and eosinophilic cytoplasm. The spindle areas may have distinctive round or epithelioid cells containing vacuoles and intracytoplasmic lumina, similar to those seen in epithelioid hemangioendothelioma. Atypia and mitoses are not prominent features. Spindle-cell hemangiomas are often partly or completely intravascular, and intravascular extension of the lesion can sometimes be seen around the main nodule (109,112). Cells that line the cavernous vascular spaces stain with von Willebrand factor, CD31, and variably with CD34. The spindle cells show variable staining with vimentin and actin, but are negative for CD34 (109,113).

Kasabach–Merritt phenomenon (KMP)-associated tumors

Kasabach–Merritt phenomenon is characterized by profound thrombocytopenia due to platelet trapping in the tumor, sometimes accompanied by microangiopathic hemolytic anemia and secondary consumption of coagulation factors. It is distinct from the consumptive coagulopathy that may develop in large venous or lymphatic malformations (114).

Kaposiform hemangioendothelioma (KHE) and tufted angioma (TA) account for the vast majority of KMP cases (115). The significant degree of clinical and histological overlap between tufted angioma and kaposiform hemangioendothelioma, and the association of these two entities with KMP suggest that TA is a milder, more superficial form of KHE (115).

Tufted angioma (TA)

Tufted angioma was first described in 1989 (116). Identical lesions had been described earlier as angioblastoma and progressive capillary hemangioma (117,118).

Clinical presentation: Approximately 15% are congenital, and most of them are present <5 years of age (119), but some cases have been reported in adults (120). There is no racial or Sex predominance. Most TAs occur on the upper trunk, neck, and shoulders, and fewer cases occur on the face, scalp, and proximal extremities. Involvement of the feet and oral mucosa has been observed in rare cases (121,122).

Tufted angioma is typically a solitary lesion, but multiple tumors have been described (123). Lesions present as enlarging pink-red, purple, or red-brown patches and plaques with superimposed papules or nodules that spread slowly, then stabilize, and rarely regress (124). The lesion generally ranges from less <1 cm to several centimeters. Tufted angioma often has a rubbery consistency, and may be painful. Tenderness and hyperhidrosis are commonly associated symptoms (125). Hypertrichosis may also be observed (126). Tufted angioma may be associated with KMP, and also with chronic consumptive coagulopathy (127).

Histology: Classically described as a poorly demarcated lesion in the dermis and subcutis, consisting of multiple discrete cannonball-like lobules of capillaries. Crescent-shaped thin-walled lymphatic vessels surround some of these lobules peripherally (Figure 1.17). A second component of lymphangioma-like anastomosed vessels is a prominent feature in some cases (128). The intervening dermis and subcutis are sometimes fibrotic, but may be histologically normal. The surrounding adnexal structures are unaffected, although hypertrophy of neighboring eccrine sweat glands can be seen (129). The pinpoint capillary lumina that form the lobules occasionally contain fibrin and platelet microthrombi. Endothelial cells may appear spindle-like at the periphery of lobules, but this is never a prominent feature. Immunohistochemically, endothelial cells are focally positive for D2–40, LYVE1, and PROX1, but less extensively than in KHE (130,131). As other vascular tumors, TA is positive for WT1 (96). Lesional endothelial cells are GLUT1 negative (95).

Kaposiform hemangioendothelioma (KHE)

Kaposiform hemangioendothelioma is most commonly seen in infancy and childhood and it is strikingly associated with KMP (150).

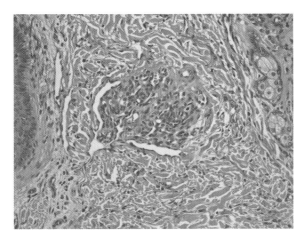

Figure 1.17 Tufted angioma. A cannon-ball lobule surrounded by a dilated lymphatic vessel.

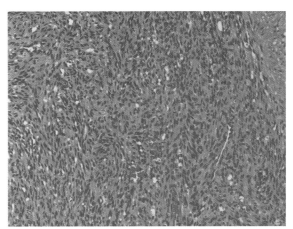

Figure 1.18 Kaposiform hemangioendothelioma. Spindle endothelial cells fascicles.

Clinical presentation: Most cases of KHE (115,132–134) present in early childhood, especially in the first two years of life, and are occasionally detected prenatally (135,136). The lesions range from superficial locally infiltrative stains and plaques to deeply seated bulky masses. The latter may occur in soft tissue of the extremities, trunk, or the head and neck, or may be diagnosed as large body cavity or retroperitoneal masses, often followed by a complicated course with KMP and adverse outcome. Skin manifestations include purpura and ecchymosis. Untreated tumors do not regress (135).

Histology: Kaposiform hemangioendothelioma are composed of infiltrative, ill-defined, frequently coalescing lobules of spindled endothelial cell fascicles (Figure 1.18; 115,132–135). The moderately plump spindle cells form elongated slit-like lumina containing erythrocytes. Nodular pericyte-rich epithelioid nests with pinpoint vascular lumina, often surround platelet-rich microthrombi. The epithelioid nodules are rich in pericytes and contain cytoplasmic hyaline globules and erythrocyte fragments. Dilated lymphatic vessels surround and intermingle with nodules, most prominently at the margins of lesions. Areas with a lobular pattern, indistinguishable from TA are sometimes seen at the periphery of the tumor. At the margin of the lesion, the spindle cells may freely infiltrate the surrounding adipose tissue and between collagen bundles, or may be encased by desmoplastic stroma. The spindled endothelial cells are positive for CD31, CD34 (95,137), and the lymphothelial markers D2–40, LYVE-1, and PROX1 (130). All endothelial cells are negative for GLUT1 and LeY antigen.

Multifocal lymphangioendotheliomatosis with thrombocytopenia (MLT)

This is a rare disorder first described in 2004 (138). Multifocal lymphangioendotheliomatosis with thrombocytopenia is characterized by a proliferation of multiple congenital and progressive vascular lesions usually associated with mild-to-moderate thrombocytopenia.

Clinical presentation: MLT involves skin and the gastrointestinal system, but it may also involve lungs, brain, spleen, bone, synovium, or muscle. Males and females are equally affected. Gastrointestinal bleeding is almost universally present and may be life threatening (139). Cutaneous lesions are flat or indurated red-brown to burgundy plaques or papules up to 5 cm present in variable numbers. Appearance of new lesions and slow progression of existing lesions, without evidence of regression, is typical (139).

Histology: Multifocal lymphangioendotheliomatosis with thrombocytopenia lesions involving the skin consist of delicate vessels scattered throughout the dermis and subcutis. They are lined by a monolayer of slightly hobnailed endothelial cells forming complex papillary projections that appear to float within the lumina. Mitoses are rare or absent. The endothelial cells show strong reactivity for CD31, CD34, and LYVE-1, and light or no staining for D2–40; they are negative for GLUT1 (138).

Papillary intralymphatic angioendothelioma/retiform hemangioendothelioma spectrum

Papillary intralymphatic angioendothelioma (PILA) and retiform hemangioendothelioma (RH) are closely related lesions considered within the group of vascular tumors known as "hemangioendotheliomas," implying that they are borderline between benign hemangiomas and conventional angiosarcomas. This reflects their ability to recur, but their limited capacity for metastasis.

It has been suggested that PILA is the juvenile variant of RH and that both tumors probably develop from lymphatic endothelial cells.

Papillary intralymphatic angioendothelioma

Papillary intralymphatic angioendothelioma, also known as Dabska tumor, is a low-grade vascular tumor of childhood (140).

Clinical presentation: PILA occurs almost exclusively in children and young adults and some cases are congenital. Most PILA originate in the skin and superficial soft tissues of head and neck, trunk, or extremities (141,142). Rarely, bone (143) and spleen (144) are affected. Typically, these are ill-defined masses of the dermis and subcutaneous tissue that may impart a violaceous hue to the overlying skin. Some arise from a *bona fide* lymphangioma or vascular malformation (145–147).

Histology: At low power, lesions resemble a vascular malformation with large, irregular, thick-walled vessels surrounded by lymphoid aggregates. Smaller lymphatic channels can also be identified. "Hobnail" endothelial cells line the blood vessels. These cells are a characteristic feature of this tumor, and the diagnosis should not be made in their absence. They are identified by their cuboidal shape, high nuclear–cytoplasmic ratio, finely stippled chromatin pattern, nuclear clefts, and cytoplasmic vacuoles. Intravascular endothelial papillary projections lined by these hobnail cells and containing a central hyaline core of accumulated basement membrane material are seen within small and large vessels. Although there is a tendency to identify a vascular tumor with intravascular endothelial tufts as a Dabska tumor, it should be remembered that endothelial tufting can be seen in other tumors, notably angiosarcoma. Thus the diagnosis of Dabska tumor is made when the other criteria, particularly the presence of hobnail endothelium, are met as well.

The endothelial cells within a Dabska tumor have an immunophenotype that mirrors normal lymphatic endothelium. They usually express von Willebrand factor, Fli1, CD31, and CD34 (staining with the first two is usually significantly less intense than with the last). They also express the lymphatic markers VEGFR3 and D2-40, and lack an actin-positive cuff of pericytes (141,148).

Dabska tumors metastasize to regional lymph nodes, but only an exceptional case has given rise to disseminated disease (140).

Retiform hemangioendothelioma (RE)

Retiform hemangioendothelioma is a superficially located tumor that occurs mainly in adults and is characterized by vessels having an elongated shape resembling the rete testis (149).

Kaposi sarcoma (KS)

Kaposi sarcoma is a low-grade malignant vascular neoplasm with four known clinical subtypes: classic, iatrogenic, AIDS-associated, and African/endemic (150,151). All clinical subtypes of KS are caused by HHV-8, also called KS-associated herpes virus, and are rarely observed in children.

Clinical presentation: Most African children who progress from latent HHV-8 infection to KS do so in the context of untreated HIV. Kaposi sarcoma lesions are characterized by multiple violaceous dermal patches, plaques, and/or nodules. Clinicopathological variants of KS include anaplastic, telangiectatic, lymphangioma-like, bullous, hyperkeratotic, keloidal, micronodular, pyogenic granuloma-like, ecchymotic, and intravascular KS (152,153). It has been suggested that certain variants, such as anaplastic KS and possibly lymphangioma-like KS, might have prognostic relevance (152). In children, cervical and oropharyngeal lymphadenopathy, and visceral involvement, respectively, are more common than cutaneous involvement.

Histology: Patch lesions can be misinterpreted at low-power magnification as some form of inflammatory dermatosis. On closer examination, a subtle vasoformative process composed of slit-like vascular spaces dissecting dermal collagen is present. The protrusion of native vascular structures into the lumina of ectatic neoplastic channels results in the characteristic "promontory" sign. A mild inflammatory infiltrate comprising lymphocytes and plasma cells, often accompanied by iron-laden macrophages, is usually noticed. In the plaque stage, numerous dissecting vascular channels containing erythrocytes occupy the dermis. Vessels are more irregular in shape and fascicles or solid sheets of spindle cells with slit-like vascular lumina and extravasated erythrocytes are demonstrated. Hyaline globules are seen within solid areas of the tumor. Mitoses are sparse and there is no significant nuclear or cytological pleomorphism. Nodular KS exhibits dermal expansion by a relatively circumscribed proliferation of neoplastic spindled cells arranged in fascicles. Erythrocytes are contained within slit-like channels between the individual spindled cells. The proliferating cells are relatively monomorphic, but some mitoses can be identified. Hyaline globules and intracytoplasmic red cells are seen more readily.

HHV-8 latent nuclear antigen-1 protein can be demonstrated by immunohistochemistry in KS. HHV-8 can also be assessed by PCR analysis in tissues processed for conventional histopathology (154). HHV-8 is not specific for KS, as the virus has been detected in other vascular and non-vascular neoplasms (155). CD31, CD34, FLI-1, and D2–40 are variably expressed in HIV- and non-HIV-related KS (156). Differential diagnosis in children includes spindle-cell hemangioma, kaposiform hemangioendothelioma, hobnail angioma, and microcystic lymphatic malformation; clinical features and absence of HHV-8 staining help in the differentiation of these lesions from KS.

Cutaneous angiosarcoma (CAS)

Cutaneous angiosarcoma is a malignant neoplasm of endothelial cells and in children appears to have a better outcome than deep soft tissues or visceral variants (157).

Clinical presentation: Cutaneous angiosarcoma is a rare tumor, which predominantly arises in the sun-exposed skin of the head and neck of adults and elderly patients. Rarely, these tumors can be seen in children, and most of them have been associated with a pre-existing condition, such as xeroderma pigmentosum, Aicardi syndrome, and radiation therapy. Most pediatric cases of angiosarcoma are seen in late childhood and adolescence; congenital and infantile angiosarcomas are very rare (157).

Cutaneous angiosarcoma in children differs significantly from that in adults. Pediatric CAS is more common in female patients, in the lower extremities, and tends to be small and unifocal (157).

Histology: Pediatric CAS shares most of the features seen in the adult form, although there seems to be a disproportionate number of purely epithelioid variants (90%) (158). Diagnostic criteria include the presence of racemose and arborizing vessels, significant cytologic atypia, and endothelial stratification or areas of solid morphology (Figure 1.19). Well-differentiated areas and poorly differentiated foci may alternate. Immunohistochemical analysis reveals endothelial markers (CD31, CD34, Ulex europaeus, and von Willebrand factor). There is variable reactivity

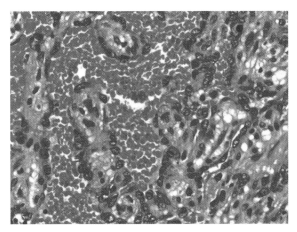

Figure 1.19 Angiosarcoma. Epitheliod atypical cells lining irregular vascular spaces.

for lymphatic markers such as VEGFR-3 and D2–40 (159,160), but human herpes virus type 8 is absent (161).

Vascular malformations

Vascular malformations are non-neoplastic lesions that result from abnormal vascular morphogenesis. These vascular anomalies are present at birth, grow proportionally with the size of the child, and do not involute spontaneously.

Based on both the primary vessel type within the lesion and its blood-flow characteristics, vascular malformations are further subdivided into distinct categories: slow-flow capillary, venous, or lymphatic malformations, and fast-flow arterial malformations.

Endothelial cells in vascular malformations are always negative for GLUT1. They are also negative for WT1 in most cases, except for the rare arterio-venous malformations (95,96).

Capillary malformation (CM)

Commonly referred to as Port-wine stains, CMs are dermal vascular anomalies that occur in about 0.3% of newborns and have an equal sex distribution. Capillary malformations must be differentiated from fading macular stains, colloquially termed "stork bite," "salmon patch," or "angel's kiss."

Clinical presentation: The appearance varies from small patches with a red to pink hue to large lesions that involve an entire limb or part of the face. Capillary malformation can appear all over the body, but are frequently present on the head and neck. Children

23

with a CM affecting the eyelids must be evaluated for Sturge–Weber syndrome. Capillary malformations tend to darken throughout life, turning a deeper shade of red or blue and may even become thicker or more nodular as the individual matures.

Histology: Capillary malformations are seldom biopsied, but when they are, they reveal an increased number of blood vessels confined to the dermis. Endothelial cells are flat and mitotically inactive. Lesion vessels are difficult to recognize in biopsies from young children, but become more visible as they progressively dilate over a period of years.

Venous malformation (VM)

Venous malformations are relatively rare congenital lesions, but are not always clinically evident at birth. Venous malformations are frequently misdiagnosed as "cavernous hemangiomas."

Clinical presentation: Venous malformations can appear all over the body and usually appear as soft, compressible, blue masses. Venous malformations may be associated with either a localized or generalized consumptive coagulopathy. Venous malformation-associated bleeding diathesis must be differentiated from Kasabach–Merritt syndrome, which occurs in infants with kaposiform hemangioendothelioma and tufted angioma, as mentioned previously.

Histology: Venous malformations are slow-flow vascular malformations composed of anomalous, ectatic, irregular venous channels with flat endothelial cells and scant mural smooth muscle. Thrombi in various stages of organization are commonly present (Figure 1.20).

Glomuvenous malformation (GVM)

Glomuvenous malformation, also known as glomangioma, is an uncommon entity with histological features of both glomus cell proliferation and venous malformation. Most cases are familial; autosomal-dominant inheritance has been demonstrated. Mutations in the glomulin gene, located on chromosome 1p22–p21, have been identified as the underlying genetic defect (162).

Clinical presentation: They appear as multiple bluish-purple nodules in the skin and mucous membranes. Glomuvenous malformations have a solid, cobble-stone-like appearance. Congenital lesions tend to grow slowly, and new lesions occur up to the age of 20. Their number varies from a few to hundreds (163). Unlike the solitary glomus tumor seen in adults (typically located subungually), they are not painful on palpation. In addition to multiple nodules, congenital, extensive plaques have been described (164). In two

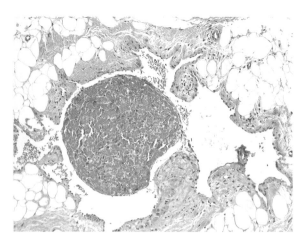

Figure 1.20 Venous malformation. Irregular venous channels with scant mural smooth muscle.

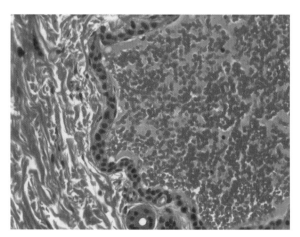

Figure 1.21 Glomuvenous malformation. Glomus cells in the wall of dilated venous channels.

cases, congenital extensive plaque-type GVM were associated with fetal pleural effusion and ascites (165).

Histology: Glomuvenous malformations are characterized by enlarged vein-like channels lined by flattened endothelium and surrounded by one or several rows of uniform, cuboidal eosinophilic glomus cells (Figure 1.21). The glomus cell component may vary widely between regions, and some microscopic fields may show only veins devoid of glomus cells, leading to a misdiagnosis of venous malformation. In keeping with their derivation from vascular smooth-muscle cells, glomus cells stain positive for vimentin and smooth-muscle cell α-actin.

Lymphatic malformations (LM)

Lymphatic malformations are developmental anomalies of the lymphatic system that result in abnormal lymphatic flow.

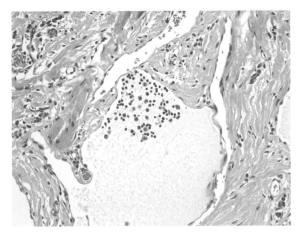

Figure 1.22 Lymphatic malformation. Dilated lymphatic channels containing proteinaceous fluid and a few lymphocytes and histiocytes.

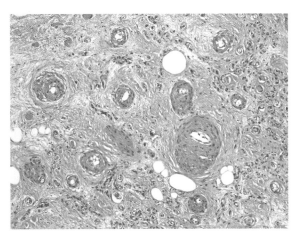

Figure 1.23 Arteriovenous malformation. Venous arterialization and increased number of reactive angiomatous capillaries.

Clinical presentation: Lymphatic malformations are present at birth and grow commensurately with the child, but in some cases they can grow suddenly, due to hemorrhage or infection. Lymphatic malformations can present as localized or diffuse masses with vesicles on the skin surface. They are frequently referred to as "lymphangiomas" and can be divided into macrocystic and microcystic types.

Histology: Biopsies and surgical specimens reveal sponge-like collections of dilated lymphatic channels containing proteinaceous fluid and a few lymphocytes and histiocytes (Figure 1.22). Mural lymphoid tissue is sometimes abundant. Different antibodies can be used to stain lymphatic endothelium: D2–40, PROX1, LYVE1, and VEGFR3, among others. Endothelial cells in LM are usually negative for CD34, but positive for CD31. Immunohistochemistry is useful to identify LM with intralesional hemorrhage, that otherwise may be mistaken for VM.

Arteriovenous malformation (AVM)

Arteriovenous malformations are fast-flow vascular lesions composed of dysmorphic arteries and veins connected directly to one another with the absence of the normal intervening capillary bed.

Clinical presentation: Arteriovenous malformations have no gender predilection, and they are more common on the head and neck. Arteriovenous malformations may be present at birth, but many cases become clinically apparent during childhood. Clinically, they can mimic a CM, but the presence of higher local temperature, a palpable thrill, or an audible bruit suggests a high-flow component. Common

symptoms include pain, overgrowth of the involved body part, ulceration, bleeding, and heart failure.

Histology: Biopsies reveal abnormal, variably composed collections of arterial and venous channels, admixed with congeries of smaller vessels. Increased venous pressure results in venous "arterialization." Endothelial cells are flat and without demonstrable mitotic activity, except in areas of reactive angiomatosis (Figure 1.23). Endothelial cells in AVM are reactive for panendothelial markers and WT1.

Non-vascular mesenchymal neoplasms

Most benign and malignant mesenchymal neoplasms affecting the skin in children are discussed in the chapter dedicated to soft tissue tumors (Chapter 11), including the most frequently seen lesions such as dermatofibroma, myofibroma/myofibromatosis, fibrous hamartoma of infancy, infantile digital fibromatosis, (referred as inclusion-bearing fibromatosis), DFSP/giant-cell fibroblastoma, etc.

Two mesenchymal lesions affecting exclusively the skin will be discussed in this section.

Dermatomyofibroma (DMF)

Rare benign fibroblastic/myofibroblastic cutaneous tumor mostly occurring in young adult women; can also be seen in pediatric patients (166).

Clinical presentation: Dermatomyofibroma appears as small, ill-defined, skin-colored, slightly hyperpigmented or erythematous plaque or nodule, usually located on the shoulder and adjacent regions,

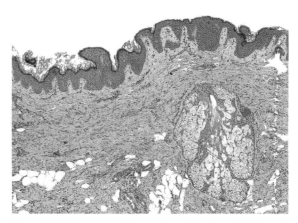

Figure 1.24 Dermatomyofibroma. Dermal fascicles of spindle cells oriented parallel to the epidermal surface.

such as the upper arm, axilla, neck, and upper trunk. Most cases are asymptomatic, but can also be slightly painful or itchy.

Histology: Composed of spindle cells with bland fusiform nuclei and weakly eosinophilic cytoplasm, arranged in fascicles or ill-defined nodules. The dermal fascicles are usually oriented parallel to the epidermal surface, while in the subcutaneous tissue they can be arranged perpendicularly (Figure 1.24). Numerous elastic fibers, sometimes enlarged and fragmented, can be present between the spindle cells. Variable expression of calponin, SMA, MSA, CD34, and CD10 has been demonstrated.

Differential diagnosis: Other myofibroblastic lesions, such as myofibromatosis, fibrous hamartoma of infancy, or smooth muscle hamartoma lack the typical parallel arrangement to the epidermis of DMF. In contrast to the fascicular pattern seen in dermatomyofibroma, dermatofibroma shows a storiform pattern, entrapment of collagen, and reduction of elastic fibers. Scars exhibit a disordered architecture, variable cellularity, increased vascularization, prominent collagenous stroma, and loss of elastic fibers.

Plaque-like CD34-positive dermal fibroma (PDF)

Very rare dermal lesion, most commonly seen in children, also known as medallion-like dermal dendrocyte hamartoma (167,168).

Clinical presentation: Positive dermal fibroma presents as a solitary, several centimeter-sized, round or oval, slightly pigmented, atrophic, and indurated plaque on the neck, trunk, and extremities. Positive

dermal fibroma is congenital and remains stable with time.

Histology: Positive dermal fibroma appears as a cellular band-like fibroblastic proliferation mostly located in the papillary and adjacent upper reticular dermis, but sometimes extending into the subcutaneous tissue. The fusiform cells stain positive for CD34 and factor XIIIa, but are negative for S100.

Differential diagnosis: The main diagnostic pitfall of PDF is atrophic congenital dermatofibrosarcoma protruberans (DFSP), due to clinical and histological similarities between them. The fusion gene *COL1A1-PDGFB* is present in most cases of DFSP, but not in PDF. Atrophic cutaneous neurofibroma can be easily ruled out based on the negative stain for S100.

Epidermal and adnexal neoplasms and cysts

Benign epidermal tumors and cysts are frequent in children. Dermoid cysts and pilomatrixomas are the most common. Some epidermal or adnexal tumors in children may be troublesome, because of potential malignancy, multiplicity, or association with genetic syndromes.

Epidermal nevi (EN)

Epidermal nevi are hamartomas (usually present at birth and due to mosaicism) characterized by hyperplasia of the epidermis and adnexal structures. These nevi may be classified into a number of variants, which are based on clinical morphology, extent of involvement, and the predominant epidermal structure in the lesion. Variants include keratinocytic nevus, nevus sebaceous, nevus comedonicus, eccrine nevus, apocrine nevus, Becker nevus, and white sponge nevus.

Keratinocytic nevus

Most keratinocytic epidermal nevi are due to activating mosaic mutations in three different genes within the keratinocyte: *FGFR3*, *PIK3CA*, and the *RAS* family. Some identical mutations are found in seborrheic keratosis.

Clinical presentation: A velvety or verrucous group of papules, usually following a linear arrangement within the lines of Blaschko, is the most common presentation. Keratinocytic nevi are frequently asymptomatic, although occasionally can be pruritic with erythema and hyperkeratosis, as in inflammatory linear verrucous epidermal nevus (ILVEN). They can appear anywhere on the skin, but are less common on the head

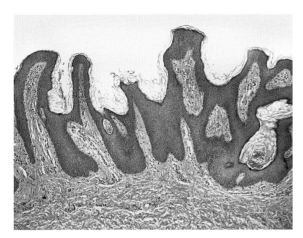

Figure 1.25 Keratinocytic nevus. The epidermis shows hyperkeratosis, acanthosis, and papillomatosis.

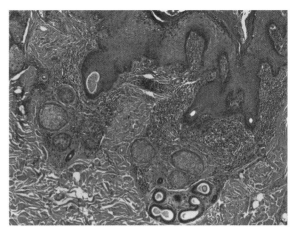

Figure 1.26 Sebaceous nevus. Sebaceous glands aberrantly placed, opening directly onto the epidermis.

and scalp. Keratinocytic epidermal nevi may present as cutaneous lesions alone or associated with neurologic and/or musculoskeletal abnormalities (epidermal nevus syndrome, Solomon syndrome; 169).

Histology: There is hyperkeratosis, acanthosis, and papillomatosis, often accompanied by hyperpigmentation of the basal cell layer (Figure 1.25). Epidermolytic hyperkeratosis may be noted in some cases showing orthokeratosis, a thickened granular layer with enlarged keratohyaline granules, and keratinocytes with perinuclear clearing and vacuolar change. Inflammatory linear verrucous epidermal nevus typically shows psoriasiform epidermal hyperplasia, vertically and horizontally alternating parakeratosis with orthokeratosis, and a predominantly intraepidermal lymphocytic inflammatory infiltrate. Other patterns include those of seborrheic keratosis (sometimes irritated or clonal) and acantholytic dyskeratosis.

Differential diagnosis: Keratinocytic nevi may clinically mimic other linear conditions such as the verrucous stage of incontinentia pigmenti, lichen striatus, linear porokeratosis, or linear lichen planus. Inflammatory linear verrucous epidermal nevus may appear histologically identical to linear psoriasis and some keratinocytic nevi can easily be confused with seborrheic keratosis. The young age of onset supports the diagnosis of ILVEN and keratinocytic nevus, as lineal psoriasis and seborrheic keratosis are not typically seen in children.

Nevus sebaceous (NS)

Nevus sebaceous is a cutaneous hamartoma in which the cellular component is mainly the sebaceous gland, although hair follicle, apocrine gland, and keratinocyte involvement is not uncommon. *RAS* family gene mosaic mutations are involved (170).

Clinical presentation: Usually present at birth as a tawny plaque on the scalp completely devoid of hair. Sometimes, a Blaschko-linear arrangement on the scalp and face is seen. Similarly to normal sebaceous glands, the abnormal glands of the nevus sebaceous are under androgenic control; thus the lesions often become clinically more conspicuous at puberty, with development of cobblestoned surface and more intense yellow or orange hue. Nevus sebaceous lesions, especially when large, may be associated with multiple internal abnormalities, similar to those reported in linear epidermal nevus syndrome.

Histology: An increase in the number of sebaceous glands is the hallmark in adolescents and adults; however, sebaceous hyperplasia can be subtle before puberty. Sebaceous glands may be aberrantly placed, such as opening directly onto the epidermis rather than into the hair follicle (Figure 1.26). Follicles may be reduced in number or abnormally shaped, immature or abortive in appearance. The epidermis shows features of keratinocytic epidermal nevus. An increased number of apocrine glands in the dermis and subcutis is another feature, but is not always present. Secondary neoplasms such as syringocystadenoma papilliferum, trichoblastoma (diagnosed in the past as basal cell carcinoma), apocrine adenomas, or other adnexal tumors may develop (171).

Dermoid cyst (DC)

Clinical presentation: Dermoid cysts appear in early infancy as round, easily mobile, cystic nodules that

27

may be located in areas of fusion (such as the midline; 172) or in typical locations, such as the eyebrow or the scalp. Dermoid cysts located on the midline of the face and scalp may be connected with the CNS.

Histology: Dermoid cysts are lined by stratified squamous epithelium that keratinizes through a granular layer. The cavity contains loose, laminated orthokeratin, and hair shafts. The presence of pilosebaceous structures within the cyst wall and hair shafts protruding into the cyst cavity differentiate them from epidermoid cysts, rarely seen in children. Smooth muscle, eccrine glands, and apocrine glands may occasionally be identified surrounding the cyst.

Pilomatrixoma

Pilomatrixoma (pilomatricoma or calcifying epithelioma of Malherbe) is a relatively common benign cutaneous adnexal neoplasm with differentiation towards the matrix and inner sheath of a normal hair follicle, as well as the hair cortex. Pilomatrixomas are one of the most common dermal and subcutaneous tumors of children.

Clinical presentation: They may appear at infancy or childhood, and usually take the form of a hard, palpable, deep dermal or subcutaneous nodule, generally located on the head, neck, or upper trunk regions; however, they may appear elsewhere. The size may range from millimeters to a few centimeters. In many cases calcification can be easily perceived. Multiple pilomatrixomas (rare) are a marker for myotonic dystrophy, and may rarely be associated with different conditions including Rubinstein–Taybi syndrome, Turner syndrome, Goldenhar syndrome, sternal cleft defects, coagulative defects, and sarcoidosis. Pilomatrixoma-like features are an occasional finding in cutaneous cysts removed from patients with Gardner syndrome.

Histology: Well-circumscribed nodules in the dermis or superficial subcutis, typically composed of basaloid (matrical) cells and shadow (ghost) cells. Basaloid cells exhibit deeply basophilic oval or round nuclei and a variable number of mitoses. Shadow cells are polygonal, eosinophilic cell remnants, with a centrally located clear area corresponding to the absent nucleus (Figure 1.27). The transition from basaloid to ghost cells is abrupt. There is often associated foreign-body-type reaction. Calcifications are common. Some pilomatrixomas contain melanophages in the stroma and dendritic melanocytes within the clusters of basaloid cells (pigmented or melanocytic variants). The

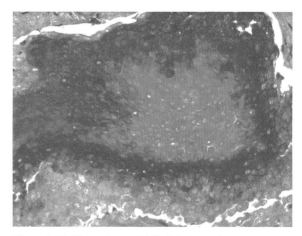

Figure 1.27 Pilomatrixoma. Calcified shadow cells.

early stage of pilomatrixomas has a higher proportion of basaloid cells, often with numerous mitoses. In a later stage, the basaloid component may be minimal or absent, and calcification or even ossification may be seen.

Trichoblastoma/trichoepithelioma

Trichoblastoma (TBL) and trichoepithelioma (TE) are rare benign follicular fibroepithelial tumors showing differentiation toward the trichoblast. Trichoepithelioma and trichoblastoma are used synonymously in the 2006 WHO classification of skin tumors.

Clinical presentation: Trichoblastoma presents as a solitary, small papule on any hair-follicle-bearing location, usually the head and the neck. They can also present as multiple centrofacial papules or nodules, particularly in Brooke–Fordyce and Brooke–Spiegler diseases. Most trichoblastomas are non-ulcerated skin-colored papules <1 cm in diameter.

Histology: Biphasic tumors composed of basaloid epithelial cells and a cellular fibrous stroma distinctly different from the surrounding normal reticular dermis (Figure 1.28). Epithelial components can show different patterns such as nodular (large and small nodules), cribriform, and columnar (desmoplastic). A typical finding is the presence of follicular papillae, which are cup-like proliferations of basaloid cells engulfing fibroblasts. Scant mitoses or apoptotic bodies can be present. Clefts between the tumor stroma and surrounding normal dermis, and stromal calcifications are common. In some cases melanocytes can be prominent within the epithelial areas.

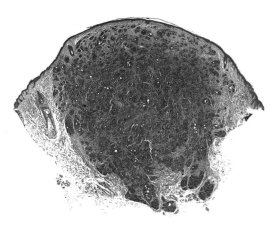

Figure 1.28 Trichoblastoma. Biphasic tumors composed of basaloid epithelial cells and a cellular fibrous stroma distinctly different from the surrounding normal reticular dermis.

Superficial lesions of TBL, usually referred to as TE, typically contain small keratocysts with infundibular keratinization and may form connections to the epidermis.

Differential diagnosis: Mainly with BCC. The presence of papillary bodies, few mitoses and clefts between the tumor stroma and surrounding normal dermis, are all features favoring trichoblastoma (173).

Syringoma

Syringomas are small, benign adnexal neoplasms composed of sweat gland eccrine epithelium within densely sclerotic stroma.

Clinical presentation: Usually multiple small, skin-colored papules around the eyelids, axilla, abdomen, and vulva.

Histology: Small, circumscribed proliferation of small dermal sweat gland ducts lined by at least two layers of flat and/or cuboidal non-atypical cells within a dense stroma of compactly arranged bundles of collagen. The cells often have eosinophilic cytoplasm, but clear cell changes are not uncommon. Some ducts have a tennis racket or tadpole configuration, and some of them show cystic changes. Lesions are usually restricted to the upper dermis.

Basal cell carcinoma

Basal cell carcinoma represents a group of malignant cutaneous tumors characterized by the presence of lobules, columns, bands, or cords of basaloid cells ("germinative cells"; 43).

Table 1.8 Predisposing factors for BCC

- Nevoid basal cell carcinoma syndrome (Gorlin)
- Bazex–Dupré–Christol syndrome
- Xeroderma pigmentosum
- Rothmund–Thompson syndrome
- Albinism
- Immunodeficiency
- Immunosuppression
- Chemotherapy
- Ionizing radiation
- Arsenic exposure
- Nevus sebaceous

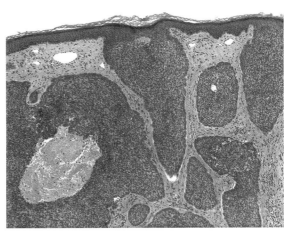

Figure 1.29 Basal cell carcinoma. Nests of basaloid cells with peripheral palisading attached to the epidermis.

Basal cell carcinoma is very uncommon in children. Although some sporadic cases have been described (174), most of them are associated with different predisposing conditions (see Table 1.8). Nevoid basal cell carcinoma syndrome is the most common underlying disorder in pediatric BCC.

Histology (Figure 1.29), immunohistochemistry, and variants of BCC are shown in Table 1.9.

Differential diagnosis: Some other follicular tumors, such as basaloid follicular hamartoma, trichoblastoma, or trichoepithelioma may be mistaken for BCC in children. Conversely, some cases of BCC have been diagnosed as follicular basaloid hamartomas (175,176).

Squamous cell carcinoma

Cutaneous SCC is a malignant neoplasm of epidermal keratinocytes in which the proliferating cells show variable squamous differentiation (66). Cutaneous SCC comprises less than 0.1% of all

Table 1.9 Histological features of BCC

Histology
- Nests or islands of basaloid cells with hyperchromatic nuclei and scant cytoplasm
- Attachment to the undersurface of the epidermis
- Numerous mitoses, sometimes atypical
- Peripheral palisading
- Clefts between tumor and surrounding stroma
- Variable dermal infiltration
- New-formed stroma distinct from the adjacent dermis
- Mucinous alteration of the tumoral stroma

Immunophenotype
- Positive for Ber-EP4, 34Be12, mNF116
- Melan-A often demonstrates melanocytes within the tumor

Variants
- Nodular (solid), Superficial, Micronodular, Morpheaform
- Other (cystic, adenoid, sclerosing, infundibulocystic, pigmented, fibroepithelial or Pinkus tumor, BCC with adnexal differentiation, basosquamous, keratotic, etc.)
- Mixed types

Differential diagnosis
- Trichoblastoma/Trichoepithelioma
- Basaloid follicular hamartoma
- Other non-melanoma skin cancers

Table 1.10 Predisposing factors for SCC

- Xeroderma pigmentosum
- Epidermolysis bullosa
- Hidrotic ectodermal dysplasia
- Albinism
- Fanconi's anemia
- Dyskeratosis congenita
- Erythropoietic porphyria
- Immunodeficiency
- Immunosuppression
- Epidermodysplasia verruciformis
- Burn scars
- Chronic infections with sinus tracts
- Chemotherapy
- Ionizing radiation
- Arsenic exposure

Table 1.11 Histological features of SCC

Histology
- Nests of atypical squamous epithelial cells arising from the epidermis
- Cells have abundant eosinophilic cytoplasm and a large, often vesicular, nucleus
- Keratinization usually present (dyskeratosis or horn pearl formation)
- Infiltrative growth pattern
- Variable stromal inflammatory reaction and desmoplasia

Immunophenotype
- Positive for 34BE12, AE1/AE3, EMA, p63, MNF116, CK5/6

Variants
- Acantholytic, Clear cell, Warty, Verrucous, Spindle cell, Desmoplastic, Lympho-epitheliomatous, etc.

Differential diagnosis
- Pseudoepitheliomatous hyperplasia
- Inflammatory dermatoses (e.g., lichen planus)
- Other malignant tumors (e.g., melanoma, lymphoma)

childhood malignancies and at most, 5% of cutaneous malignancies (177).

Ultraviolet radiation and DNA-repair disorders (XP, Fanconi's anemia, etc.) represent the most common predisposing factor for SCC in children. Other predisposing conditions are listed in Table 1.10.

The principal precursor of cutaneous SCC is actinic keratosis (AK), which in children is very rare, and if present in childhood and adolescence should prompt an evaluation for an underlying DNA-repair problem, particularly XP.

Clinical presentation: Usually a non-healing, scaly, crusted, or verrucous, indurated papule or plaque on a sun-exposed skin area (177).

Histology: Histological and immunohistochemical features (Figure 1.30), differential diagnosis and variants of SCC are shown in Table 1.11.

Hematopoietic neoplasms

Cutaneous lymphomas and leukemias

Primary cutaneous lymphomas are rare in children and are mostly represented by mycosis fungoides and the CD30+ lymphoproliferative disorders, lymphomatoid papulosis (178) and anaplastic large T-cell lymphoma (ALCL; 179). More rarely, a wide spectrum of cutaneous lymphomas can be diagnosed in children, among

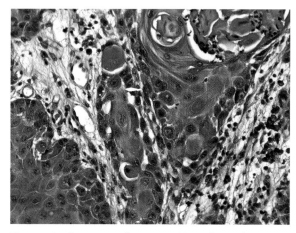

Figure 1.30 Squamous cell carcinoma. Nests of atypical squamous epithelial cells arising from the epidermis with dyskeratosis.

them "panniculitis-like" T-cell lymphoma, small-medium pleomorphic T-cell lymphoma, natural killer (NK)/T-cell lymphoma of the nasal type, hydroa vacciniforme-like T-cell lymphoma, follicle center cell lymphoma, lymphomatoid granulomatosis, marginal zone B-cell lymphoma, etc. (180). Lymphoblastic lymphoma, a common pediatric tumor most frequently seen in mediastinal locations and usually showing a T-cell phenotype, can also present as a primary skin disorder, especially when it has a B-cell derivation (181).

Cutaneous lymphoma in children should be differentiated from benign skin disorders that may simulate them. In particular, mycosis fungoides and lymphomatoid granulomatosis in this age group may present with clinicopathologic features reminiscent of pityriasis alba, vitiligo, pityriasis rosea, and PLEVA.

Secondary involvement of the skin by systemic lymphomas and acute or chronic leukemias is sometimes the first manifestation of the disease in children. Cutaneous lesions can precede the bone marrow and blood involvement in leukemia. Clinical and phenotypic features of childhood leukemias and systemic lymphomas are discussed in Chapter 7.

Mycosis fungoides (MF)

Mycosis fungoides is a peripheral, epidermotropic, low-grade non-Hodgkin T-cell lymphoma.

Clinical presentation: Mycosis fungoides is characterized by sequential appearance of patches, plaques, and tumors. Patches are circumscribed lesions with discoloration, without palpable infiltration of the skin. Plaques usually evolve out of patches and present with palpable infiltration. Tumors exhibit an exophytic growth and tend to ulcerate. Extracutaneous spread can be seen in advanced stages of the disease. Rare clinical variants, such as hypopigmented MF, pagetoid reticulosis, granulomatous slack skin and MF-associated follicular mucinosis, have been reported in children (182).

Histology: Band-like aggregates of atypical lymphocytes are seen within the superficial dermis and invading the epidermis as single cells and small clusters (Pautrier microabscesses). Solitary lymphocytes aligned along the dermal–epidermal junction are sometimes recognized. Atypical lymphocytes have convoluted contours with folded nuclear membranes (cerebriform appearance). Patches and plaques show pronounced epidermotropism, but in more advanced nodular lesions the malignant T-cells often lose this epidermotropic tendency, grow deeply into the dermis, and eventually spread systemically. The number of large lymphocytes (more than four times the size of a small lymphocyte) is prognostically relevant. Large cell transformation (more than 25% large lymphocytes) portends a poor prognosis. Spongiosis or Civatte bodies are not features of MF. Prototypical lesions of MF show an increase in CD4:CD8 ratio. The immunophenotype of classic MF is CD3(+), CD2(+), CD4(+), TCR beta(+), CD45 RO+, but some cases can be CD8+/CD4–, CD8+/CD4+, or CD4–/CD8–. In many cases a monoclonal rearrangement of the T-cell receptor gene can be demonstrated by PCR; however, the lack of detection of a T-cell clone in histologically subtle patch lesions does not exclude the diagnosis, since false-negative results occur in approximately 40% of early MF.

Lymphomatoid papulosis (LyP)

Lymphomatoid papulosis is a chronic recurrent T-cell CD30+ lymphoproliferative skin disease with self-regressing papulo-nodular skin lesions and atypical lymphoid cells in a polymorphous inflammatory background.

Clinical features: Lymphomatoid papulosis is characterized by disseminated asymptomatic papules and/or nodules, which regress spontaneously after a few weeks. Typically, the lesions occur in crops and are in different stages of evolution. The most commonly affected sites include the trunk and proximal extremities; however, lesions may be seen on the face, palms, soles, and scalp. Localized forms of LyP have also been reported in the literature (183).

Histology: Three classic histological subtypes are recognized. Type A is the most common histological variant; it is characterized by large CD30 atypical cells intermingled with a prominent mixed inflammatory infiltrate (Figure 1.31). The large tumor cells exhibit convoluted nuclei with one or more prominent nucleoli. Type B is characterized by smaller atypical cells with hyperchromatic and cerebriform nuclei resembling the atypical lymphocytes in MF. Type C is characterized by sheets of anaplastic large cells, histologically indistinguishable from ALCL. A variant of lymphomatoid papulosis simulating primary cutaneous aggressive epidermotropic CD8+ cytotoxic T-cell lymphoma and referred to as type D LyP has been recently characterized (184). Large cells in types A and C are strongly positive for CD30 and also express T-cell markers. CD30-positive cells are almost always absent in type B LyP.

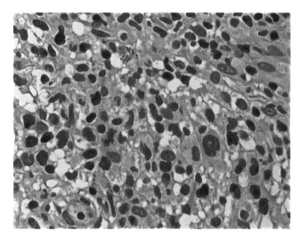

Figure 1.31 Lymphomatoid papulosis. Scattered atypical cells in a background of mixed inflammation.

Differential diagnosis: Type A LyP may show overlap with PLEVA and a clear separation between both entities is not always possible (178). CD30-positive cells can be seen in reactive conditions, such as hypersensitivity reactions from arthropod bites or drugs; the presence of clusters of CD30+ atypical cells favors LyP. Mycosis fungoides, ALCL, and aggressive epidermotropic CD8+ cytotoxic T-cell lymphoma should be differentiated from types B, C, and D, respectively.

Primary cutaneous anaplastic large-cell lymphoma (C-ALCL)

Cutaneous anaplastic large-cell lymphoma is a neoplasm composed of large atypical lymphocytes showing expression of CD30 antigen by the majority of tumor cells.

Clinical presentation: Lesions are usually solitary nodules, tumors, or plaques that frequently ulcerate or become necrotic. Spontaneous regression may be seen in approximately 25% of the patients and approximately 20% have multifocal disease. Involvement of regional lymph nodes is sometimes seen.

Histology: A dermal nodular infiltrate composed of dense cohesive sheets of large atypical CD30-positive cells comprises the majority of the lesional cell population (more than 75%). Acanthosis and secondary epidermal changes with exocytosis or ulceration are commonly seen (Figure 1.32). Eosinophils and/or neutrophils may be numerous. Cutaneous anaplastic large-cell lymphoma is almost always negative for anaplastic-lymphoma-related tyrosine kinase (ALK). Rare cases of ALK-positive anaplastic large-cell lymphomas limited to the skin have been reported in children. These cases behave similarly to ALK-negative C-ALCL (185).

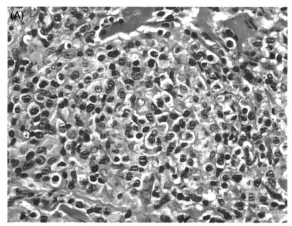

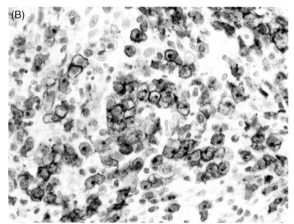

Figure 1.32 Anaplastic large-cell lymphoma. Diffuse infiltration of the skin by atypical cells (A) showing positivity for CD30 (B).

Differential diagnosis: Cutaneous anaplastic large-cell lymphoma should be differentiated from Type C LyP and systemic ALK-positive ALCL. Clinical features need to be considered, as histological features can overlap.

Mastocytosis

This is a heterogeneous group of disorders characterized by abnormal growth and accumulation of mast cells in one or more organ systems (186). Most patients have indolent cutaneous mastocytosis that may regress spontaneously. A minority of patients, usually adults, have systemic mastocytosis that rarely may be highly aggressive (187).

Clinical presentation: Mastocytosis in children is mostly a skin disorder. Solitary lesions, sometimes called mastocytoma, appear as yellow-orange plaques that easily urticate and develop blisters. Mastocytomas are often present at birth. Multiple skin lesions, in the form

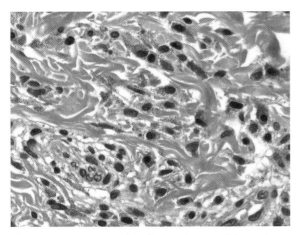

Figure 1.33 Mastocytosis. Spindle-shaped mast cells in a patient with urticarial pigmentosa.

of macules, papules, and small nodules, with color ranging from tan-brown to yellowish, are often referred to as urticaria pigmentosa. Typically, these lesions urticate after vigorous rubbing, a feature called Darier's sign.

Genetics: Mastocytosis is a benign clonal disease, due to autoactivating mutations of c-KIT in mast cells and sometimes other bone-marrow cell lines. Rare kindreds with familial mastocytosis have germline c-KIT mutations. These patients may also have gastrointestinal stromal tumors (GISTs; 188,189).

Histology: Mast cells in mastocytosis tend to accumulate perivascularly, mainly in the superficial dermis, but may extend into the deep reticular dermis and subcutaneous fat. The histologic picture in urticaria pigmentosa or solitary mastocytoma varies from a subtle increase in the numbers of spindle-shaped mast cells, to large numbers of tightly packed, rounded mast cells in the upper to mid-dermis (Figure 1.33). Variable fibrosis, edema, and small numbers of eosinophils may also be present. Metachromatic mast-cell granules are demonstrated on Giemsa and toluidine blue. Mast cells express CD45, CD117, and HLA-DR.

Differential diagnosis: When there are eosinophils, dermal hypersensitivity reactions, parasitosis, or arthropod bites are the main differential diagnoses. Inflammatory dermatosis with increased mast cells may simulate mastocytosis. Unequivocal diagnosis of cutaneous mastocytosis requires the demonstration of aggregates of mast cells within the dermis.

Histiocytosis

The histiocytoses are a heterogeneous group of proliferative disorders of the macrophage-monocyte lineage. The most common types of histiocytosis in children fall within two categories: Langerhans-cell histiocytosis (LCH) and non-Langerhans-cell types. In the former, a reactive proliferation of Langerhans cells may cause variable symptoms, ranging from limited skin involvement, to a severe systemic disease that eventually can be fatal. In the latter there are a number of entities representing macrophage or dermal dendrocyte proliferations, often with cell lipidization, leading to overlapping manifestations.

Langerhans cell histiocytosis (LCH)

Langerhans cell histiocytosis is a clonal disorder with systemic spread, characterized by proliferation of dendritic cells bearing morphologic and phenotypic markers of Langerhans cells (LC).

Clinical presentation: Langerhans cell histiocytosis most commonly affects newborns and young infants. The skin lesions usually consist of discrete papules, with a pearly color and a purpuric hue, usually located on the scalp, back, abdomen, and groin. They show thick, yellowish scales that, when lesions coalesce, provide a seborrheic dermatitis-like appearance, mainly on the scalp and retroauricular region. A bright red erythema on the large folds of the neck and groin is also characteristic of LCH. Mucosal involvement may also ensue. Skin lesions may be the only manifestation of the disease, or there may be multiple organ involvement, mainly in bones, liver, lungs, bone marrow, and gastrointestinal tract. Congenital reticulohistiocytosis of Hashimoto and Pritzker is a self-healing variant, characterized by discrete fleshy nodules often with central crusting, affecting different areas of the skin surface.

Histology: Fully developed papules have a dense band-like infiltrate of the superficial dermis obscuring the dermal–epidermal junction, showing epidermotropism and microabscess formation. Langerhans cells are characterized by large, pale, folded, lobulated, or reniform nuclei, and abundant, eosinophilic, or amphophilic cytoplasm (Figure 1.34). In Hashimoto–Pritzker disease, LCs show a reticulocytic appearance with abundant eosinophilic cytoplasm. The band-like infiltrate may contain variable numbers of eosinophils, lymphocytes, macrophages, neutrophils, plasma cells, and extravasated erythrocytes. Langerhans-cell histiocytosis expresses CD1a, Langherin, CD4, and S-100 protein. Macrophage markers are usually negative, but can be co-expressed in some cases. Birbeck granules can be identified on electron microscopy. Histology does not predict biologic behavior.

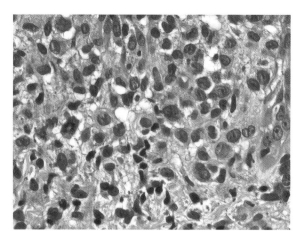

Figure 1.34 Langerhans-cell histiocytosis. A dense infiltrate of Langerhans cells showing reniform nuclei.

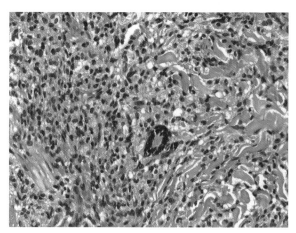

Figure 1.35 Juvenile xanthogranuloma. A mature lesion showing foamy histiocytes and Touton giant cells.

Differential diagnosis: Florid reactive Langerhans-cell hyperplasia may be seen in different dermatoses, such as atopic dermatitis, contact dermatitis, PLEVA, scabies, and others (190). In LCH, cells typically form dense clusters, whereas in reactive hyperplasia, LCs tend to be more dispersed. Strict clinical–pathologic correlation is important in order to avoid misdiagnosis. Langerhans cell histiocytosis may also be confused with non-Langerhans histiocytes, mastocytosis, leukemias, and melanocytic lesions. Nuclear morphology and immunophenotype are helpful diagnostic features.

Juvenile xanthogranuloma (JXG)

Juvenile xanthogranuloma is a benign, self-healing proliferation of non-Langerhans lipid-laden histiocytes, typically seen in children.

Clinical presentation: Juvenile xanthogranuloma is one of the most common tumors in children. The typical presentation consists of a solitary papule or small nodule on any skin location. The orange or yellow appearance is due to lipidization, and usually develops later. Eventually, JXG fades leaving slight skin atrophy. Multiple lesions of JXG ranging from very few to hundreds may be seen; in these cases, systemic involvement of JXG lesions on the liver, CNS, eyes, lungs, and virtually every organ is possible, and should be ruled out (191). Multiple JXG may also be associated with multiple café-au-lait spots and neurofibromatosis. Juvenile xanthogranuloma and LCH can rarely co-exist in the same patient (192). Agminated or clustered JXG has also been reported (193). Benign cephalic histiocytosis (BCH) is considered by some authors to be an early form of JXG. BCH is a self-limited eruption that typically affects infants and young children, and presents as multiple, small, reddish to yellow, macules and papules, limited to the head and upper body.

Histology: Juvenile xanthogranuloma presents as non-encapsulated nodular dermal aggregates of small-to intermediate-sized macrophages. The nuclei are small, round, ovoid, or indented, with inconspicuous nucleoli. With time, the macrophage cytoplasm becomes laden with lipid and appears foamy. Mature lesions contain foamy cells, foreign-body giant cells and Touton giant cells, mainly distributed in the superficial dermis and on the nodule's edge (Figure 1.35). Lymphocytes, plasma cells, neutrophils, and eosinophils are usually present within the infiltrate. Mitoses can be readily found in non-lipidized early lesions. Macrophages in JXG demonstrate strong, granular, cytoplasmic staining for CD68. They are frequently positive for Factor XIIIa, HAM56 and CD4. Juvenile xanthogranuloma is negative for CD1a and Langherin, and for S100 protein in most cases.

Histologically the lesions seen in BCH are indistinguishable from JXG.

Metastasic infiltration of the skin

Leukemias and lymphomas represent a large proportion of metastatic disease in the skin in children (see Chapter 7). Cutaneous or subcutaneous metastasis of non-hematopoietic malignancies in children and adolescents are rare, but may be the first manifestation of the disease.

The tumors most likely to metastasize to the skin in children are neuroblastoma and rhabdomyosarcoma (194,195).

Infants and neonates with neuroblastoma can present with multiple dark blue cutaneous metastases, the so-called "blueberry muffin baby" (196). These nodules may blanch centrally and develop an erythematous halo for several minutes or hours following palpation (194,197,198). Other conditions associated with a "blueberry muffin baby" include infections (TORCH), hematologic dyscrasias (199), or metabolic disorders (200).

Rhabdomyosarcoma, the most common soft-tissue sarcoma in children, may be primary in the skin (201), but can also metastasize to the skin (202,203). Other sarcomas, such as primitive neuroectodermal tumor (PNET), malignant rhabdoid tumor, and osteogenic sarcoma, may also give cutaneous metastasis.

Tumors that have rarely been reported to metastasize to the skin in pediatric patients, include melanoma, choriocarcinoma, malignant paraganglioma, colonic adenocarcinoma, and nasopharyngeal carcinoma (204).

References

1. Alsaad KO, Ghazarian D. My approach to superficial inflammatory dermatoses. J. Clin. Pathol. 2005;**58**(12):1233–41.

2. Paller AS. Clinical features of atopic dermatitis. Clin. Rev. Allergy. 1993;**11**(4):429–46.

3. Elias PM, Eichenfield LF, Fowler JF, Horowitz P, McLeod RP. Update on the structure and function of the skin barrier: Atopic dermatitis as an exemplar of clinical implications. Semin. Cutan. Med. Surg. 2013;**32**(2 Suppl 2):S21–4.

4. Eichenfield LF, Ellis CN, Mancini AJ, Paller AS, Simpson EL. Atopic dermatitis: epidemiology and pathogenesis update. Semin. Cutan. Med. Surg. 2012;**31**(3 Suppl):S3–5.

5. Mercy K, Kwasny M, Cordoro KM, Menter A, et al. Clinical manifestations of pediatric psoriasis: results of a multicenter study in the United States. Pediatr. Dermatol. 30(4):424–8.

6. Crowson AN, Magro CM, Mihm MC. Interface dermatitis. Arch. Pathol. Lab. Med. 2008;**132**(4):652–66.

7. Léauté-Labrèze C, Lamireau T, Chawki D, Maleville J, Taïeb A. Diagnosis, classification, and management of erythema multiforme and Stevens–Johnson syndrome. Arch. Dis. Child. 2000;**83**(4):347–52.

8. Harr T, French LE. Toxic epidermal necrolysis and Stevens–Johnson syndrome. Orphanet J. Rare Dis. 2010;5:39.

9. Markus JR, Carvalho VO, Lima MN et al. The relevance of recognizing clinical and morphologic features of pityriasis lichenoides: clinicopathological study of 29 cases. Dermatol. Pract. Concept. 2013;**3**(4):7–10.

10. López-Villaescusa MT, Hernández-Martín A, Colmenero I, Torrelo A. Pityriasis lichenoides in a 9-month-old boy. Actas Dermosifiliogr. 2013;**104**:829–30.

11. Fisler RE, Saeb M, Liang MG, Howard RM, McKee PH. Childhood bullous pemphigoid: A clinicopathologic study and review of the literature. Am. J. Dermatopathol. 2003;**25**(3):183–9.

12. Venning VA. Linear IgA disease: clinical presentation, diagnosis, and pathogenesis. Dermatol. Clin. 2011;**29**(3):453–8, ix.

13. Weiss PF. Pediatric vasculitis. Pediatr. Clin. North Am. 2012;**59**(2):407–23.

14. Carlson JA, Chen K-R. Cutaneous vasculitis update: small vessel neutrophilic vasculitis syndromes. Am. J. Dermatopathol. 2006;**28**(6):486–506.

15. Carlson JA. The histological assessment of cutaneous vasculitis. Histopathology. 2010;**56**(1):3–23.

16. Thornsberry LA, English JC. Etiology, diagnosis, and therapeutic management of granuloma annulare: An update. Am. J. Clin. Dermatol. 2013;**14**(4):279–90.

17. Grogg KL, Nascimento AG. Subcutaneous granuloma annulare in childhood: clinicopathologic features in 34 cases. Pediatrics. 2001;**107**(3):E42.

18. Torrelo A, Hernández A. Panniculitis in children. Dermatol. Clin. 2008;**26**(4):491–500, vii.

19. Polcari IC, Stein SL. Panniculitis in childhood. Dermatol. Ther. 23(4):356–67.

20. Requena L. Normal subcutaneous fat, necrosis of adipocytes and classification of the panniculitides. Semin. Cutan. Med. Surg. 2007;**26**(2):66–70.

21. Segura S, Pujol RM, Trindade F, Requena L. Vasculitis in erythema induratum of Bazin: A histopathologic study of 101 biopsy specimens from 86 patients. J. Am. Acad. Dermatol. 2008;**59**(5):839–51.

22. Hogeling M, Meddles K, Berk DR, et al. Extensive subcutaneous fat necrosis of the newborn associated with therapeutic hypothermia. Pediatr. Dermatol. **29**(1):59–63.

23. Akcay A, Akar M, Oncel MY, et al. Hypercalcemia due to subcutaneous fat necrosis in a newborn after total body cooling. Pediatr. Dermatol. **30**(1):120–3.

24. Mahé E, Girszyn N, Hadj-Rabia S, et al. Subcutaneous fat necrosis of the newborn: A systematic evaluation of risk factors, clinical manifestations, complications and outcome of 16 children. Br. J. Dermatol. 2007;**156**(4):709–15.

25. Bellew SG, Quartarolo N, Janniger CK. Childhood warts: An update. Cutis. 2004;**73**(6):379–84.

26. Silverberg NB. Human papillomavirus infections in children. Curr. Opin. Pediatr. 2004;**16**(4):402–9.

27. Chen X, Anstey A V, Bugert JJ. Molluscum contagiosum virus infection. Lancet Infect. Dis. 2013;**13**(10):877–88.

28. Lee R, Schwartz RA. Pediatric molluscum contagiosum: reflections on the last challenging poxvirus infection, Part 1. Cutis. 2010;**86**(5):230–6.

29. Lee R, Schwartz RA. Pediatric molluscum contagiosum: reflections on the last challenging poxvirus infection, Part 2. Cutis. 2010;**86**(6):287–92.

30. Layegh P, Moghiman T, Ahmadian Hoseini SA. Children and cutaneous leishmaniasis: A clinical report and review. J. Infect. Dev. Ctries. 2013;**7**(8):614–7.

31. Koçarslan S, Turan E, Ekinci T, Yesilova Y, Apari R. Clinical and histopathological characteristics of cutaneous Leishmaniasis in Sanliurfa City of Turkey including Syrian refugees. Indian J. Pathol. Microbiol. **56**(3):211–5.

32. Swick BL. Polymerase chain reaction-based molecular diagnosis of cutaneous infections in dermatopathology. Semin. Cutan. Med. Surg. 2012;**31**(4):241–6.

33. Rivers JK, Frederiksen PC, Dibdin C. A prevalence survey of dermatoses in the Australian neonate. J. Am. Acad. Dermatol. 1990;**23**(1):77–81.

34. Reyes-Múgica M, Beckwith M, Etchevers H. Etiology of congenital melanocytic nevi and other related conditions. In: Marghoob A, Grinchik J, Sccope A, Dusza S, editors, *Nevogenesis*, New York. Springer, 2012:69–72.

35. Krengel S, Scope A, Dusza SW, Vonthein R, Marghoob AA. New recommendation for the categorization of cutaneous features of congenital melanocytic nevi. J. Am. Acad. Dermatol. 2013;**68**(3):441–51.

36. Wyatt a J, Hansen RC. Pediatric skin tumors. *Pediatr. Clin. North Am.* 2000;**47**(4):937–63.

37. Castilla EE, da Graça Dutra M, Orioli-Parreiras IM. Epidemiology of congenital pigmented naevi: I. Incidence rates and relative frequencies. Br. J. Dermatol. 1981;**104**(3):307–15.

38. Tannous ZS, Mihm MC, Sober AJ, Duncan LM. Congenital melanocytic nevi: clinical and histopathologic features, risk of melanoma, and clinical management. J. Am. Acad. Dermatol. 2005;**52** (2):197–203.

39. Hale EK, Stein J, Ben-Porat L, *et al.* Association of melanoma and neurocutaneous melanocytosis with large congenital melanocytic naevi – results from the NYU-LCMN registry. Br. J. Dermatol. 2005;**152** (3):512–7.

40. Mark GJ, Mihm MC, Liteplo MG, Reed RJ, Clark WH. Congenital melanocytic nevi of the small and garment type. Clinical, histologic, and ultrastructural studies. Hum. Pathol. 1973;**4**(3):395–418.

41. Barnhill RL, Fleischli M. Histologic features of congenital melanocytic nevi in infants 1 year of age or younger. J. Am. Acad. Dermatol. 1995;**33**(5 Pt 1):780–5.

42. Rhodes AR, Silverman RA, Harrist TJ, Melski JW. A histologic comparison of congenital and acquired nevomelanocytic nevi. Arch. Dermatol. 1985;**121** (10):1266–73.

43. LeBoit PE. Burg G, Weeden D, Sarasin A. *World Health Organization Classificationof Tumours. Pathology and Genetics of Skin Tumours.* (Internet). IARC Press Lyon: 2006. Available from: http://www.iarc.fr/en/publications/ pdfs-online/pat-gen/bb6/BB6.pdf (accessed May 2014).

44. Phadke PA, Rakheja D, Le LP, *et al.* Proliferative nodules arising within congenital melanocytic nevi: A histologic, immunohistochemical, and molecular analyses of 43 cases. Am. J. Surg. Pathol. 2011;**35** (5):656–69.

45. Spitz S. Melanomas of childhood. Am. J. Pathol. 1948;**24**(3):591–609.

46. Akyürek M, Kayikçioğlu A, Ozkan O, *et al.* Multiple agminated Spitz nevi of the scalp. Ann. Plast. Surg. 1999;**43**(4):459–60.

47. Böer A, Wolter M, Kneisel L, Kaufmann R. Multiple agminated Spitz nevi arising on a café au lait macule: review of the literature with contribution of another case. Pediatr. Dermatol. 2001;**18**(6):494–7.

48. Bullen R, Snow SN, Larson PO, *et al.* Multiple agminated Spitz nevi: report of two cases and review of the literature. Pediatr. Dermatol. 1995;**12**(2):156–8.

49. Hueso L, Hernández A, Torrelo A, Colmenero I, Zambrano A. (Agminated Spitz nevi on a hyperpigmented macule). Actas Dermosifiliogr. **99** (1):69–72.

50. Levy RM, Ming ME, Shapiro M, *et al.* Eruptive disseminated Spitz nevi. J. Am. Acad. Dermatol. 2007;**57**(3):519–23.

51. Fass J, Grimwood RE, Kraus E, Hyman J. Adult onset of eruptive widespread Spitz's nevi. J. Am. Acad. Dermatol. 2002;**46**(5 Suppl):S142–3.

52. Kamino H, Flotte TJ, Misheloff E, Greco MA, Ackerman AB. Eosinophilic globules in Spitz's nevi. New findings and a diagnostic sign. Am. J. Dermatopathol. 1979;**1**(4):319–24.

53. Walsh N, Crotty K, Palmer A, McCarthy S. Spitz nevus vs. spitzoid malignant melanoma: An evaluation of the current distinguishing histopathologic criteria. Hum. Pathol. 1998;**29**(10):1105–12.

54. Busam KJ, Barnhill RL. Pagetoid Spitz nevus. Intraepidermal Spitz tumor with prominent pagetoid spread. Am. J. Surg. Pathol. 1995;**19**(9):1061–7.

55. Requena C, Botella R, Nagore E, *et al.* Characteristics of spitzoid melanoma and clues for differential diagnosis

with Spitz nevus. Am. J. Dermatopathol. 2012;**34** (5):478–86.

56. Lyon VB. The spitz nevus: review and update. Clin. Plast. Surg. 2010;**37**(1):21–33.

57. Bergman R, Dromi R, Trau H, Cohen I, Lichtig C. The pattern of HMB-45 antibody staining in compound Spitz nevi. Am. J. Dermatopathol. 1995;**17**(6):542–6.

58. Kanter-Lewensohn L, Hedblad MA, Wejde J, Larsson O. Immunohistochemical markers for distinguishing Spitz nevi from malignant melanomas. Mod. Pathol. 1997;**10**(9):917–20.

59. Palazzo J, Duray PH. Typical, dysplastic, congenital, and Spitz nevi: A comparative immunohistochemical study. Hum. Pathol. 1989;**20**(4):341–6.

60. Ribé A, McNutt NS. S100A6 protein expression is different in Spitz nevi and melanomas. Mod. Pathol. 2003;**16**(5):505–11.

61. Li LX, Crotty KA, McCarthy SW, Palmer AA, Kril JJ. A zonal comparison of MIB1-Ki67 immunoreactivity in benign and malignant melanocytic lesions. Am. J. Dermatopathol. 2000;**22**(6):489–95.

62. Blokx WAM, van Dijk MCRF, Ruiter DJ. Molecular cytogenetics of cutaneous melanocytic lesions – diagnostic, prognostic and therapeutic aspects. Histopathology. 2010;**56**(1):121–32.

63. Gerami P, Li G, Pouryazdanparast P, et al. A highly specific and discriminatory FISH assay for distinguishing between benign and malignant melanocytic neoplasms. Am. J. Surg. Pathol. 2012;**36** (6):808–17.

64. Spatz A, Calonje E, Handfield-Jones S, Barnhill RL. Spitz tumors in children: A grading system for risk stratification. Arch. Dermatol. 1999;**135**(3):282–5.

65. Barnhill RL, Argenyi ZB, From L, et al. Atypical Spitz nevi/tumors: lack of consensus for diagnosis, discrimination from melanoma, and prediction of outcome. Hum. Pathol. 1999;**30**(5):513–20.

66. Barnhhill R. Childhood melanoma. In: LeBoit P, Burg G, Weedon D, Sarasain A, editors, *World Health Organisation Classification of Tumours: Pathology and Genetics of Skin Tumours.* Lyon: IARC Press; 2006;84–5.

67. Smith KJ, Barrett TL, Skelton HG, Lupton GP, Graham JH. Spindle cell and epithelioid cell nevi with atypia and metastasis (malignant Spitz nevus). Am. J. Surg. Pathol. 1989;**13**(11):931–9.

68. Ludgate MW, Fullen DR, Lee J, et al. The atypical Spitz tumor of uncertain biologic potential: A series of 67 patients from a single institution. Cancer. 2009;**115** (3):631–41.

69. Ferrara G, Argenziano G, Soyer HP, et al. The spectrum of Spitz nevi: A clinicopathologic study of 83 cases. Arch. Dermatol. 2005;**141**(11):1381–7.

70. Sau P, Graham JH, Helwig EB. Pigmented spindle cell nevus: A clinicopathologic analysis of ninety-five cases. J. Am. Acad. Dermatol. 1993;**28**(4):565–71.

71. Sagebiel RW, Chinn EK, Egbert BM. Pigmented spindle cell nevus. Clinical and histologic review of 90 cases. Am. J. Surg. Pathol. 1984;**8**(9):645–53.

72. Zembowicz A, Phadke PA. Blue nevi and variants: An update. Arch. Pathol. Lab. Med. 2011;**135**(3):327–36.

73. Mills O, Messina JL. Pediatric melanoma: A review. Cancer Control. 2009;**16**(3):225–33.

74. Hill SJ, Delman K a. Pediatric melanomas and the atypical spitzoid melanocytic neoplasms. Am. J. Surg. 2011;**203**(6):761–7.

75. McElearney ST, Dengel LT, Vaughters ABR, Patterson JW, McGahren ED, Slingluff CL. Neonatal congenital malignant melanoma with lymph node metastasis. J. Clin. Oncol. 2009;**27**(16):2726–8.

76. Huynh PM, Grant-Kels JM, Grin CM. Childhood melanoma: update and treatment. Int. J. Dermatol. 2005;**44**(9):715–23.

77. Valenzano Menada M, Moioli M, Garaventa A, et al. Spontaneous regression of transplacental metastases from maternal melanoma in a newborn: case report and review of the literature. Melanoma Res. 2010;**20**(6):443–9.

78. Boddie AW, Smith JL, McBride CM. Malignant melanoma in children and young adults: effect of diagnostic criteria on staging and end results. South. Med. J. 1978;**71**(9):1074–8.

79. Ferrari A, Bono A, Baldi M, et al. Does melanoma behave differently in younger children than in adults? A retrospective study of 33 cases of childhood melanoma from a single institution. Pediatrics. 2005;**115** (3):649–54.

80. Neier M, Pappo A, Navid F. Management of melanomas in children and young adults. J. Pediatr. Hematol. *Oncol.* 2012;**34** Suppl 2:S51–4.

81. Pappo AS. Melanoma in children and adolescents. Eur. J. Cancer. 2003;**39**(18):2651–61.

82. Strouse JJ, Fears TR, Tucker MA, Wayne AS. Pediatric melanoma: risk factor and survival analysis of the surveillance, epidemiology and end results database. J. Clin. Oncol. 2005;**23** (21):4735–41.

83. Linabery AM, Ross JA. Trends in childhood cancer incidence in the U.S. (1992–2004). Cancer. 2008;**112** (2):416–32.

84. Hamm H, Höger PH. Skin tumors in childhood. Dtsch. Arztebl. Int. 2011;**108**(20):347–53.

85. Whiteman DC, Valery P, McWhirter W, Green AC. Risk factors for childhood melanoma in Queensland, Australia. Int. J. Cancer. 1997;**70**(1):26–31.

86. Downard CD, Rapkin LB, Gow KW. Melanoma in children and adolescents. Surg. Oncol. 2007;**16**(3):215–20.

87. Gimotty PA, Botbyl J, Soong S-J, Guerry D. A population-based validation of the American Joint Committee on Cancer melanoma staging system. J. Clin. Oncol. 2005;**23**(31):8065–75.

88. Landi MT, Bauer J, Pfeiffer RM, *et al.* MC1R germline variants confer risk for BRAF-mutant melanoma. Science. 2006;**313**(5786):521–2.

89. Barnhill RL. Childhood melanoma. Semin. Diagn. Pathol. 1998;**15**(3):189–94.

90. Barnhill RL, Flotte TJ, Fleischli M, Perez-Atayde A. Cutaneous melanoma and atypical Spitz tumors in childhood. Cancer. 1995;**76**(10):1833–45.

91. Livestro DP, Kaine EM, Michaelson JS, *et al.* Melanoma in the young: differences and similarities with adult melanoma: A case-matched controlled analysis. Cancer. 2007;**110**(3):614–24.

92. Bruder E, Alaggio R, Kozakewich HPW, *et al.* Vascular and perivascular lesions of skin and soft tissues in children and adolescents. Pediatr. Dev. Pathol. 2012;**15**(1 Suppl):26–61.

93. Mulliken JB, Glowacki J. Hemangiomas and vascular malformations in infants and children: A classification based on endothelial characteristics. Plast. Reconstr. Surg. 1982;**69**(3):412–22.

94. Gonzalez-Crussi F, Reyes-Mugica M. Cellular hemangiomas ("hemangioendotheliomas") in infants. Light microscopic, immunohistochemical, and ultrastructural observations. Am. J. Surg. Pathol. 1991;**15**(8):769–78.

95. North PE, Waner M, Mizeracki A, Mihm MC. GLUT1: A newly discovered immunohistochemical marker for juvenile hemangiomas. Hum. Pathol. 2000;**31**(1):11–22.

96. Trindade F, Tellechea O, Torrelo A, Requena L, Colmenero I. Wilms tumor 1 expression in vascular neoplasms and vascular malformations. Am. J. Dermatopathol. 2011;**33**(6):569–72.

97. Berenguer B, Mulliken JB, Enjolras O, *et al.* Rapidly involuting congenital hemangioma: clinical and histopathologic features. Pediatr. Dev. Pathol. **6**(6):495–510.

98. Enjolras O, Mulliken JB, Boon LM, *et al.* Noninvoluting congenital hemangioma: A rare cutaneous vascular anomaly. Plast. Reconstr. Surg. 2001;**107**(7):1647–54.

99. Picard A, Boscolo E, Khan ZA, *et al.* IGF-2 and FLT-1/VEGF-R1 mRNA levels reveal distinctions and similarities between congenital and common infantile hemangioma. Pediatr. Res. 2008;**63**(3):263–7.

100. Imperial R, Helwig EB. Verrucous hemangioma. A clinicopathologic study of 21 cases. Arch. Dermatol. 1967;**96**(3):247–53.

101. Trindade F, Torrelo A, Requena L, *et al.* An immunohistochemical study of verrucous hemangiomas. J. Cutan. Pathol. 2013;**40**(5):472–6.

102. Tennant LB, Mulliken JB, Perez-Atayde AR, Kozakewich HPW. Verrucous hemangioma revisited. Pediatr. Dermatol. **23**(3):208–15.

103. Pagliai KA, Cohen BA. Pyogenic granuloma in children. Pediatr. Dermatol. **21**(1):10–3.

104. Browning JC, Eldin KW, Kozakewich HPW, Mulliken JB, Bree AF. Congenital disseminated pyogenic granuloma. Pediatr. Dermatol. **26**(3):323–7.

105. Gordón-Núñez MA, de Vasconcelos Carvalho M, Benevenuto TG, *et al.* Oral pyogenic granuloma: A retrospective analysis of 293 cases in a Brazilian population. J. Oral Maxillofac. Surg. 2010;**68**(9):2185–8.

106. Shields JA, Mashayekhi A, Kligman BE, *et al.* Vascular tumors of the conjunctiva in 140 cases. Ophthalmology. 2011;**118**(9):1747–53.

107. Baselga E, Wassef M, Lopez S, *et al.* Agminated, eruptive pyogenic granuloma-like lesions developing over congenital vascular stains. Pediatr. Dermatol. **29**(2):186–90.

108. Hoeger PH, Colmenero I. Vascular tumours in infants. Part I: benign vascular tumours other than infantile haemangioma. Br. J. Dermatol. 2013 Oct 1; doi: 10.1111/bjd.12650 (Epub ahead of print).

109. Fletcher CD, Beham A, Schmid C. Spindle cell haemangioendothelioma: A clinicopathological and immunohistochemical study indicative of a non-neoplastic lesion. Histopathology. 1991;**18**(4):291–301.

110. Imayama S, Murakamai Y, Hashimoto H, Hori Y. Spindle cell hemangioendothelioma exhibits the ultrastructural features of reactive vascular proliferation rather than of angiosarcoma. Am. J. Clin. Pathol. 1992;**97**(2):279–87.

111. Weiss SW, Enzinger FM. Spindle cell hemangioendothelioma. A low-grade angiosarcoma resembling a cavernous hemangioma and Kaposi's sarcoma. Am. J. Surg. Pathol. 1986;**10**(8):521–30.

112. Perkins P, Weiss SW. Spindle cell hemangioendothelioma. An analysis of 78 cases with reassessment of its pathogenesis and biologic behavior. Am. J. Surg. Pathol. 1996;**20**(10):1196–204.

113. Fukunaga M, Ushigome S, Nikaido T, Ishikawa E, Nakamori K. Spindle cell hemangioendothelioma: An immunohistochemical and flow cytometric study of six cases. Pathol. Int. 1995;**45**(8):589–95.

114. Cohen MM. Vascular update: morphogenesis, tumors, malformations, and molecular dimensions. Am. J. Med. Genet. A. 2006;**140**(19):2013–38.

115. Enjolras O, Wassef M, Mazoyer E, *et al.* Infants with Kasabach-Merritt syndrome do not have "true" hemangiomas. J. Pediatr. 1997;**130**(4):631–40.

116. Jones EW, Orkin M. Tufted angioma (angioblastoma). A benign progressive angioma, not to be confused with Kaposi's sarcoma or low-grade angiosarcoma. J. Am. Acad. Dermatol. 1989;**20**(2 Pt 1):214–25.

117. Nakagawa K. Case report of angioblastoma of the skin. Nippon Hifuka Gakkai Zasshi. 1949;**59**:92–4.

118. Macmillan A, Champion RH. Progressive capillary haemangioma. Br. J. Dermatol. 1971;**85**(5):492–3.

119. Heagerty AH, Rubin A, Robinson TW. Familial tufted angioma. Clin. Exp. Dermatol. 1992;**17**(5):344–5.

120. Hebeda CL, Scheffer E, Starink TM. Tufted angioma of late onset. Histopathology. 1993;**23**(2):191–3.

121. Fukunaga M. Intravenous tufted angioma. APMIS. 2000;**108**(4):287–92.

122. Kleinegger CL, Hammond HL, Vincent SD, Finkelstein MW. Acquired tufted angioma: A unique vascular lesion not previously reported in the oral mucosa. Br. J. Dermatol. 2000;**142**(4):794–9.

123. Maronn M, Chamlin S, Metry D. Multifocal tufted angiomas in 2 infants. Arch. Dermatol. 2009;**145**(7):847–8.

124. Ishikawa K, Hatano Y, Ichikawa H, Hashimoto H, Fujiwara S. The spontaneous regression of tufted angioma. A case of regression after two recurrences and a review of 27 cases reported in the literature. Dermatology. 2005;**210**(4):346–8.

125. Suarez SM, Pensler JM, Paller AS. Response of deep tufted angioma to interferon alfa. J. Am. Acad. Dermatol. 1995;**33**(1):124–6.

126. Herron MD, Coffin CM, Vanderhooft SL. Tufted angiomas: variability of the clinical morphology. Pediatr. Dermatol. **19**(5):394–401.

127. Osio A, Fraitag S, Hadj-Rabia S, *et al.* Clinical spectrum of tufted angiomas in childhood: A report of 13 cases and a review of the literature. Arch. Dermatol. 2010;**146**(7):758–63.

128. Sadeghpour M, Antaya RJ, Lazova R, Ko CJ. Dilated lymphatic vessels in tufted angioma: A potential source of diagnostic confusion. Am. J. Dermatopathol. 2012;**34**(4):400–3.

129. Ban M, Kamiya H, Kitajima Y. Tufted angioma of adult onset, revealing abundant eccrine glands and central regression. Dermatology. 2000;**201**(1):68–70.

130. Le Huu AR, Jokinen CH, Rubin BP, *et al.* Expression of prox1, lymphatic endothelial nuclear transcription factor, in Kaposiform hemangioendothelioma and tufted angioma. Am. J. Surg. Pathol. 2010;**34**(11):1563–73.

131. Arai E, Kuramochi A, Tsuchida T, *et al.* Usefulness of D2-40 immunohistochemistry for differentiation between kaposiform hemangioendothelioma and tufted angioma. J. Cutan. Pathol. 2006;**33**(7):492–7.

132. North PE, Waner M, Buckmiller L, James CA, Mihm MC. Vascular tumors of infancy and childhood: beyond capillary hemangioma. Cardiovasc. Pathol. **15**(6):303–17.

133. Lyons LL, North PE, Mac-Moune Lai F, *et al.* Kaposiform hemangioendothelioma: A study of 33 cases emphasizing its pathologic, immunophenotypic, and biologic uniqueness from juvenile hemangioma. Am. J. Surg. Pathol. 2004;**28**(5):559–68.

134. Sarkar M, Mulliken JB, Kozakewich HP, Robertson RL, Burrows PE. Thrombocytopenic coagulopathy (Kasabach-Merritt phenomenon) is associated with Kaposiform hemangioendothelioma and not with common infantile hemangioma. Plast. Reconstr. Surg. 1997;**100**(6):1377–86.

135. Enjolras O, Mulliken JB, Wassef M, *et al.* Residual lesions after Kasabach-Merritt phenomenon in 41 patients. J. Am. Acad. Dermatol. 2000;**42**(2 Pt 1):225–35.

136. Walsh MA, Carcao M, Pope E, Lee K-J. Kaposiform hemangioendothelioma presenting antenatally with a pericardial effusion. J. Pediatr. Hematol. Oncol. 2008;**30**(10):761–3.

137. Debelenko L V, Perez-Atayde AR, Mulliken JB, *et al.* D2-40 immunohistochemical analysis of pediatric vascular tumors reveals positivity in kaposiform hemangioendothelioma. Mod. Pathol. 2005;**18**(11):1454–60.

138. North PE, Kahn T, Cordisco MR, *et al.* Multifocal lymphangioendotheliomatosis with thrombocytopenia: A newly recognized clinicopathological entity. Arch. Dermatol. 2004;**140**(5):599–606.

139. Maronn M, Catrine K, North P, *et al.* Expanding the phenotype of multifocal lymphangioendotheliomatosis with thrombocytopenia. Pediatr. Blood Cancer. 2009;**52**(4):531–4.

140. Dabska M. Malignant endovascular papillary angioendothelioma of the skin in childhood. Clinicopathologic study of 6 cases. Cancer. 1969;**24**(3):503–10.

141. Fanburg-Smith JC, Michal M, Partanen TA, Alitalo K, Miettinen M. Papillary intralymphatic angioendothelioma (PILA): A report of twelve cases of a distinctive vascular tumor with phenotypic features of lymphatic vessels. Am. J. Surg. Pathol. 1999;**23**(9):1004–10.

142. Neves RI, Stevenson J, *et al*. Endovascular papillary angioendothelioma (Dabska tumor): underrecognized malignant tumor in childhood. J. Pediatr. Surg. 2011;**46**(1):e25–8.

143. McCarthy EF, Lietman S, Argani P, Frassica FJ. Endovascular papillary angioendothelioma (Dabska tumor) of bone. Skeletal Radiol. 1999;**28**(2):100–3.

144. Rodgers B, Zeim S, Crawford B, *et al*. Splenic papillary angioendothelioma in a 6-year-old girl. J. Pediatr. Hematol. *Oncol*. 2007;**29**(12):808–10.

145. Emanuel PO, Lin R, Silver L, *et al*. Dabska tumor arising in lymphangioma circumscriptum. J. Cutan. Pathol. 2008;**35**(1):65–9.

146. Argani P, Athanasian E. Malignant endovascular papillary angioendothelioma (Dabska tumor) arising within a deep intramuscular hemangioma. Arch. Pathol. Lab. Med. 1997;**121**(9):992–5.

147. Quecedo E, Martínez-Escribano JA, Febrer I, *et al*. Dabska tumor developing within a preexisting vascular malformation. Am. J. Dermatopathol. 1996;**18**(3):302–7.

148. Fletcher C, Unni K, Mertens F. Tumors of soft tissue and bone. *World Health Organization Classification of Tumours*. Lyon: IARC Press; 2002:163–77.

149. Calonje E, Fletcher CD, Wilson-Jones E, Rosai J. Retiform hemangioendothelioma. A distinctive form of low-grade angiosarcoma delineated in a series of 15 cases. Am. J. Surg. Pathol. 1994;**18**(2):115–25.

150. Sahin G, Palanduz A, Aydogan G, *et al*. Classic Kaposi sarcoma in 3 unrelated Turkish children born to consanguineous kindreds. Pediatrics. 2010;**125**(3):e704–8.

151. Abbas AAH, Jastaniah WA. Extensive gingival and respiratory tract Kaposi sarcoma in a child after allogenic hematopoietic stem cell transplantation. J. Pediatr. Hematol. *Oncol*. 2012;**34**(2):e53–5.

152. Cossu S, Satta R, Cottoni F, Massarelli G. Lymphangioma-like variant of Kaposi's sarcoma: clinicopathologic study of seven cases with review of the literature. Am. J. Dermatopathol. 1997;**19**(1):16–22.

153. Grayson W, Pantanowitz L. Histological variants of cutaneous Kaposi sarcoma. Diagn. Pathol. 2008;**3**(1):31.

154. Pak F, Pyakural P, Kokhaei P, *et al*. HHV-8/KSHV during the development of Kaposi's sarcoma: evaluation by polymerase chain reaction and immunohistochemistry. J. Cutan. Pathol. 2005;**32**(1):21–7.

155. Pantanowitz L, Pinkus GS, Dezube BJ, Tahan SR. HHV8 is not limited to Kaposi's sarcoma. Mod. Pathol. 2005;**18**(8):1148; author reply 1149–50.

156. Rosado FGN, Itani DM, Coffin CM, Cates JM. Utility of immunohistochemical staining with FLI1, D2–40, CD31, and CD34 in the diagnosis of acquired immunodeficiency syndrome-related and non-acquired immunodeficiency syndrome-related Kaposi sarcoma. Arch. Pathol. Lab. Med. 2012;**136**(3):301–4.

157. Deyrup AT, Miettinen M, North PE, *et al*. Pediatric cutaneous angiosarcomas: A clinicopathologic study of 10 cases. Am. J. Surg. Pathol. 2011;**35**(1):70–5.

158. Deyrup AT, McKenney JK, Tighiouart M, Folpe AL, Weiss SW. Sporadic cutaneous angiosarcomas: A proposal for risk stratification based on 69 cases. Am. J. Surg. Pathol. 2008;**32**(1):72–7.

159. Kahn HJ, Bailey D, Marks A. Monoclonal antibody D2-40, a new marker of lymphatic endothelium, reacts with Kaposi's sarcoma and a subset of angiosarcomas. Mod. Pathol. 2002;**15**(4):434–40.

160. Folpe AL, Veikkola T, Valtola R, Weiss SW. Vascular endothelial growth factor receptor-3 (VEGFR-3): A marker of vascular tumors with presumed lymphatic differentiation, including Kaposi's sarcoma, kaposiform and Dabska-type hemangioendotheliomas, and a subset of angiosarcomas. Mod. Pathol. 2000;**13**(2):180–5.

161. Lasota J, Miettinen M. Absence of Kaposi's sarcoma-associated virus (human herpesvirus-8) sequences in angiosarcoma. Virchows Arch. 1999;**434**(1):51–6.

162. Brouillard P, Boon LM, Mulliken JB, *et al*. Mutations in a novel factor, glomulin, are responsible for glomuvenous malformations ("glomangiomas"). Am. J. Hum. Genet. 2002;**70**(4):866–74.

163. Glick SA, Markstein EA, Herreid P. Congenital glomangioma: case report and review of the world literature. Pediatr. Dermatol. 1995;**12**(3):242–4.

164. Mallory SB, Enjolras O, Boon LM, *et al*. Congenital plaque-type glomuvenous malformations presenting in childhood. Arch. Dermatol. 2006;**142**(7):892–6.

165. Goujon E, Cordoro KM, Barat M, *et al*. Congenital plaque-type glomuvenous malformations associated with fetal pleural effusion and ascites. Pediatr. Dermatol. 2011;**28**(5):528–31.

166. Tardío JC, Azorín D, Hernández-Núñez A, *et al*. Dermatomyofibromas presenting in pediatric patients: clinicopathologic characteristics and differential diagnosis. J. Cutan. Pathol. 2011;**38**(12):967–72.

167. Kutzner H, Mentzel T, Palmedo G, *et al*. Plaque-like CD34-positive dermal fibroma ("medallion-like dermal dendrocyte hamartoma"): clinicopathologic, immunohistochemical, and molecular analysis of 5 cases emphasizing its distinction from superficial, plaque-like dermatofibrosarcoma protuberans. Am. J. Surg. Pathol. 2010;**34**(2):190–201.

168. Rodríguez-Jurado R, Palacios C, Durán-McKinster C, *et al*. Medallion-like dermal dendrocyte hamartoma: A new clinically and histopathologically distinct lesion. J. Am. Acad. Dermatol. 2004;**51**(3):359–63.

169. Solomon LM, Fretzin DF, Dewald RL. The epidermal nevus syndrome. Arch. Dermatol. 1968;**97**(3):273–85.

170. Happle R. Nevus sebaceus is a mosaic RASopathy. J. Invest. Dermatol. 2013;**133**(3):597–600.

171. Cribier B, Scrivener Y, Grosshans E. Tumors arising in nevus sebaceus: A study of 596 cases. J. Am. Acad. Dermatol. 2000;**42**(2 Pt 1):263–8.

172. Bellet JS. Developmental anomalies of the skin. Semin. Perinatol. 2013;**37**(1):20–5.

173. Tebcherani AJ, de Andrade HF, Sotto MN. Diagnostic utility of immunohistochemistry in distinguishing trichoepithelioma and basal cell carcinoma: evaluation using tissue microarray samples. Mod. Pathol. 2012;**25**(10):1345–53.

174. Landau JM, Moody MN, Goldberg LH, Vergilis-Kalner IJ. An unusual presentation of idiopathic basal cell carcinoma in an 8-year-old child. Pediatr. Dermatol. 2012;**29**(3):379–81.

175. Ackerman AB. Nevoid basal cell carcinoma syndrome vs. generalized basaloid follicular hamartoma syndrome. J. Cutan. Pathol. 2009;**36**(5):603; author reply 604.

176. Ramos-Ceballos FI, Pashaei S, Kincannon JM, Morgan MB, Smoller BR. Bcl-2, CD34 and CD10 expression in basaloid follicular hamartoma, vellus hair hamartoma and neurofollicular hamartoma demonstrate full follicular differentiation. J. Cutan. Pathol. 2008;**35**(5):477–83.

177. Burgdorf W, Gerami P, Yan A. Bening and malignant tumors. In: Schachner L, Hansen R, editors. *Pediatric Dermatology* 4th edn. Maryland Heights, MO: Mosby Elsevier; 2011:1181–216.

178. Martorell-Calatayud A, Hernández-Martín A, Colmenero I, *et al.* (Lymphomatoid papulosis in children: report of 9 cases and review of the literature). Actas Dermosifiliogr. 2010;**101**(8):693–701.

179. Santiago-et-Sánchez-Mateos D, Hernández-Martín A, Colmenero I, *et al.* Primary cutaneous anaplastic large cell lymphoma of the nasal tip in a child. Pediatr. Dermatol. 2010;**28**(5):570–5.

180. Zambrano E, Mejía-Mejía O, Bifulco C, Shin J, Reyes-Múgica M. Extranodal marginal zone B-cell lymphoma/maltoma of the lip in a child: case report and review of cutaneous lymphoid proliferations in childhood. Int. J. Surg. Pathol. 2006;**14**(2):163–9.

181. Kahwash SB, Qualman SJ. Cutaneous lymphoblastic lymphoma in children: report of six cases with precursor B-cell lineage. Pediatr. Dev. Pathol. 2002;**5**(1):45–53.

182. Tsianakas A, Kienast AK, Hoeger PH. Infantile-onset cutaneous T-cell lymphoma. Br. J. Dermatol. 2008;**159**(6):1338–41.

183. Torrelo A, Colmenero I, Hernández A, Goiriz R. Persistent agmination of lymphomatoid papulosis. Pediatr. Dermatol. 2009;**26**(6):762–4.

184. Saggini A, Gulia A, Argenyi Z, *et al.* A variant of lymphomatoid papulosis simulating primary cutaneous aggressive epidermotropic CD8+ cytotoxic T-cell lymphoma. Description of 9 cases. Am. J. Surg. Pathol. 2010;**34**(8):1168–75.

185. Oschlies I, Lisfeld J, Lamant L, *et al.* ALK-positive anaplastic large cell lymphoma limited to the skin: clinical, histopathological and molecular analysis of 6 pediatric cases. A report from the ALCL99 study. Haematologica. 2013;**98**(1):50–6.

186. Valent P, Horny HP, Escribano L, *et al.* Diagnostic criteria and classification of mastocytosis: A consensus proposal. Leuk. Res. 2001;**25**(7):603–25.

187. Valent P, Akin C, Sperr WR, *et al.* Mastocytosis: pathology, genetics, and current options for therapy. Leuk. Lymphoma. 2005;**46**(1):35–48.

188. Fett NM, Teng J, Longley BJ. Familial urticaria pigmentosa: report of a family and review of the role of KIT mutations. Am. J. Dermatopathol. 2013;**35**(1):113–6.

189. Huss S, Künstlinger H, Wardelmann E, *et al.* A subset of gastrointestinal stromal tumors previously regarded as wild-type tumors carries somatic activating mutations in KIT exon 8 (p.D419del). Mod. Pathol. 2013;**26**(7):1004–12.

190. Drut R, Peral CG, Garone A, Rositto A. Langerhans cell hyperplasia of the skin mimicking Langerhans cell histiocytosis: A report of two cases in children not associated with scabies. Fetal Pediatr. Pathol. 2010;**29**(4):231–8.

191. Torrelo A, Juarez A, Hernández A, Colmenero I. Multiple lichenoid juvenile xanthogranuloma. Pediatr. Dermatol. 2009;**26**(2):238–40.

192. Pérez-Gala S, Torrelo A, Colmenero I, *et al.* (Juvenile multiple xanthogranuloma in a patient with Langerhans cell histiocytosis). Actas Dermosifiliogr. 2006;**97**(9):594–8.

193. Messeguer F, Agustí-Mejias A, Colmenero I, Hernández-Martin A, Torrelo A. Clustered Juvenile Xanthogranuloma. Pediatr. Dermatol. 2012.

194. Maher-Wiese VL, Wenner NP, Grant-Kels JM. Metastatic cutaneous lesions in children and adolescents with a case report of metastatic neuroblastoma. J. Am. Acad. Dermatol. 1992;**26**(4):620–8.

195. De la Luz Orozco-Covarrubias M, Tamayo-Sanchez L, Duran-McKinster C, *et al.* Malignant cutaneous tumors in children. Twenty years of experience at a large pediatric hospital. J. Am. Acad. Dermatol. 1994;**30**(2 Pt 1):243–9.

196. Van Erp IF. Cutaneous metastases in neuroblastoma. Dermatologica. 1968;**136**(4):265–9.

197. Hawthorne HC, Nelson JS, Witzleben CL, Giangiacomo J. Blanching subcutaneous nodules in neonatal neuroblastoma. J. Pediatr. 1970;**77**(2):297–300.

198. Lucky AW, McGuire J, Komp DM. Infantile neuroblastoma presenting with cutaneous blanching nodules. J. Am. Acad. Dermatol. 1982;**6**(3):389–91.

199. Mehta V, Balachandran C, Lonikar V. Blueberry muffin baby: A pictoral differential diagnosis. Dermatol. Online J. 2008;**14**(2):8.

200. Steiner LA, Ehrenkranz RA, Peterec SM, *et al.* Perinatal onset mevalonate kinase deficiency. Pediatr. Dev. Pathol. 2011;**14**(4):301–6.

201. Brecher AR, Reyes-Mugica M, Kamino H, Chang MW. Congenital primary cutaneous rhabdomyosarcoma in a neonate. Pediatr. Dermatol. 2003;**20**(4):335–8.

202. Nesbit ME. Advances and management of solid tumors in children. Cancer. 1990;**65**(3 Suppl):696–702.

203. Wiss K, Solomon AR, Raimer SS, *et al.* Rhabdomyosarcoma presenting as a cutaneous nodule. Arch. Dermatol. 1988;**124**(11):1687–90.

204. Isaacs H. Cutaneous metastases in neonates: A review. Pediatr. Dermatol. 2011;**28**(2):85–93.

Gastrointestinal tract

Marie-Anne Brundler, Paula Borralho, Riitta Karikoski,
Paola Domizio, and Marta C. Cohen

Esophagus

Congenital malformations

Esophageal atresia (EA) and tracheo-esophageal fistula (TEF)

The esophagus develops from the embryonal early foregut when it differentiates into the ventral respiratory and the dorsal digestive tract. The process of separation of the trachea and esophagus remains largely unclear (1). It is suggested that TEF results from an incomplete division of the ventral and dorsal parts of the foregut, thus forming an abnormal connection between the trachea and the esophagus. The cranial end of the esophagus may form a blind pouch or EA with or without a fistula into the trachea. Five types of esophageal atresia are recognized (Figure 2.1). The most common variant is proximal atresia with a distal TEF, occurring in 85% of cases (2). There can be a missing segment of esophagus, and the lower esophageal section may also form a fistula into the trachea. It is thought that a combination of genetic and environmental factors plays a role in the etiology of foregut anomalies (2). Esophageal atresia can occur in isolation, but approximately half of the cases are associated with other anomalies, which are usually in the midline.

Clinical features: Esophageal atresia and TEF are one of the relatively common malformations, occurring approximately in 1 in 3500 births (3). These malformations are life threatening and require emergency surgery in the neonatal period (4). The neonate presents with choking, cyanosis, dyspnea, and cough at first feeds. The surgical treatment consists of either joining the esophageal ends or using a jejunal interposition technique in a small minority, and closing the fistula to the trachea. Prenatal presentation may include polyhydramnios.

Complications: After EA repair in infancy, gastro-esophageal reflux (GER) and esophageal dysmotility, as well as respiratory problems are common and will extend into adulthood (5). With increasing age, development of columnar cell metaplasia in the esophageal squamous epithelium is more likely. Gastric or intestinal metaplasia (Barrett's metaplasia) develops in about 15% of patients, within a time window of about 10 years (6). Endoscopical follow-up with biopsies is the best way to detect these changes. Esophageal cancer has been described in a small number of young adults treated for EA. Adults with a history of repaired EA have significantly more respiratory symptoms, asthma, and allergies when compared with the general population (7).

Histology: The esophageal mucosa in EA and in repaired TEF shows non-specific features of submucosal fibrosis and thinning of the muscularis propria. Gastroesophageal reflux is usually a sequela of a repaired atresia and thus, features of esophagitis or Barrett's esophagus may be seen. The trachea adjacent to the TEF may show non-specific inflammation and occasionally squamous metaplasia of the respiratory epithelium.

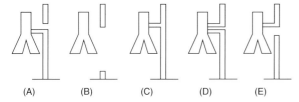

| | | | | |
| (A) | (B) | (C) | (D) | (E) |

Figure 2.1 Classification of esophageal atresia: the different types are illustrated in decreasing order of frequency. The commonest type (A) shows a proximally blind ending esophagus and a distal tracheo-esophageal fistula.

Malformation syndromes associated with EA/TEF: VACTERL/VATER (Vertebral defects, Anal atresia, Cardiac defects, Tracheo-esophageal fistula, Renal malformations, and Limb defects) is the most common condition associated with EA or TEF. The incidence is estimated at approximately 1 in 10 000 to 40 000 live-born infants. The management of patients is surgical correction of anomalies (8).

Other syndromes that can present with EA or TEF include (9,10): Feingold (oculo-digito-esophago-duodenal) syndrome (caused by a dominant mutation in the MYCN gene), anophthalmia-esophageal-genital syndrome (caused by mutations in SOX2), VACTERL-H (associated with X-linked and recessive forms of hydrocephalus), Fanconi syndrome and CHARGE syndrome (Coloboma, Heart defect, Atresia of choanae, Retarded growth, Genital anomaly, and Ear anomaly) caused by mutations of CHD7. Trisomies 18 and 21 are significant risk factors for EA and TEF. The 22q11 deletion syndrome may show clinically overlapping features with VACTERL association. In addition to the above, offsprings of diabetic mothers show a two- to threefold increase in malformations, which include EA.

Esophagitis

This refers to the presence of inflammation of the esophageal mucosa. It can be due to various causes, which can broadly be grouped into: (a) infectious and (b) non-infections. Esophageal involvement in inflammatory bowel disease is discussed separately (see below).

Infectious esophagitis

This group of esophagitis is far less common than non-infectious causes. The organisms most frequently involved in infectious esophagitis in children are *Candida albicans*, herpes simplex virus (HSV) and cytomegalovirus. Children with primary or secondary immunosuppression are at higher risk of developing infectious esophagitis. Other less common organisms include viruses such as Epstein–Barr virus, varicella zoster virus, and human immunodeficiency virus, and fungus strains such as *Aspergillus* and *Mucor*.

Candida is a commensal organism in the gastrointestinal tract. Esophagitis due to *Candida* sp. has a characteristic endoscopic appearance, presenting with patchy white plaques that cover a very friable erythematous mucosa (11). Histologically, the esophageal mucosa in candidiasis shows necrotic debris and

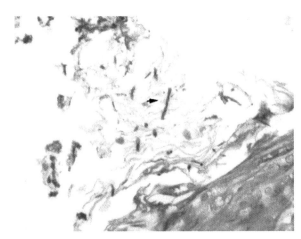

Figure 2.2 Esophagitis showing pseudohyphae corresponding to *Candida albicans* (arrow) (PAS stain × 60).

inflammatory cells mixed with pseudohyphae and budding yeasts (Figure 2.2). The fungus is better demonstrated with PAS (periodic acid–Schiff stain) or Gomori's silver stain.

Herpes simplex virus esophagitis is a well-recognized infection in the immunocompromised host, although it is occasionally described in the immunocompetent patient (12,13). Conditions that increase the risk of HSV esophagitis include: human immunodeficiency virus infection, chemotherapy, diabetes, leukemia or lymphoma, and transplantations (bone marrow, stem cell, and solid organs). Fever, odynophagia, and retrosternal pain of acute onset are the most common symptoms. Endoscopy shows an erythematous mucosa with ulcers. Biopsies should be taken from the margins of the ulcer. Histological examination reveals acute inflammation and superficial erosions and/or ulcerations of the epithelium. Intranuclear inclusions are reported in about half of cases (14). Immunohistochemistry against HSV is useful in confirming the diagnosis.

Polymerase chain reaction (PCR) *in-situ* hybridization (ISH) and immunohistochemistry are also helpful in the diagnosis of infectious esophagitis caused by viruses.

Non-infectious esophagitis
Gastro-esophageal reflux (GER)

Gastro-esophageal reflux disease (GERD) in children is a condition that develops when persistence of reflux of stomach contents causes symptoms and/or complications (15). The diagnosis of GERD is established on a combination of clinical symptoms, endoscopy, histology, and pH studies. The estimated prevalence

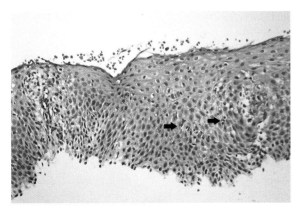

Figure 2.3 Esophagitis showing basal-cell hyperplasia, increased intraepithelial lymphocytes, papillary elongation, and intraepithelial eosinophils (arrows) (H&E × 10).

using esophageal pH monitoring is 11.7% in infants and 5.4% in children aged 0–9 years (16).

Clinical features: Symptoms include apnea, irritability, crying, fussing or arching back, weight loss, pain, dysphagia, and blood loss (17–21). Pediatric patients at risk of GERD include those with neurodevelopmental delay, repaired esophageal atresia, prematurity, and chronic respiratory diseases. Incompetence of the esophageal sphincter, delayed gastric emptying, or increased abdominal pressure are likely underlying mechanisms.

Endoscopic features of GER include erosions, ulcerations, exudates, and strictures (Figure 2.3). In rare cases GER is complicated by the development of Barrett's esophagus and adenocarcinoma (20). Gastroesophageal reflux usually affects the distal 5 cm of the esophageal mucosa. Proximal extension occurs with increasing severity of the reflux. As the involvement usually is patchy, multisite biopsy and serial sections of the biopsies should be done.

Histology: The mucosa of the distal esophagus shows (17,21,22) (Figure 2.3):

- Basal cell hyperplasia: >3 cell layers; nuclear enlargement; increased mitotoses
- Basal cell spongiosis
- Papillary elongation: the papillae reach the upper third of the mucosa
- Papillary hyperplasia
- Increased number of cytotoxic T-cell lymphocytes, ("squiggle" cells): > 6 /HPF
- Frequent intraepithelial eosinophils: usually <15/HPF

More severe cases may also show mucosal break, either through the muscularis mucosae into the submucosa (ulceration) or through the epithelium into the lamina propria and muscularis mucosae, but not into the submucosa (erosion) (22).

A degree of basal cell hyperplasia, as well as papillary hyperplasia and papillary elongation is common at the distal esophageal mucosa and should not be over-interpreted as esophagitis (23,24).

Eosinophilic esophagitis (EE)

Also known as allergic esophagitis, EE is a recently recognized clinico-pathological entity that preferentially affects young adults. Patients are predominantly males (3:1 ratio), presenting with dysphagia in the presence of a normal barium swallow, and normal esophageal acid exposure on 24-hour pH monitoring (25). The endoscopy may be normal or shows furrowing, white patches, and trachealization of the affected esophagus (25,26).

The incidence of EE is on the rise, (4.5/100 000 children in the North of England) (26). Eosinophilic esophagitis is a chronic interleukin (IL)-5-driven inflammatory disorder in which the etiology seems to be linked to a combination of allergic and immunologic responses (27,28).

Clinical features: The symptoms include vomiting, regurgitation, nausea, epigastric pain, heartburn, food aversion, food bolus obstruction, allergies, dysphagia, and failure to thrive (26,27,29–32).

The endoscopic appearance is characterized by a ring-like esophagus ("trachealization"), with longitudinal linear furrows, friability of the mucosa and/or multiple small white papules suggestive of candidiasis (33,34).

The histological marker is the presence of severe eosinophilia restricted to the esophageal mucosa in patients in whom GERD has been excluded by normal pH monitoring, and failure to respond to high-dose proton-pump inhibitor therapy (29, 35,36). Characteristically, the proximal esophagus is more severely affected than the distal esophagus. Therefore, the intraepithelial eosinophils are more numerous in the proximal biopsy.

Histology: The main features are (26,30,37,38) (Figure 2.4):

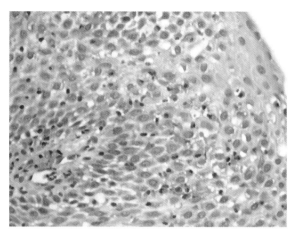

Figure 2.4 Eosinophilic esophagitis showing basal-cell hyperplasia, dilated intercellular spaces and up to 46 eosinophils/high power field (H&E × 40).

- ≥ 15 eosinophils/ HPF in the esophageal mucosa without involvement of other parts of the gastrointestinal tract
- Microabscesses: groups containing > 4 eosinophils preferentially located near the surface of the mucosa
- Spongiosis (due to accumulation of fluid)
- Basal cell hyperplasia: proliferation and thickening of the basal cell layer representing ≥ 30% of mucosal thickness
- Papillary elongation: the papillae reach the upper third of the mucosa and represent ≥ 70% of mucosal thickness. Increased number of intraepithelial T-cells ("squiggle cells") > 6/HPF
- Epithelial cell vacuolation: clear vacuoles in the cytoplasm
- Increased number of mast cells and mast cell degranulation
- Fibrosis of the lamina propria

The sole presence of ≥ 15 intraepithelial eosinophils/ HPF is not enough evidence to diagnose EE. In fact, one-third of patients with esophageal eosinophilia present the so-called "overlap" syndrome, characterized by histological features suggestive of EE and abnormal pH studies. Although the symptoms usually improve with proton-pump inhibitors, occasionally these need to be combined with treatment for EE (26).

Lymphocytic esophagitis

The hallmark of lymphocytic esophagitis is the presence of intraepithelial lymphocytosis with peripapillary distribution, associated with basal cell hyperplasia and intercellular edema. There is no neutrophilic or eosinophilic infiltrate. It has been described in the young, and in association with Crohn's disease; the incidence and clinical-pathological features have yet to be clearly defined (39).

Caustic esophagitis

Ingested caustic substances are usually alkaline household or garden substances. In addition, "pill-induced" esophagitis is associated with the ingestion of certain drugs and accounts for many cases of erosive esophagitis. To date, more than 70 drugs have been reported to induce esophageal disorders. Antibacterials such as doxycycline, tetracycline, and clindamycin are the offending agents in more than 50% of cases (40). A pill might be retained in the esophagus as the result of esophageal dysmotility, stricture, or impaction (18). The histology shows erosions, acute mucosal inflammation, and ulceration, with variable degrees of eosinophilic infiltrate. Perforation of the esophagus is a complication seen in cases with severe injury.

Involvement in inflammatory bowel disease (IBD)

Esophageal involvement is more commonly seen in CD than in ulcerative colitis (UC). Granulomas may be identified in the lamina propria, although they are not obligatory. More recently, lymphocytic esophagitis has been described in association with CD (for further discussion of upper GI manifestations in IBD see below).

Strictures

An esophageal stricture is a narrowing of the esophagus. The majority are acquired and the consequence of severe GERD, or less commonly caustic esophagitis or infectious esophagitis that has caused esophageal ulcers (18).

Clinical features: Usual symptoms include food impaction, difficulty swallowing solids or liquids, dysphagia, odynophagia, and cough. If the stricture is severe and/or long standing, choking and weight loss may be present. Endoscopically, esophageal strictures present as a narrow lumen lined by pale, usually non-inflamed, mucosa.

Histology: The hallmark is the presence of fibrosis of the esophageal wall, accompanied by a variable degree of inflammation that does not usually involve the muscularis propria.

Barrett esophagus (BE)

Barrett esophagus is a preneoplastic condition caused by chronic GERD, which predisposes to the development of esophageal adenocarcinoma. BE is the result of an adaptive response of the surface mucosa to long-standing acid reflux, replacing the normal esophageal squamous epithelium with the columnar epithelium diagnostic of the condition (41–43). The term "metaplasia" is defined as a change of one adult cell type to another, both in adults (44) and children (45,46).

Clinical features: Barrett esophagus has a male predominance (43). Co-morbidities include neurological impairment, chronic lung disease (in particular cystic fibrosis), obesity, repaired esophageal atresia, and chemotherapy-treated malignancies (17,43). The reported prevalence in children with GERD varies between 0.3% and 4.8%, much lower than in adults.

In children, BE is usually present in short segments. This difference may be explained by the fact that the development of BE is related to the duration of GERD (the longer the duration of GERD the higher the number of patients developing BE) (47). On endoscopy velvety red mucosa is seen.

Histology: The hallmark of BE is the presence of specialized intestinal columnar metaplasia containing goblet cells. As goblet cell numbers are age-dependent, these are less numerous in children than in adults (48). The British Society of Gastroenterology defines BE as "a segment of columnar metaplasia (whether intestinalized or not) of any length, visible endoscopically above the gastro-oesophageal junction and confirmed or corroborated histologically" (49). However, the American Society of Gastroenterology requires the presence of goblet cells to diagnose BE (50).

Different types of columnar epithelium in the esophagus have been described: gastric cardia-type, gastric fundic-type, and intestinal metaplastic-type with goblet cells. The latter type may be subdivided into those with or without brush border (i.e., small bowel subtype or large colon subtype) (42,43). Although all three types often co-exist in BE, it is recognized that only the intestinal metaplastic epithelium has malignant potential (17,41–43). Goblet cells in BE have a characteristic shape, with an expanded apical portion, the nucleus at the base, and cytoplasmic acid mucin positive for Alcian blue at pH 2.5 (43) (Figure 2.5).

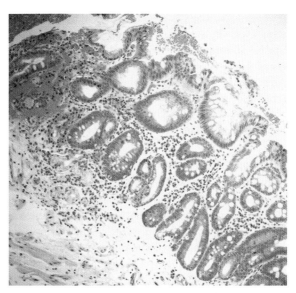

Figure 2.5 Intestinal metaplasia with presence of goblet cells in a case of Barrett esophagus (H&E × 20).

Esophageal malignancies

Esophageal cancer is rare in children and is limited to isolated case reports (51,52). These belong to two major types: squamous cell carcinoma and adenocarcinoma. Presenting symptoms include difficulty swallowing, weight loss, cough, and vomiting. The histological features are similar to the adult counterpart.

Stomach

Congenital malformations

Pyloric stenosis (PS)

In PS there is obstruction of the gastric outflow due to thickened pyloric smooth muscle.

Clinical features: Idiopathic hypertrophic pyloric stenosis (IHPS) is not uncommon among neonates, affecting 2:1000. It has a striking male predominance. Non-bilious projectile vomitus is the first symptom of the disease, where a palpable firm pyloric muscle mass can be found. Abdominal ultrasound is diagnostic. The treatment is surgical with pyloromyotomy (53). The etiology of isolated IHPS in neonates is still unknown. There is an increased familial risk, but no genetic association has been found (54,55). Idiopathic hypertrophic pyloric stenosis may be associated with Cornelia de Lange and Smith–Lemli–Opitz syndrome. The gastric mucosa may show foveolar cell hyperplasia, adding to gastric outlet problems (56).

Histology: Biopsies are rarely taken, but then histology will show cellular smooth muscle with plump nuclei. Additional biopsies of the gastric mucosa may reveal hyperplasia of foveolar cells and parietal cells. An increase in desmin staining may point towards structural immaturity of the pyloric muscle (57) and a decrease of GFAP might indicate poor innervation, but these features are not diagnostic.

Heterotopic (ectopic) pancreas

Ectopic pancreatic tissue has no anatomical, neural, or vascular connection to the normal pancreas. Also called aberrant or accessory pancreas, heterotopic pancreas is most commonly found in the stomach, duodenum, and jejunum, although it can occur anywhere in the alimentary tract. Pancreatic heterotopia is uncommon, occurring in 0.6–13%. Rarely, these heterotopias may occur as double or multiple (58). Although usually asymptomatic, it may also cause obstruction of the gastric outlet. Complications include bleeding and inflammation (59). In the small bowel heterotopic pancreatic tissue may form a lead point for intussusception (60).

Macroscopy: Heterotopic pancreas presents as a submucosal mass with a central dimple corresponding to the opening of the pancreatic duct.

Histology: Pancreatic tissue in a lobular arrangement with either exocrine pancreas only, or also including endocrine islets. In some cases only the ductal component without acini or islets, is represented. Occasionally pancreatitis is seen.

Gastritis

Infectious gastritis

Infectious causes of gastritis include: *Helicobacter pylori*, *Helicobacter heilmannii*, pyogenic bacteria (*Streptococcus* and *Staphylococcus* spp.), *Mycobacterium tuberculosis*, *Mycobacterium avium*, cytomegalovirus, herpes simplex virus, *Candida albicans*, and other fungi. Amongst these *H. pylori* is by far the most common cause. Herpes and fungal infections are exceedingly rare and mostly seen in the immunocompromised child.

Helicobacter pylori: Gram-negative, curved-shaped, flagellated bacillus that has been linked with chronic gastritis, and gastric and duodenal ulcers, and is associated with a higher risk of gastric carcinoma and lymphoma in adults. In children, *H. pylori* has a worldwide distribution, being more prevalent in under-developed countries, poorer socioeconomic groups, children with mental disabilities, and among teenagers, with a high prevalence among family members of infected patients.

Available tests for the diagnosis of *H. pylori* infection include endoscopy with biopsy, culture, urease test, urea breath test, PCR, stool antigen tests, and serology. Histological confirmation of gastritis and detection of *H. pylori* organisms in the biopsy remains the diagnostic gold standard in children. Detection of *H. pylori* antigens in the stool is a reliable non-invasive test for eradication of *H. pylori* (61).

Histology: Acute gastritis characterized by neutrophilic inflammation; antral erosions are rare. *H. pylori*-associated chronic gastritis (HpCG) in children usually presents as a pangastritis, with antrum, cardia, and body affected in that order of severity (62). There is an inflammatory cell infiltrate composed of lymphoid cells, lymphoid follicles with expanded germinal centers, plasma cells, and a variable number of neutrophils (63). In its active form, the neutrophilic infiltrate characteristically involves the proliferative area of the gastric mucosa, at the level of the glandular necks (Figure 2.6) (63,64). The presence of lymphoid

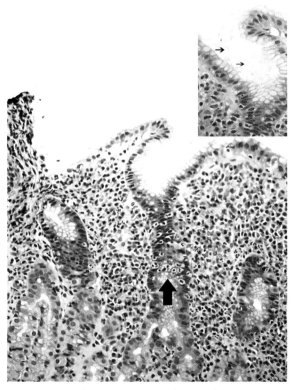

Figure 2.6 Antral gastric mucosa with features of chronic active inflammation, which characteristically affects the glandular necks (arrow) (H&E × 40). Inset: 4μ curved bacilli seen on the surface mucosa (arrows) (H&E × 60).

follicles, characteristic of the chronic stages of the gastritis, is responsible for the nodularity of the antral mucosa at endoscopy (63). This pattern of gastritis is called follicular gastritis.

The presence of sulfomucin-containing cells has been described in patients with long-standing HpCG. It has been speculated that this finding may represent a "minimal" form of incomplete intestinal metaplasia (65). Although atrophic gastritis has not been described in children, the presence of focal stellate areas of fibrosis, indicating loss of individual glandular units has been described in children with long-standing HpCG (66).

Helicobacter heilmannii: This animal pathogen with a characteristic corkscrew appearance may infect the human stomach with much the same acute (not chronic) effects as *H. pylori*.

Viruses: Herpes virus and cytomegalovirus (CMV) can produce acute erosive gastritis; CMV additionally causes an unusual lesion in the childhood stomach – so-called Ménetrier disease with striking foveolar hyperplasia. Herpes virus and CMV infections may occur in immunocompromised and immunocompetent patients. The presenting symptoms include nausea, vomiting, and hematemesis. Intranuclear eosinophilic inclusions and smaller intracytoplasmic inclusions are typical of CMV. This is associated with a patchy acute inflammatory infiltrate in the lamina propria.

Ménetrier disease (hypertrophic gastropathy) is uncommon in children. It usually is an acute and self-limiting condition. Presenting symptoms include abdominal pain, weight loss, peripheral edema due to hypoalbuminemia. and protein-losing gastropathy. Histologically, it is characterized by enlarged gastric folds associated with mucous cell hyperplasia, foveolar elongation, glandular atrophy, and reversal of the normal pit-to-gland ratio (67). Gastric cytomegalovirus infection is confirmed in a third of the cases by immunohistochemistry and PCR (67–69).

Non-infectious gastritis

Lymphocytic gastritis (LG)

Lymphocytic gastritis (LG) is a morphologic entity characterized by a significant increase in the number of intraepithelial lymphocytes (IELs) in the surface and foveolar epithelium of the gastric mucosa (70). The normal number of IELs in the gastric mucosa is < 1 per 5 epithelial cells. However, in LG this usually exceeds 25 per 100 epithelial cells (62) (Figure 2.7).

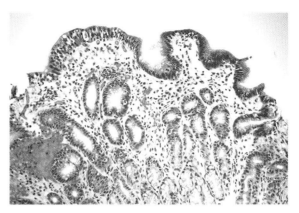

Figure 2.7 Intraepitelial lymphocytes (>25/100 epithelial cells) infiltrate the gastric mucosa in a case of lymphocytic gastritis (H&E × 20)

Clinical features: Endoscopically, LG usually shows varioliform gastritis with thickened mucosal folds bearing small nodules and surface erosions (70).

Lymphocytic gastritis is seen in association with celiac disease, *H. pylori* infection, gastric malignancies, CD, and Ménetrier disease (62,71). The prevalence of LG in pediatric patients with celiac disease ranges between 10 and 45% (72). Patients with LG tend to have a longer exposure to gluten, and to present with more severe disease (by clinical and histological measures) (71,72). The IELs possibly reflect a systemic immune activation in these patients.

Histology: Commonly seen in the antrum and sometimes also involving the body, LG is characterized by marked infiltration of the gastric surface and foveolar epithelium by T-lymphocytes and accompanying chronic inflammation in the lamina propria. The IELs are CD3 and CD8-T lymphocytes (72,73).

Vasculitis

Henoch–Schönlein purpura, an IgA-mediated small-vessel vasculitis, and polyarteritis nodosa may affect the entire gastrointestinal tract, causing colicky abdominal pain and bleeding. On endoscopy, the mucosa shows punctate hemorrhagic lesions or erosions, which usually indicate underlying leukocytoclastic vasculitis. The vasculitis, however, may not be seen in superficial biopsies (62).

Autoimmune gastritis

This is a relatively rare disease, but represents the most frequent cause of pernicious anemia in temperate climates in adult patients (73). An increased prevalence of autoimmune gastritis is reported in children with autoimmune disorders such as thyroiditis and type 1 diabetes (62). Gastric biopsies show chronic, predominantly fundic, inflammation, with loss of specialized glands. Antibodies against parietal cells are the serological hallmark of autoimmune gastritis.

Atrophic gastritis

Atrophy is defined by the loss of glands in the gastric mucosa. The severity of glandular loss is graded as mild, moderate, or severe, as described in the Sydney System score (74). Gastric atrophy usually develops on a background of chronic gastritis, hence the term atrophic gastritis, and is accompanied by intestinal metaplasia carrying an increased risk of gastric cancer. Although rare, it may be encountered in children with long-standing *H. pylori* infection (64,66,75).

Eosinophilic gastritis (EG)

Eosinophilic gastritis is an inflammatory condition with an immunologic pathogenesis. Primary EG is thought to be the consequence of an altered immunological response of the digestive mucosa to potential airborne or food allergens in genetically predisposed individuals (76). The incidence of EG is on the rise and shows familial clustering. Other segments of the gastrointestinal tract can also be involved. Significant (secondary) eosinophilic inflammation may also be seen in patients with collagen vascular, parasitic infections, or IBD, or may be due to drug-induced or caustic injury (76,77).

Clinical features: The clinical presentation of primary EG is variable and includes abdominal pain, bleeding, vomiting, weight loss, and diarrhea (77).

Histology: In the stomach, EG affects mainly the antrum with a mucosal eosinophilic infiltrate, which involves the surface and foveolar epithelium and is accompanied by variable degree of edema and erosions (76,77). Plasma cells, neutrophils, and regenerative features are frequently seen. An infiltration of >30 eosinophils per high-power field in at least five HPFs, exhibiting signs of eosinophilic degranulation and extending to the muscularis mucosa or submucosa, are histological indicators of EG (77). The inflammation may affect the mucosa, muscularis, and/or serosa. The mucosal type causes protein loss, the muscular form presents with dysmotility, and the unusual serosal eosinophilia with ascites (76,77).

Chronic granulomatous disease (CGD)

Chronic granulomatous disease is a rare primary defect of the innate immune system leading to recurrent or chronic infections and persistent granulomatous inflammation as phagocytes are unable to kill ingested microorganisms. Chronic granulomatous disease is caused by mutations in any one of four genes that encode the subunits of phagocyte NADPH oxidase, the enzyme that generates microbicidal (and pro-inflammatory) oxygen radicals (78). Autosomal recessive or X-linked inheritance are documented. The mutations lead to a defect in the burst of oxygen consumption that normally accompanies phagocytosis in myeloid cells (79).

Clinical features: Chronic granulomatous disease in most cases is diagnosed in infancy and the lungs are most frequently affected. Other common manifestations include lymphadenitis, superficial and deep abscesses, dermatitis, and gastro-intestinal symptoms. In the stomach, Chronic granulomatous disease shows a predilection for the antrum causing narrowing and gastric outlet obstruction.

Histology: Chronic granulomatous disease is characterized by the presence of ill-formed granulomas or individual histiocytes intermixed with lymphocytes and eosinophils. The presence of numerous pigmented macrophages in association with such inflammation should raise suspicion of the diagnosis (80).

The differential diagnosis includes other causes of granulomatous gastritis such as CD, tuberculosis, sarcoidosis, and Langerhans-cell histiocytosis (62).

Diagnosis: The diagnosis is confirmed by the NBT test (phorbol-myristate acetate-stimulated nitroblue tetrazolium). This shows percentage values of stained neutrophils close to zero in affected cases, close to 100 in normal subjects, and intermediate (usually 20–80) in females heterozygous for the X-linked form (81).

Chemical gastropathy

Drug/chemical lesions predominately affect the pre-pyloric region. The mucosa shows reactive changes as a consequence of chronic bile reflux or non-steroid inflammatory drug ingestion. This pauci-inflammatory lesion is far more common in adult patients, but can also occur in children.

Histology: The histopathologic features include mucosal edema, congestion, smooth muscle stranding in the lamina propria, and foveolar hyperplasia with a corkscrew appearance in the most severe forms. The foveolar epithelium characteristically shows reactive nuclear features and reduction of mucin. The

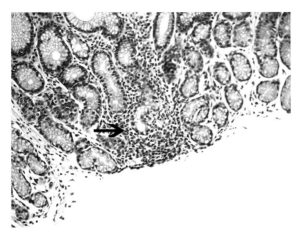

Figure 2.8 Focally enhanced gastritis in a patient with Crohn's disease. A small collection of lymphocytes surrounds gastic crypts (arrow) (H&E × 20).

epithelial changes occur with little background chronic inflammation (62).

Crohn's disease

Crohn's disease-associated gastritis is characterised by the presence of patchy, acute inflammation with possible gastric pit or glandular abscesses, commonly on a background of lymphoid aggregates. The occurrence of small collections of lymphocytes and histiocytes surrounding a small group of gastric foveolae or glands, often with infiltrates of neutrophils, is called focally enhanced gastritis (82). Non-caseating granulomas are seen in one-third of cases with Crohn's disease (Figure 2.8).

Gastric inflammation may also be present in ulcerative colitis, but the pattern of focal active inflammation is less commonly encountered (for more detailed discussion of upper GI changes in IBD see below).

Tumors

Polyps

These can be categorized as non-neoplastic and neoplastic (83,84).

Non-neoplastic polyps that can present in infancy include:

Hyperplastic polyp: These are associated with chronic inflammation in the setting of *H. pylori* gastritis. They present as sessile or pedunculated polyps less than 2 cm in diameter (84). Histologically they are characterized by a proliferation of hyperplastic foveolar cells lining elongated pits.

Fundic gland polyps: Present in children with familial adenomatous polyposis (FAP) syndrome or develop following administration of proton pump inhibitors for GER or dyspepsia (67). In the setting of FAP the fundic polyps arise from mutations of the APC gene. They may be solitary or multiple, and present as small transparent sessile polyps, located in the body and fundus (84). On microscopy, they are characterized by dilatation of the fundic glands with protrusion of the cytoplasm of the parietal cells into the dilated gland lumen. There is accompanying parietal cell hyperplasia; the fundic glands appear lined by cells with a serrated rather than a smooth border (67,84). Characteristically there is no accompanying inflammation or edema.

Hamartomatous polyps: Clinical, genetic, and histologic features are discussed in more detail below.

Peutz–Jeghers polyps present in the setting of Peutz–Jeghers syndrome (PJS). The hallmark of these polyps is the presence of branching fascicles of smooth muscle accompanying hyperplastic fovcolar epithelium.

Juvenile polyps in the stomach usually occur in the context of the juvenile polyposis syndrome. Histologically they are characterized by cystic dilated glands with variable chronic inflammation of the intervening stroma and surface ulceration.

Polyps in Cowden syndrome are of juvenile or hyperplastic type.

Neoplastic polyps: Adenomatous polyps are rare in children and occur mainly in patients with FAP.

Gastric neoplasms

Malignant gastric tumors are rare in children (see WHO Classification (83) in Table 2.1).

Of these, the most frequent epithelial malignancy is the diffuse gastric carcinoma seen in the context of the familial hereditary syndrome with germline mutations in the E-cadherine gene (83). Patients with other cancer predisposition syndromes such as Li–Fraumeni and FAP have also an increased risk of developing gastric carcinoma at an early age (83). Mesenchymal tumors of the stomach in children include inflammatory myofibroblastic tumor and gastrointestinal stromal tumor (GIST).

Hereditary diffuse gastric carcinoma (HDGC)

This is an autosomal-dominant cancer syndrome presenting with diffuse gastric and lobular breast cancer (85). It is caused by heterozygous germline mutation in

Table 2.1 Epithelial tumors

Premalignant lesions	Adenoma
Carcinoma	Adenocarcinoma and its subtypes (including undifferentiated carcinoma)
Neuroendocrine neoplasms	Carcinoid, neuroendocrine carcinoma, mixed adenoneuroendocrine carcinoma, serotonin- and gastrin-producing tumors
Mesenchymal tumors	Glomus tumor, granular cell tumor, leiomyoma, plexiform fibromyxoma, schwannoma, inflammatory myofibroblastic tumor, gastrointestinal stromal tumor, Kaposi sarcoma, leiomyosarcoma, synovial sarcoma
Lymphomas	
Secondary tumors	

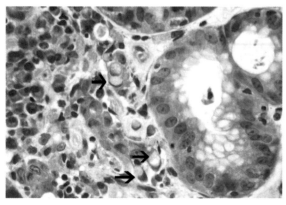

Figure 2.9 Signet-ring-cell carcinoma showing cells with large mucin-filled vacuole distending the cytoplasm (arrows) in a 15-year-old with Lynch syndrome (H&E × 40).

the tumor-suppression gene E-cadherin (CDH1; 192090) on chromosome 16q22 (86). The mutations in CDH1 have high penetrance and confer more than 80% lifetime risk of developing gastric cancer (89). In addition to gastric cancer, up to 60% of female mutation carriers develop lobular carcinoma of the breast, and some carriers may develop colorectal cancer (86). Specific diagnostic criteria for HDGC have been developed by the International Gastric Cancer Linkage Consortium (87).

Signet ring cells, which characterize HDGC, are defined by the presence of a large vacuole filled with mucin, which distends the cytoplasm and displaces the nucleus to the periphery (Figure 2.9). Early histological features of HDGC are the presence of multifocal foci of invasive and or *in situ* signet ring cell carcinoma. Invasive signet ring cell carcinomas can show mucin pooling and desmoplasia.

The use of histochemical stains for neutral mucins may be useful for the detection or confirmation of carcinoma *in situ*. There is reduced or absent E-cadherin immunoexpression in early invasive gastric carcinomas, contrasting with the normal membranous E-cadherin expression in adjacent non-neoplastic mucosa (88).

Although unusual, signet ring cell carcinoma can present in patients with Lynch syndrome (associated with mutations of MSH2, MLH1, MSH6, EPCAM, or PMS2) (83).

Gastrointestinal stromal tumor (GIST)

Clinical presentation and genetics: Gastrointestinal stromal tumors are rare connective tissue tumors that show similar differentiation patterns to the interstitial cells of Cajal. Underlying activating mutations in the KIT or PDGFRA proto-oncogenes are common in adult patients, but rarely seen in GISTs occurring in children and adolescents (89,90).

Most of the gastric GISTs in younger patients (< 20 years) are associated with loss of function mutations in the SDH gene (91). In addition to sporadic cases, this includes those associated with Carney triad or Carney–Stratakis syndrome. Multiple GISTs are commonly seen in neurofibromatosis type 1, though they rarely present in childhood.

Presenting symptoms in children include iron-deficiency anemia, abdominal pain, vomiting, and a palpable mass.

Macroscopy: Gastric GIST may present as a polyp, a mural nodule, or a large mass (90–92).

Histology: Gastrointestinal stromal tumors can be classified into three main types: spindle cell type (70%), epithelioid type (20%), and mixed spindle and epithelioid cell type (10%) (92). Gastrointestinal stromal tumors occurring in connection with Carney triad or Carney–Stratakis syndrome are mostly of the epitheliod type.

Immunohistochemistry shows positivity for c-KIT (CD117) in 95% of cases. Other markers that show a positive reaction include CD34 (70%) and SMA (40%). Recently, immunohistochemical staining for the DOG1.1 antibody has been shown to be a highly specific marker for GISTs, including pediatric and KIT antigen-negative tumors (93).

All GISTs carry a malignant potential; the relative risk of intra-abdominal dissemination and liver metastasis is primarily dependent on tumor size and mitotic activity (90). The National Institutes of Health (NIH) consensus classification system, based on tumor size and mitotic count, is commonly used to assess patient prognosis after surgical resection (94).

Small bowel

Congenital malformations

Atresia and stenosis

Small bowel atresia is a congenital malformation characterized by interruption of the intestinal lumen, which does not allow the intestinal contents to be propelled forward to the large intestine. In stenosis the lumen is significantly narrowed, but not totally obstructed.

Atresia and stenosis of the intestine are thought to be caused by a mesenteric vascular accident *in utero*, which may result from hernia, mid-gut volvulus associated with intestinal malrotation (95) or intussusception, producing aseptic necrosis and resorption of the necrotic bowel. A volvulus is caused when the intestine twists around the root of the mesentery.

Other suggested mechanisms leading to atresia include a failure of recanalization of the embryonal intestine and intrauterine meconium peritonitis leading to perforation and bowel atresia (96,97). Gastroschisis is associated with small bowel atresia in 10–20% of cases (98).

Although atresia may occur in any portion of the intestine, the duodenum, proximal jejunum, and distal ileum are most commonly affected (99,100). Atresia of the colon is very rare.

Classification: The classification of intestinal atresia (101) is schematically illustrated in Figure 2.10. A short segment of necrosis may produce only stenosis or a membranous web occluding the lumen (type I atresia). This is the most common finding in the duodenum where an associated pancreas annulare contributes to obstruction in 30% of cases. Bowel length is usually preserved. The occurrence of a more extensive infarct during fetal development may leave a fibrous cord between the two bowel loops (type II atresia), or the proximal and distal bowel may be completely separated with a V-shaped defect in the mesentery (type IIIa atresia). Multiple atresias occur in 10% of cases (type IV). In the type III variant (type IIIb), commonly called apple-peel or Christmas-tree atresia, there is a blind-ending proximal jejunum;

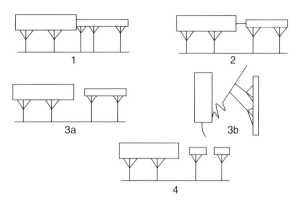

Figure 2.10 Classification of intestinal atresia: schematic representation of different types (adapted from Grosfeld *et al.* 101).

absence of a long length of mid small bowel, and the terminal ileum is coiled around its tenuous blood supply from an ileocolic vessel.

Clinical features: The symptoms are those of bowel obstruction: bilious vomiting, abdominal distension, and failure to have a bowel movement on the first days of life. An intrauterine volvulus or small bowel atresia may be suspected in cases with polyhydramnios. In these cases the so-called "double bubble" in prenatal ultrasound is characteristic of duodenal atresia (102). Postnatal imaging studies will show the blockage level and the dilated proximal loops of intestine. Intestinal atresia is a surgical emergency. At operation a continuous bowel lumen is created by resecting the atretic bowel followed, if possible, by end-to-end anastomosis. In multiple atresia or when there is more extensive bowel necrosis, notably in cases associated with gastroschisis or volvulus, this may lead to the loss of a significant length of small bowel and at worst be complicated by short-bowel syndrome and total parenteral nutrition requirements (which in turn could lead to hepatic complications). Intestinal transplantation may be required (103). The length of the remaining small bowel correlates with survival (103,104).

Intestinal atresia should be excluded in any case of gastroschisis and omphalocele where the small bowel lies outside the abdominal cavity *in utero* as in these cases the blood supply to the gut may be compromised. Jejunoileal atresia is associated with gastroschisis in 16% and with omphalocele in 1.5% of the cases. Of patients with distal small bowel or colonic atresia, 12% show cystic fibrosis documented by sweat chloride determinations (100).

Small bowel atresia shows an incidence of 1:10 000 in patients with a normal karyotype. Duodenal atresia is associated with trisomy 21 in 24–30% of cases, other associations include cardiac anomalies and maternal diabetes (99,100).

The syndrome of hereditary multiple gastrointestinal atresias is characterized by multiple atresias from pylorus to rectum (105). Histological appearances suggest a failure of recanalization of the embryonic intestinal lumen. This autosomal recessive syndrome has an invariably fatal course.

Histology: The atretic segment shows a tiny or occluded lumen. In multiple intestinal atresia there can be multiple small lumina surrounded by a separate mucosa and muscularis mucosae (101,106). There may be fragmentation of muscularis mucosae and multiple cysts (106). Thickening of the proximal small bowel muscularis propria with reduced expression of α-SMA and disruption of the network of interstitial cells of Cajal has been noted (107–109). Also a decrease of neuronal cells can occur at the proximal segment of duodenal atresia (109). Segmental defects in intestinal musculature may be seen (110). An intrauterine intussusception can present as a polypoid lesion (111) and the proximal mucosa may show pseudodysplastic regenerative changes (112).

Meckel's diverticulum

Meckel's diverticulum (Figure 2.11) results from the failure of the omphalomesenteric (or vitelline) duct to obliterate during the fifth week of fetal development. It is a diverticulum of small intestine that contains all the normal layers of the intestinal wall. Approximately half the cases contain heterotopic tissue, most commonly gastric fundic type mucosa and in rare cases heterotopic pancreas (113). Omphalomesenteric or vitelline duct remnants can also be found in the

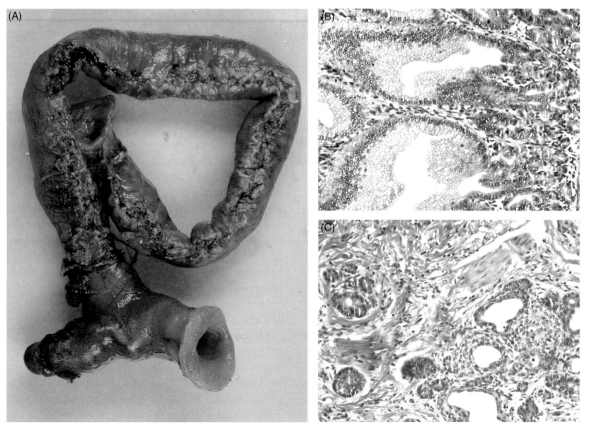

Figure 2.11 Meckel's diverticulum: (A) The diverticulum may act as a lead point for intussusception, as in this case, and result in bowel ischemia, requiring more extensive bowel resection. Gastric (B), and less commonly, pancreatic (C) heterotopia are seen on microscopic examination (H&E × 20).

umbilicus. They manifest usually in infancy or early childhood as granular reddish, and in some cases secreting umbilical lesions.

Clinical features: Meckel's diverticulum occurs in about 2% of the population (113). It can be asymptomatic and an incidental finding at surgery or post-mortem. When symptomatic it represents a diagnostic challenge to the clinician (114). Presenting symptoms in children include bleeding per rectum, intestinal obstruction, peritonitis, and intussusception, appendicitis- like symptoms, upper abdominal complaints, nausea, and vomiting. An ultrasound scan may reveal the diverticulum, whereas a Meckel's technetium 99m scan is more helpful, but its positivity depends on the presence of gastric heterotopic mucosa where it accumulates. The latter is present in only about 50% of cases (113). In the newborn, perforation of a Meckel's diverticulum often mimics necrotizing enterocolitis (115). Surgical treatment for an asymptomatic diverticulum may be a diverticulectomy, whereas a diseased diverticulum is removed with intestinal resection (116,117).

Macroscopy: Meckel's diverticulum arises on the antimesenteric border and 90% of cases are located within 90 cm of the ileocoecal valve (113). It is a short 2–4 cm long wide-mouthed diverticulum, which may show perforation or ulceration.

Histology: The diverticulum is lined by ileal mucosa; in about 50% of cases there is heterotopic gastric fundic-type mucosa. As this is acid producing there may be associated ulceration causing hemorrhage or even perforation. Rarely, the heterotopia may be of pancreatic tissue that can also cause ulcerations due to alkaline secretions. Colonic heterotopic epithelium has also been reported. Meckel's

diverticulum may also show inflammation and gangrenous necrosis (118).

Umbilical omphalomesenteric or vitelline duct remnants typically present as polypoid lesions that are covered at least partly by ectopic small intestinal mucosa, and contain smooth muscle in their core.

Duplication cysts

Intestinal duplications are rare developmental anomalies that can be found anywhere along the gastrointestinal tract (119). Most arise in the small intestine (approx. 45%), in particular the terminal ileum. Less commonly they occur in colon and rectum (20%), duodenum, pylorus, duodenum, and oesophagus (5–7%, each).

Clinical features: Duplication cysts may be identified on prenatal ultrasound, or become clinically manifest from birth until adulthood. Presenting symptoms include abdominal pain, vomiting, gastrointestinal obstruction, hemorrhage due to ulceration, or a palpable abdominal mass. Colonic or rectal duplications can present with perianal, urinary tract, or intestinal fistula (120,121). Other described symptoms are obstruction or prolapse of the mass. Associated anomalies include anal atresia, genitourinary malformations (duplications), and vertebral anomalies (119). Multiple short-segment duplications of the intestine (small or large) may also be present.

Macroscopy: The duplication can be an independent duplicate bowel, but more commonly it shares the muscular layer with the normal bowel. Duplications are either tubular or cystic. They may connect to the native intestine through an opening at one end of the structure, or be completely separate. The cyst may be filled with mucus (Figure 2.12).

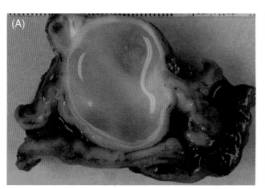 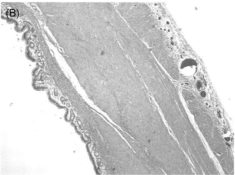

Figure 2.12 Intestinal duplication cyst: this mucus-filled non-communicating cyst is located in the wall of the terminal ileum (A). Microscopic examination (B) reveals the layers normally present in the intestinal tract; mucosa, muscularis mucosae, submucosa and muscularis propria (H&E × 20).

Histology: Duplications share the general layout of the gastrointestinal tract. The lining mucosa, depending on the location of the duplication, is of foregut, small intestinal, or colonic type. Heterotopic gastric mucosa may be identified and complicated by ulceration and may also show heterotopic pancreatic tissue.

Protracted diarrhea of infancy

Protracted diarrhea of infancy describes a complex of symptoms without designating their cause. The diarrhea starts from birth or in early infancy, is non-infectious and may be so severe that patients require parenteral nutritional support to survive. In contrast to acute diarrheal illnesses, which are common, and in most cases infectious in origin, diarrhea of longer duration (>2–4 weeks) and greater severity is rare.

Examination of endoscopic mucosal biopsies forms part of the diagnostic work-up of patients with protracted diarrhea (122).

Classification of underlying causes: Conditions causing protracted diarrhea are classified in various ways. Based on the microscopic appearance of the small intestinal biopsy they can be divided into those showing a normal villous crypt architecture and those with an abnormal villous crypt axis, i.e. showing villous blunting, with or without associated crypt hyperplasia (see Table 2.2). In a small number of conditions, specific abnormalities are identifiable by light microscopy or ultrastructurally.

The clinical presentation and the type of diarrhea also provide important clues to the underlying cause (see Table 2.3).

Osmotic diarrhea results from the presence of poorly absorbed solutes in the gut and typically resolves with bowel rest or removal of the causative agent. Congenital carbohydrate transport and enzymatic disorders commonly present with osmotic diarrhea. Secretory diarrhea may be either primary or secondary to severe mucosal injury. It results in impaired water or electrolyte absorption.

Conditions presenting with specific abnormalities identifiable by light microscopy or ultrastructural examination of the small intestinal biopsy are discussed in more detail below.

Neuro-endocrine cell dysgenesis

Definition: Neuro-endocrine (or enteroendocrine) cell dysgenesis is characterized by absence or extreme scarcity of intestinal neuro-endocrine cells secondary to mutations in the transcription factor neurogenin-3 gene (123) that controls differentiation of epithelial stem cells in the gut and pancreas into endocrine cells, through activation of NEUROD1 (124). The exact pathogenetic mechanisms leading to diarrhea are still poorly understood.

Clinical presentation: These patients present with low birth weight and severe congenital malabsorptive diarrhea with hyperchloremic metabolic acidosis. Type 1 diabetes develops later in childhood (124).

Histology: The villous architecture in most reported cases is described as normal. Absence of neuro-endocrine cells is demonstrated by immunohistochemical staining for chromogranin (123).

Table 2.2 Villous architecture in protracted diarrhea of infancy

Normal villous architecture	Villous blunting
Congenital transport defects or enzyme deficiencies	Infectious/post infectious enteropathy
Enteroendocrine cell deficiency	Food sensitivity/allergic enteropathies (cow milk, soy protein, gluten)
Short gut (post NEC or gastroschisis)	Autoimmune or immunodeficiency associated enteropathies
Motility disorders	Microvillous inclusion disease
Paraneoplastic diarrhea (neuroblastoma)	Tufting enteropathy
	Phenotypic diarrhea
	Idiopathic

Table 2.3 Clinical signs that are helpful in the differential diagnosis of protracted diarrhea

Type of diarrhea
Polyhydramnios, low birth weight
Abnormal growth, failure to thrive, malnutrition
Extra-intestinal involvement (endocrine organs, liver, kidney)
Phenotypic abnormalities/dysmorphic features
Immunodeficiency

Microvillous inclusion disease (MVID)

Clinical presentation: Patients typically present at or shortly after birth with very severe watery diarrhea and show no improvement with fasting. Without appropriate fluid and nutritional management longer-term survival beyond infancy is unlikely without small bowel transplantation. In late-onset microvillous inclusion disease, patients present at around 2 months of age and diarrhea usually is less severe (125,126). Extraintestinal manifestations (cholestastic liver disease and Fanconi syndrome) are described in a small number of patients post small bowel transplantation (127).

Genetics: Loss of function mutations in the *MYOB5* gene were recently identified in patients with MVID. This gene encodes an actin-based motor protein

Myosin Vb, which is thought to play a role in establishing and maintaining cell polarity (128,129).

Histology: On light microscopic examination, the intestinal mucosa shows variable villous blunting, a deficient brush border, and subapical PAS-positive inclusions. These can also be visualized using alkaline phosphatase or immunohistochemical staining for CD10 or carcinoembryonic antigen (CEA). Electron microscopy shows a disorganized brush border, microvillous inclusions, and increased dense apical granules and lysosomes (Figure 2.13) (130). These ultrastructural changes are thought to result from abnormal trafficking or assembly of apical membrane components (128,129).

Atypical microvillous inclusion disease refers to cases of early or late onset that present with atypical ultrastructural findings.

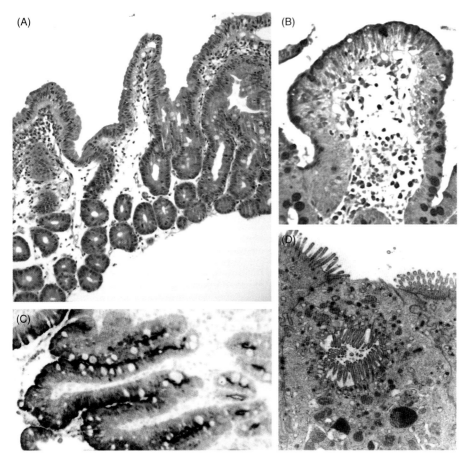

Figure 2.13 Microvillous inclusion disease: (A) Villous atrophy may be incomplete (H&E × 10). (B) Subapical inclusions are demonstrated by PAS staining (PAS × 20) or (C) immunohistochemical staining for CD10 (× 20), and Microvillous inclusions (D) are confirmed by electron microscopy.

Tufting enteropathy

Clinical presentation: Patients present within the first weeks of life with watery diarrhea that decreases with fasting, malabsorption, and failure to thrive. Clinical improvement, or less severe diarrhea and malabsorption are reported in some patients over time (131). Extra-intestinal manifestions documented in patients with tufting enteropathy include skeletal anomalies, choanal atresia, anal defects, and punctate keratitis (132).

Genetics: Abnormal cell–cell adhesion and cell–extracellular matrix interaction have been implicated in the pathogenesis of tufting enteropathy. More recently, mutations in the EpCAM gene were identified (133,134). Penetrance seems variable. A case of syndromic tufting enteropathy was found to harbor a SPINT2 mutation, otherwise described in congenital sodium diarrhea (135).

Histology: The intestinal biopsy in typical cases shows villous atrophy and epithelial tufts composed of closely packed tear-drop-shaped epithelial cells. Inflammation is not generally prominent (136). Loss of expression of EpCAM in intestinal cells of affected patients can be demonstrated by immunohistochemical staining. This observation is of particular diagnostic interest when tufts are not seen or are very sparse (Figure 2.14).

Phenotypic diarrhea: trichohepatoenteric syndrome

Clinical presentation: Diarrhea is of early neonatal onset and severe. In addition to characteristic facial features (prominent forehead and cheeks, flat broad nasal bridge, hypertelorism), patients show abnormal fragile woolly appearing hair, developmental delay, and immunodeficiency (low immunoglobulins, poor antibody response to vaccines). Hepatic involvement, cardiac anomalies, and a dual platelet population (including macro platelets) is seen in a subset of patients (137,138).

Genetics: Recently, mutations in the TTC37 (ski3) and the SKIVL2 gene were identified (139,140). The Ski complex is a multiprotein complex required for exosome-mediated RNA surveillance, regulation of normal mRNA, and decay of non-functional mRNA.

Histology: No specific epithelial abnormality is identifiable in the small bowel mucosa. Villous atrophy in most cases is mild, as is associated inflammation (139). Hair shaft (trichorrhexis nodosa) and pigmentary abnormalities are found in a majority of affected individuals (137).

Autoimmune and immunodeficiency associated enteropathies

A wide spectrum of inflammatory and architectural changes is seen in immunodeficiency associated and autoimmune or immune-mediated enteropathies, all of which can clinically present with protracted diarrhea. Prominent crypt apoptosis, villous atrophy, intraepithelial lymphocytosis, lamina propria eosinophilia, and loss of goblet or Paneth cells are amongst the morphological features described in these conditions. Enteropathic (celiac disease-like), graft-vs.-host-disease and IBD-like patterns have been described. Different patterns may be observed in a given condition (141–143). Anti-enterocyte or anti-goblet cell antibodies may be demonstrated, but their pathogenetic role remains unclear.

Gluten-sensitive enteropathy and food allergies rarely lead to severe protracted diarrhea. A specific diagnosis is supported or confirmed by the presence of specific autoantibodies (tTG, goblet cell, or enterocyte antibodies), abnormal lymphocyte counts or subsets, abnormal immunoglobulin levels, or demonstration of specific gene mutations (e.g., FOXP3 in IPEX, TTC37 in trichohepatoenteric syndrome) (139,144).

Other causes of protracted diarrhea in infancy

Occasionally protracted diarrhea develops in the course of a severe (viral) gastroenteritis. When

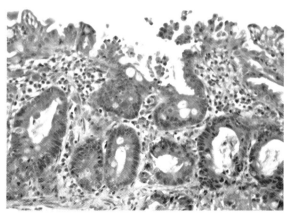

Figure 2.14 Tufting enteropathy characterized by severe villous atrophy and epithelial tufts (H&E × 20). Loss of staining for EpCAM can be demonstrated by immunohistochemistry.

reviewing biopsies of patients with underlying immunodeficiencies or patients receiving immunosuppressive drugs, the possibility of (concurrent) opportunistic infections, including EBV infection and Epstein–Barr virus (EBV)-driven lymphoproliferations, needs to be considered and investigated accordingly. In rare instances diarrhea may be a manifestation of a neoplastic process, either through direct involvement of the gut, e.g., in Langerhans-cell histiocytosis, or representing a paraneoplastic phenomenon, as in patients with neuroblastoma.

Celiac disease

Celiac disease or gluten-sensitive enteropathy is an immune-mediated disorder caused by exposure of genetically susceptible individuals to α-gliadin contained in gluten-rich cereals such as wheat, rye, and barley. The diagnosis of CD is based on a combination of intestinal and extraintestinal gluten-dependent symptoms, demonstration of celiac-specific antibodies (IgA anti-tissue transglutaminase (tTG), IgA anti-endomysium (EMA), or anti-α-gliadin antibodies (used in patients with IgA deficiency)), identification of HLA-DQ2 and/or HLA-DQ8 haplotype, and presence of characteristic changes on intestinal biopsy (145,146).

The recently issued guidelines of the European Society of Gastroenterology Hepatology and Nutrition (ESPGHAN) challenge the requirement for confirmation of celiac disease by duodenal biopsy in all patients with suspected disease (146). They propose that biopsy is omitted in symptomatic patients with tTG antibody levels >10 times the upper limit of normal and who in addition are anti-EMA and HLA-DQ2- and/or HLA-DQ8- positive as there is a high likelihood of villous atrophy.

Treatment consists of a gluten-free diet. This leads to normalization of symptoms and serological parameters. Gluten challenge or re-biopsy are no longer routinely advised to confirm a diagnosis of celiac disease.

Clinical presentation: Classic presenting symptoms are those of malabsorption, and include diarrhea, steatorrhea, abdominal bloating, poor weight gain, stunted growth, fatigue, anaemia, and/or osteopenia. The prevalence of classic celiac disease in childhood is estimated at 0.5–1% and is highest in the white population (146).

More widespread use of serological testing has led to the recognition of a wider spectrum of clinical presentations and consequently an increase in the incidence of celiac disease. The classic presentation remains predominant in young patients. Atypical presentations and clinically asymptomatic (silent) disease are more commonly encountered in older children (147,148). Atypical presentations include abdominal pain, isolated stunted growth or short stature, iron-deficiency anaemia, and metabolic bone disease.

Endoscopic examination of the duodenum characteristically shows scalloping and absence of duodenal folds.

Genetics: The histocompatibility genes HLA-DQ2 and HLA-DQ8 are the major predisposing haplotypes. They are found in about 30–40% of the white population, but only 1% will go on to develop celiac disease. Increased prevalence is documented in first-degree relatives of patients with celiac disease (up to 30%), in diabetes mellitus type 1 and other autoimmune disorders (between 3–12%), trisomy 21, Turner and Willams syndromes (0.5–9.5%) (146).

Histology: The microscopic changes of CD vary considerably in severity, may be patchy and in a small proportion of individuals are confined to the duodenal bulb (149). It is therefore recommended that separate biopsies are obtained by upper endoscopy from the duodenal bulb (at least one) and the second or third portion of duodenum (at least four biopsies) (146).

The characteristic microscopic features of untreated gluten-sensitive enteropathy include villous atrophy (total or partial), crypt hyperplasia with prominent mitotic activity, increased numbers of intraepithelial lymphocytes and lamina propria lymphoid cells (150) (Figure 2.15). Enterocyte damage with cytoplasmic vacuolation, nuclear disorganization, cuboidal shape of cells, and loss of goblets cells is often prominent. Active, neutrophilic inflammation is not uncommon, especially in younger children with a flat mucosa, and may involve lamina propria or crypts (151).

Crypt hyperplasia precedes the development of villous atrophy (150). Normal villi are between two and three times the height of crypts. Increased numbers of intraepithelial lymphocytes (IEL) were originally defined as > 40 IEL per 100 surface or upper crypt enterocytes, but subsequently lower cut-offs of between 20–25 IEL were proposed (152–154). It has been suggested that an even distribution of intraepithelial

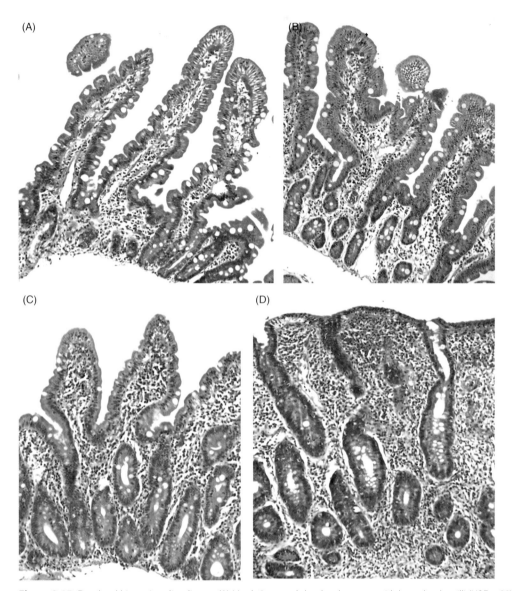

Figure 2.15 Duodenal biopsy in celiac disease: (A) Marsh 0: normal duodenal mucosa with long slender villi (H&E × 20); (B) Marsh 1: intraepithelial lymphocytes are increased, villi are preserved, and crypt hyperplasia is not seen (H&E ×20); (C) Marsh 3a: there is mild villous atrophy and crypt hyperplasia (H&E ×20); (D) Marsh 3c: severe villous atrophy is present (H&E × 20).

lymphocytes along the side of the villi or loss of the normal decrescendo pattern and clustering of intraepithelial lymphocytes in the tip region could provide a clue to a diagnosis of celiac disease in patients with normal villous architecture (155). Most of the intraepithelial lymphocytes are CD3 positive and represent activated CD8+ cytotoxic T-cells (156). Immunohistochemical stains may facilitate identification and quantification of intraepithelial lymphocytes, but are not mandatory for the diagnosis.

Classification of celiac disease: See Table 2.4
The "atrophic" pattern in the Marsh classification (type 4), was thought to be a consequence of severe malnutrition (150). The revised, widely used Marsh–Oberhuber classification further subdivides the type 3 pattern to reflect the degree of villous atrophy (154,156). A simplified classification system proposed by Corazza (153) distinguishes three patterns; Grade A/type 1 with normal villi, Grade B1/ type 2 pattern with partial villous atrophy, and

Table 2.4 Histologic classification of celiac disease (adapted from 150,153,154,156)

Marsh			Modified Marsh–Oberhuber classification			Corazza
	Pattern		IEL count*	Crypt hyperplasia	Villous atrophy	
Marsh 0	Normal		<30	Not present	Not present	
Marsh 1	Infiltrative		>30	Not present	Not present	
Marsh 2	Hyperplastic		>30	Present	Not present	Grade A/type 1
Marsh 3	Destructive	3a	>30	Present	Mild	
		3b	>30	Present	Marked	Grade B1/type 2
		3c	>30	Present	Total	Grade B2/type 3
Marsh 4	Atrophic		>30	Not present, atrophic	Present	

*IEL count = number of intraepithelial lymphocytes per 100 epithelial cells

Table 2.5 Differential diagnosis of celiac disease in children

	Intraepithelial lymphocytosis	Architectural changes	Other features
Other food allergies (e.g., soy protein, cow milk, fish)	+	+/–	Eosinophils
Inflammatory bowel disease	+	+/–	Granulomas
Giardiasis, Cryptosporidiosis	+	+/–	Giardia, Cryptosporidia
Graft-vs.-host-disease	+	+/–	Crypt apoptosis
Autoimmune enteropathy	+	+	Eosinophils, crypt apoptosis, loss of goblet or Paneth cells
Immune deficiency associated (e.g., CVID, IPEX)	+	+	Crypt apoptosis
Post infectious enteropathy	+	+	
Tufting enteropathy	-	+/–	Epithelial tufts, loss of EpCam expression OR spint2
Microvillous inclusion disease	-	+	Microvillous inclusions

Modified from Dickson (154)

Grade B2/type 3 with total villous atrophy. Intraepithelial lymphocytes are increased in all three patterns.

Differential diagnosis: The above-described histological changes are not specific to celiac disease. Similar findings can be observed in a variety of other conditions (Table 2.5).

Necrotizing enterocolitis (NEC)

Necrotizing enterocolitis affects primarily the small intestine of premature infants. It is characterized by hemorrhagic necrosis of the mucosa and the deeper bowel wall, which, in severe cases, leads to perforation. The necrosis is accompanied by inflammation and bacterial invasion of the intestinal wall. The pathogenesis is multifactorial. Historically it was believed that ischemic injury to the immature gastrointestinal tract was the main factor. More recent data suggest that a primary hypoxic–ischemic event is unlikely in premature infants, contrary to intestinal necrosis in term infants or spontaneous (isolated) intestinal perforation (157,158). Increased intestinal permeability, bacterial translocation, activation of the cytokine cascade, damage from free radicals, and an unbalanced immune response of the immature gut have been put forward as potential etiological factors (159,160).

Clinical presentation: Necrotizing enterocolitis occurs in 1–5% of all neonatal intensive care admissions and in 5–10% of all very low birth weight (> 1500 g) infants. In spite of effective modern neonatal intensive care the incidence of NEC has not decreased. Full-term neonates account for 5–25% of the cases. The latter are associated with congenital heart disease, perinatal asphyxia, and maternal cocaine use, or complicate gastroschisis, volvulus, and malrotation (159,161). Clinical symptoms may be vague, including apnoea, bradycardia, lethargy, and temperature instability. There may be emesis, bloody stools, abdominal distension, and tenderness. Occasionally there is abdominal wall discoloring. Laboratory investigations may show signs of infection or coagulation abnormalities (157). On imaging, findings include those of ileus, air in the intestinal wall (pneumatosis intestinalis), free air in the abdominal cavity and occasionally in the portal vein (162). In the early stages, clinical management is conservative with bowel rest and intensive support. Surgical therapy is needed in patients whose disease progresses despite medical therapy. Indeed, NEC is the most common surgical abdominal emergency in the newborn (163). Necrotizing enterocolitis remains the leading cause of morbidity in the premature baby and has a mortality rate of 20–40%. Sequelae can be serious in survivors. They include strictures, intestinal malabsorption, short-gut syndrome, and chronic liver disease associated with parenteral nutrition.

Macroscopy: The resected bowel shows dusky dark-reddish discoloration, variably extensive, often patchy, transmural necrosis, and possibly perforation. The regions most often affected are terminal ileum and caecum. To spare the intestinal length surgical margins are usually macroscopically affected.

Histology: The mucosa is hemorrhagic with preserved villi or shows hemorrhagic infarction destroying the mucosal architecture (Figure 2.16). Necrosis can extend through the muscularis propria to the peritoneal surface and cause perforation. Inflammation may be slight; accompanying peritonitis may be seen. It is important to look for the presence of ganglion cells, as in a full-term infant NEC may be the presenting symptom of Hirschsprung's disease.

Volvulus

Intestinal volvulus or torsion may develop *in utero*, in the neonatal period, or later in life. Midgut volvulus usually is a complication of intestinal malrotation and

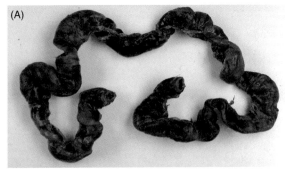

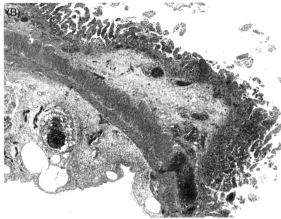

Figure 2.16 Necrotizing enterocolitis: the bowel appears dusky, with hemorrhage and focal thinning of the small bowel wall (A). Microscopy (B) shows hemorrhagic mucosal necrosis and focal pneumatosis. Inflammation is sparse (H&E × 20).

incomplete or non-fixation of the gut. Torsion of cecum, transverse colon, splenic flexure, or sigmoid can be a manifestation of excessive bowel length/ redundant bowel. A volvulus may also be the presenting symptom of cystic fibrosis (CF), particularly if associated with atresia or meconium impaction.

The clinical presentation is usually acute, with associated systemic symptoms and shock. It is often preceded by recurrent low-grade symptoms and commonly associated with intestinal dysmotility and constipation.

The macroscopic and histologic features are those of hemorrhagic necrosis and infarction of the intestinal wall.

Polyps and tumors

Gastrointestinal polyps and tumors can be divided into neoplastic and non-neoplastic lesions.

There are essentially four types of neoplastic lesions affecting the small intestine: epithelial tumors or polyps, carcinoid neuroendocrine tumors, lymphomas, and mesenchymal tumors. Although the small intestine represents 75% of the length of the alimentary tract, only 1–2% of all gastrointestinal neoplasms develop in the small bowel. Non-neoplastic juvenile or retention polyps account for the vast majority of polypoid lesions in the gastrointestinal tract (164), while non-Hodgkin's lymphoma (NHL) is the most common malignancy.

Sporadic polyps and polyposis syndromes

Polyps are the principal cause of hematochezia. They may also remain asymptomatic or manifest with intussusception, abdominal pain, protein-losing enteropathy, or diarrhea.

The polyps are either neoplastic, hyperplastic, inflammatory, or hamartomatous in nature and can present as isolated lesions or in the context of a polyposis syndrome.

In the pediatric age group, sporadic non-syndromic non-neoplastic polyps are most common. Adenomatous polyps affect mainly the duodenum and the large bowel, and occur as a manifestion of FAP and its variants.

Hamartomatous polyps and polyposis syndromes

Juvenile polyps

The isolated juvenile polyp is the commonest polypoid lesion identified in children. "Juvenile" refers to the histological type and not to the age of onset of the polyp. Sporadic solitary juvenile polyps occur mainly in the colorectum, in approximately 2% of the pediatric population, and are not associated with an increased risk of gastrointestinal cancer (164).

Genetics: Juvenile polyposis syndrome (JPS) is defined by juvenile polyps occurring throughout the gastrointestinal tract, with five or more juvenile polyps in the colorectum, or any number of juvenile polyps and a positive family history of juvenile polyposis (165,166). This autosomal dominant syndrome predisposes individuals to develop cancer. About 50–60% of JPS patients have a germline mutation in the *SMAD4*, *BMPR1A*, or *PTEN* genes (167,168).

Clinical presentation: Juvenile polyposis syndrome shows three different clinical presentations: one form with extensive intestinal involvement leading to diarrhea, malnutrition, and increased susceptibility to infection; another form limited to the colon and easily confused with familial polyposis; and a third form where there is involvement of the stomach, intestines, and colon, easily mistaken for PJS (169). These

last two forms appear to be variable expressions of the same disease, as patients of both presentations have been reported to segregate according to a dominant mode in the same family (167).

A recent cancer risk analysis calculated a cumulative lifetime risk for colorectal cancer in JPS of 39%, and a relative risk of colorectal cancer of 34% (170,171). The relative risk appears greatest when adenomatous foci are present.

In addition to JPS, juvenile polyps are seen in PTEN hamartoma syndromes (Cowden's disease, Bannayan–Riley–Ruvalcaba syndrome), Gorlin–Goltz syndrome, and Cronkhite–Canada syndrome.

Macroscopy: Juvenile polyps vary in size from 5 mm to 50 mm, and typically have a spherical, lobulated, and pedunculated appearance, with a smooth surface and surface erosion.

Histology: Juvenile polyps are considered hamartomas, i.e. arise from abnormal patterning of the gut mucosa (172). Microscopically, they are characterized by an abundance of edematous lamina propria with inflammatory cells (lymphocytes, plasma cells, eosinophils, and polymorphs) and cystic dilated glands lined by cuboidal to columnar epithelium with reactive changes (Figure 2.17). The surface frequently is ulcerated and the lamina propria may contain dilated vessels and some smooth muscle.

Juvenile polyps in JPS appear histologically similar to sporadic juvenile polyps, although syndromic polyps often have a frond-like growth pattern more similar to polyps in Peutz–Jeghers, with less stroma, fewer dilated glands and more proliferative smaller glands (173). In addition, polyps in JPS may contain adenomatous foci not found in sporadic juvenile polyps.

Differential diagnosis: The distinction between a true inflammatory polyp and a juvenile polyp is often difficult. There is considerable overlap of microscopic features. There also is some overlap with polyps in PJS, although cystic glands are not usually present in PJS. In addition, the smooth muscle in juvenile polyps lacks the arborizing pattern characteristic of Peutz–Jeghers polyps.

Peutz–Jeghers syndrome

Peutz–Jeghers syndrome is inherited in an autosomal-dominant pattern, with a variable and incomplete penetrance (165,166). The incidence is

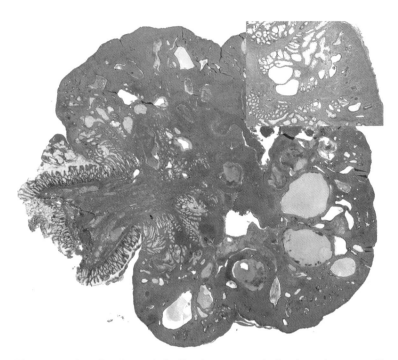

Figure 2.17 Juvenile polyp: cystically dilated crypts are set in abundant edematous or fibrotic inflammatory stroma (H&E × 2). Inset: surface ulceration is common.

estimated at 1 in 30 000–200 000. In most cases there is an underlying germline deletion in the LKB-1 (STK11) gene. *De novo* mutations occur in about 25% of cases. PJS consists of gastrointestinal hamartomatous polyps and pigmented macules in the mucous membranes and skin. Small, dark-colored spots usually develop within the first year of life, on the lips, around and inside the mouth, near the eyes and nostrils, and around the anus. Small bowel polyps most commonly develop in the jejunum and ileum, and manifest with intussusception and obstruction, chronic bleeding, and abdominal pain. Affected individuals are at significantly increased risk of developing cancer in various other organs. The Peutz–Jeghers polyps themselves carry a very low risk of malignant transformation.

Macroscopy: Polyps occur most commonly in the jejunum and ileum. The number of polyps is variable and they can be sessile or pedunculated, ranging from a few millimeters to several centimeters in diameter. They can be solitary, or can occur in clusters, at times carpeting the entire mucosal surface (174).

Histology: The polyps show a characteristically branched or "frond-like" architecture with a core of stromal tissue and mature smooth muscle, which is surrounded by hyperplastic epithelial tissue with a near normal appearance (174). Small intestinal polyps consist of crypts and villi of varying lengths lined by cells normally present within small bowel mucosa (enterocytes, Paneth cells, goblet cells, and argentaffin cells) (Figure 2.18). Inflammation is not usually present. The surface, as with other polypoid lesions, may be ulcerated, and regenerative epithelial changes may be observed.

Differential diagnosis: Especially small Peutz–Jegher polyps can be difficult to differentiate from juvenile polyps. However, they do not usually show an inflamed lamina propria or contain cystically dilated glands.

PTEN hamartoma syndromes

Germline mutations in the tumor-suppressor gene *PTEN* have been implicated in two rare autosomal dominant hamartoma syndromes that exhibit some clinical overlap, Cowden syndrome (CS), and Bannayan–Riley–Ruvalcaba syndrome (BRRS). The incidence is around 1 in 200 000. Polyps are limited to the terminal ileum and colon. The risk of gastrointestinal cancer is very low (165,166).

Hamartomatous polyps are the most prevalent polypoid lesions in PTEN hamartoma syndrome. Other types of polyps encountered include ganglioneuromatous or inflammatory polyps.

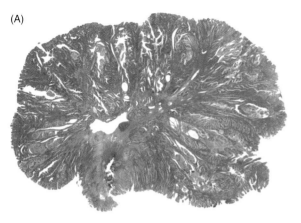

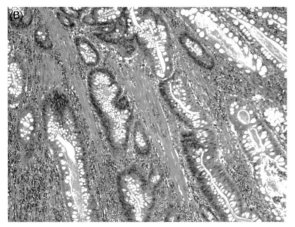

Figure 2.18 (A) Peutz–Jeghers polyp: typically shows a frond-like or arborising architecture (H&E × 2). (B) Higher magnification shows strands of smooth muscle and hyperplastic intestinal epithelium (H&E ×20).

Hereditary mixed polyposis syndrome (HMPS)

Hereditary mixed polyposis syndrome is very rare and characterized by multiple bowel polyps of differing histological types (165,166). Mutations in the *BRMP1* gene and a large gene duplication involving the *GREM1* locus, respectively, were recently identified (175). Interestingly, these genetic pathways also seem involved in tumorigenesis in juvenile polyposis. The relative risk of gastrointestinal cancer is significantly increased in patients with HMPS. Polyps show differing or composite histologic features, and include tubulovillous or serrated adenomas and juvenile polyps with dysplastic crypts, or combinations of hyperplastic and adenomatous elements.

Adenomyomatous polyps

Adenomyoma of the gastrointestinal tract is a rare benign tumor-like lesion, that is also referred to as myoepithelial hamartoma, adenomyomatous hamartoma, or foregut choristoma (176). In children, most of the cases are found in the gastric antrum or in the duodenum. Presenting symptoms include pyloric outlet obstructions. Rare cases are reported in the proximal small bowel or terminal ileum, where they may manifest with intussusception (177). These latter lesions may represent a variant of pancreatic heterotopia. Adenomyoma or adenomyomatous hyperplasia of the ampullary region is a tumor-like lesion of extrahepatic bile ducts that occurs mainly in the adult (178).

Macroscopy: Adenomyoma of the GI tract presents as an intramural or protruding polypoid nodule covered by mucosa. The diameter of adenomyoma in reported cases ranges from 0.6 cm to 4.5 cm.

Histology: Adenomyomas of the small intestine occupy mainly the submucosa and often extend into the muscularis propria (176,177). The lesion consists of variably dilated glandular structures surrounded by interlacing smooth muscle bundles. The glandular structures are typically lined by biliary or foregut-type epithelium with basally oriented nuclei.

Diagnosis on endoscopic biopsies is usually difficult, because the lesion primarily occupies the submucosa. The differential diagnosis includes duplication cysts and other hamartomatous polyps.

Adenomatous polyps

Adenomatous polyps or adenocarcinoma in children, especially in the small bowel, are exceedingly rare and should raise the suspicion of an underlying syndrome, notably FAP.

Inflammatory myofibroblastic tumor

Inflammatory myofibroblastic tumor (IMFT) is a spindle-cell proliferation with a distinctive fibro-inflammatory and even pseudosarcomatous appearance (179). Inflammatory myofibroblastic tumor is now considered by many a true neoplasm, with some cases showing aggressive behavior. A gene rearrangement involving the ALK1 gene with activation of the ALK receptor tyrosine kinase gene is found in about 50% of cases, mostly in children.

Clinical presentation: Inflammatory myofibroblastic tumors present as a mass in the wall of the stomach, the intestine, or the mesentery that eventually causes intestinal obstruction. General symptoms (fever, anaemia) are common.

Macroscopy: Typically, IMFT is a well-circumscribed but non-encapsulated lobulated lesion that may be polypoid and protrude into the bowel lumen.

Histology: As their counterpart in the soft tissues (see Chapter 12).

Carcinoid/neuroendocrine tumors

Gastrointestinal neuroendocrine tumors are rare in children. They mostly are benign carcinoid tumors (well-differentiated neuroendocrine tumors according to WHO) that arise in the tip of the appendix (180). Metastatic disease is exceedingly rare in tumors of < 2 cm, and surgical appendicectomy is considered sufficient in such cases, provided the margins are clear. Small intestinal neuroendocrine tumors are very uncommon. They derive from two separate embryonic divisions, the forgut (duodenum) and the midgut (jejunum and ileum).

Clinical presentation: Neuroendocrine or carcinoid tumors in children are mostly an incidental finding. Bulky tumors and carcinoid syndrome are rarely observed in children.

Macroscopy: In the gastrointestinal tract, neuroendocrine tumors develop deep in the mucosa and extend into the underlying submucosa and the mucosal surface, eventually bulging into the intestinal lumen. They typically have a yellow or tan appearance.

Histology: Carcinoid tumors are characterized by the presence of small, uniformly stained clear cells, with moderate amounts of finely granular cytoplasm. The cells are typically arranged in a solid, trabecular, insular, or organoid pattern, and surrounded by thin layers of stroma (Figure 2.19). Strong staining for chromogranin and synaptophysin is characteristic. Focal cytokeratin staining is also present.

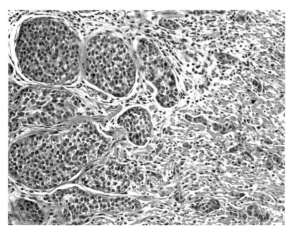

Figure 2.19 Carcinoid tumor: nests and trabecules of small uniform cells with finely granular cytoplasm infiltrate the smooth muscle of the appendiceal wall (H&E × 20).

The WHO classification scheme (181), divides neuroendocrine tumors into three prognostic groups (well-differentiated tumors of benign or uncertain behavior, well-differentiated neuroendocrine carcinoma, and poorly differentiated neuroendocrine carcinoma), depending on location, size, differentiation, mitotic count, Ki-67 index, vascular invasion, and metastasis.

Lymphoid polyps and tumors

Lymphoid hyperplasia

Lymphoid hyperplasia is a common finding, especially in the terminal ileum of small children and occasionally can form polypoid masses and cause intussusception or intestinal obstruction.

Intestinal lymphoma

Non-Hodgkin lymphomas are the most frequent intestinal malignancy in children (182).

Burkitt's type lymphoma, the commonest extranodal lymphoma in the pediatric age group, shows a predilection for the terminal ileum and the ileocecal region (183–185). There is a well-established relationship between EBV infection and the pathogenesis of both endemic and sporadic Burkitt's lymphoma (186).

Clinical presentation: Most patients present with involvement of the ileocecal area. Symptoms include abdominal pain, bowel obstruction, torsion, or intussusception. Some patients have ascites or present with a clinical picture of acute appendicitis or peritonitis.

Burkitt's lymphoma is significantly more common in sub-Saharan Africa than in other parts of the world, accounting for approximately one half of all childhood cancers in that region. Its incidence also appears to be higher in Latin America, North Africa, and the Middle East than it is in the United States or Europe.

Genetics: The hallmark of Burkitt's lymphoma is (8;14)(q24;q32) translocation, which is observed in approximately 80% of patients.

Macroscopy: Intestinal lymphoma usually presents as an ulcerated polypoid mass, frequently located in the ileocecal region.

Histology: The histological pattern and the immunoprofile vary according to the lymphoma subtype. Burkitt's lymphoma is defined in the updated WHO classification (2008) as a B-cell lymphoma with an extremely high proliferation rate (187). The typical Burkitt's lymphoma (Figure 2.20) is composed of sheets of medium-sized lymphoid cells with basophilic cytoplasm, intermingled with large histiocytes with

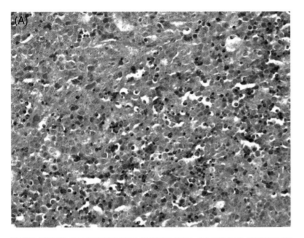

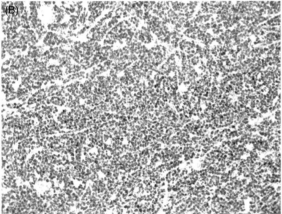

Figure 2.20 Burkitt's lymphoma: apoptosis (A) is prominent (H&E × 40); (B) > 95% of tumor cells stain with Ki67 (× 20).

cytoplasmic debris responsible for a typical "starry-sky" pattern. Numerous mitotic figures and apoptotic bodies are present. The cells usually express B-cell markers (CD10+/bcl2−/Bcl6+) and have a proliferative index ≥ 95%. The latter is a powerful parameter to distinguish Burkitt's lymphoma (including atypical BL) from diffuse large B-cell lymphoma (187).

Colon

Congenital malformations: atresia and stenosis

Colonic atresia is very rare, accounting for no more than 1% of all intestinal atresias. Colonic atresia or stenosis may be congenital or acquired. The diagnosis may be delayed as the obstruction lies distally in the bowel. It occurs most often in the right colon where the marked discrepancy of atretic ends presents a

technical challenge to establish bowel continuity thus necessitating hemicolectomy (188). Perforation may complicate colonic atresia and may occur before surgical decompression of the obstructed colon or postoperatively. The mortality can be as high as 19%. Colonic atresia or perforation may be associated with Hirschsprung's disease (189). Congenital atresia and acquired colonic stricture in older patients has been reported in association with cystic fibrosis (190).

Histology: The atretic segment may show fibrosis, septal formation, and tiny or absent lumen. It is most important to check for the presence of ganglion cells in the normal bowel wall of the resected specimen to exclude Hirschsprung's disease.

Intestinal pseudo-obstruction

Intestinal pseudo-obstruction refers to a heterogeneous group of primary and secondary disorders of gut motility, which are far less common in the pediatric age group (191). Patients with intestinal pseudo-obstruction show symptoms and signs suggesting bowel obstruction, but true mechanical obstruction of the gut is not identified.

Classification: Disorders of gut motility can broadly be divided into disorders of the gastro-intestinal autonomous nervous system (visceral neuropathies) and of the gastrointestinal smooth muscle (visceral myopathies). Primary conditions represent intrinsic disorders. They may be familial or non-familial, congenital or acquired, localized or more extensive. Involvement of other hollow viscera, ocular musculature, or syndromic features characterize some of these conditions. Secondary pseudo-obstruction is less commonly encountered in children when compared to adults. It may arise as a direct manifestation of a systemic disorder involving the smooth muscle or the enteric nervous system, or complicate a systemic disorder.

Clinical presentation: Symptoms vary, depending on the severity of the condition. Chronic constipation, abdominal distension and pain, paradoxical diarrhea, and soiling are common. Failure to thrive and malnourishment is seen in severe cases. Patient with intestinal pseudo-obstruction often undergo repeat procedures to exclude an underlying mechanical obstruction or to alleviate symptoms by placing a stoma or resect lengths of affected bowel.

Histology: With the exception of Hirschsprung's disease, full-thickness biopsies are required for diagnosis. The intestinal smooth muscle and the intestinal nerve plexus are assessed on H&E-stained paraffin sections. Connective tissue stains (Masson's trichrome), immunohistochemical stains for smooth-muscle contractile proteins (e.g., α-smooth muscle actin, muscle actin, desmin, caldesmon), and neural markers (e.g., neurofilaments, S-100, calretinin, CD117/c-kit), electron microscopy, and enzyme histochemical staining for acetylcholinesterase can provide useful additional information to assist in the identification or confirmation of a myopathic or neural disorder (192–194).

Hirschsprung's disease (HD)

Hirschsprung's disease (or intestinal aganglionosis) is a congenital developmental disorder of the intestinal autonomous nervous system caused by a failure of neural crest cells to migrate to the gut. It is defined by a total absence of ganglion cells in the submucosal and myenteric plexus, starting from the distal rectum, with variable typically contiguous proximal extension of the aganglionic segment.

Clinical presentation: Approximately 1:5000 liveborn infants are affected. Boys are about four times more commonly affected then girls. Most patients present in the first six months of life with obstructive symptoms, failure to pass meconium, abdominal distension, and bilious vomiting. Patients with extensive small bowel involvement usually show severe failure to thrive and are dependent on parenteral nutrition or possibly small bowel transplantation to survive. Refractory chronic constipation and abdominal distension are the main complaints in older infants and children. In rare cases a diagnosis of HD is not established until adulthood. Delayed diagnosis of HD, particularly in the neonatal period, may result in serious or life-threatening complications, such as toxic megacolon and NEC. Abdominal X-ray and barium enema typically show a distal narrow bowel segment and proximal bowel distension.

Genetics: At least 10 different susceptibility genes have so far been identified. Autosomal recessive and autosomal dominant inheritance is documented with variable penetrance in syndromic and nonsyndromic forms. Genetic syndromes associated with HD include MEN-2A and neurofibromatosis type 1. Chromosomal anomalies are found in about 12% of cases, most commonly trisomy 21 (195–197).

Classification: Involvement of the distal rectum is seen in all cases of HD. Depending on the proximal extension HD is further classified as follows:

- Classical or short segment disease (about 80% of cases): rectum and sigmoid colon
- Long segment disease (about 15%): extension to proximal large bowel
- Total colonic aganglionosis (about 5%): entire large bowel, and variable length of terminal ileum
- Total intestinal aganglionosis (< 5%): severest form, entire large and small bowel ultra-short segment (controversial): ≤ 2 cm of the distal rectum

Treatment: The definite treatment of HD (except for cases with extensive small bowel involvement) consists of the resection of the aganglionic bowel segment and anastomosis of the proximal ganglionic bowel to the distal end. Type and site of anastomosis varies depending on the technique used (Soave, Duhamel, or Swenson). The corrective procedure is performed in one stage or preceded by placement of a stoma (two-step procedure) as an open or laprascopically assisted transanal procedure. Choice of procedure and time of surgery largely depend on local surgical practice. Complications such a sepsis, enterocolitis, or massive distension of the proximal bowel may necessitate emergency placement of a stoma.

Reported short- and long-term post-operative complications are similar for each procedure and include recurrent enterocolitis, obstructive symptoms, and constipation (198). Anastomotic stricture (199), pull-through at the level of the transitional zone (200), hypoganglionic or dysganglionic bowel proximal to the aganglionic segment (201,202), acquired aganglionosis (203), and skip lesions (204) are potential causes of persistent obstructive symptoms.

Macroscopy: Typically, the resected aganglionic bowel is much narrower than the proximal ganglionic bowel, which may become significantly dilated. The transition zone may be identifiable macroscopically by its funnel shape.

Histology: Rectal biopsies are done for diagnostic purposes and intraoperative seromuscular biopsies are done to confirm the localization of ganglionic intestine. The resected specimen also requires a special approach.

Rectal suction biopsy: The diagnosis of HD is confirmed on rectal suction biopsies in infants or surgical ("strip") biopsies in older children. The diagnostic criteria are summarized in Table 2.6. The microscopic features are illustrated in Figure 2.21.

Absence of ganglion cells is a reliable feature provided the biopsy: (1) has been taken from at least

Table 2.6 Diagnostic criteria for Hirschsprung's disease

Diagnosis	Ganglion cells (serial sections, H&E)	Hypertrophic submucosal nerves (> 40 μm)	Acetylcholinesterase staining pattern	Calretinin-positive nerve fibers
Normal gut	Present	No	Normal	Present
Hirschsprung disease	Absent	Yes, but not always	Abnormal or normal	Absent
Long segment HD	Absent	No	Normal	Absent
Ultra-short	Absent	Variable	Abnormal	Probably absent (further data required)
Low biopsy	Rare or absent	Absent	Normal	Present
Uncertain	Present, mature	Absent	Abnormal	Present
	Present, immature	Absent	Normal or abnormal	Present

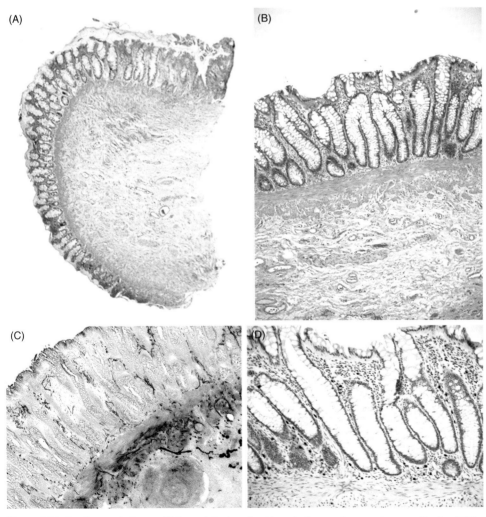

Figure 2.21 Hirschsprung's disease: (A) A good-sized suction biopsy is illustrated at scanning magnification (H&E × 2); (B) Thickened nerves without ganglion cells are identified at higher magnification (H&E × 20); (C) Increased acetylcholinesterase (× 20) and (D) absence of calretinin positive delicate nerve twigs (× 20).

1–1.5 cm above the anorectal junction (thereby avoiding the physiologically hypoganglionic zone of the most distal rectum), (2) is of sufficient size and well preserved, and (3) a large enough number of sections is examined (205). The biopsies should be ≥ 2–3 mm and contain similar amounts of mucosa and submucosa, the tissue well preserved and not crushed or hemorrhagic. It may require 100 or more consecutive (serial) sections at a thickness of 3–5 μm to identify ganglion cells on H&E-stained sections.

Presence of adjunct features such as hypertrophic (> 40 μm) submucosal nerves and an abnormal acetylcholinesterase (AchE) staining pattern help to confirm a diagnosis of HD. These features, however, are not seen in all cases and are typically absent in long-segment HD. Loss of calretinin expression in mucosal and submucosal nerves correlates strongly with aganglionosis and interpretation of the staining pattern appears more consistent than that of the AChE staining (206,207). In a normal ganglionic bowel the AchE staining will reveal no or very sparse delicate AchE positive fibers in the muscularis mucosae. Abundant coarse and strongly positive fibers are seen in HD in the muscularis mucosae and thicker intensely positive nerves in the immediately underlying submucosa, with variable presence of AchE-positive fibers in the lamina propria. Often a gradient is appreciable with respect to the staining intensity, which tends to be strongest in the submucosa. Potential pitfalls in the interpretation of rectal biopsies include identification of immature ganglion cells and an abnormal or equivocal AChE staining pattern in ganglionic biopsies, or the absence of ganglion cells in a suboptimal or low biopsy. In normal ganglionic bowel calretinin stain is seen as thin fibers in the lamina propria. Mast cells stain positive with calretinin and may be seen in aganglionic bowel; unless thin fibers are present, this should not be considered positive.

Reliable and reproducible diagnostic criteria for ultra-short HD (defined as extending 2 cm or less) are yet to be established. Similarly, it is unclear how these patients should best be managed.

Intraoperative diagnosis: Seromuscular biopsies are performed to ensure that the stoma or bowel anastomosis is placed in the ganglionic bowel and with enough distance to the transitional zone. The latter represents a short irregularly delineated segment (3 cm or less) of bowel that forms the interface between aganglionic and normally ganglionic bowel (208). Seromuscular biopsies should be of sufficient size (1 cm at least) and include both muscle layers to facilitate orientation and appropriate identification of ganglion cells on a small number of frozen sections. Often multiple biopsies are taken along the length of the colon to map the transition zone or identify potential skip lesions. A diagnosis of total colonic aganglionosis cannot reliably be based on examination of the appendix alone, as this approach fails to identify potential skip lesions (204). Intraoperative assessment of the proximal margin of the resected bowel to determine the percentage of bowel circumference that contains ganglion cells is performed in some institutions. It may reduce the frequency of obstructive systems following surgery (209).

Examination of the pull through resection specimen: The resection specimen (variable lengths of colon and rectum from the definitive corrective operation) is examined to confirm the diagnosis of HD, to determine the length of the aganglionic segment, and to map the transitional zone (interface between aganglionic and ganglionic segment). This can be achieved by submitting consecutive transverse sections or, more frequently, by taking sequential longitudinal sections of the whole resected gut. Depending on the surgical approach used, the specimen will be full-thickness throughout (Duhamel and Swenson), or will consist at the distal end of a sleeve of mucosa and submucosa only, while the rest of the segment is full-thickness (Soave).

Intestinal neuronal dysplasia (IND)

The concept of IND as a pathological correlate of intestinal pseudo-obstruction is fraught with controversy since its original description (210). The main reason for this is the lack of reproducibility of diagnostic criteria on rectal biopsies as opposed to Hirschsprung disease (211), and repeated revision of diagnostic criteria (212–214).

Intestinal hypoganglionosis

Reduced numbers of ganglion cells and reduced or small nerve ganglia in the myenteric and submucosal plexus characterize intestinal hypoganglionosis (205). A diagnosis of hypoganglionosis is difficult to establish on suction biopsies and when changes in numbers are subtler. Hypoganglionosis is most commonly recognized in the transition zone of Hirschsprung's disease. Rare cases of primary intestinal hypoganglionosis are reported, but it is unclear whether these represent a distinct condition or a variant of Hirschsprung disease.

Hypoganglionosis and aganglionosis may be acquired and develop secondary to ischemic bowel necrosis (NEC, gastroschisis), intestinal infection (HSV, Chagas disease), or complicate intestinal inflammatory disorders (CD, paraneoplastic or autoimmune ganglionitis).

Visceral myopathies

Primary visceral myopathies are very rare and characterized by smooth muscle atrophy and fibrosis. Myocyte vacuolation, nuclear changes, and loss of expression of smooth muscle contractile proteins are inconstant features. Clinically (i.e. drugs) or morphologically identifiable causes such as ischemia or inflammation should have been excluded.

Colitis

The interpretation of colonic biopsies displaying inflammatory changes (colitis) can be challenging since the colorectal mucosa has a limited repertoire of morphologic responses to various injurious agents. Histological reaction patterns within the colon are not disease-specific and only a few processes have defined diagnostic features. Many of the various histological patterns reflect severity and duration of the disease, rather than its cause, and therefore have to be correlated with clinical and endoscopic/macroscopic features to be conclusive. The importance of dialog between the pathologist and gastroenterologist is emphasized.

Common histological patterns include acute colitis, with and without features of pseudomembranous or ischemic colitis, as opposed to chronic colitis (with and without crypt destruction). Less common patterns include eosinophilic colitis, graft-vs.-host disease, chronic mucosal prolapse, and non-specific or idiopathic ulcer.

Eosinophilic conditions affecting the colon

Eosinophilic disorders of the gut are classified as either primary or secondary. Primary eosinophilic colitis is uncommon and occurs in the absence of an identifiable cause for eosinophilia. The colon can be involved, together with other parts of the gut (in the context of eosinophilic gastroenteritis) or exclusively (215).

Eosinophilic colitis (EC) or allergic colitis is characterized by inflammatory changes in the rectum and colon as a result of immune-mediated reactions to ingested foreign proteins. It more commonly affects infants and adolescents, and most infantile cases are thought to be due to allergy to soy protein or cow's milk protein. Yet, interestingly, eosinophilic colitis has been reported to occur more often in infants that are exclusively breastfed (probably as a result of the maternal diet). Diarrhea, which can be bloody, is the classic presentation. Symptoms may include abdominal pain, anorexia, and weight loss. Most affected infants lack constitutional symptoms and are otherwise healthy. Peripheral blood eosinophilia and stool eosinophils may be present (216).

Macroscopy: The colonoscopy is non-specific, including erythema and loss of vascularity, friability, and nodularity.

Histology: Increased numbers of clustering eosinophils are noted within the lamina propria while the architecture is preserved (Figure 2.22). Despite the absence of consensus criteria, a threshold of > 20 eosinophils per HPF has been used (216). Other useful features include infiltration of surface and crypt epithelium, and of the muscularis mucosae, by eosinophils. Involvement of other segments of the gastrointestinal mucosa should suggest a diagnosis of eosinophilic gastroenteritis. Clinicopathological correlation and exclusion of secondary causes of gastrointestinal eosinophilia are important, as the described features are non-specific.

Acute infectious colitis

This refers to an inflammatory condition triggered by a potentially identifiable infectious cause. It is usually self-limiting and resolves within 2–4 weeks or less, without residual inflammation or recurrent

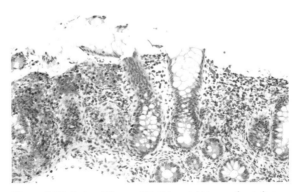

Figure 2.22 Eosinophilic proctitis; this rectal biopsy of an infant shows a heavy infiltrate of eosinophils and eosinophil degranulation (H&E × 20).

symptoms. Since a proportion of cases return a negative culture, the term "acute infectious-type colitis" or "acute self-limiting colitis" is commonly used to refer to patients who present with a transient diarrheal illness, with biopsy findings similar to those with an identifiable infectious etiology, but in whom no pathogen is identified. Acute infectious colitis is infrequently seen by pathologists. Hence, features are discussed only very broadly.

Although the ability to detect infectious processes in tissue sections has grown exponentially with the advent of new techniques, such as histochemical and immunohistochemical stains, *in situ* hybridization and PCR, the most valuable and least expensive diagnostic tool is the dialog with the gastroenterologist. Appropriate clinical information, including specific symptoms, endoscopic findings, travel history, and immune status are essential to the successful interpretation of gut biopsies.

The pathological diagnosis of GI infections depends on the recognition of several features, which include specific tissue reactions and cytopathic effects, as well as particular pathogenic agents (217,218). The histologic picture infections produce can be grouped into a limited number of patterns, reflecting mechanisms of injury and disease duration:

1. None or very mild histological changes
2. Focal active colitis pattern: acute self-limited colitis/acute, non-crypt destructive colitis
3. Crypt destructive colitis pattern, with regenerative changes and distortion mimicking IBD
4. Diagnostic features specific of a causative agent (pseudomembranes, granulomas, or viral inclusions).

Microscopic colitis

Microscopic colitis (MC) typically presents with chronic, watery, non-bloody diarrhea with normal endoscopy findings, but abnormal inflammatory histopathological findings. It is mainly a condition of the elderly, uncommon in children (219).

Histologically, MC is a form of chronic colitis that combines a non-crypt-destructive histological pattern with a chronic inflammatory process.

Lymphocytic colitis is characterized by an increase in surface and crypt intraepithelial lymphocytes. A threshold of > 20 per 100 enterocytes has been suggested (normal is < 5 per 100 enterocytes) (220). The presence of epithelial injury, including loss of the

normal columnar shape, mucin depletion, and an attenuated or syncytial appearance of the surface epithelium is commonly noted. The lamina propria has increased cellularity due to lymphocytes and plasma cells.

In collagenous colitis a characteristic thick collagen (> 10 μm) band is present beneath the surface epithelium, which does not extend down the sides of the crypts.

Neutropenic enterocolitis (NE)

NE or thyplitis is clinically defined by the triad of neutropenia, abdominal pain, and fever, and is considered a life-threatening gastrointestinal complication of profound neutropenia (frequently secondary to acute leukemia and lymphoma, or after getting combined chemotherapy). The exact pathogenesis is unclear, but there is probably an association of mucosal damage, bacterial invasion, and ischemia (221). The process preferentially involves the cecum.

Macroscopically, the changes range from mucosal erythema to areas of hemorrhagic necrosis or diffuse transmural hemorrhagic necrosis. On histology, a severe necrotizing colitis with edema and vasculitis can be seen. The process typically starts from the superficial mucosa and progressively involves the deep crypts, as seen in ischemic colitis. In severe cases there is transmural necrosis. There is a striking paucity of inflammatory cells, with absence of neutrophils. Numerous bacteria are usually present overlying the damaged epithelium (222).

Inflammatory bowel disease (IBD)

The descriptive term "inflammatory bowel disease" (IBD) is generally applied to the idiopathic varieties, UC and CD. The pathologist's opinion is often considered the final arbiter in the diagnosis and classification of IBD, but judgement may be hampered by the considerable histological overlap. Accurate diagnosis, particularly in biopsy specimens, thus relies on a multidisciplinary approach – with clinical, radiological, and endoscopic input – perhaps even more so than with other intestinal diseases. Although IBD in children and adolescents is similar in many essential features to adult IBD, failure to recognize differences may lead to diagnostic confusion or uncertainty. It is these features that will be particularly emphasized in this section.

In past years, both the European and North American Societies for Pediatric Gastroenterology,

Hepatology, and Nutrition have issued recommendations regarding the work-up and diagnosis of IBD in children and adolescents (23,24). These aim: (1) to standardize the diagnostic work-up of patients with suspected IBD, (2) to define evidence-based criteria for diagnosis and classification of IBD in children, and (3) to allow collection of uniform phenotypic data on patients ≤ 18 years with newly diagnosed IBD, based on resources available.

Ulcerative colitis (UC)

The incidence of UC in Western countries is 1–2 per 100 000 children (225–228). The most common age group to be affected is adolescents; approximately 10–18% of children are under 10 years old and about one-third of these are aged five or less at time of diagnosis. The male-to-female ratio is roughly equal. In most cases, UC is a chronic disease characterized by periods of exacerbation and remission; less commonly there is a single attack, a continuous unremitting pattern, or acute fulminant disease with colonic dilatation.

Sites and pattern of involvement: Ulcerative colitis is primarily a mucosal disease that begins in the rectum and extends proximally in continuity to involve all or part of the remaining colon. Compared to adults, children tend to have more extensive disease at initial presentation (229,230). When presenting with proctitis alone, children are more than twice as likely as adults to subsequently develop proximal extension of disease (50% vs. 10–30%) (231,232). A proportion of patients with total colitis, but not usually with left-sided colitis alone, have inflammation of the terminal ileum extending 5–25 cm from the ileocecal valve. This so-called "backwash" ileitis is more common in children (39%) (233,234) than adults (18%) (235). It may cause diagnostic confusion with CD, particularly in mucosal biopsies.

The appendix is involved in approximately 56% of children with UC (236), but this does not usually lead to symptomatic appendicitis, as the inflammatory process remains confined to the mucosa. The appendix, ascending colon and cecum can be involved in so-called "skip" lesions (237), involvement of the latter being termed a "cecal patch" (238,239).

Macroscopy: The pathological features form a spectrum that parallels the variability in clinical course. In contrast to CD, active, resolving, and quiescent phases are recognized, reflecting the typical clinical pattern of exacerbation and remission.

The macroscopic appearances vary considerably according to the phase of the disease and its severity. Most resections are carried out for severe active disease or chronic continuous disease unresponsive to medical treatment.

In long-standing disease, the affected bowel is contracted and narrowed. This shortening is particularly severe in the distal large bowel. Smooth tubular strictures can occur due to muscular thickening rather than fibrosis. The mucosal changes may involve a variable length of large bowel in continuity. The transition from diseased to normal mucosa is usually gradual. The disease process may vary in stage or severity in different parts of the bowel, thus giving the impression of segmental involvement. The most common pattern is quiescent or healing disease in the rectum – induced, for example, by local treatment – with active disease in the proximal colon.

The involved mucosa in the early stages may appear simply granular and hyperemic, but with progression of the disease there is usually some degree of ulceration. In the quiescent phase, the mucosa generally has a featureless bland or atrophic appearance. Polypoid change is common in UC, particularly following severe disease. If healing occurs, the polyps may remain as evidence of past disease, so-called "colitis polyposa." This most commonly affects the proximal colon, leaving the rectum relatively spared. In some cases of chronic unremitting disease, lymphoid follicular hyperplasia causes a multiple diffuse polyposis-like appearance.

Rarely patients with UC have a fulminant episode, either as a first attack or in an acute relapse (acute fulminant colitis or "toxic megacolon"). The mucosa is extensively ulcerated with intervening mucosal islands showing intense congestion. Single or multiple perforations may be apparent with evidence of peritonitis on the external surface. The transverse or sigmoid colon becomes dilated and thin-walled. The distal sigmoid and rectum are often spared in fulminant disease and, as a consequence, diagnostic changes may not be evident on sigmoidoscopy or rectal biopsy. This is potentially misleading, particularly during a first attack.

Histology: The abnormalities in UC are confined to the mucosa. The deeper layers of the bowel wall are almost never involved unless there is deep ulceration. The histological findings usually correlate well with the endoscopic and macroscopic appearances. Thus, the histology varies with the phase and severity of the clinical disease in a similar manner to the gross

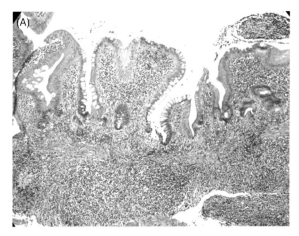

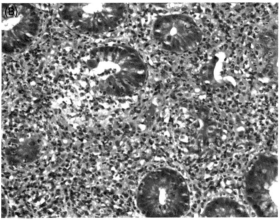

Figure 2.23 Ulcerative colitis: (A) There is severe distortion of the crypt architecture with villous transformation. The mucosa shows marked plasmacytosis and small basal lymphoid aggregates are identified (H&E × 10). (B) Cryptolytic inflammation with pericryptal collections of histiocytes (pericryptal or crypotlytic granuloma) is illustrated in (H&E ×40).

pathology. Characteristic microscopic features have been defined for each of the recognized phases of disease. In all phases, the inflammatory infiltrate is almost exclusively mucosal (Figure 2.23).

Active phase: Characteristically there is a diffuse inflammatory cell infiltrate that fills and expands the lamina propria. This, together with variable edema and capillary congestion, gives the impression of mucosal thickening and imparts an undulating or low villiform pattern to the surface.

The inflammatory infiltrate, which comprises plasma cells, lymphocytes, and neutrophils, mast cells, and eosinophils, is in most cases distributed evenly throughout the lamina propria. Variability in intensity of the inflammation can result in a somewhat patchy distribution. A band of plasma cells and

lymphocytes is almost always present in the basal part of the lamina propria, separating the bases of crypts from the underlying muscularis mucosae. Neutrophils are most conspicuous in the lumina of crypts, forming crypt abscesses. The number of crypt abscesses is variable. In some cases of long-standing active disease, hyperplasia of mucosal lymphoid follicles occurs, accompanied by crypt atrophy. This feature is particularly prominent in the rectum, giving rise to so-called follicular proctitis.

The inflammatory damage to crypts produces a combination of degenerative and regenerative changes in the crypt epithelium. Depletion of goblet cell mucin is a characteristic feature and is most pronounced when the inflammatory infiltrate is intense. The crypts lose their regular architecture and become branched, distorted, and eventually shortened. In some cases, a histiocytic and giant-cell reaction occurs around damaged crypts and spilled mucin. This is also referred to as cryptolytic or peri-cryptal granuloma and should be distinguished from true granulomas that are never seen in UC. Small surface erosions to large areas of deep ulceration with a tendency for tunneling beneath marginal mucosa may be seen. The associated inflammation spreads into the submucosa and deeper layers.

Resolving phase: Regenerative features predominate and the inflammatory infiltrate subsides. The neutrophil component of the inflammatory infiltrate diminishes first. Plasma cells and lymphocytes are the last to disappear and their distribution often becomes focal. In some cases, there may be an apparent excess of eosinophils, but this is most likely due to persistence of these cells in a resolving inflammatory reaction (240).

Quiescent phase (disease in remission): The hallmarks of the quiescent phase are variable crypt atrophy and architectural distortion. Rarely, the mucosa regenerates so well that it is indistinguishable from normal. In most cases, however, the crypts are reduced in number, more widely separated, and frequently branched. Shortening of crypts may leave an apparent gap between the crypt bases and the muscularis mucosae. The goblet cell population is normal at this stage and the mucosal surface predominantly flat. Paneth cells, which in the normal colon are restricted to the vicinity of the ileocecal valve, may be seen in any part of the colon or rectum. They are usually located at the bases of crypts and are occasionally numerous. The inflammatory infiltrate completely resolves and the lamina propria may have an unusually empty appearance, suggesting a reduced cellular component. The muscularis mucosae often becomes hypertrophied with splitting of fibers, particularly in the rectum, where it is normally thickest. Repeated episodes of activity may cause a multilayered muscularis mucosae, which may be responsible for the tubular strictures observed in some long-standing cases.

Acute fulminant colitis: Unlike classical UC, the ulceration in acute fulminant colitis tends to be widespread and deep, involving submucosa and muscularis propria. In addition, the associated inflammatory infiltrate is often transmural. The deep muscle layers show myocytolysis, edema, and intense vascular congestion, and areas of incipient or established perforation may be present in the thinned bowel wall. In some cases, the muscle damage results in longitudinal splitting of the muscularis propria, which superficially resembles the fissuring of CD. Features that point towards UC rather than CD are flask-shaped rather than fissuring ulcers, diffuse inflammation of the mucosa between and around the ulcers with no normal areas, and transmural inflammation that is limited to the ulcer bases with any lymphoid infiltrates being diffuse rather than follicular.

Unusual patterns of ulcerative colitis: In most children with untreated UC, colonic biopsies at presentation show the classical features described above, namely diffuse mucosal chronic inflammation, basal plasmacytosis, active inflammation with crypt abscesses, and crypt abnormalities such as atrophy and distortion. Typically, these findings are similar in pattern and severity in all involved areas.

Up to a quarter of children, however, do not show this classical pattern (229,241,242). Instead 21% show patchy rather than diffuse inflammation, 23% show relative rectal sparing, and 3% have a completely normal rectum (229). In addition, children are less likely than adults to show features of chronicity, such as crypt atrophy and crypt architectural distortion.

The reason for these differences is unclear, but it has been suggested that this may be due to shorter disease duration prior to their initial diagnostic procedure, resulting in less time for histological features to become established. Awareness of these atypical features is crucial to avoid erroneously labeling a child as having CD. Relative rectal sparing and patchy colitis at initial biopsy do not necessarily indicate CD, unless other corroborative evidence (e.g., granulomas) is present.

Upper alimentary tract involvement in ulcerative colitis: Although UC is classically regarded as involving the colon only, several studies have shown that histological abnormalities in the upper alimentary tract are not uncommon in patients with UC (243–245). Most of these studies have been done in children, but this may just reflect the fact that upper GI endoscopy and biopsy are more frequently performed in children than adults with suspected IBD.

The most common site of pathology is the stomach (69–80%), followed by the esophagus (28–50%) and duodenum (23–27%). The commonest pattern at all three sites is mild patchy chronic inflammation, with up to half of cases showing mild activity as well. Focal destructive (or enhanced) gastritis is rarely seen in UC (246). Severe active chronic inflammation, particularly with ulceration, should prompt reconsideration of the diagnosis.

Crohn's disease (CD)

In Western countries, childhood CD is more common than UC, the incidence ranging from 1.3–5 per 100 000 children (226–228,247). Similar to UC, the peak incidence is in adolescence, with approximately 10% of children aged less than 10 at the time of diagnosis. The episodes of remission and relapse that characterize UC tend to be less clear-cut in children with CD, and the presenting symptoms are more variable.

Sites and pattern of involvement: Crohn's disease classically can affect any part of the alimentary tract from mouth to anus, including several areas simultaneously. In both children and adults, the ileum is the site most commonly involved. In a large study of CD in Scottish children, 30% of patients had disease confined to the ileum, 38% had concomitant ileal and colonic involvement, and 28% had colitis alone (243). Similar findings were reported by others (249). Anal involvement occurs in 25% of patients with ileal disease and in 75% with colonic disease, and may be the presenting feature (250). Some 5% of patients with anorectal disease will not have lesions in the proximal bowel. Pancolitis is more common, whilst structuring and fissuring disease are less common in children and adolescents when compared to adults.

The appendix is involved by CD in up to 50% of children who undergo colonic resection or right hemicolectomy (236). In a small number of children, granulomatous appendicitis without overt involvement of other parts of the alimentary tract is the initial presenting feature of CD. In such cases, differentiation from other causes of granulomas in the appendix can be difficult (251). All children with granulomatous appendicitis should be followed up clinically, preferably with biopsies of their intestinal tract, to determine whether or not there is evidence of Crohn's disease elsewhere (252).

Macroscopy: Appearances are basically similar at all levels of the alimentary tract. One of the most characteristic features is the presence of "skip" lesions with multiple, well-demarcated segments of disease separated by macroscopically normal bowel. In some cases, however, only a single area of bowel is involved, most commonly the terminal ileum. The length of the affected segments varies considerably from a few centimeters to 25 cm or more. Diffuse involvement of long segments of small or large intestine may also occur, most commonly in the form of total or pancolitis.

The affected bowel is almost always thickened and often resembles a hosepipe. The peritoneal surface is pale and granular, with fibrinous exudates or fibrous adhesions, which matt together adjacent loops of bowel. In many cases, the mesenteric fat spreads or "creeps" over the entire circumference of the bowel wall, virtually burying the affected segment (fat wrapping). A variable degree of stenosis is found in the affected segment according to the amount of fibrosis present; occasionally the bowel lumen is reduced to the size of a narrow probe. With significant stricture formation, subacute intestinal obstruction may develop, sometimes associated with dilatation of the proximal unaffected bowel.

The luminal surface shows a variety of changes, the most common being ulceration, "cobblestoning," and stricture formation. The ulcers start as tiny pinpoint hemorrhagic lesions or well-defined shallow erosions with a white base, so-called aphthoid ulcers. A characteristic feature of Crohn's ulcers is their tendency to fissuring. Transmural fissuring ulcers in conjunction with serosal inflammation predispose to the formation of abscesses, sinuses, and fistulae, but perforation and peritonitis are uncommon. The cobblestone pattern is produced by intercommunicating linear or fissuring ulcers that delineate islands of mucosa, raised above the surface by submucosal edema and inflammation. Mucosal polyps are occasionally seen in CD as a result of inflammation, granulation tissue, or mucosal regeneration.

Colorectal and anal Crohn's disease: Crohn's disease may affect any part of the colon or rectum,

causing a pancolitis, a segmental colitis that often spares the rectum, or an apparently isolated proctitis (253). The cobblestone pattern is unusual in the large intestine and the picture is more frequently one of serpiginous or longitudinal ulceration with strictures. Foci of mucosal hyperemia may be present, but the intense mucosal congestion characteristic of UC is seldom seen. Anal disease takes the form of chronic fissures, complex fistulae, anal ulceration, edematous skin tags, and recurrent perianal abscesses (254).

Histology: The most consistent histological feature is the presence of transmural inflammation in the form of focal lymphocytic aggregates of variable size (Figure 2.24). These are found in all layers of the bowel wall, but are particularly evident in the submucosa and serosal fat. Some of the aggregates resemble lymphoid follicles with prominent germinal centers.

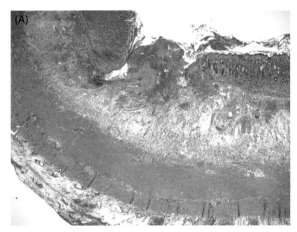

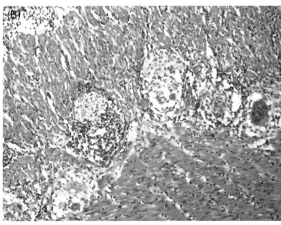

Figure 2.24 Crohn's disease: (A) Transmural inflammation with lymphoid modules lined up like rosary beads (H&E × 20) and (B) epitheloid granulomas (H&E × 40).

The hallmark of CD is the granuloma. In the context of IBD, granulomas are a key diagnostic feature, but are present in only two-thirds of resected specimens (250,255) and a smaller proportion of mucosal biopsies (see below). They occur throughout the bowel wall, often distributed along lymphatic channels or perivascular tissues, and also involve regional lymph nodes. Some granulomas are "naked," but more often they are associated with a mantle of lymphocytes. The granulomas have a variable appearance, ranging from rather loose collections of epithelioid macrophages through sarcoid-like densely cellular aggregates to larger tuberculoid granulomas with Langhans-type multinucleate giant cells. Small foci of central necrosis and clusters of neutrophils or eosinophils are occasionally present, but areas of caseous necrosis, characteristic of tuberculosis, are not seen.

Granulomas vary considerably in number, size, and location, and with the patient's age and duration of the disease. In children prevalence of granulomas is twice that of adults (256); the highest number of granulomas is found in the rectum and decreases proximally. Also, the number of granulomas diminishes with increasing duration of the disease.

Fissuring ulcers, which may not be visible to the naked eye, are usually evident microscopically on examination of bowel resections. They extend for a variable distance through the bowel wall and may show complex branching. Complete penetration of the bowel wall is often seen in conjunction with abscess formation in the serosal fat. Aphthoid ulcers representing punched-out areas of shallow ulceration usually situated above a mucosal lymphoid follicle may be demonstrated on resection specimens and mucosal biopsies.

The submucosa is usually edematous and contains dilated lymphatics and blood vessels. Fibrosis, which may be present throughout the bowel wall, is usually maximal in the submucosa. Neuronal hyperplasia may affect the myenteric plexus, but can also be seen in the submucosa where it produces a branching network of nerve fibers associated with fibrosis. Periarteritis or vasculitis is seen in a small proportion (5–10%) of cases (250,255).

Granulomas apart, the mucosal changes in CD are variable. The distribution of the inflammatory infiltrate is patchy, reflecting the discontinuous macroscopic involvement. Lymphocytes are the main constituents of the infiltrate and are often located in the basal part of the lamina propria; plasma cells and neutrophils are less conspicuous. There is often focal cryptitis; crypt abscesses are fairly common, but never dominate the picture. Crypt architecture and the goblet cell population are usually well preserved, even in the presence of considerable inflammation. The crypts maintain their length and the surface epithelial cells show only minor degenerative changes. Crypt branching may occur, particularly adjacent to ulcers, but this is not a prominent feature.

Anal lesions of CD show focal lymphocytic infiltrates with variable numbers of granulomas in the subepithelial tissues. The infiltrates are often dense and perivascular, and the granulomas may have small foci of necrosis but caseation is not seen. Foreign body granulomas associated with implanted fecal or foreign material are common in many types of anal disease and should be distinguished from true Crohn's-type granulomas.

Upper alimentary tract involvement in Crohn's disease: Asymptomatic involvement of the upper alimentary tract, assessed by endoscopy and/or biopsy, has been reported in 40–100% of children with established CD (257,258), a figure that is higher than in adults (246). Rarely, the upper alimentary tract can be involved in isolation, but is more likely to be affected in children with concomitant ileal and colonic disease (257).

The most common site of involvement is the stomach, followed by the duodenum and esophagus. The inflammation at all sites is most often described as non-specific active chronic inflammation, often with focal erosion or ulceration. This pattern does not reliably distinguish between CD and other causes of gastritis, particularly *H. pylori*-associated gastritis, or even UC-associated gastritis (244,245). Conversely, the pattern of more patchy periglandular or "focally enhanced gastritis" (246), is much more common in CD than in *H. pylori*-associated gastritis (2%) and UC-associated gastritis (20%). When this type of gastritis is present, particularly if granulomas are present as well, a diagnosis of CD can be made with a reasonable degree of confidence in a proportion that again is higher than in adults. Interestingly, in up to 35% of children with CD, the stomach is the only site where granulomas are found in the entire alimentary tract (245). The ileal and colonic biopsies in these children not infrequently show non-specific inflammation alone and it is only because their gastric biopsies contain granulomas that a definite diagnosis is possible. This phenomenon provides further evidence for the need to take routine upper alimentary tract biopsies in children with suspected IBD, even in the absence of upper intestinal tract symptoms.

Indeterminate colitis: IBD unclassifiable

The difficulty in distinguishing between colonic CD and UC, particularly in mucosal biopsies, has troubled pathologists and clinicians alike since Crohn's colitis was first described more than five decades ago. In resection specimens, features that favor CD over UC are involvement of the anus and perianal region, segmental distribution of lesions, fissuring and cobblestoning character of the ulceration, and transmural inflammatory infiltrates. There remain, however, approximately 5–10% of cases in which it is not possible to make a definitive diagnosis despite examination of the surgical specimen. These cases are labeled indeterminate colitis or IBD-U (unclassifiable).

The term "colitis indeterminate" was originally coined (259) to describe the 10–20% of colectomies for IBD, which could not be confidently classified as UC or CD from examination of the resection specimen. In about half of these cases, the clinical and radiological features, in conjunction with pre- and postoperative biopsy histology, later enabled a definite diagnosis to be made. Nowadays, the term is applied more widely and includes all cases with endoscopic, radiographic, or histological evidence of IBD confined to the colon, but without fulfilment of diagnostic criteria for UC or CD (260). In one pediatric series (261), indeterminate colitis accounted for 23% of all cases of IBD. In another, 14% of children with a diagnosis of IBD presenting over a 12-year period had indeterminate colitis at presentation (249).

It is unclear at present whether indeterminate colitis is an entity distinct from UC and CD or whether it merely represents a provisional classification until further information establishes a definite diagnosis. Several studies in adults have shown that patients with indeterminate colitis are unlikely to show features of CD in the long term (262,263), while a significant proportion eventually develop features of UC in the rectal stump. On the other hand, in a pediatric series (261), 4 of 59 children with a diagnosis of indeterminate colitis were re-classified as having CD within two years of presentation, while none developed features of UC.

Polyps and tumors

Polyps and polyposis syndromes

Polyps can occur sporadically or be a manifestation of a polyposis syndrome. Diagnostic criteria including microscopic features are discussed in detail earlier in this chapter. Accurate classification of polyps is important to determine the possibility of an associated hereditary cancer syndrome where lifelong cancer surveillance is crucial to disease prevention. To achieve this, the pathologist will have to be informed of the number of polyps, their location and endoscopic appearance, and the family history.

The *sporadic*, usually single benign *juvenile polyp* is by far the commonest childhood intestinal polyp a surgical pathologist will see, occurring in about 2% of the pediatric population (166). It is a hamartomatous polyp with a prominent inflammatory stroma and epithelial lined, often cystically distended, glands. Most solitary polyps are found in the left colon and rectum (264).

The presenting symptoms include rectal bleeding, abdominal pain, sometimes intussusception, and intestinal obstruction. It is not unusual for the polyp to autoamputate and be passed in stools (265). Solitary juvenile polyps do not need any further surveillance.

The colon is commonly involved in JPS (266). Syndromic juvenile polyps often are larger and multilobulated and have an increased amount of epithelial component compared with stroma. They may harbor small areas of dysplasia of glandular epithelium, but also frankly adenomatous foci can be found (267). Therefore it is recommended that all polyps from a JPS colectomy specimen should be subjected to histopathological examination (268). Juvenile polyps with dysplasia may be interpreted as adenoma if the cystic component is overlooked.

Adenomas are formed by a proliferation of dysplastic crypt epithelium either forming pedunculated or sessile tumors or even flat, non-raised adenomas. There is progressive nuclear stratification and loss of cell polarity. Uncontrolled proliferation of dysplastic epithelium will lead eventually to development of adenocarcinoma within the adenoma. The occurence of even a solitary adenoma in a child should alert the pathologist to the possibility of *FAP*. This is an autosomal dominantly inerited syndrome caused by a mutation in the adenomatous polyposis coli (APC) gene. It occurs in approximately 1:8000 live births and is the most common inherited polyposis syndrome (269). The adenomas can cause symptoms in the first decade, but mainly are detected in the second decade of life. Almost all patients will develop colorectal carcinoma within 10 years of diagnosis if they are not treated in time. Clinical follow-up and genetic counselling for the family are thus mandatory. Extraintestinal manifestations in FAP include osteomas, dental abnormalities, skin lesions, and congenital hypertrophy of the retinal pigment epithelium, which occur along with desmoids-type fibromas in soft tissue or the abdominal cavity in Gardner's syndrome. Extracolonic malignancies may also include hepatoblastoma, or a brain tumor (glioblastoma or medulloblastoma) when the eponym Turcot's syndrome has been used.

Macroscopic and histological features: Colectomy specimens from FAP patients typically show hundreds to thousands of polypoid adenomas. Histology shows tubular and later tubulovillous adenomas with increasing degree of dysplasia and eventually invasive adenocarcinoma.

Differential diagnosis: Dysplastic changes in other (hamartomatous) polyps must be differentiated from true adenomas of FAP to reach the correct genetic diagnosis.

Stromal polyps: They arise from mesenchymal or other components of the bowel wall, i.e. nerve, muscle, lymphoid tissue, fatty tissue, and endothelium.

Neurofibromatosis 1 (NF1), also known as von Recklinghausen's disease, and *multiple endocrine hyperplasia type 2B (MEN 2B)*, can affect the bowel with numerous submucosal neurofibromas. Neurofibromatous polyps may cause dyspepsia, abdominal pain, and hemorrhage. Ganglioneuromatous polyps may be linked to vasoactive intestinal peptide production with associated watery diarrhea (270). The polyps show the histology typical of a neurofibroma, whereas mature ganglion cells are found in ganglioneuromas. Positive S-100 immunostain will confirm the diagnosis.

Malignant tumors

Colorectal adenocarcinoma

Clinical presentation: Adenocarcinoma is uncommon in children when compared to adults, but represents the most frequent malignant neoplasm in the colorectum in children and adolescents. It has been reported in children as young as nine months of age. Patients usually present with abdominal pain, anemia-altered bowel habits, and/or weight loss. Hematochezia

or rectal bleeding has also been reported, as well as palpable masses or fullness in the abdomen (271).

Genetics: Most colorectal adenocarcinomas in children are sporadic, but may also arise in the setting of predisposing conditions, such as gastrointestinal polyposis syndromes, non-polyposis familial cancer syndromes (HNPCC), and IBD, although carcinoma is very unusual in the setting of IBD in children (272).

Macroscopy: Tumors are similarly distributed between the left and right colon, sigmoid colon, or rectum. Grossly, pediatric colonic adenocarcinomas resemble their adult counterparts, except that they are more likely to have a gelatinous appearance, as mucinous tumors are particularly frequent in pediatric age. Mucinous tumors seem to be equally common in the right and left colon.

Histology: While most tumors in adults are moderately or well differentiated, the majority of colorectal adenocarcinomas in children are poorly differentiated mucinous tumors, sometimes including some signet-ring cells, or comprising exclusively signet-ring cells (271–273). Pre-existing dysplastic lesions can be found adjacent to adenocarcinomas with non-mucinous tumor histology. Rarely neuroendocrine differentiation is reported (272). Mucinous adenocarcinomas have a poorer prognosis than ordinary adenocarcinomas, with a greater tendency to invade and develop distant metastasis.

Patients with HNPCC lack mutations of the APC gene, but may show loss of expression of MSH2, MLH1, MSH6, or PMS2 (274). This is a useful tool to direct subsequent molecular studies in search of an underlying germline mutation in a DNA mismatch-repair gene. Molecular testing should also be performed for KRAS mutations (codons 12 and 13) to identify patients with metastatic disease who are likely to benefit from therapy with anti-EGFR (epidermal growth factor receptor) monoclonal antybodies (cetuximab and panitumumab).

References

1. Metzger R, Wachowiak R, Kluth D. Embryology of the early gut. Semin. Pediatr. Surg. 2011;**20**(3):136–44.

2. Felix JF, Keizer R, van Dooren MF, *et al.* Genetics and developmental biology of oesophageal atresia and tracheo-oesophageal fistula: lesson from mice relevant for paediatric surgeons. Pediatr. Surg. Int. 2004;**20**(10):731–6

3. Depaepe A, Dolk H, Lechat MF. The epidemiology of tracheo-oesophageal fistula and oesophageal atresia

in Europe. EUROCAT Working Group. Arch. Dis. Child. 1993;**68**:743–8.

4. Kinottenbelt G, Skinner A, Seefeleder C. Tracheo-oesophageal fistula (TOF) and oesophageal atresia (OA) Best Pract. Res. Clin. Anaesthesiol. 2010;**24**(3) 387–401.

5. Sistonen SJ, Pakarinen MP, Rintala RJ. Long-term results of esophageal atresia: Helsinki experience and review of literature. Pediatr. Surg. Int. 2011;**27**(11):1141–9.

6. Burjonrappa SC, Youssef S, St-Vil D. What is the incidence of Barnett's and gastric metaplasia in esophageal atresia/tracheoesophageal fistula (EA/TEF) patients? Eur. J. Pediatric. Surg. 2011;**21**(1):25–9.

7. Sistonen S, Malmberg P, Malmström K, *et al.* Repaired oesophageal atresia: respiratory morbidity and pulmonary function in adults. Eur. Respir. J. 2010;**36**(5):1106–12.

8. Solomon BD. VACTERL/VATER association. Orphanet. J. Rare Dis. 2011;**16**:6–56.

9. Shaw-Smith C. Oesophageal atresia, tracheo-oesophageal fistula and the VACTERL association. Review of genetics and epidemiology. J. Med. Gen. 2006;**43**:545–54.

10. Cox PM, Gibson RA, Morgan N, *et al.* VACTERL with hydrocephalus in twins due to Fanconi anaemia (FA): mutation in the FAC gene. Am. J. Med. Genet. 1997;**68**:86–90

11. Lopez Dupla M, Sanz PM, Garcia VP, *et al.* Clinical, endoscopic, immunologic, and therapeutic aspects of oropharyngeal and esophageal candidiasis in HIV-infected patients: A survey of 114 cases. Am. J. Gastroenterol. 1992;**87**:1771–6.

12. Rodrigues F, Brandão N, Duque V, *et al.*, Herpes Simplex Virus Esophagitis in Immunocompetent Children. JPGN 2004; **39**: 560–3.

13. Cohen MC, Drut R. Herpetic esophagitis: A retrospective analysis of two paediatric cases. Arch. Arg. Pediatr. 1996;**94**:98–101.

14. Galbraith J, Shafran S. Herpes simplex esophagitis in the immunocompetent patient: report of four cases and review. Clin, Infect, Dis, 1992;**14**:894–901.

15. Sherman PM, Hassall E, Fagundes-Neto U, *et al.* A Global, Evidence-Based Consensus on the Definition of Gastroesophageal Reflux Disease in the Pediatric Population. Am. J. Gastroenterol. 2009;**104**:1278–95.

16. Gold BD. Epidemiology and management of gastro-oesophageal reflux in children. Aliment. Pharmacol. Ther. 2004; **19** (Suppl. 1): 22–7.

17. Dahms B, Qualman SJ (eds). *Gastrointestinal Diseases.* Perspectives in Pediatric Pathology, Vol **20**. Basel: Karger 1997:14–34.

18. Ruchelli ED, Liacouras ChA. Esophageal disorders in childhood. In: Russo P, Ruchelli E, Piccoli D, editors, *Pathology of Pediatric Gastrointestinal and Liver Disease,* New York: Springer, 2004.

19. Salvatore S, Hauser B, Vandemaele K, *et al.* Gastroesophageal reflux disease in infants: how much is predictable with questionnaires, pH-metry, endoscopy and histology? JPGN 2005;**40**:210–15.

20. Kahrilas PJ. Diagnosis of symptomatic gastroesophageal reflux disease. Am. J. Gastroenterol. 2003;**98**:S15–23.

21. Shub MD, Ulshen MH, Hargove ChB, *et al.* Esophagitis: A frequent consequence of gastroesophageal reflux in infancy. J. Pediatr. 1985;**107**:881–4.

22. Ridell RH. The biopsy diagnosis of gastroesophageal reflux disease, "carditis," and Barrett's esophagus, and sequelae of therapy. Am. J. Surg. Pathol. 1996;**20** Suppl 1:S31–50.

23. Ismail-Beigi F, Horton PF, Pope CE. Histological consequences of gastroesophageal reflux in man. Gastroenterol. 1970;**58**:163–74.

24. Tobey NA, Carson JL, Alkiek RA, *et al.* Dilated intercellular spaces: A morphological feature of acid reflux-damaged human esophageal epithelium. Gastroenterol. 1996;**111**:1200–5.

25. Atwood SEA, Smyrk TC, Demeester TR, *et al.* Esophageal eosinophilia with dysphagia. A distinct clinicopathologic syndrome. Dig. Dis. Sci. 1993;**38**:109–16.

26. Cohen MC, Rao P, Thomson M, *et al.* Eosinophils in the oesophageal mucosa: Clinical, pathological and epidemiological relevance in children: A cohort study. BMJ. Open 2012;**2**(1):e000493.

27. Straumann A, Spichtin H-P, Bucher KA, *et al.* Eosinophilic esophagitis: red on microscopy, white on endoscopy. Digestion 2004;**70**:109–16.

28. Liacouras CA, Wenner WJ, Brown K, *et al.* Primary eosinophilic esophagitis in children: Successful treatment with oral corticosteroids. J. Pediatr. Gastroenterol. Nutr. 1998; **26**:380–5.

29. Markowitz JE, Liacouras CA. Eosinophilic esophagitis. Gastroenterol. Clin. North Am. 2003;**32**:949–66.

30. Rothenberg ME. Eosinophilc gastrointestinal disorders (EGID). J. Allergy Clin. Immunol. 2004;**113**:11–28.

31. Lim JR, Gupta SK, Croffie JM, *et al.* White specks in the esophageal mucosa: An endoscopic manifestation of non-reflux eosinophilic esophagitis in children. Gastrointest. Endosc. 2004;**59**:835–8.

32. Fox VL, Nurko S, Furuta GT. Eosinophilic esophagitis: It's not just kid's stuff. Gastrointestinal Endosc. 2002;**56**:260–70.

33. Orenstein SR, Shalaby T, Di Carlo L, *et al.* The spectrum of pediatric eosinophilic esophagitis beyond infancy: A clinical series of 30 children. Am. J. Gastroenterol. 2000;**95**:1422–30.

34. Cury EK, Schraibman V. Eosinophilic infiltration of the esophagus: gastroesophageal reflux vs. eosinophilic esophagitis in children- discussion on daily practice. J. Pediatr. Surg. 2004;**39**(Suppl): e4–7.

35. Dellon ES, Aderoju A, Woosley JT, *et al.* Variability in diagnostic criteria for eosinophilic esophagitis: A systematic review. Am. J. Gastroenterol. 2007;**102**:1–14.

36. Furuta G, Liacouras CA, Collins MH, *et al.* Eosinophilic esophagitis in children and adults: A systematic review and consensus recommendations for diagnosis and treatment. Gastroenterology 2007;**133**:1342–63.

37. Mueller S, Neureiter D, Aigner T, *et al.* Comparison of histological parameters for the diagnosis of eosinophilic oesophagitis vs. gastro-oesophageal reflux disease on oesophageal biopsy material. Histopathology 2008;**53**:676–84.

38. Lai Al, Giris G, Liang Y, *et al.* Diagnostic criteria for eosinophilic esophagitis: A 5-year retrospective review ina pediatric population. J. Ped. Gastr. Nutr. 2009;**49**:63–70.

39. Ebach DR, Vanderheyden AD, Ellison JM, *et al.* Lymphocytic esophagitis: A possible manifestation of pediatric upper gastrointestinal Crohn's disease. Inflamm. Bowel Dis. 2011;**17**(1):45–9.

40. Jaspersen D. Drug-induced oesophageal disorders: pathogenesis, incidence, prevention and management. Drug Saf. 2000;**22**:237–49.

41. Pensabene L, Cohen MC, Thomson M. Clinical implications of molecular changes in pediatric Barrett's Esophagus. Curr. Gastroenterol. Rep. 2012;**14**(3):253–61.

42. Maltby EL, Dyson MJ, Wheeler MR, *et al.* Molecular abnormalities in pediatric Barrett's esophagus: Can we test for potential of neoplastic progression? Pediatr. Dev. Pathol. 2010;**13**:310–17.

43. Cohen MC, Dhandapani A, Gell M, *et al.* Pediatric columnar lined esophagus (CLO) vs Barrett's esophagus: Is it the time for a consensus definition? Ped. Develop. Pathol. 2009;**12**:116–26.

44. Sharma P, McQuaid K, Dent J, *et al.* A critical review of the diagnosis and management of Barrett's esophagus: the AGA Chicago Workshop. Gastroenterol. 2004;**127**(1):310–30.

45. Hassall E. Barrett's esophagus: new definitions and approaches in children. J. *Pediatr.* Gastroenterol. Nutr. 1993;**16**(4):345–64.

46. Hassall E. Barrett's esophagus: congenital or acquired? Am. J. Gastroenterol. 1993;**88**(6):819–24.

47. Jeurnink SM, van Herwaarden-Lindeboom MY, Siersema PD, *et al.* Barrett's esophagus in children: does it need more attention? Dig. Liver Dis. 2011;**43**(9):682–7.

48. Qualman SJ, Murray RD, McClung HJ, *et al.* Intestinal metaplasia is age related in Barrett's esophagus. Arch. Pathol. Lab. Med. 1990;**114**(12):1236–40.

49. British Society of Gastroenterology. Guidelines for the diagnosis and management of Barrett's columnar-lined oesophagus. 2005; http://www.bsg.org.uk (accessed May 2014).

50. Wang KK, Sampliner RE. Updated guidelines for the diagnosis, surveillance and therapy of Barrett's esophagus. Am. J. Gastroenterol. 2008;**103**(3):788–97.

51. Issaivanan M, Redner A, Weinstein T, *et al.* Esophageal carcinoma in children and adolescents. J. Pediatr. Hematol. Oncol. 2012;**34**:63–7.

52. Steven MJ, Fyfe AH, Raine PA, *et al.* Esophageal adenocarcinoma: A long-term complication of congenital diaphragmatic hernia? J. Pediatr. Surg. 2007;**42**(7):E1–3.

53. Niedzilski J, Kobielski A, Sokal J, *et al.* Accuracy of sonographic criteria in the decision for surgical treatment in infantile hypertrophic pyloric stenosis. Arch. Med. Sci. 2011;**7**(3):508–11.

54. Peeters B, Benninga MA, Hennekam RC. Infantile hypertrophic pyloric stenosis-genetics and syndromes. Nat. Rev. Gastroenterol. Hepatol. 2012;**9**(11):646–60.

55. Everet KV, Chioza BA, Georgula C, *et al.* Genome-wide high-density SNP-based linkage analysis of idiopathic hypertrophic pyloris stenosis identifies loci on chromosomes 11q14.q22 and xq23. Am. J. Hum. Gen. 2008;**82**:756–62.

56. Tan HL, Blythe A, Kirby CP, *et al.* Gastric foveolar cell hyperplasia and its role in postoperative vomiting in patients with infantile hypertrophic pyloric stenosis. Eur. J. Pediatr. Surg. 2009;**19**(2):76–8.

57. Guarino N, Shima H, Puri P. Structural immaturity of the pylorus muscle in infantile hypertrophic pyloric stenosis. Pediatr. Surg. Int. 2000;**16**(4):282–4.

58. Kalkan IH, Öztas E, Beyazit Y, *et al.* An unusual case of double heterotopic pancreatic tissues in the same location. J. Pancreas 2012;**13**(2):243–4.

59. Trifan A, Tarcoveanu E, Danclu M, *et al.* Gastric heterotopic pancreas: An unusual case and review of the literature. J. Gastrointestin. Liver Dis. 2012;**21**(2):209–12.

60. Abel R, Keen CE, Bingham JB, *et al.* Heterotopic pancreas as lead point in intussusception: A new variant of vitellointestinal tract malformation. Pediatr. Dev. Pathol. 1999;**2**(4):367–70.

61. Koletzko S, Jones NL, Goodman KJ, *et al.* H. pylori Working Groups of ESPGHAN and NASPGHAN. Evidence-based guidelines from ESPGHAN and NASPGHAN for Helicobacter pylori infection in children. J. Pediatr. Gastroenterol. Nutr. 2011;**53**(2):230–43.

62. Dimmick J, Jevon G. Gastritis and gastropathies of childhood. In Russo P, Ruchelli E, Piccoli D, editors, *Pathology of Pediatric Gastrointestinal and Liver Disease*. New York: Springer; 2004.

63. Riddell RH. Pathobiology of *Helicobacter pylori* infection in children. Can. J. Gastroenterol. 1999;**14**:599–603.

64. Cohen M, Cueto Rua E, Balcarce N, *et al.* Testing the utility of the Sydney System in *Helicobacter Pylori* associated gastritis in children. Acta Gastroent. Latinoamer. 2000;**30**:35–40.

65. Cohen MC, Cueto Rua E, Balcarce N, *et al.* Sulfomucins in *Helicobacter pylori*-associated chronic gastritis in children. Is this incipient intestinal metaplasia? JPGN 2000;**31**:63–7.

66. Cohen MC, Quijano G, Drut R. Stellate scars in *Helicobacter pylori*-associated chronic gastritis. Is this atrophic gastritis? Acta Gastroenter. Latinoamer. 2001;**31**:411–16.

67. Eber ChR. The gastrointestinal tract. In Stocker JT, Dehner LP, Husain AN, editors, *Stocker & Dehner's Pediatric Pathology*, third edn. Philadelphia: Walter Kluwer, Lippincott, Willams & Wilkins; 2011.

68. Di Nardo G, Oliva S, Aloi M, *et al.* A pediatric non-protein losing Menetrier's disease successfully treated with octreotide long acting release. World J. Gastroenterol. 2012;**18**:2727–9.

69. Blackstone MM, Mittal MK. The edematous toddler: A case of pediatric Ménétrier disease. Pediatr. Emerg. Care. 2008;**24**:682–4.

70. Haot J, Wallez L, Jouret-Mourin A, *et al.* La gastrite a lymphocytes: une nouvelle entite? Acta Endosc. 1985;**15**:187–8.

71. Bhatti TR, Jatla M, Verma R, *et al.* Lymphocytic gastritis in pediatric celiac disease. Ped. Dev. Pathol. 2011;**14**:280–3.

72. Feeley KM, Heneghan MA, Stevens FM, *et al.* Lymphocytic gastritis and coeliac disease: evidence of a positive association. J. Clin. Pathol. 1988;**51**:207–10.

73. Sepulveda A, Patil M. Practical approach to the pathological diagnosis of gastritis. Arch. Pathol. Lab. Med. 2008;**132**:1586–93.

74. Stolte M, Meining A. The updated Sydney system: classification and grading of gastritis as the basis of diagnosis and treatment. Can. J. Gastroenterol. 2001;**15**:591–8.

75. Hoepler W, Hammer K, Hammer J. Gastric phenotype in children with Helicobacter pylori infection undergoing upper endoscopy. Scand. J. Gastroenterol. 2011;**46**:293–8.

76. Khan S, Orenstein SR. Eosinophilic gastroenteritis. Gastroenterol. Clin. North Am. 2008;**37**:333–48.

77. Lucendo AJ, Arias A. Eosinophilic gastroenteritis: An update. Expert Rev. Gastroenterol. Hepatol. 2012;**6**:591–601.

78. Heyworth PG, Cross AR, Curnutte JT. Chronic granulomatous disease. Curr. Op. Immunol. 2003;**15**:578–84.

79. van den Berg JM, van Koppen E, Ahlin A, *et al.* Chronic granulomatous disease: the European experience. PLoS ONE 2009;**4**:e5234.

80. Levine S, Smith VV, Malone M, *et al.* Histopathological features of chronic granulomatous disease (CGD) in childhood. Histopathology 2005;**47**:508–16.

81. Finn A, Hadzic N, Morgan G. Prognosis of chronic granulomatous disease. ADC 1990;**65**:942–5.

82. Xin W, Greenson JK. The clinical significance of focally enhanced gastritis. Am. J. Surg. Pathol. 2004;**28**:1347–51.

83. Lauwers GY, Carneiro F, Graham DY, *et al.* Tumours of the stomach. In: Bosman FT, Carneiro F, Hruban RH, Theise ND, editors, *WHO Classification of Tumours of the Digestive System*. Lyon: International Agency for Research on Cancer, 2010.

84. Goddard AF, Badreldin R, Pritchad DM, *et al.* The management of gastric polyps. Gut 2010;**59**:1270–6.

85. Carneiro F, Charlton A, Huntsman, DG. Hereditary diffuse gastric cancer. In: Bosman FT, Carneiro F, Hruban RH, Theise ND, editors, *WHO Classification of Tumours of the Digestive System*. Lyon: International Agency for Research on Cancer, 2010.

86. http://www.OMIM.org/entry/137215 (accessed May 2014).

87. Fitzgerald RC, Hardwick R, Huntsman *et al.* Hereditary diffuse gastric cancer: updated consensus guidelines for clinical management and directions for future research. J. Med. Genet. 2010;**47**:436–4.

88. Chu PG, Weiss LM. Immunohistochemical characterization of signet-ring cell carcinomas of the stomach, breast, and colon. Am. J. Clin. Pathol. 2004;**121**:884–92.

89. Rink RL, Godwin AK. Clinical and molecular characterisation of gastrointestinal stromal tumours in the pediatric and young adult population. Curr. Oncol. Rep. 2009;**11**(4):314–21.

90. Miettinen M, Lasota J, Sobin LH. Gastrointestinal stromal tumours of the stomach in children and young

adults: A clinicopathologic, immunohistochemical and molecular genetic study of 44 cases with long term-follow up and review of the literature. Am. J. Surg. Pathol. 2005;**29**(10):1373–81.

91. Miettinen M, Wang ZF, Sarlomo-Rikala M, *et al*. Succinate dehydrogenase-deficient GISTs: A clinicopathologic, immunohistochemical, and molecular study of 66 gastric GISTs with predilection to young age. Am. J. Surg. Pathol. 2011;**35**(11):1712–21.

92. Miettinen M, Lasota J. Gastrointestinal stromal tumours: review on morphology, molecular pathology, prognosis and differential diagnosis. Arch. Pathol. Lab. Med. 2006;**130**(10);1466–78.

93. Liegl B, Hornick JL, Corless Ch L. Monoclonal antibody DOG1.1 shows higher sensitivity than KIT in the diagnosis of gastrointestinal stromal tumors, including unusual subtypes. Am. J. Surg. Pathol. 2009;**33**:437–46.

94. Joensuu H. Risk stratification of patients diagnosed with gastrointestinal stromal tumor. Hum. Pathol. 2008;**39**:1411–19.

95. Steffensen TS, Gilbert-Barnes E, DeStefano KA, *et al*. Midgut volvulus causing fetal demise in utero. Fetal Pediatr. Pathol. 2008;**27**(4–5):223–31.

96. Puri P, Guiney EJ, Carroll R. Multiple gastrointestinal atresias in three consecutive siblings: observations on pathogenesis. J. Pediatr. Surg. 1985:**20**(1):22–4.

97. Shen-Schwarz S, Fitko R. Multiple gastrointestinal atresias with imperforate anus: pathology and pathogenesis. Am. J. Med. Genet. 1990;**36**(4):451–5.

98. Phillips JD, Raval MV, Redden C, *et al*. Gastroschisis, atresia, dysmotility: surgical treatment strategies for a distinct clinical entity. J. Ped. Surg. 2008;**43**(12):2208–13.

99. Dalla Vecchia LK, Grosfeld JL, West KW, *et al*. Intestinal atresia and stenosis: A 25-year experience with 277 cases. Arch. Surg. 1998;**133**(5):490–7.

100. Best KE, Tennant PW, Addor MC, *et al*. Epidemiology of small intestinal atresia in Europe: A registry based study. Arch. Dis. Child. Fetal. Neonatal Ed. 2012;**97**(5): F353–8.

101. Grosfeld JL. Ballantine TV, Shoemaker R. Operative mangement of intestinal atresia and stenosis based on pathologic findings. J. Pediatr. Surg. 1979;**14**(3):368–75.

102. Pariente G, Landau D, Aviram M, *et al*. Prenatal diagnosis of a rare sonographic appearance of duodenal atresia: report of 2 cases and literature review. J. Ultrasound Med. 2012;**31**(11):1829–33.

103. Thakur A, Chiu C, Quitros-Tejeira RE, *et al*. Morbidity and mortality of short bowel syndrome in infants with abdominal wall defects. Am. Surg. 2002;**68**:75–9.

104. Cowan KN, Puligandia PS, Laberge JM, *et al*. Canadian Pediatric Surgery Network. The gastroschisis prognostic score: reliable outcome prediction of gastroschisis. J. Pediatr. Surg. 2012;**47**(6):1111–7.

105. Bilodeau A, Prasil P, Cloutier R, *et al*. Hereditary multiple intestinal atresia: thirty years later. J. Pediatr. Surg. 2004;**39**(5):726–30.

106. Kao KJ, Fleischer R, Bradford WD, *et al*. Multiple congenital septal atresias of the intestine: histomorphologic and pathogenetic implications. Pediatr. Pathol. 1983;**1**(4):443–8.

107. Gfoerer S, Fiegel H, Ramachandran P, *et al*. Changes of smooth muscle contractile filaments in small bowel atresia. World J. Gastroenterol. 2012;**18**(24):3099–104.

108. Masumoto K, Suita S, Taguchi T. The occurence of unusual smooth muscle bundles expressing α-smooth muscle actin in human intestinal atresia. J. Pediatr. Surg. 2003;**38**(2):161–6.

109. Alatas FS, Masumoto K, Esumi G, *et al*. Significance of abnormalities in systems proximal and distal to the obstructed site of duodenal atresia. J. Pediatr. Gastroenterol. Nutr. 2012;**54**(2):242–7.

110. Budhiraja S, Jaiewal TS, Sen R. Ileal atresia with segmental defect of intestinal musculature. Indian J. Pediatr. 2004;**7**(2):177–9.

111. Hayashida Y, Ikeda K, Hashimoto N. Histological study of intestinal atresia due to intrauterine intussusception. Z. Kinderchir. 1984;**39**(2):106–9.

112. Fujimoto M, Sakashita H, Hattori K, *et al*. Pseudodysplastic regenerative mucosa associated with congenital ileal atresia. Pathol. Int. 2011;**61**(11).691–3.

113. Martin JP, Connor PD, Charles K. Meckel's diverticulum. Am. Fam. Physician 2000;**61**(4):1037–42.

114. Menezes M, Tareen F, Saeed A, *et al*. Symptomatic Meckel's diverticulum in children: A 16-year review. Pediatr. Surg. Int. 2008;**24**(5):575–7.

115. Khan A, de Waal K. Pneumoperitoneum in a micropremie: Not always NEC. Case Rep. Pediatr. 2012;**2012**:295657.

116. Tauro L, Martis JJ, Menezes LT, *et al*. Clinical profile and surgical outcome of Meckel's diverticulum. J. Indian Med. Assoc. 2011;**109**(7):489–90.

117. Williams RS. Management of Meckel's diverticulum. Br. J. Surg. 1981;**68**:477–80.

118. Ben Brahim E, Jouini R, Aboulkacem S, *et al*. Gastric heterotopia: clinical and histological study of 12 cases. Tunis. Med. 2011;**89**(12):935–9.

119. Iyer CP, Mahour GH. Duplications of the alimentary tract in infants and children. J. Pediatr. Surg. 1995;**30**(9):1267–70.

120. Jackson KL, Peche WJ, Rollins MD. An unusual presentation of rectal duplication cyst. Int. Surg. Case Rep. 2012;**3**(7):314–5.

121. Jellali MA, Mekki M, Saad J, et al. Perinatal colonic duplication associated with anal atresia. J. Pediatr. Surg. 2012;**47**(6):e19–23.

122. Sherman PM, Mitchell DJ, Cutz E. Neonatal enteropathies: defining the causes of protracted diarrhea of infancy. J. Pediatr. Gastroenterol. Nutr. 2004;**38**(1):16–26.

123. Cortina G, Smart CN, Farmer DG, et al. Enteroendocrine cell dysgenesis and malabsorption, a histopathologic and immunohistochemical characterization. Hum. Pathol. 2007;**38**(4):570–80.

124. Wang J, Cortina G, Wu SV, et al. Mutant neurogenin-3 in congenital malabsorptive diarrhea. N. Engl. J. Med. 2006;**355**(3):270–80.

125. Ruemmele FM, Schmitz J, Goulet O. Microvillous inclusion disease (microvillous atrophy). Orphanet. J. Rare Dis. 2006;**1**:22.

126. Ruemmele FM, Jan D, Lacaille F, et al. New perspectives for children with microvillous inclusion disease: early small bowel transplantation. Transplantation 2004;**77**(7):1024–8.

127. Golachowska MR, van Dael CM, Keuning H, et al. MYO5B mutations in patients with microvillus inclusion disease presenting with transient renal Fanconi syndrome. J. Pediatr. Gastroenterol. Nutr. 2012;**54**(4):491–8.

128. Müller T, Hess MW, Schiefermeier N, et al. MYO5B mutations cause microvillus inclusion disease and disrupt epithelial cell polarity. Nat. Genet. 2008;**40**(10):1163–5.

129. Ruemmele FM, Müller T, Schiefermeier N, et al. Loss-of-function of MYO5B is the main cause of microvillus inclusion disease: 15 novel mutations and a CaCo-2 RNAi cell model. Hum. Mutat. 2010;**31**(5):544–51.

130. Davidson GP, Cutz E, Hamilton JR, et al. Familial enteropathy: A syndrome of protracted diarrhea from birth, failure to thrive, and hypoplastic villus atrophy. Gastroenterology 1978;**75**(5):783–90.

131. Lmale J, Coulomb A, Dubern B, et al. Intractable diarrhea with tufting enteropathy: A favorable outcome is possible. J. Pediatr. Gastroenterol. Nutr. 2011;**52**(6):734–9.

132. Goulet O, Salomon J, Ruemmele F, et al. Intestinal epithelial dysplasia (tufting enteropathy). Orphanet. J. Rare Dis. 2007;**20**(2):20.

133. Sivagnanam M, Mueller JL, Lee H, et al. Identification of EpCAM as the gene for congenital tufting enteropathy. Gastroenterology 2008;**135**(2):429–37.

134. Sivagnanam M, Schaible T, Szigeti R, et al. Further evidence for EpCAM as the gene for congenital tufting enteropathy. Am. J. Med. Genet. A. 2010;**152A**(1):222–4.

135. Sivagnanam M, Janecke AR, Müller T, et al. Case of syndromic tufting enteropathy harbors SPINT2 mutation seen in congenital sodium diarrhea. Clin. Dysmorphol. 2010;**19**(1):48.

136. Reifen RM, Cutz E, Griffiths A-M, et al. Tufting enteropathy: A newly recognized clinicopathological entity associated with refractory diarrhea in infants. J. Pediat. Gastroent. Nutr. 1994;**18**:379–85.

137. Fabre A, André N, Breton A, et al. Intractable diarrhea with "phenotypic anomalies" and tricho-hepato-enteric syndrome: two names for the same disorder. Am. J. Med. Genet. A. 2007;**143**(6):584–8.

138. Fabre A, Martinez-Vinson C, Goulet O, et al. Syndromic diarrhea/Tricho-hepato-enteric syndrome. Orphanet. J. Rare Dis. 2013 Jan 9;**8**:5.

139. Hartley JL, Zachos NC, Dawood B, et al. Mutations in TTC37 cause trichohepatoenteric syndrome (phenotypic diarrhea of infancy). Gastroenterology 2010;**138**(7):2388–98, 2398.e1–2.

140. Fabre A, Charroux B, Martinez-Vinson C, et al. SKIV2L mutations cause syndromic diarrhea, or trichohepatoenteric syndrome. Am. J. Hum. Genet. 2012;**90**(5):689–92.

141. Lachaux A, Loras-Duclaux I, Bouvier R. Autoimmune enteropathy in infants. Pathological study of the disease in two familial cases. Virchows Arch. 1998;**433**(5):481–5.

142. Russo PA, Brochu P, Seidman EG, et al. Autoimmune enteropathy. Pediatr. Dev. Pathol. 1999;**2**(1):65–71.

143. Murch SH, Fertleman CR, Rodrigues C, et al. Autoimmune enteropathy with distinct mucosal features in T-cell activation deficiency: the contribution of T cells to the mucosal lesion. J. Pediatr. Gastroenterol. Nutr. 1999;**28**(4):393–9.

144. Patey-Mariaud de Serre N, Canioni D, Garvousse S, et al. Digestive histopathological presentation of IPEX syndrome. Mod. Pathol. 2009;**22**(1):95–102.

145. Hill DI, Dirks MH, Liptak GS, et al. North American Society for Pediatric Gastroenterology, Hepatology and Nutrition. Guideline for the diagnosis and treatment of celiac disease in children: recommendations of the North American Society for Pediatric Gastroenterology, Hepatology and Nutrition. J. Pediatr. Gastroenterol. Nutr. 2005;**40**(1):1–19.

146. Husby S, Koletzko S, Korponay-Szabó IR, et al. European Society for Pediatric Gastroenterology, Hepatology, and Nutrition guidelines for the diagnosis

of coeliac disease. J. Pediatr. Gastroenterol. Nutr. 2012;**54**(1):136–60.

147. Ravikumara M, Tuthill DP, Jenkins HR. The changing clinical presentation of Coeliac disease. Arch. Dis. Child. 2006;**91**(12):969–71.

148. McGowan KE, Castiglione DA, Butzner JD. The changing face of childhood celiac disease in North America: impact of serological testing. Pediatrics 2009;**124**(6):1572–8.

149. Bonamico M, Mariani P, Thanasi E, *et al.* Patchy villous atrophy of the duodenum in childhood celiac disease. J. Pediatr. Gastroenterol. Nutr. 2004;**38**(2):204–7.

150. Marsh MN. Grains of truth: evolutionary changes in small intestinal mucosa in response to environmental antigen challenge. Gut. 1990;**31**(1):111–14.

151. Moran CJ, Kolman OK, Russell GJ, *et al.* Neutrophilic infiltration in gluten-sensitive enteropathy is neither uncommon norinsignificant: Assessment of duodenal biopsies from 267 pediatric and adult patients. Am. J. Surg. Pathol. 2012;**36**(9):1339–45.

152. Antonioli DA. Celiac disease: A progress report. Mod. Pathol. 2003;**16**(4):342–6.

153. Corazza GR, Villanacci V. Coeliac disease. J. Clin. Pathol. 2005;**58**(6):573–4.

154. Dickson BC, Streutker CJ, Chetty R. Coeliac disease: An update for pathologists. J. Clin. Pathol. 2006;**59**(10):1008–16.

155. Goldstein NS, Underhill J. Morphologic features suggestive of gluten sensitivity in architecturally normal duodenal biopsy specimens. Am. J. Clin. Pathol. 2001;**116**(1):63–71.

156. Oberhuber G, Vogelsang H, Stolte M, *et al.* Evidence that intestinal intraepithelial lymphocytes are activated cytotoxic T cells in celiac disease but not in giardiasis. Am. J. Pathol. 1996;**148**(5):1351–57.

157. Thompson AM, Bizzarro MJ. Necrotizing enterocolitis in newborns: pathogenesis, prevention and management. Drugs 2008;**68**(9):1227–38.

158. Young CM, Kingma SD, Neu J. Ischemia-reperfusion and neonatal intestinal injury. J. Pediatr. 2011;**158**(2 Suppl):e25–8.

159. Berman L, Moss RL. Necrotizing enterocolitis: An update. Semin. Fetal Neonatal. Med. 2011;**16**(3):145–50.

160. Wu S, Caplan M, Lin HC. Necrotizing enterocolitis: old problem with new hope. Peadiatr. Neonatol. 2012;**53**(3):156–63.

161. Ng S. Necrotizing enterocolitis in the full term neonate. J. Pediatr. Child. Health. 2001;**37**(1):1–4.

162. Tooke L, Alexander A, Hoen A. Extensive portal venous gas without obvious pneumatosis intestinalis in a pretem infant with necrotizing enterocolitis. J. Pediatr. Surg. 2012;**47**(7):1463–5.

163. Dominguez KM, Moss RL. Necrotizing enterocolitis. Clin. Perinatol. 2012;**39**(2):387–401.

164. Durno CA. Colonic polyps in children and adolescents. Can. J. Gastroenterol. 2007;**21**(4):233–9.

165. Calva D, Howe JR. Hamartomatous polyposis syndromes. Surg. Clin. North Am. 2008;**88**(4):779.

166. Schreibman IR, Baker M, Amos C, *et al.* The hamartomatous polyposis syndromes: A clinical and molecular review. Am. J. Gastroenterol. 2005;**100**(2):476–90.

167. Calva-Cerqueira D, Chinnathambi S, Pechman B, *et al.* The rate of germline mutations and large deletions of SMAD4 and BMPR1A in juvenile polyposis. Clin. Genet. 2009;**75**:79–85.

168. Delnatte C, Sanlaville D, Mougenot JF. Contiguous Gene Deletion within Chromosome Arm 10q Is Associated with Juvenile Polyposis of Infancy, Reflecting Cooperation between the BMPR1A and PTEN Tumor-Suppressor Genes. Am. J. Hum. Genet. 2006;**78**:1066–74.

169. Sachatello CR, Griffen WO Jr. Hereditary polypoid diseases of the gastrointestinal tract: A working classification. Am. J. Surg. 1975;**129**(2):198–203.

170. Howe JR, Mitros FA, Summers RW. The risk of gastrointestinal carcinoma in familial juvenile polyposis. Ann. Surg. Oncol. 1998;**5**:751–6.

171. Brosens LA, van Hattem A, Hylind LM, *et al.* Risk of colorectal cancer in juvenile polyposis. Gut 2007;**56**:965–7.

172. Brosens LA, Langeveld D, van Hattem WA, *et al.* Juvenile polyposis syndrome. World J. Gastroenterol. 2011;**17**(44):4839–44.

173. Aaltonen LA, Jass JR, Howe JR. Juvenile Polyposis. In: Hamilton SR, Aaltonen LA, editors, *Pathology and Genetics of Tumours of the Digestive System.* Lyon: IARC Press; 2000: 130–2.

174. Lowichik A, Jackson WD, Coffin CM. Gastrointestinal polyposis in childhood: clinicopathologic and genetic features. Pediatr. Dev. Pathol. 2003;**6**(5):371–91.

175. Jaeger E, Leedham S, Lewis A, *et al.* Hereditary mixed polyposis syndrome is caused by a 40-kb upstream duplication that leads to increased and ectopic expression of the BMP antagonist GREM1. Nat. Genet. 2012;**44**(6):699–703.

176. Chan YF, Roche D. Adenomyoma of the small intestine in children. J. Pediatr. Surg. 1994;**29**(12):1611–2.

177. Takahashi Y, Fukusato T. Adenomyoma of the small intestine. World J. Gastrointest. Pathophysiol. 2011;**2**(6):88–92.

178. Handra-Luca A, Terris B, Couvelard A, *et al.* Adenomyoma and adenomyomatous hyperplasia of the Vaterian system: clinical, pathological, and new immunohistochemical features of 13 cases. Mod. Pathol. 2003;**16**(6):530–6.

179. Coffin CM, Watterson J, Priest JR, *et al.* Extrapulmonary inflammatory myofibroblastic tumor (inflammatory pseudotumor). A clinicopathologic and immunohistochemical study of 84 cases. Am. J. Surg. Pathol. 1995;**19**(8):859–72.

180. Neves GR, Chapchap P, Sredni ST, *et al.* Childhood carcinoid tumors: description of a case series in a Brazilian cancer center. Sao Paulo Med. J. 2006;**124**(1):21–5.

181. Klimstra DS, Modlin IR, Coppola D, *et al.* The pathologic classification of neuroendocrine tumors: A review of nomenclature, grading, and staging systems. Pancreas 2010;**39**(6):707–12.

182. Ladd AP, Grosfeld JL. Gastrointestinal tumors in children and adolescents. Semin. Pediatr. Surg. 2006;**15**:37–47.

183. Berry CL, Keeling JW Gastrointestinal lymphoma in childhood. J. Clin. Pathol. 1973;**3**:459–63.

184. Takahashi H, Hansmann ML. Primary gastrointestinal lymphoma in childhood (up to 18 years of age). J. Cancer Res. Clin. Oncol. 1990;**116**:190–6.

185. Lewin K, Ranchod M, Dorfman RF. Lymphomas of the gastrointestinal tract. A study of 117 cases presenting with gastrointestinal disease Cancer, 1978,**42**:693–70.

186. Cohen M, De Matteo E, Narbaitz M, *et al.* Epstein Barr virus presence in pediatric diffuse large B-cell lymphoma reveals a particular association and latency patterns. Analysis of viral role in tumor microenvironment. Int. J. Cancer 2013;**132** (7):1572–80.

187. Chuang SS, Ye H, Du MQ, *et al.* Histopathology and immunohistochemistry in distinguishing Burkitt lymphoma from diffuse large B-cell lymphoma with very high proliferation index and with or without a starry-sky pattern: A comparative study with EBER and FISH. Am. J. Clin. Pathol. 2007;**128**(4):558–64.

188. England RJ, Scammel S, Murthi GV. Proximal colonic atresia: is right hemicolectomy inevitable? Pediatr. Surg. Int. 2011;**27**(10):1059–62.

189. Komuro H, Urita Y, Hori T, *et al.* Perforation of the colon in neonates. J. Pediatr. Surg. 2005;**40**(12):1916–9.

190. Yap TS, Jiwane A, Belessis Y, *et al.* Colonic atresia presenting as neonatal bowel obstruction in cystic fibrosis. J. Pediatr. Gastroenterol. Nutr. 2012;**58** (4):e37–8.

191. Rudolph CD, Hyman PE, Altschuler SM, *et al.* Diagnosis and treatment of chronic intestinal pseudo-obstruction in children: report of consensus workshop. J. Pediatr. Gastroenterol. Nutr. 1997;**24**:102–12.

192. Smith VV, Milla PJ. Histological phenotypes of enteric smooth muscle disease causing functional intestinal obstruction in childhood. Histopathology 1997;**31**:112–22.

193. Streutker CJ, Huizinga JD, Campbell F, *et al.* Loss of CD117 (c-kit)- and CD34-positive ICC and associated CD34-positive fibroblasts defines a subpopulation of chronic intestinal pseudo-obstruction. Am. J. Surg. Pathol. 2003;**27**:228–35.

194. Amiot A, Cazals-Hatem D, Joly F, *et al.* The role of immunohistochemistry in idiopathic chronic intestinal pseudoobstruction (CIPO): A case-control study. Am. J. Surg. Pathol. 2009;**33**:749–58.

195. Parisi MA, Kapur RP. Genetics of Hirschsprung disease. Curr. Opin. Pediatr. 2000;**12**:610–7.

196. Kapur RP. Practical pathology and genetics of Hirschsprung's disease. Semin. Pediatr. Surg. 2009;**18**:212–23.

197. Mundt E, Bates MD. Genetics of Hirschsprung disease and anorectal malformations. Semin. Pediatr. Surg. 2010;**19**:107–17.

198. Niramis R, Watanatittan S, Anuntkosol M, *et al.* Quality of life of patients with Hirschsprung's disease at 5 – 20 years post pull-through operations. Eur. J. Pediatr. Surg. 2008;**18**:38–43.

199. Langer JC. Repeat pull-through surgery for complicated Hirschsprung's disease: indications, techniques, and results. J. Pediatr. Surg. 1999;**34**:1136–41.

200. Farrugia MK, Alexander N, Clarke S, *et al.* Does transitional zone pull-through in Hirschsprung's disease imply a poor prognosis? J. Pediatr. Surg. 2003;**38**:1766–9.

201. Friedmacher F, Puri P. Residual aganglionosis after pull-through operation for Hirschsprung's disease: A systematic review and meta-analysis. Pediatr. Surg. Int. 2011;**27**:1053–7.

202. Schulten D, Holschneider AM, Meier-Ruge W. Proximal segment histology of resected bowel in Hirschsprung's disease predicts postoperative bowel function. Eur. J. Pediatr. Surg. 2000;**10**(6):378–81.

203. Cohen MC, Moore SW, Neveling U, *et al.* Acquired aganglionosis following surgery for Hirschsprung's disease: A report of five cases during a 33-year experience with pull-through procedures. Histopathology 1993;**22**:163–8.

204. Kapur RP. Contemporary approaches toward understanding the pathogenesis of Hirschsprung disease. Pediatr. Pathol. 1993;**13**(1):83–100. Erratum in: Pediatr. Pathol. 1993;13(1):270.

205. Kapur RP. Hirschsprung disease and other enteric dysganglionoses. Crit. Rev. Clin. Lab. Sci. 1999;**36**:225–73.

206. Barshack I, Fridman E, Goldberg I, *et al.* The loss of calretinin expression indicates aganglionosis in Hirschsprung's disease. J. Clin. Pathol. 2004;**57**:712–6.

207. Kapur RP, Reed RC, Finn LS, *et al.* Calretinin immunohistochemistry vs. acetylcholinesterase histochemistry in the evaluation of suction rectal biopsies for Hirschsprung Disease. Pediatr. Dev. Pathol. 2009;**12**:6–15.

208. White FV, Langer JC. Circumferential distribution of ganglion cells in the transition zone of children with Hirschsprung disease. Pediatr. Dev. Pathol. 2000;**3**:216–22.

209. Boman F, Sfeir R, Priso R, *et al.* Advantages of intraoperative semiquantitative evaluation of myenteric nervous plexuses in patients with Hirschsprung disease. J. Pediatr. Surg. 2007;**42**:1089–94.

210. Meier-Ruge WA, Bruder E, Kapur RP. Intestinal neuronal dysplasia type B: one giant ganglion is not good enough. Pediatr. Dev. Pathol. 2006;**9**:444–52.

211. Koletzko S, Jesch I, Faus-Kebetaler T, *et al.* Rectal biopsy for diagnosis of intestinal neuronal dysplasia in children: A prospective multicentre study on interobserver variation and clinical outcome. Gut 1999;**44**:853–61.

212. Kapur RP. Neuronal dysplasia a controversial pathological correlate of intestinal pseudo-obstruction. Am. J. Med. Genet. A 2003;**122A**:287–93.

213. Martucciello G, Pini Prato A, Puri P, *et al.* Controversies concerning diagnostic guidelines for anomalies of the enteric nervous system: A report from the fourth International Symposium on Hirschsprung's disease and related neurocristopathies. J. Pediatr. Surg. 2005;**40**:1527–31.

214. Kapur RP. Developmental disorders of the enteric nervous system. Gut 2000;**47** Suppl 4:81–3; discussion 87.

215. Odze, RD, Wershil BK, Leichtner AM, *et al.* Allergic colitis in infants. J. Pediatr. 1995:**126**(2);163–70.

216. Machida HM, Catto Smith AG, Gall DG, *et al.* Allergic colitis in infancy: clinical and pathologic aspects. J. Pediatr. Gastroenterol. Nutr. 1994;**19**:22–6.

217. Carpenter HA, Talley NJ. The importance of clinicopathological correlation in the diagnosis of inflammatory conditions of the colon: histological patterns with clinical implications. Am. J. Gastroenterol. 2000;**95**(4):878–96.

218. Khor TS, Fujita H, Nagata K, *et al.* Biopsy interpretation of colonic biopsies when inflammatory bowel disease is excluded. J. Gastroenterol. 2012;**47**(3):226–48.

219. El-Matary W, Girgis S, Huynh H, *et al.* Microscopic colitis in children. Dig. Dis. Sci. 2010;**55**(7):1996–2001.

220. Pardi DS, Kelly CP. Microscopic colitis. Gastroenterology 2011;**140**:1155–65.

221. Fike FB, Mortellaro V, Juang D, *et al.* Neutropenic colitis in children. J. Surg. Res. 2011;**170**(1):73–6.

222. Fenoglio-Preiser CM, Noffsinger AE, Stemmermann GN, Lantz PE, Listrom MB, Rilke FO. The nonneoplastic lesions of the colon. In *Gastrointestinal Pathology: An Atlas and Text*. Philadelphia: Lippincott – Raven;1999: 763–908.

223. IBD Working Group of the European Society for Paediatric Gastroenterology, Hepatology and Nutrition. Inflammatory bowel disease in children and adolescents: recommendations for diagnosis – the Porto criteria. J. Pediatr. Gastroenterol. Nutr. **41**(1):1–7.

224. Bousvaros A, Antonioli DA, Colletti RB, *et al.* Differentiating ulcerative colitis from Crohn disease in children and young adults: report of a working group of the North American Society for Pediatric Gastroenterology, Hepatology, and Nutrition and the Crohn's and Colitis Foundation of America. J. Pediatr. Gastroenterol. Nutr. 2007;**44**(5):653–74.

225. Bentsen BS, Moum B, Ekbom A. Incidence of inflammatory bowel disease in children in southeastern Norway – A prospective population-based study 1990–94. Scand. J. Gastroenterol. 2002;**37**:540–5.

226. Lindberg E, Lindquist B, Holmquist L, *et al.* Inflammatory bowel disease in children and adolescents in Sweden, 1984–1995. J. Pediatr. Gastroenterol. Nutr. 2000;**30**:259–64.

227. Kugathasan S, Judd RH, Hoffmann RG, *et al.* Epidemiologic and clinical characteristics of children with newly diagnosed inflammatory bowel disease in Wisconsin: A statewide population-based study. J. Pediatr. 2003;**143**:525–31.

228. Sawczenko A, Sandhu BK, Logan RFA, *et al.* Prospective survey of childhood inflammatory bowel disease in the British Isles. Lancet 2001;**357**:1093–4.

229. Glickman JN, Bousvaros A, Farraye FA, *et al.* Pediatric patients with untreated ulcerative colitis may present initially with unusual morphologic findings. Am. J. Surg. Path. 2004;**28**:190–7.

230. Nixon JB, Riddell RH. Histopathology of ulcerative colitis. In Allan RN, *et al.*, editors, *Inflammatory Bowel Disease*. Edinburgh: Churchill Livingstone; 1990:247–62.

231. Hyams J, Davis P, Lerer T, *et al.* Clinical outcome of ulcerative proctitis in children. J. Pediatr. Gastroenterol. Nutr. 1997;**25**:149–52.

232. Powell-Tuck J, Ritchie JK, Lennard-Jones JE. The prognosis of idiopathic proctitis. Scand. J. Gastroenterol. 1977;**12**:727–32.

233. Alexander F, Sarigol S, DiFiore J, *et al.* Fate of the pouch in 151 pediatric patients after ileal pouch anal anastomosis. J. Pediatr. Surg. 2003;**38**:78–82.

234. Laghi A, Borrelli O, Paolantonio P, *et al.* Contrast enhanced magnetic resonance imaging of the terminal ileum in children with Crohn's disease. Gut 2003;**52**:393–7.

235. Heuschen UA, Hinz U, Allemeyer EH, *et al.* Backwash ileitis is strongly associated with colorectal carcinoma in ulcerative colitis. Gastroenterology 2001;**120**:841–7.

236. Kahn E, Markowitz J, Daum F. The appendix in inflammatory bowel disease in children. Mod. Pathol. 1992;**5**:380–3.

237. Kroft SH, Stryker SJ, Rao MS. Appendiceal involvement as a skip lesion in ulcerative colitis. Mod. Pathol. 1994;**7**:912–4.

238. Dendrinos K, Cerda S, Farraye FA. The "cecal patch" in patients with ulcerative colitis. Gastrointest. Endosc. 2008;**68**:1006–7.

239. D'Haens G, Geboes K, Peeters M, *et al.* Patchy cecal inflammation associated with distal ulcerative colitis: A prospective endoscopic study. Am. J. Gastroenterol. 1997;**92**:1275–9.

240. Talbot IC, Price AB. Ulcerative collitis. In Talbot IC, Price AB, editors, *Biopsy Pathology in Colorectal Disease.* London: Chapman and Hall; 1987: 117–34.

241. Washington K, Greenson JK, Montgomery E, *et al.* Histopathology of ulcerative colitis in initial rectal biopsy in children. Am. J. Surg. Pathol. 2002;**26**:1441–9.

242. Robert ME, Tang L, Hao LM. Patterns of inflammation in mucosal biopsies of ulcerative colitis – Perceived differences in pediatric populations are limited to children younger than 10 years. Am. J. Surg. Pathol. 2004;**28**:183–9.

243. Ruuska T, Vaajalahti P, Arajärvi P, *et al.* Prospective evaluation of upper gastrointestinal mucosal lesions in children with ulcerative colitis and Crohn's disease. J. Pediatr. Gastroenterol. Nutr. 1994;**19**(2):181–6.

244. Tobin JM, Sinha B, Ramani P, *et al.* Upper gastrointestinal mucosal disease in pediatric Crohn disease and ulcerative colitis: A blinded, controlled study. J. Pediatr. Gastroenterol. Nutr. 2001;**32**:443–8.

245. Abdullah BA, Gupta SK, Croffie JM, *et al.* The role of esophagogastroduodenoscopy in the initial evaluation of childhood inflammatory bowel disease: A 7-year study. J. Pediatr. Gastroenterol. Nutr. 2002;**35**:636–40.

246. Oberhuber G, Puspok A, Oesterreicher C, *et al.* Focally enhanced gastritis: a frequent type of gastritis in patients with Crohn's disease. Gastroenterology 1997;**112**:698–706.

247. Hildebrand H, Finkel Y, Grahnquist L, *et al.* Changing pattern of paedia tric inflammatory bowel disease in northern Stockholm 1990–2001. Gut 2003;**52**:1432–4.

248. Barton JR, Ferguson A. Clinical features, morbidity and mortality of Scottish children with inflammatory bowel disease. Q. J. Med. 1990;**75**:423–39.

249. Evans CM, Walker-Smith JA. Inflammatory bowel disease in children. In Allan RN, *et al.*, editors, *Inflammatory Bowel Disease.* Edinburgh: Churchill Livingstone, 1990: 523–46.

250. Morson BC, Dawson IMP, Day DW. Crohn's disease. In Morson BC, Dawson IMP, editors, *Gastrointestinal Pathology.* Oxford: Blackwell Scientific Publishers, 1990: 258–76.

251. Bass JA, Goldman J, Jackson MA, *et al.* Pediatric crohn disease presenting as appendicitis: differentiating features from typical appendicitis. Eur. J. Pediatr. Surg. 2012;**22**:274–8.

252. Dudley TH, Jr., Dean PJ. Idiopathic granulomatous appendicitis, or Crohn's disease of the appendix revisited. Hum. Pathol. 1993;**24**:595–601.

253. Lockhart-Mummery HE, Morson BC. Crohn's disease (regional enteritis) of the large intestine and its distinction from ulcerative colitis. Gut 1960;**1**:87–105.

254. Markowitz J, Daum F, Aiges H, *et al.* Perianal disease in children and adolescents with Crohn's disease. Gastroenterology 1984;**86**:829–33.

255. Thompson H. Histopathology of Crohn's disease. In Allan RN, *et al.*, editors, *Inflammatory Bowel Diseases.* Edinburgh: Churchill Livingstone, 1990: 263–85.

256. Schmitz-Moormann P, Schag M. Histology of the lower intestinal tract in Crohn's disease of children and adolescents. Multicentric paediatric Crohn's disease study. Pathol. Res. Pract. 1990;**186**:479–84.

257. Lenaerts C, Roy CC, Vaillancourt M, *et al.* High incidence of upper gastrointestinal tract involvement in children with Crohn disease. Pediatrics 1989;**83**:777–81.

258. Schmidt-Sommerfeld E, Kirschner BS, Stephens JK. Endoscopic and histologic findings in the upper gastrointestinal tract of children with Crohn's disease. J. Pediatr. Gastroenterol. Nutr. 1990;**11**:448–54.

259. Price AB. Overlap in the spectrum of non-specific inflammatory bowel disease – "colitis indeterminate". J. Clin. Pathol. 1978;**31**:567–77.

260. Chong SK, Blackshaw AJ, Boyle S, *et al.* Histological diagnosis of chronic inflammatory bowel disease in childhood. Gut 1985;**26**:55–9.

261. Hildebrand H, Fredrikzon B, Holmquist L, *et al.* Chronic inflammatory bowel disease in children and adolescents in Sweden. J. Pediatr. Gastroenterol. Nutr. 1991;**13**:293–7.

262. Wells AD, McMillan I, Price AB, *et al.* Natural history of indeterminate colitis. Br. J. Surg. 1991;**78**:179–81.

263. Pezim ME, Pemberton JH, Beart RW, *et al.* Outcome of "indeterminant" colitis following ileal pouch-anal anastomosis. Dis. Colon Rectum 1989;**32**:653–8.

264. Gupta SK, Fitzgerald JF, Croffie JM, *et al.* Experience with juvenile polyps in North American children: the need for pancolonscopy. Am J. Gastroenterol 2001;**96**(6):1695–7.

265. Wang LC, Lee HC, Yeung CY, Chan WT, Jiang CB. Gastrointestinal polyps in children. Pediatr. Neonatol. 2009;**50**(5):196–201.

266. Geboes K, Hertogh G, van Caillie M, *et al.* Non-adenomatous colorectal polyposis syndromes. Curr. Diagn. Pathol. 2007;**13**;479–89.

267. Daniels J, Montgomery E. Non-neoplastic colorectal polyps. Curr. Diagn. Pathol. 2007;**13**:467–478.

268. Vaiphei K, Thapa BR. Juvenile polyposis (coli) -high incidence of dysplastic epithelium. J. Pediatr. Surg. 1997;**32**(9);1287–90.

269. Alkhouri N, Franciosi JP, Mamula P. Familial adenomatous polyposis in children and adolesents. J. Pediatr. Gastroenterol. Nutr. 2010;**51**(6):727–32.

270. Moon SB, Park KW, Jung SE, *et al.* Vasoactive intestinal polypeptide producing ganglioneuromatosis involving the entire colon and rectum. J. Pediatr. Surg. 2009;**4**(3):e19–21.

271. Hill DA, Furman WL, Billups CA, *et al.* Colorectal carcinoma in childhood and adolescence: A clinicopathologic review. J. Clin. Oncol. 2007;**25**(36):5808–14.

272. Ferrari A, Rognone A, Casanova M, *et al.* Colorectal carcinoma in children and adolescents: the experience of the Istituto Nazionale Tumori of Milan, Italy. Pediatr. Blood Cancer. 2008;**50**(3):588–93.

273. Karnak I, Ciftci AO, Senocak ME, *et al.* Colorectal carcinoma in children. J. Pediatr. Surg. 1999 Oct;**34**(10):1499–504.

274. Bodas A, Pérez-Segura P, Maluenda C, *et al.* Lynch syndrome in a 15-year-old boy. Eur. J. Pediatr. 2008;**167**:1213–15.

Chapter 3

Hepatobiliary system and pancreas

Jens Stahlschmidt, Eumenia Castro, and Dolores López-Terrada

The pancreas and liver provide integral functions in the digestive and metabolic homeostasis of the body. After the skin, the liver is the largest organ of the body with central immune and metabolic functions, including the storage and release of nutrients and the neutralization and elimination of toxic substances. It is currently one of the few organs for which an artificial temporary biochemical back-up is not available. It is obvious that dysfunction of these organs causes significant morbidity and mortality.

Development of the liver, biliary tract, and pancreas

The developmental key stages of the liver, pancreas, and bile duct system are briefly outlined to facilitate the understanding of pathological features encountered in surgical pathology practice.

The development of the liver and biliary tract begins in the fourth week post-conception, with the formation of the endodermally derived hepatic diverticulum or liver bud from the ventral surface of the foregut. The cranial portion of the hepatic diverticulum grows into the mesoderm of the septum transversum to form to the liver and intrahepatic bile ducts, whereas the gallbladder and extrahepatic biliary tree originate from the caudal portion of the hepatic diverticulum (Figure 3.1) (1,2). The paired vitelline veins incorporate into the hepatic primordium and form primitive sinusoids. They also supply hematopoietic, sinusoidal endothelial, and Kupffer cells. Once the basic framework is established, the liver grows rapidly and extends beyond the limitations of the septum transversum. After the 6th week of development the liver is an important hematopoietic organ, with increased activity in the first and second trimester.

Hematopoiesis is extravascular within the lobules (predominately erythropoiesis) and in portal tracts (predominately granulocytopoiesis). Hematopoietic foci are still identifiable postnatally and persist in pathological conditions, including hepatic neoplasms.

The common bile duct, the major intrahepatic hilar ducts, and the gallbladder develop from the caudal portion of the hepatic diverticulum and appear as distinct structures by the 5th week post-conception. The larger bile ducts at the porta hepatis are fully formed by 16 weeks' gestation. The most cranial portions of the hepatic ducts appear in continuity with the converging ductules at the hepatic hilum and developing intrahepatic ducts. Intrahepatic bile duct formation is a centrifugal process starting from the hilum.

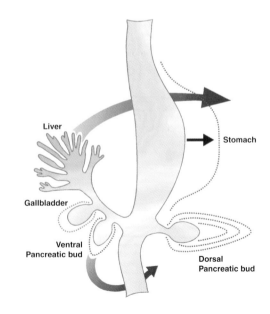

Figure 3.1 Diagram representing hepatic, biliary duct, and pancreatic development from the foregut.

Essentials of Surgical Pediatric Pathology, ed. Marta C. Cohen and Irene Scheimberg. Published by Cambridge University Press.
© Cambridge University Press 2014.

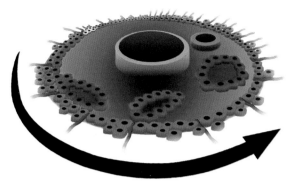

Figure 3.2 Diagram representing interlobular bile duct development (anticlockwise). Arrest in an early stage of development will result in ductal plate malformation. Central vessel: Portal vein with adjacent anteriole. Adapted from Ruchelli ED. In: Russo P, Ruchelli E and Picolli DA (eds), Pathology of Pediatric Gastrointestinal and Liver Disease, Springer, 2004, p 192. (3)

The biliary epithelium of the intrahepatic ducts derives from precursor bipotential hepatoblasts, which are in contact with the portal mesenchyme (2). These develop a collarette of low cuboidal epithelial cells, which become progressively incorporated into the portal mesenchyme (Figure 3.2). Arrest in an early stage of development will result in ductal plate malformation.

Only after approximately 38 weeks, the expected normal bile duct/portal tract ratio of 0.9 or higher is achieved. The maturation of functional hepatocytes, and the formation and differentiation of a biliary network connected to extrahepatic bile ducts continues after birth.

The pancreas is an unpaired organ located in the left superior retroperitoneum. It is principally an epithelial organ that includes both exocrine and endocrine elements. It develops during the fourth to fifth weeks of gestation (4,5) from two distinct foregut diverticula: the ventral pancreatic diverticulum, which derives from the proximal liver diverticulum, and a dorsal diverticulum, which forms from an evagination opposite the liver and ventral pancreatic diverticulum. The subsequent rotation of the duodenum to the right, positions the ventral pancreatic diverticulum posteriorly where it fuses with the dorsal pancreatic diverticulum. The pancreatic development involves an endodermal-mesenchymal induction and differentiation process. The pancreatic acinar cells, constituents of the islet cells and epithelia of the intra- and extrapancreatic duct, are endodermally derived (6). These are supported by mesenchymal tissue elements derived from the splanchnic mesodermal anlage that enveloped the pancreatic bud. The mesenchyme induces branching and cell differentiation. Trypsin, chymotrypsin, and lipase levels increase during

intrauterine life, with levels near normal by birth, while amylase and lipase levels increase slowly during the first year of life. Zymogen granules are evident at 12 weeks' gestation (5).

Microscopic anatomy of the liver, biliary tract, and pancreas

Microanatomy of the liver

The histological units of the liver comprise lobules and portal tracts. The close relationship between the angio architecture with liver cell plates and portal tracts, results in a relatively uniform, almost bland histological appearance. This simple pattern does not reflect the metabolic complexity of the liver, with no single model being sufficient to explain hepatic function satisfactorily. For the histopathologist current pragmatic models to conceptualize hepatic function include the almost hexagonal classic lobule and the hepatic acinus (7), with its three zones centered around the portal venule (with zone I closest to the portal vein, receiving a maximum amount of nutrients and oxygen, and zone III centered around the central vein, with the least amount of nutrients and oxygen).

The developed portal tract comprises two afferent vessels and a bile duct. From here, the smallest branches of the portal venous system, the interlobular venules, empty directly into sinusoids. Approximately 90% of the hepatic blood flow derives from the portal venous system, which is nutrient rich, but oxygen poor. The remainder derives from the hepatic arterioles (8). The hepatic portal arteriole supplies the portal vein branches, the interlobular bile ducts, as well as the interstitial tissue of the portal tracts. Approximately 70–80% of portal arterioles are accompanied by interlobular bile ducts. The interlobular bile duct epithelia express cytokeratins 7 and 19 and rest on a fairly regular PAS-D positive basement membrane. Larger portal tracts contain nerve fibers and also lymphatic channels, which are usually collapsed and not visible. Not all constituents of the portal tract are present in each tract. In the newborn period portal tracts may harbor foci of extramedullary granulocytic hematopoiesis.

The lobules are composed of polygonal hepatocytes. Up to 4–5 years of age hepatocytes are arranged as twinned hepatocyte cords. Hepatocytes label for cytokeratins 8 and 18 and hepatocyte paraffin 1 (Hep Par 1). Vacuolated nuclei can be seen until adolescence and are usually found periportally. Sinusoids usually appear empty in a needle biopsy, but can contain erythropoietic foci in the newborn. They are lined by specialized CD 31-positive endothelium. They are separated from the hepatocytes by the space of Disse, which contains pit and stellate cells. Both cell types are inconspicuous in the normal liver. Kupffer cells lie within the sinusoids and become markedly hyperplastic after parenchymal damage, even if the latter is not so obvious in its extent in a biopsy, and in storage disorders.

Bile canaliculi are formed by the apical surfaces of adjacent hepatocytes. They label with polyclonal carcinoembryonic antigen (CEA) or CD10 (neutral endopeptidase) antibodies. Physiological expression is only achieved after two years of age and labeling remains absent in Alagille syndrome (9).

Microanatomy of the pancreas

The mature pancreas comprises three morphologically and functionally distinct tissues that are derived from cells within the embryonic foregut endoderm (10). Nearly 90% of the pancreas is composed of acinar cells, which synthesize and secrete digestive enzymes for food processing. They are arranged in a ring of single polygonal cells surrounding a minute central lumen. The individual acinar cells have basally located nuclei and apical granular eosinophilic cytoplasm, rich in zymogen granules, which stain positive with periodic acid–Schiff (PAS) stain, resistant to diastase digestion. The endocrine tissue is organized into islets composed of α, β, δ, PP, and ε cells, which produce the hormones glucagon, insulin, somatostatin, pancreatic polypeptide, and ghrelin, respectively. The endocrine pancreas regulates broad aspects of metabolism, especially glucose homeostasis. The pancreatic ductal tissue is a branched tubular tree that serves as the conduit for transporting enzymes synthesized in the acinar tissue to the duodenum. It is subdivided in five portions according to the anatomical location and increasing caliber: centroacinar, intercalated, intralobular large, interlobular small, and main ducts. They are lined by cuboidal epithelium with minimal variation in the cell morphology according to the segmental subdivision (10).

Liver biopsy in children

Assessment of the liver histology is essential for diagnosis, evaluation, and management of numerous pediatric disorders. Liver biopsies should always be interpreted in combination with laboratory and clinical parameters. Indications of liver biopsy in children have been evolving with the implementation of new diagnostic methods, including new liver imaging techniques, and disease biomarkers. Current indications include neonatal cholestasis (Table 3.1), most commonly associated with extrahepatic biliary atresia, α-1 antitrypsin deficiency, Alagille syndrome, and metabolic liver disorders including familial intrahepatic cholestatic syndromes, glycogen storage diseases, Wilson disease, mitochondrial respiratory chain disorders, cystic fibrosis, and other rare ones. Other indications include acute liver failure, hepatitis (before initiating therapy), autoimmune hepatitis, sclerosing cholangitis, neonatal hemochromatosis, and non-alcoholic fatty liver disease. Liver biopsies are also required for the diagnosis of most liver masses/tumors, after liver transplantation (11), and may also be indicated in children with abnormal liver tests of unknown etiology (12).

There are several liver biopsy techniques and routes that can be used in pediatric patients (11), and the choice will depend on the clinical assessment of the patient and the best method to minimize risks. Pediatric biopsies are handled in a similar way to adult biopsies, with some differences, depending on the institutions. Clinical history and communication with the clinicians should take place before the biopsy is submitted in order to plan the handling of the biopsy (13). The biopsy should be received fresh in the laboratory and gross aspects such as liver parenchymal color, fragmentation of the specimen, and size of the biopsy should be recorded. While small biopsies can be of diagnostic value when dealing with a tumor, in

Table 3.1 Histological features associated with neonatal cholestasis etiologies (cholestasis and giant-cell formation may be seen in several of the etiologies listed below). (Adapted from reference number 66.)

Etiology	Microscopic features
Biliary atresia (extrahepatic)	Ductal cholestasis, portal/periportal fibrosis, ductular reaction
Paucity of intrahepatic ducts	Loss of interlobular bile ducts (duct/hepatic artery ratio <1)
Neonatal hepatitis	Portal/lobular mononuclear inflammation, apoptotic bodies
Metabolic	Fibrosis/cirrhosis, steatosis, Kupffer cell accumulation
Parenteral nutrition	Fibrosis/cirrhosis, ductular reaction

other cases, such as hepatitis, an optimal liver biopsy specimen should measure between 20 and 25 mm long and/or contain more than 11 complete portal tracts (13). These new standards have been established to decrease interobserver error, and decrease sampling error due to potential heterogeneity of liver disease (13). Frozen tissue might be a priority for the diagnosis of infections, whereas a sample should routinely be sent for electron microscopy for cholestatic and metabolic disorders (14).

Required stains include hematoxylin-eosin, trichrome, and PAS with and without diastases. These are useful to address common diagnostic problems such as the stage of fibrosis in chronic hepatitis, documenting the presence of cirrhosis, disorders of the biliary tract, and tumor histogenesis. Periodic acid–schiff stain staining can also assist in the diagnosis of glycogen storage disease, α1-antitrypsin deficiency, and fungal infections. The presence of glycogen can be confirmed by using PAS stain with diastase. Trichrome stain is mainly used to assess fibrosis, and also to highlight intracytoplasmic material such as Mallory hyaline and hepatocyte ground-glass change. Orcein, copper, and iron stains are used to highlight deposits and accumulations in the liver (13).

Immunostains such as cytokeratin 7 and 19 may be useful to demonstrate ductular reaction, and CD56 to demonstrate proliferation of hepatic progenitor cells (15), particularly in injured livers (16). In addition, cytokeratin stains may confirm the absence of bile ducts in Alagille. Other immunostains are useful in the evaluation of viral hepatitis antigen, diagnosis of α-1 antitrypsin, and liver tumors. *In situ* hybridization and Reverse transciptase polymerase chain reaction (RT-PCR) can be performed in frozen specimens to identify viral infection. Extracted DNA may also be needed for inherited metabolic disease testing.

Electron microscopy may be useful in the diagnosis of metabolic disorders (17), familial intrahepatic cholestasis (18), mitochondrial and peroxisomal diseases (19), and infections, such as the identification of viral particles in cases of fulminant acute hepatitis (20).

Metabolic disorders

Inherited metabolic diseases involving the liver are rare, but manifold, and only a small selection of these entities will be discussed here. Biopsies for suspected cases should be carefully planned and an additional fresh, snap-frozen liver biopsy should be obtained to perform additional molecular tests. If there is suspicion of a glycogen storage disorder or cystinosis, alcohol fixation should be considered.

Metabolic diseases may affect the liver at different ages and cause variable morphological changes, with some diverse metabolic disorders showing rather similar morphological changes. However, the recognition of basic histological patterns may at least narrow down or exclude certain diagnoses (21–23). In all cases clinical correlation including imaging studies is essential. Recognized light-microscopic lesional patterns in metabolic disorders include hepatitic, cholestatic, cirrhotic, ductopenic, neoplastic, steatotic, and storage (see Table 3.2).

Patterns

Hepatitic pattern

The changes seen in the neonatal period include neonatal giant-cell hepatitis (NGCH; aka idiopathic neonatal hepatitis). These are varied, but the following features are usually present: lobular disarray with multinucleate giant cells and hepatocyte loss, variable neoductular proliferation, bile plugging, canalicular and hepatocellular bilirubinostasis, hepatocyte drop-out, persistent extramedullary hematopoiesis, and inflammatory cell infiltrates in portal tracts (Figure 3.3A). The overall lobular architecture remains intact and there is no, or only mild, portal fibrosis. It is crucial to exclude the possibility of an obstructive cholangiopathy, i.e. due to biliary atresia, which is usually associated with portal edematous changes and neoductular proliferations, some of which contain bile plugs. Fatty changes may suggest galactosemia or fructose intolerance (23). NGCH is not a specific diagnosis and emphasizes the need to perform an appropriate clinical work-up to reach a final diagnosis. Older children show the classic hepatitic pattern seen in adults.

Cholestatic pattern

A cholestatic pattern may be associated with a hepatitic pattera and can be seen in a wide range of disorders, such as in extrahepatic biliary atresia, Byler disease, α-1 antitrypsin deficiency, or total parenteral nutrition (TPN). It may later persist as bland canalicular or hepatocellular cholestasis.

Cirrhotic pattern

Genetic disorders can progress rapidly to cirrhosis. *In utero* insults may result in a cirrhotic pattern at birth such as in neonatal hemochromatosis. Other examples include tyrosinemia, α-1 antitrypsin deficiency, bile-acid synthesis disorders, progressive familial intrahepatic cholestasis (PFIC) types II and III, Alagille syndrome, and others.

Table 3.2 Histological patterns associated with metabolic conditions (21-24)

Condition	Hepatitic	Cholestatic	Cirrhotic	Ductopenic	Steatotic	Storage	Neoplastic
Gaucher disease	X		X			X	
α-1 Antitrypsin deficiency	X	X	X	X	X		X
Fructosemia	X	X			X		
Galactosemia	X	X	X		X		X
mtDNA depletion disorder	X	X			X		
Fatty acid oxidation disorder					X		
Neonatal hemochromatosis	X						
Niemann–Pick disease	X	X	X			X	
Cystic fibrosis	X	X	X	X	X		
PFIC type I				X			X
PFIC types II and III	(type II)		X				X
Bile acid disorder	X	X					
Oxidative phosphorylation disorder			X		X		
Glycogen storage III and IV			X			X	
Glycogen storage I, III				X		X	
Peroxisomal disorder	X	X	X	X	X	X	
Urea cycle disorder					X		
Organic acidurias					X		
Tyrosinemia	X	X	X				

(PFIC: progressive familial intrahepatic cholestasis)

Steatotic pattern

Fatty change can be divided into macro- and microvesicular steatosis. In the former the nucleus is displaced to the membrane of the cytoplasm by a clearly identifiable vacuole, whereas in microvesicular fatty change the nucleus remains central (Figure 3.3B). Examples include mitochondrial fatty oxidation defects, Wilson disease, glycogen storage disorders types I and III, galactosemia, and others.

Ductopenic pattern

There is progressive loss of intralobar ducts with cholestasis, with or without a hepatitic pattern (Figure 3.3C). Examples include α-1 antitrypsin deficiency, cystic fibrosis, Alagille syndrome, neonatal sclerosing cholangitis, and others.

Neoplastic pattern

Adenomas, regenerative nodules, and hepatocellular carcinoma are described as a complication of cirrhosis. In particular, tyrosinemia shows an association with early development of hepatocellular carcinoma (23). Other conditions include certain glycogen storage disorders, α-1 antitrypsin deficiency, galactosemia, PFIC, and others.

Storage pattern

Depending on the enzyme defect, this causes enlargement of hepatocytes and/or macrophages, or of biliary

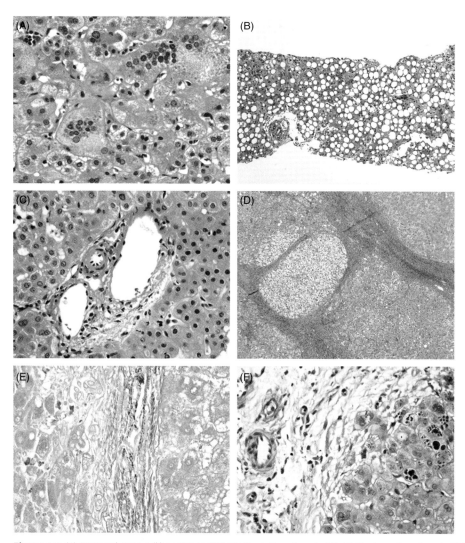

Figure 3.3 (A): Neonatal giant-cell hepatitis (× 400). (B): Steatotic pattern (× 50). (C): Ductopenic pattern (× 400). (D): Cirrhotic pattern in Wilson disease (× 50). (E): Wilson disease – copper-associated protein mainly in Kupffer cells. Note different distribution of copper in the nodules (× 400, Shikata stain). (F): Periportal PAS-diastase-resistant hepatocellular globules in α-1 antitrypsin deficiency (× 400).

epithelial cells, with or without disturbance of the sinusoidal architecture. Examples are the mucopoly-saccharides (types I–III), glycogen storage disorders, and others.

Selected diseases

Wilson disease

Clinical features: Wilson disease is an autosomal recessive disorder with an incidence of 1:30 000–100 000. More than 300 different mutations of the ATP7B gene, located on the long arm of chromosome 13, and responsible for Wilson disease, have been described (25).

The liver contains the highest amount of copper, predominately as ceruplasmin, and is responsible for its secretion. The newborn liver contains approximately 50% of the entire copper body storage; this drops to about 8% at around three months and remains stable afterwards. Symptoms of the disease are usually not recognizable before the age of six years, with a mean age at diagnosis of between 11 and 16 years, presenting with either acute or fulminant liver failure. Clinical tests for Wilson disease, including ophthalmic, renal, and neurological assessment, biochemical tests (including 24 hour urine copper evaluation), and copper assessment of fresh liver tissue, assist in the diagnosis.

Histopathology: There is a range of histological patterns. The earliest changes, seen in screening biopsies of family members, are non-specific and include micro- and macrovesicular fatty changes, with increased periportal glycogenated hepatocyte nuclei. Acute presentation with severe liver dysfunction shows severe hepatitis with hepatocyte ballooning degeneration, syncytial giant cell changes, Mallory's hyaline, and/or fine to broad portal fibrosis, resulting in cirrhosis (usually macronodular). A hepatitic pattern can predominate with irregular portal mononuclear inflammatory cell infiltrates and areas of spotty liver cell necrosis. Increased hepatocellular and Kupffer cell copper-associated protein may be seen, although in the cirrhotic stage its distribution can be uneven (Figure 3.3D–E). Rhodamine is better for copper evaluation (26).

Differential diagnosis: This includes chronic hepatitis, mainly autoimmune hepatitis. It should be noted that chronic exogenous copper poisoning can lead to an increased liver copper content and subsequent cirrhosis, similar to that seen in Wilson disease. The condition, designated as Indian childhood cirrhosis, results from copper-contaminated milk (see cirrhosis section). In the Western World soft water from copper-containing water systems may cause similar liver changes when exposed to during the newborn period (27).

α-1 Antitrypsin deficiency

Clinical features: This is an autosomal recessive disorder characterized by low serum levels of α-1 antitrypsin. Prevalence for severe α-1 antitrypsin deficiency (PiZZ) homozygosity is approximately 1:3500 worldwide, but most prevalent in Scandinavia (28). It represents the most common genetic cause of neonatal liver disease, and about 75% of newborns may present with a prolonged icteric period.

Histopathology: Features include cholestatic giant-cell hepatitis similar to that seen in extrahepatic biliary atresia. There may be features of advanced bile duct loss. On occasions, children may present with cirrhosis (21). The PAS-D-resistant periportal hepatocellular inclusions require time to accumulate and are only visible after four months of age (Figure 3.3F).

Differential diagnosis: The differential diagnosis of cytoplasmic eosinophilic inclusions includes Mallory bodies (differentiated using antibodies for ubiquitin, cytokeratins, and p62), megamitochondria (PAS-D negative), and fibrinogen bodies (PAS-D negative).

Lysosomal storage disorders

Lysosomes are membrane-bound vacuoles in the cytoplasm of the monocyte–macrophage system cells, but also in epithelial tissues that contain hydrolytic enzymes, either within membranes or their matrix. Defects in various enzymes will result in accumulation of their substrates. In evaluating liver biopsies, determining the cell type or types involved, in combination with enzyme activity studies (performed on frozen sections), and characterization of accumulated substrates, may be helpful in the diagnosis. Electron microscopy is also an important tool to characterize these disorders (29,30).

Several lysosomal storage disorders are briefly outlined below.

Sphingolipidoses

These are characterized by accumulation of gangliosides, glycosphingolipids, and sphingomyelin, the following affecting the liver:

Glucocerebrosidosis (Gaucher disease): Swollen, sometimes massively enlarged foamy Kupffer cells and portal macrophages, weakly PAS positive.

Sphingomyelin-lipidosis (Niemann–Pick disease): Initially enlarged, microvesicular change in Kupffer cells which, with disease progression also involves hepatocytes. Fat stains may be positive. In type C, perisinusoidal fibrosis may be prominent, together with hepatic acinar formations (31).

GM1 – Gangliosidosis: Characterized by foamy Kupffer and portal macrophages, lymphocytes, and hepatocytes. In the juvenile form (Fabry's disease) there are PAS-diastase positive vacuoles in hepatocytes, endothelial cells, and Kupffer cells.

Metachromatic leukodystrophy: Usually presents with a small gallbladder and with foamy macrophages either in the gallbladder mucosa or the portal tract and hepatocytes.

Wolman disease: There is foamy vacuolization of lymphocytes and Kupffer cells; expanded portal tracts by foamy macrophages. Steatosis may be present. Characteristically there are adrenal calcifications.

Oligosaccharidoses

α-Mannosidosis: There is non-specific perisinusoidal fibrosis and steatosis. The hepatocytes show typically PAS-negative vacuoles. In aspartyl glucosaminuria hepatocytes contain variable-sized vacuoles, which are partly PAS positive. Fucosidosis reveals vacuolar change of hepatocytes, Kupffer cells, and biliary epithelial cells.

Mitochondrial fatty acid oxidation defects

This group of disorders comprises nine subtypes. Many of those will show a secondary depletion of carnitine. A common feature of these disorders is hepatocellular micro- and/or macrovesicular steatosis. In some cases, this may be associated with fibrosis, such as in long-chain acyl-CoA dehydrogenase. Many of these disorders can present as sudden unexpected death in infancy (32). Acylcarnitine studies are diagnostic tools.

Neonatal hemochromatosis

Neonates with this condition usually present with acute liver failure, including ascites, hypoglycaemia, bleeding disorders, and anemia. The liver shows advanced focal or confluent parenchymal loss, together with nodular regenerative changes and eventual cirrhosis. A lip biopsy to detect iron in labial salivary glands may aid in the diagnosis. No single gene defect has been identified so far. An association with the alloimmune form of hepatitis is described (33).

Pathology of the biliary system

Intra- and extrahepatic biliary tract disorders

Processes that interfere with bile formation or flow through the intra- and extrahepatic biliary tree will result in cholestatic liver disease. Unfortunately, many cholestatic liver diseases (including those that interfere with bile formation), as well as infections, metabolic, genetic disorders, and others may share similar histological features, and differentiating between intra- and extrahepatic causes of cholestasis can be challenging. The differential diagnosis in newborns and infants is broader than in older children (Table 3.3).

Hepatic fibrocytic diseases

Ductal plate malformation (DPM)

Remodeling of the ductal plate is a prerequisite for the formation of the various hierarchical orders of intrahepatic bile ducts. Arrest or lack of ductal plate remodeling results in ductal plate malformations (DPM) (34,35) (see Figure 3.2). The congenital diseases

associated with DPM include, but are not limited to, congenital hepatic fibrosis, autosomal dominant polycystic kidney disease (ADPKD), autosomal recessive polycystic kidney disease (ARPKD), Caroli's disease, Caroli's syndrome, and von Meyenburg complexes.

Ductal plate malformations are identified in cases of ARPKD, and are a defining histological feature of congenital hepatic fibrosis. Ductal plate malformation has also been identified in ADPKD, and occasionally in extrahepatic biliary atresia (the so-called *fetal form*). Abnormal development of the ductal plate is often accompanied by cystic disorders of the kidney. Mutations of the *PKHD1* gene have been identified as causing ARPKD.

The relationship between ARPKD and congenital hepatic fibrosis is not entirely clear. Some investigators propose that congenital hepatic fibrosis and ARPKD represent a single disorder with a wide spectrum of phenotypic manifestations, as all show features of DPM (Figure 3.4A). Others propose that they are distinct disorders with phenotypically similar bile duct lesions.

Congenital hepatic fibrosis

The characteristic lesion of congenital hepatic fibrosis is DPM, associated with increased fibrosis that links portal areas. This can be diffuse, but also confined to one lobe or a liver segment. As a result, needle core biopsies may be unreliable for diagnosis and several biopsies may be necessary. Abnormal duct profiles have the tendency to increase and dilate with age, and later complications include cholangitis, calculi, portal hypertension, and cholangiocarcinoma (usually in adults). Microscopically, the portal tracts are enlarged by connective tissue and contain marginal, partly dilated bile duct profiles. Normal interlobular ducts in the center of portal tracts are missing.

Caroli's disease: congenital dilatation of large intrahepatic bile ducts

The pure type shows ectasia of intrahepatic bile ducts without other hepatic pathology. This type is not inheritable. The second is the combined type, which encompasses Caroli's disease associated with lesions of congenital hepatic fibrosis (Caroli's syndrome), and has been associated with an autosomal dominant inheritance.

Autosomal dominant polycystic kidney disease

This is the most common hereditary kidney disease (frequency 1 in 500–1000), compared to autosomal

Table 3.3 Histological features associated with neonatal liver diseases

Etiology	Histological features	Helpful additional information
Extrahepatic biliary atresia	Interface ductular reaction; ductular cholestasis, portal and periportal edema and infiltrate neutrophils, portal fibrosis	CK 19 and 7 highlights ductular reaction
Paucity of intrahepatic bile ducts	Syndromic: Alagille syndrome Canalicular cholestasis, chronic periportal cholestasis, small bile ducts scanty or absent, slight inflammation Non-syndromic: α-1 antitrypsin deficiency, cytomegalovirus infection, idiopathic adulthood ductopenia	CK19 and 7 confirm the absence of bile ducts Jagged 1 gene mutation; facial, vertebral anomalies and other malformations Positive immunohistochemical stain for: cytomegalovirus (CMV), A-1 antitrypsin
Idiopathic neonatal hepatitis	More pronounced giant-cell transformation, portal and lobular mononuclear infiltrate, apoptotic bodies, less prominent ductular reaction	Iron, copper, infectious CMV immunostains
Metabolic disorders	Steatosis, variable storage products in the liver cells and Kupffer cells (20)	Genetic testing, electron microscopy
Neonatal hemochromatosis	Hepatocellular necrosis, giant-cell transformation, iron in periportal hepatocytes, fibrosis and nodular formation (31)	Pitfall: normal iron deposition in the neonatal liver; secondary iron overload after transfusions (iron in Kupffer cells)
α-1 Antitrypsin	Periportal accumulation of hyaline globules positive for α-1 antitrypsin immunohistochemical stain	Genetic testing Pitfall: The characteristic globules might not be present until the age of 3–4 months
Parenteral nutrition	Ductular reaction, portal fibrosis or cirrhosis,	Main differential: Sepsis, biliary obstruction
Hyperbilirubinemias	Gilbert syndrome: histological normal Dubin–Johnson Progressive familial cholestatic syndromes	Stainable iron in hepatocytes Dark, large pigment in perivenular hepatocytes Absent immunohistochemistry stain for BSEP and MDR3 protein in the canaliculi

recessive polycystic kidney disease (frequency 1 in 20 000) (36) (see Chapter 9). Liver cysts can sometimes be identified in affected fetuses and infants, located close to portal tracts and lined by biliary-type epithelium.

Isolated hepatic polycystic disease

These are clinically and histologically indistinguishable from ADPKD with no obvious renal cysts. The condition is characterized by numerous intrahepatic cysts ranging from 1 cm or more without any previous history of infection or trauma. The genetic cause is now known; the condition usually affects adults only (37).

Ductal plate malformation in malformation syndromes

Ductal plate malformation changes are seen in association with other syndromes, including:

- Meckel–Gruber syndrome (cystic dysplasia of kidneys, postaxial polydactyly, and occipital encephalocele)
- Jeune syndrome (asphyxiating thoracic dystrophy)
- Cystic lesions in pancreas and kidney and DPM in liver
- Ivemark syndrome
- Bardet–Biedl syndrome.

Extrahepatic biliary atresia (BA)

BA is an extremely rapid progressive cholangiopathy of infancy with obstruction of extrahepatic bile ducts at the time of diagnosis, affecting 1 in 5000–8000 live births. The etiology is unknown and its pathogenesis is poorly defined (38). Some epidemiological studies have suggested geographical clustering, seasonal variations, and an association with advanced maternal age, increased parity, or viral infection.

General features: Infants usually present with a triad of jaundice (conjugated hyperbilirubinemia), acholic stools, and dark-colored urine. Most cases present in infants with atypically jaundice-free interval afterbirth (*perinatal* form). Up to 15–30% of affected infants have an earlier onset of jaundice, often present at birth and accompanied by non-hepatic congenital malformation (*embryonic/congenital* or *fetal* form of biliary atresia). Splenic abnormalities (mainly polysplenia, and less frequently asplenia) have been reported in 8–12% of infants (also known as "biliary atresia splenic malformation," BASM syndrome). Timeliness of the diagnosis (as well as other factors) and successful bile flow after portoenterostomy improved long-term outcome. Proposed mechanisms in the development of

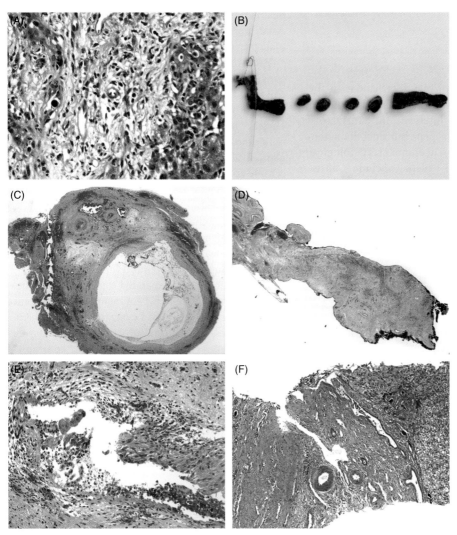

Figure 3.4 Biliary tract disorders: (A) Ductal plate malformation in congenital hepatic fibrosis. Note the absence of the portal vein (× 100). (B) Atropic extrahepatic biliary tree with suture-orientated portal plate resection margin and atrophic gallbladder. (C) Gallbladder in extrahepatic biliary atresia: extensive surface epithelial denudation (× 20). (D) Portal tract in extrahepatic biliary atresia with edema and marginal ductular proliferation containing bile plugs (× 200). (E) Epithelial denudation in a bile duct and stromal fibroinflammation in the portal-plate resection margin in extrahepatic biliary atresia (× 100). (F) Section of a portal-plate margin with no obvious bile-duct structures in extrahepatic biliary atresia; note circumferential ink as an orientation aid.

BA include exposure to environmental toxins, defects in fetal/prenatal circulation, defects in biliary morphogenesis, viral infection, and inflammation. The persistence of ductal plate raises the possibility that abnormal mesenchymal support and faulty remodeling of hilar ducts may be important pathogenetic factors in early stages of the disease. Several viruses have been implicated in the pathogenesis of BA including CMV, human papilloma virus, human herpes simplex virus type 6, Ebstein–Barr virus, reovirus, and rotavirus. Treatment options include portoenterostomy to restore flow between the resected fibrotic extrahepatic biliary tree and the patent intrahepatic ducts. If successful this procedure will extend the time to liver transplantation.

Histology: Kasai divided atresia of extrahepatic biliary ducts into the following main categories:

TYPE I: atresia of the common bile duct (CBD) with intact bile duct segments adjacent to the liver

TYPE IIA: atresia of the common hepatic duct +/– atresia of the CBD

TYPE IIB: atresia of all main branches of the extrahepatic system

TYPE III: atresia of the hepatic and cystic duct without any dilated cystic hilar ducts, which are all atretic (considered as non-correctable and representing 90% of cases).

In the past, the presence of bile duct fistulas in the portal plate resection margin was regarded as central to the success of surgical intervention. Satisfactory drainage is achieved if portal plate bile duct diameters are between 100 and 200 μm in diameter. Histological features at the portal plate include fibro-inflammation with bile ducts/bile-duct fistulas showing loss of epithelium. Focal metaplasia of the remaining biliary epithelium can be present. Correct orientation and embedding of portal plate resection specimens, after inking the margin, is crucial to assess bile ductules closest to the margin (Figure 3.5).

Liver biopsies usually display characteristically prominent portal tracts showing edema, variable inflammation, and fibrosis, as well as neoductules with characteristic focal bile plugs (Figure 3.4B–D). The lobules may show features of cholestatic giant-cell hepatitis. Additional features may include increased extramedullary hematopoiesis, canalicular, and hepatocellular cholestasis, ballooning degeneration, and giant-cell transformation of hepatocytes. Progressive loss of intrahepatic ducts is noted in untreated cases as early as five to six months (Figure 3.4E–F).

Choledochal cyst (CC)

The frequency is approximately 1 in 150 000 live births, although incidences have been reported as 1 in 13 500 births in the United States, and up to 1 in 1000 in the Asian population. There is an unexplained female to male preponderance, commonly reported as 3–4:1.

Classification: Choledochal cysts are believed to be congenital and are most often diagnosed during early childhood, though some patients can present in adolescence or even late adulthood. The pathogenesis is unclear but considered mechanisms include bile reflux, obstruction of the distal biliary tree, in particular and abnormal pancreatobiliary duct junction, and ectopic location of the papilla of Vater (39). Many patients have an elevated γGT and approximately 50% have elevations of bilirubin. Ultrasound studies are the most useful diagnostic tools. Choledochal cysts have been associated with malignancies, most commonly adenocarcinoma, squamous carcinoma, rhabdomyosarcomas, and carcinoid tumors.

Todani *et al.* (40) expanded a previous classification by Alonso-Lej *et al.* (41) to include the occurrence of intrahepatic cysts. Type I cysts (approximately 50–80% of cases) have been subsequently subclassified into three types (A–C). The second most common is type IV cysts with 15–35% of cases, and type V with approximately 20%. Some authors regard type I and type IVA cysts as simple variations of the same disease, all type I cysts having some intrahepatic dilatation.

Histology: Histological sections reveal increased dense connective tissue with interspersed smooth muscle, often with a denuded epithelium and hardly any inflammation. Mucosal hyperplasia and papillary neoplasia of the biliary tree have been reported in choledochal cysts. Examination of liver biopsy reveals similar changes to those seen in biliary atresia.

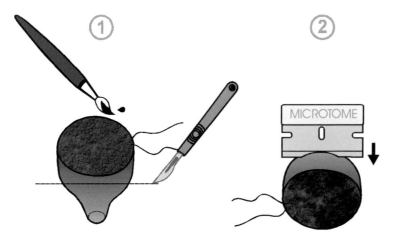

Figure 3.5 Processing of a portal-plate resection specimen. After inking the resection margin, correct orientation for embedding is crucial to assess bile ductules closest to the margin.

Neonatal sclerosing cholangitis

Neonatal sclerosing cholangitis may represent a forme fruste of biliary atresia. Typical beading of the extrahepatic biliary tree on cholangiography has been described. Debray *et al.* (42) and Batres *et al.* (43) have described sclerosing cholangitis in a neonatal subset. In the majority of patients, bridging fibrosis or cirrhosis was present in the first biopsy. There is some indication that the severity of histological findings at diagnosis does not necessarily predict disease progression. In children, primary sclerosing cholangitis is associated with inflammatory bowel disease in up to half of the cases (43).

Secondary causes of sclerosing cholangitis

Secondary causes of sclerosing cholangitis includes a variety of diverse conditions such as:

- Immune deficiencies
- Langerhans-cell histiocytosis
- Choledochal lithiasis
- Hodgkin's disease
- Cystic fibrosis
- Post-biliary surgery
- Ischemia
- Sclerosing cholangitis in association with genetic syndromes.

In Langerhans-cell histiocytosis, the liver biopsy may not show any atypical histiocytic infiltrates, and diagnosis rests on characteristic infiltrates in other organ sites, such as skin.

Spontaneous idiopathic perforation of bile duct in infancy

This is a rare disease, usually occurring between 1 and 20 weeks of age. The pathogenesis is unclear, and associations with congenital stenosis, acquired obstruction, and congenital weakness of the biliary tract with pancreatic reflux, have been proposed. The defect is commonly found at the junction of the cystic and common bile ducts.

Intrahepatic bile duct paucity

Bile duct paucity is characterized by absence or marked decrease in the number of interlobular bile ducts, with fewer than 0.5 bile ducts for each portal tract. A lower value is commonly seen in infants before 30 weeks of gestation.

Arteriohepatic dysplasia (syndromic paucity of the intrahepatic bile ducts – Alagille syndrome)

Alagille syndrome is an autosomal dominant inherited multisystem developmental disorder due to defects in Notch pathway signaling, most commonly due to mutations in the *JAG1* gene (ALGS type 1), and to a smaller degree, to *NOTCH2* mutations (ALGS type 2) (44). The expression is highly variable, with a consequently wide range of clinical features. Patients usually present with cholestasis, increased serum levels of alkaline phosphatase and γGT. Serum cholesterol levels may be markedly increased, and patients may present with xanthomas. Other clinical manifestations seen in patients with Alagille syndrome, including ocular, facial, and skeletal (vertebral) features, can be helpful to achieve a clinical diagnosis.

Histology: Proliferation of bile ducts has been reported in initial, neonatal, biopsies of patients with Alagille syndrome mimicking extrahepatic biliary obstruction. Evidence of bile duct damage may be present, together with hepatocellular giant-cell hepatitis, increased extramedullary hematopoiesis, and intralobular cholestasis. Portal tracts are usually not expanded. Late histological changes include portal expansion and fibrosis. Bile ductular proliferations at this stage are usually absent. Canalicular and apical biliary epithelial CD10 labeling is normally acquired by two years of age, but remains absent in children with Alagille syndrome (9).

Non-syndromic bile duct paucity

Most cases of non-syndromic paucity are acquired due to infections, immune-mediated injury, inflammation, drugs, or graft-vs.-host disease. Some cases remain without a diagnosis or may represent familial cholestatic syndromes.

Hepatitis

Liver biopsy is mostly utilized in hepatitis when there is uncertainty about the diagnosis and to grade the severity of the liver disease. Biopsy is especially valuable in cases of overlap syndromes and atypical clinical presentation.

Neonatal hepatitis

The neonatal liver reacts to different etiological factors with a non-specific hepatitis-like picture, so-called neonatal hepatitis or giant-cell neonatal hepatitis (45). The histological findings are very similar, regardless of the cause, consisting of variable degrees of hepatocyte swelling and multinucleation, cholestasis, and lobular and portal inflammation (46). Table 3.3 describes the main entities and their prevalent histological features; however, it should be noted that the diagnosis is not always straightforward, as there is often considerable overlap and the main diagnostic features can sometimes be absent or less prominent in the biopsy.

Infectious hepatitis

Viral hepatitis

Liver biopsy in patients with viral hepatitis B and C has been used to grade and stage the activity and chronicity of the disease, rather than for diagnosis. In children, biopsy is recommended in most hepatitis B patients with compensated liver disease before initiation of therapy (47). The histological features are similar to those seen in adults and consist of portal and lobular inflammation, interface hepatitis, and distinctive eosinophilic, ground-glass PAS-diastase-resistant cytoplasmic inclusions in hepatocytes (48). Positive immunohistochemical stains for hepatitis B surface (cytoplasmic) and core (nuclear) antigens are helpful in the differential diagnosis with other entities with similar hepatitic features.

The diagnosis of chronic hepatitis C is no longer based on liver histology, but on serological and virological tests (45). However, liver biopsy remains the gold standard for assessing the severity of inflammation and fibrosis in chronic hepatitis C (46). The histopathological features are these of lymphoid follicles in the portal tracts, damaged interlobular bile ducts, lobular activity, including acidophil bodies, steatosis, and, less frequently, granulomas. In the latter course of the disease, the histological features are less pronounced, with increased fibrosis and nodularity of the parenchyma (48,49).

Rare infections and parasitic diseases of the liver

Amebiasis is the disease caused by the enteric-dwelling protozoan parasite *Entamoeba histolytica* that primarily lives in the colon as a harmless commensal (50). It is usually acquired by contaminated water consumption, but single reports in the literature show acquired infection by liver transplantation (51). Amebic liver abscess is the most common extraintestinal complication of colonic amebiasis, and it can be complicated by rupture, migration to adjacent organs, or, rarely, vascular thrombosis (50,52).

Fascioliasis is a zoonosis caused by *Fasciola hepatica* (common liver fluke). It is endemic in the southeast Mediterranean area, but uncommon in other areas (53). Clinical signs are usually non-specific, but

include hypereosinophilia. In the liver, infection is characterized by irregular nodular lesions in periportal areas with an eosinophilic-rich inflammatory reaction, followed by fibrosis and cirrhosis (53).

Toxocariasis is a parasitic infection caused by *Toxocara canis* or *Toxocara cati*. It is distributed worldwide (54). Liver is the main organ affected by toxocara infection, typically with multiple eosinophilic infiltrates and rare abscess formation (54).

Schistosomiasis is most often caused by *Schistosoma mansoni* infection and continues to be a significant cause of parasitic morbidity and mortality worldwide, and in endemic areas such as Africa, the Middle East, the Caribbean, Brazil, Venezuela, and Suriname (55,56). In some regions of Africa, the Middle-east and Asia, portal hypertension is caused most frequently by *Schistosoma japonicum* (57). *Schistosoma* infection invariably results in egg-induced granulomas surrounded by concentric fibrosis localized in the portal space (55). This leads to presinusoidal block, inducing severe portal hypertension without affecting the hepatic lobule (55).

Herpes simplex virus infection

Herpes infection is one of the causes of acute liver failure in children, occurring most frequently in the neonatal period, or in the setting of malnutrition and immunodeficiency. The characteristic histological features include haphazardly distributed areas of hepatocellular necrosis associated with multinucleated cells with intranuclear basophilic viral inclusions (58). When the necrosis is too extensive, immunohistochemical stain might add to the diagnosis. The differential diagnosis includes other viral hepatitis and tumoral necrosis, as well as drug toxicity such as acetaminophen poisoning, which produces similar features, with the caveat that necrosis is usually more extensive and confluent, instead of the punch-out pattern seen in herpes infection (59).

Cytomegalovirus (CMV) infection

Cytomegalovirus infection is usually asymptomatic or self-limited. Severe forms are more frequent in the setting of congenital transmission or immunosuppression. Disease involving only the liver could be fatal. Characteristic histopathological findings are small aggregates of neutrophils centered by an infected hepatocyte with the diagnostic cytoplasmic and nuclear inclusion body (60). Cytomegalovirus is the leading viral infection after solid organ transplantation (60), acquired from both donor infection and from community exposure, and has been reported as causing marked ductopenia and vanishing bile duct syndrome in transplanted patients (61).

Echinococcus infection

Cystic echinococcosis is caused by the infestation with the larvae of tapeworms of the genus *Echinococcus*. It is endemic in Europe, especially in the regions surrounding the Mediterranean Sea (62). By image, echinococcosis causes unilocular cysts or multiloculated fluid-filled cysts that may show the "snow-flakes" sign, reflecting free-floating protoscoleces (hydatid-sand) within the cyst cavity. Detached or ruptured membranes, solid-looking pseudotumor and calcification are usually found in degenerate, dying cysts. The histological picture is that of a hepatitic pattern with granulomatous inflammation surrounding a central necrotizing eosinophilic exudate (63). The treatment is surgical resection of the cyst and complications include biliary fistulas, postoperative cholangitis, infection of the residual cavity, and anaphylactic reactions due to cyst rupture (64). Differential diagnoses include other mass-forming lesions in the liver, with a cystic component, such as embryonal sarcomas (65).

Autoimmune hepatitis

Autoimmune hepatitis is characterized by inflammatory liver histology, circulating autoantibodies, and increased levels of immunoglobulins, in the absence of a known etiology (66). Two types of childhood autoimmune hepatitis are recognized according to serology. Type 1 is characterized by positive smooth-muscle antibody and/or antinuclear antibody, whereas type 2 is characterized by the presence of antibodies to liver–kidney microsome type 1 (66). The spectrum of clinical manifestations is wide and ranges from asymptomatic disease to acute hepatitis, or even acute liver failure. Histological findings of interface hepatitis, lymphoplasmacytic infiltration, perivenular hepatocyte necrosis, pseudorosetting, and hepatocellular damage with acidophil bodies are the most characteristic. The differential diagnosis includes among others, sclerosing cholangitis, which can present with autoantibodies and similar histological features.

Cirrhosis

Many agents that cause cirrhosis in adults can cause it in children, including viral infections, as well as

metabolic disorders, other genetic disorders (rare familial forms), and Wilson's disease, or may be cryptogenic. The possibility of autoimmune hepatitis should always be considered in young women with cirrhosis. A rare form of pediatric cirrhosis has been described in young Indian children, sometimes with a familial incidence and associated with increased copper ingestion (67). In these patients hepatocellular swelling is followed by ballooning, Mallory body formation, necrosis, fibrosis, and acute inflammation, without steatosis. Hepatocytes accumulation of copper and copper-associated protein and very small nodular cirrhosis ("micro-micronodular cirrhosis") are characteristic (68).

Tumors of the liver

Liver cancer is rare in children, representing approximately 1% of all pediatric malignancies and accounting for 6–8% of all congenital tumors. The typical age of presentation varies, depending on the tumor type (69), but most common malignant liver tumors in children are of hepatocellular origin, hepatoblastoma during infancy, and hepatocellular carcinoma in older children and adolescents. Other relatively common pediatric liver tumors include benign vascular tumors (13%), mesenchymal hamartomas and sarcomas (6%, each), and benign lesions, such as adenomas and focal nodular hyperplasia (2%, each) (70; Table 3.4) The majority of pediatric liver tumors present as asymptomatic palpable masses in children presenting with an enlarged abdomen. Abdominal pain, anorexia, weight loss, vomiting, and diarrhea are also common symptoms at diagnosis.

Hepatoblastoma (HB)

HB is the most common liver cancer in children and is usually diagnosed during the first three years of life (71,72). Most HBs are sporadic and their etiology is not presently known. An increase in the incidence of HB during the last two decades, along with a significantly higher rate of HB among low and very low birth weight infants, has been reported (73). HB has also been associated with constitutional genetic abnormalities, malformations, familial cancer syndromes (familial adenomatous polyposis, Beckwith–Wiedemann syndrome), and metabolic disorders (glycogen storage diseases types I and IV) (74).

Table 3.4 Most common pediatric liver tumors by age at presentation. (Adapted from 129.)

Age	Malignant	Benign
Infancy	Hepatoblastoma Rhabdoid tumor Yolk sac tumor Langerhans-cell histiocytosis Megakaryoblastic leukemia Metastatic neuroblastoma	Hemangioendothelioma Mesenchymal hamartoma Vascular malformation Teratoma
Early childhood (1–3 y)	Hepatoblastoma Rhabdomyosarcoma	Hemangioendothelioma Mesenchymal hamartoma Inflammatory myofibroblastic tumor
Mid-childhood (3–10 y)	Hepatocellular carcinoma Embryonal sarcoma Angiosarcoma	Adenoma Focal nodular hyperplasia Angiomyolipoma
Adolescence (10–16 y)	Fibrolamellar/HCC Nested stromal epithelial tumor Lymphoma (Hodgkin's) Leiomyosarcoma	Adenoma Focal nodular hyperplasia Nodular regenerative hyperplasia Biliary cystadenoma

Macroscopic features: HBs are generally large multinodular expansile masses, well demarcated, but not encapsulated. Gross appearance is usually variegated, and ranges depending of the various microscopic components present (Figure 3.6), often including areas of necrosis, hemorrhage, and gritty areas where osteoid is present, particularly after chemotherapy.

Histology: Microscopically, HB frequently displays a combination of epithelial and sometimes mesenchymal patterns that may resemble developmental stages of the liver. These patterns range from primitive undifferentiated cells, to immature hepatocytes, other epithelial types, or heterotopic (heterologous) tissue types such as osteoid, or neuroectodermal derivates. Histologic classification schemes are used to categorize HBs into either epithelial or mixed types, as well as into a variable number of subtypes (70,75,76; Table 3.5). Clinical associations of different histologic HB subtypes lead to the incorporation of histopathology as a parameter for risk stratification of these patients (77,79). Resectable patients with favorable histology (pure fetal HB with low mitotic activity) survive with surgery alone, while patients with tumors demonstrating unfavorable histology (i.e. small cell), usually recur, and have a poor prognosis (78).

Immunohistochemistry is being increasingly used in the diagnosis and classification of hepatoblastoma subtypes. A limited panel using α-fetoprotein (AFP), glypican-3, beta-catenin, glutamine synthetase, vimentin, cytokeratin (pankeratin), Hep-Par1, and INI1 is presently the most useful in this setting (76). Immunohistochemical stains used in biopsy or resection specimens are especially useful in postchemotherapy specimens to identify the persistence of tumor.

Genetics: A number of acquired genetic changes, including cytogenetic and epigenetic abnormalities, have been reported in HB. Conventional cytogenetic analysis usually demonstrates karyotypes with a limited number of numerical and or structural chromosomal abnormalities in approximately 50% of HBs analyzed, with trisomies of chromosomes 2, 8, and 20 being the most frequent. Unbalanced translocations involving chromosome 1 (1q), some cases carrying a t(1;4) translocation or other translocations involving chromosome 1, as well as other structural abnormalities, have also been reported (80–82). Recent and ongoing HB molecular studies have started to elucidate the common underlying abnormalities in these tumors. Expression and miRNA profiling have identified prognostic groups of tumors and gene signatures that may be useful to further clinically stratify these patients (83,84).

Hepatocellular carcinoma (HCC)

Hepatocellular carcinoma is the second most common primary malignant tumor of the liver in children. It accounts for approximately 20% of all malignant pediatric liver tumors (70), mostly affecting children older than 10 years of age, and representing the majority (87%) of liver cancers diagnosed in adolescents (85). Presenting symptoms are similar to those described for HB, and AFP elevation is also commonly used as a tumor marker (86).

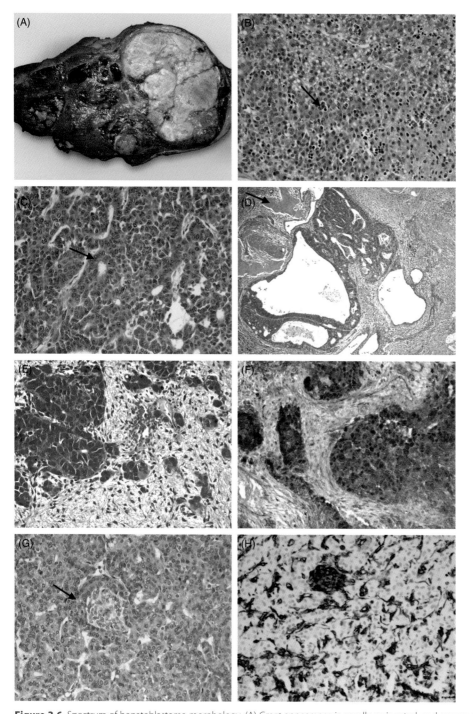

Figure 3.6 Spectrum of hepatoblastoma morphology. (A) Gross appearance is usually variegated, and ranges depending of the various microscopic components present often including areas of necrosis and hemorrhage, particularly after chemotherapy. (B–H) Microscopically the tumor displays a combination of epithelial and mesenchymal patterns. (B) The fetal component is characterized by dense and light areas comprising medium-sized cells with hyperchromatic, round, bland nuclei and abundant eosinophilic intermixed with cells with a clearer vacuolized cytoplasm. Foci of extramedullary hematopoieses (arrow) are consistently associated with the fetal areas and are a helpful feature in differentiating tumor from normal liver (HE ×40). (C) The embryonal component is made up of sheets of tumor cells with larger, more vesicular, angulated nuclei and scant cytoplasm, often organized in primitive-looking tubules (arrow) (HE × 40). (D–E). The mesenchymal component of the tumor is composed of heterotopic (heterologous) tissue types, such as osteoid (D, HE × 20, arrow) intermixed with sheets of spindle cells (E, HE × 40, arrow). (F) β-catenin immunohistochemical stain shows positive nuclear and cytoplasmic stain in the epithelial component (PAP × 40). (G) Hepatoblastoma, small-cell component is composed of smaller undifferentiated nest (arrow) of dyscohesive cells surrounded by the epithelial component of the tumor (PAP × 40). (H) The small-cell component is positive for vimentin, whereas the epithelial tumor cells are negative (PAP × 40).

Table 3.5 Consensus classification of pediatric liver tumors. (Adapted from 74.)

Hepatocellular	
Benign and tumor-like conditions	Hepatocellular adenoma (adenomatosis) Focal nodular hyperplasia Macroregenerative nodule
Premalignant lesions	Dysplastic nodules
Malignant	Hepatoblastoma *Epithelial variants* – Pure fetal with low mitotic activity – Fetal, mitotically active – Pleomorphic, poorly differentiated – Embryonal – Small cell undifferentiated – Epithelial mixed, (any/all above) – Cholangioblastic – Macrotrabecular pattern *Mixed epithelial and mesenchymal* (with/without teratoid features) Hepatocellular carcinoma (classic and fibrolamellar) Hepatocellular neoplasm NOS
Biliary	
Benign	Bile duct adenoma /hamartoma, other
Malignant	Cholangiocarcinoma Combined (hepatocellular-cholangiocarcinoma)
Uncertain origin	Malignant rhabdoid tumor Nested epithelial stromal tumor
Mesenchymal tumors	
Benign	Vascular tumors (infantile hemangioma) Mesenchymal hamartoma Pecoma
Malignant	Embryonal sarcoma Rhabdomyosarcoma Vascular tumors (angiosarcoma, epithelioid hemangioendothelioma)
Other malignancies	Germ-cell tumors (teratoma, yolk sac tumor) Desmoplastic small round-cell tumor Ewing's/PNET
Metastatic (and secondary)	Solid tumors (neuroblastoma, Wilms, other) Acute myeloid leukemia (M7)

Hepatocellular carcinoma is more prevalent in children living in hepatitis B endemic regions (Africa and South-East Asia) (87), often acquired perinatally. Other common etiological factors associated with adult HCC are not relevant to pediatric HCC. Underlying liver disease and cirrhosis are much less common in pediatric than in adult HCC patients (88). Constitutional, genetic, and metabolic abnormalities are more frequently associated with HCC in countries with low HBV rates, including hereditary tyrosinemia type 1 (89,90) and glycogen storage diseases (91,92). Familial adenomatous polyposis (FAP), is also associated with pediatric HCC (93,94) as well as neurofibromatosis, ataxia-telangiectasia (95–98), and Fanconi's anemia (99). Hepatocellular carcinoma has also been described in children with cirrhotic livers following parenteral nutrition (100), and in patients with familial cholestatic syndromes, including Alagille syndrome (101), and extrahepatic biliary atresia (102).

Macroscopy: Hepatocellular carcinoma is often diagnosed at advanced stages involving both lobes of the liver, but can also present as a solitary, non-encapsulated mass. The cut surface is sometimes bile-stained, with necrosis and hemorrhage. Vascular spread is common, and extrahepatic metastases are often to the lungs and rarely to the brain, via the hepatic veins (103).

Histology: Microscopic features of pediatric HCC are similar to those seen in adults (71,104) and can be classified according to histological grade into well-differentiated, moderately differentiated, poorly differentiated, and undifferentiated types (103,106). Grading can also be done by nuclear features alone or in combination with microvascular invasion (71). The most common architectural pattern in well- and moderately differentiated HCC is the trabecular pattern. Pseudoglandular, acinar, and solid patterns can also be present. Neoplastic hepatocytes usually display prominent, hyperchromatic nuclei, and eosinophilic, granular, or clear cytoplasm, containing glycogen, fat, Mallory bodies, or other inclusions.

The fibrolamellar variant constitutes a distinctive clinical and histological variant of HCC that occurs almost exclusively in adolescents and young adults (77,104,107,108). It characteristically presents in patients without cirrhosis, hepatitis, metabolic, or other underlying chronic liver disease. They are well-circumscribed, firm masses with characteristic radiating fibrous septa, resembling focal nodular hyperplasia, with a characteristic microscopic appearance that consists of cords and nests of large neoplastic hepatocytes with granular oncocytic cytoplasm, separated by dense hyalinized collagen bands (Figure 3.7A,B). Children with fibrolamellar HCC do not have a better prognosis as they do not respond any differently to current therapeutic regimens than patients with typical HCC at a similar stage (109).

Immunohistochemical stains may be useful to differentiate HCC from other tumor types. Approximately 90% of HCCs demonstrate HepPar-1 (hepatocyte paraffin 1) and glypican 3 (GPC3). AFP is usually elevated in the patient's serum, and focally present in the tumor cells (108). Hepatocytes express cytokeratins 8 and 18, while biliary epithelium expresses CK7, CK19, CK8, and CK18, but aberrant cytokeratin expression in tumor cells limits the use of these antibodies for tumor classification (111). CD34 immunostaining of the sinusoids can be helpful to distinguish well-differentiated HCC from regenerative nodules, but not from adenomas (112).

Differential diagnosis: The most common differential diagnosis is HB and, rarely, metastatic lesions. Cytologic atypia and nuclear pleomorphism, although they may be variable, are usually more prominent in HCC, while other features of HB, such as co-existence of histologic patterns, extramedullary hematopoiesis,

and mesenchymal components, are not usually seen in HCC. Hepatic adenomas in older children may be challenging to differentiate from well-differentiated HCC, and from focal nodular hyperplasia, particularly in small biopsies. Adenomas may be multiple, such as those seen in patients with glycogen storage disorders. Immunohistochemical staining for proliferation markers such as Ki67 or endothelial markers (CD34) may be diagnostically useful (113,114). Fibrolamellar HCC can be clinically and radiographically difficult to differentiate from focal nodular hyperplasia, due to the typical central scar, but can be easily differentiated by its distinctive histologic features.

Genetics: Pediatric HCC is a rare, heterogeneous disease, and very little is understood regarding how genetic predisposition, metabolic disorders, cholestasis, or potential exposures during infancy and childhood may represent carcinogenic factors in these tumors. Genetic studies of adult HCC have demonstrated multiple chromosomal abnormalities, predominantly losses, most commonly of chromosomes 17p, 13q, 9p, 6q, and 16p, in contrast to HB usually displaying few chromosomal changes, and commonly trisomies (115). Chromosomal instability has been reported in HCCs associated with hepatitis B virus infection. Fibrolamellar carcinomas with abnormal karyotypes appear to behave more aggressively than cases with normal karyotypes (116). Recent studies have also identified critical signaling pathways involved in hepatocarcinogenesis, mostly in hepatitis-associated HCC, including the P53 pathway, mitogen-activated protein kinase (MAPK), Wnt/β-catenin, epidermal growth factor (EGF), and transforming growth factor-β(TGFβ) pathways (117,118). Adult HCC gene-expression profiling studies have specifically identified differences between clinical HCC subtypes (115,119–121). Unfortunately, most of these studies aimed to investigate adult HCC, and is not clear how much of what we have learned from these applies to pediatric patients.

Hepatocellular neoplasm NOS

Recent histopathology consensus reviews of pediatric liver tumors of patients enrolled in large international prospective clinical studies (76) identified a minority of pediatric hepatocellular tumors that are difficult to classify, sometimes sharing features of both HB and HC. These lesions, which will not fit into other known categories included in the current consensus

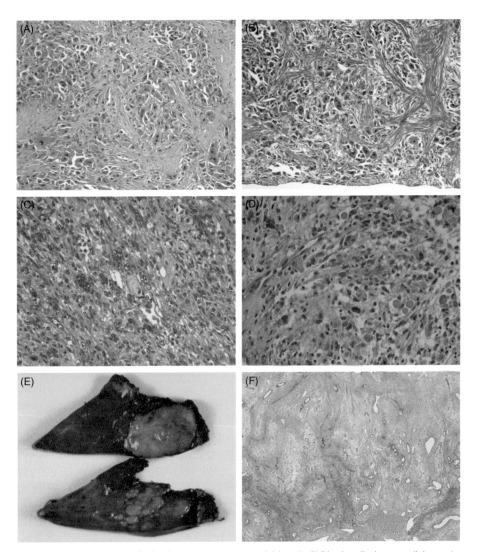

Figure 3.7 Histopathology of other hepatic tumors seen in children. (A–B) Fibrolamellar hepatocellular carcinoma is characterized by cells with increase-sized, pleomorphic nuclei with visible nucleoli and abundant, deep-eosinophilic cytoplasm embedded in a prominent fibrous stroma, highlighted by a trichrome stain (HE × 20, Masson Trichrome × 20). (C–D). Undifferentiated sarcoma characterized by enlarged, spindly-looking cells with pleomorphic, often multinucleated vesicular nuclei in a loose edematous background. Note the multiple intracytoplasmic, eosinophilic inclusion (HE × 40). (E–F) Mesenchymal hamartoma. (E) Grossly, the tumor is a solid, tan, non-encapsulated, bulging mass that compresses the adjacent liver parenchyma. (F) Histologically, it shows multiple irregular bile ducts encased in fibromyxoid connective tissue.

classification, may therefore be classified as hepatocellular neoplasm NOS (not otherwise specified) until a precise nosological assignment is possible.

Transitional liver cell tumor (TLCT) of older children and adolescents had been described (122). These were difficult to classify tumors containing HB-like cells, cells resembling those of HCC, so-called "intermediate cell forms," and multinucleated giant cells, and some expressed β-catenin, with a mixed nuclear and cytoplasmic expression pattern. The term, transitional, was proposed based on the hypothesis that the

tumor cell might be between a hepatoblast and a hepatocyte. Tumors with these features are included under the provisional category of hepatocellular neoplasm NOS under the current classification.

Hepatocellular adenoma

Hepatocellular adenomas are benign proliferations of mature hepatocytes that sometimes may be challenging to distinguish from regenerative nodules, fibronodular hyperplasia, and HCC. These lesions are composed of cells larger than normal hepatocytes that may show a moderate degree of nuclear pleomorphism, growing in larger clusters without portal tracts or bile ducts. Adenomas have been associated with estrogen and androgen therapy, and may also demonstrate peliosis. Some adenomas display severe steatosis or show an alcoholic hepatitis-like histology. Molecular genetic features and immunostaining have been described to subclassify adenomas (121) based on their histology and biology.

Fibronodular hyperplasia (FNH)

Fibronodular hyperplasia is another benign lesion characterized by a radial scar containing bile ducts along with ducts at the periphery of nodular, bland hepatocytic proliferations that needs to be distinguished from adenoma. FNH may be found in patients with glycogen storage disease type 1a and may also occur in children with vascular lesions, such as cavernous transformation of the portal vein or its absence, or following systemic chemotherapy for non-hepatic cancer (123).

Nested stromal epithelial tumor

Nested stromal epithelial tumor of the liver (125,126), also termed desmoplastic nested spindle-cell tumor of the liver (127) is a rare hepatic neoplasm of older children and young adolescents. This tumor may present a variable clinical prognosis, with rare recurrences and metastatic cases reported, and is sometimes associated with Cushing syndrome (128). Microscopically, these tumors are composed of nests of cytokeratin 8-positive, Hepar1-negative epithelial cells, surrounded by smooth-muscle actin-positive spindle cells, calcifications, and osteoid formation. This pattern is suggestive of aberrant epithelial–mesenchymal transition and resembles the morphology of the liver bud. Rarely epithelial cells express ACTH (123) and corticotropin-releasing hormone.

Undifferentiated (embryonal) sarcoma

Embryonal sarcoma, the most common sarcoma of the liver in children, is characterized by poorly differentiated spindle or myxoid cells containing eosinophilic cytoplasmic globules, and showing marked pleomorphism and nuclear atypia (129; Figure 3.7C, D). Other patterns, including hemangiopericytomatous and fibro-histiocytosis-like growth patterns may also be present. A characteristic diffuse pattern of infiltration that tends to spare bile ducts and may

even render them cystic is shared with other sarcomas growing in the liver.

Mesenchymal hamartoma (MH)

MH are often cystic lesions lined with a single layer of cuboidal or flat epithelium, containing a plasma transudate, and surrounded by collagenous or myxoid stroma. These are almost always well-circumscribed, solitary lesions. An interesting association has been reported between these benign lesions and embryonal sarcomas (129–131,132), with MH occurring most commonly in infancy and ES in children older than 10 years of age.

Vascular tumors

Infantile hemangiomas or hemangioendotheliomas (HE) account for more hepatic masses than any other condition. This common benign neoplasia in children was originally designated as hemangioendothelioma type 1 (133) and replaced by "infantile hemangioma" to designate the proliferative lesion of infants often associated with cutaneous lesions that usually regresses spontaneously (134). Only rarely do HE fail to regress or respond to medical therapy, necessitating transplantation (135). Hemangioendothelioma are composed of bland proliferations of small vascular channels lined by endothelium. Some may have cavernous vessels with fibrosis and/or calcification, and be associated with congestive failure. Differential diagnosis includes arteriovenous malformations (which show no Glut1 antibody expression) (136) and HB or adenomas, as HE may appear solid, without significantly increased blood flow by imaging, and in some cases present with elevated serum AFP, leading to misinterpretation (137).

Angiosarcomas may rarely occur in children, usually arising *de novo*, although rare cases preceded by benign hemangiomatous hamartomas and hemangiomas have been reported (135). Epithelioid hemangioendothelioma (EHE) is a malignancy of intermediate malignant potential, very rarely diagnosed in children (138).

Other rare pediatric liver tumors

Rhabdomyosarcomas involving the biliary tract may also be seen in young children (139). They may display a botryoid pattern of growth and cystic bile ducts, and also features of embryonal rhabdomyosarcoma, with rare cross-striations present. *Malignant rhabdoid tumors* are characterized by discohesive round cells with prominent nucleoli and both cytokeratin and vimentin intermediate filaments (140). *Inflammatory myofibroblastic tumors* may present in the liver as spindle-cell proliferations associated with an inflammatory infiltrate containing plasma cells, lymphocytes, and eosinophils, with myxoid degeneration and necrosis that may resemble granulation tissue. Patients may present with obstructive jaundice when these lesions involve the liver hilum (75). *Germ-cell tumors (GCT)* may also occur in the liver of young infants, including yolk sac tumors, choriocarcinomas, or teratomas. These components can also be part of an HB (141). Hepatic GCT shows histological features identical to other sites, and may present with increased serum AFP and β-HCG. Endocrine tumors, primary *carcinoids* of the liver also occur infrequently (142,143) and need to be differentiated from teratoid HBs, which may also contain cells expressing markers such as chromogranin and serotonin.

Metastatic tumors such as neuroblastoma, Wilms' tumor, desmoplastic small-cell tumor, rhabdomyosarcoma, pancreatoblastoma, and lymphoma can be mistaken for poorly differentiated variants of HB. *Megakaryoblastic leukemia* can be challenging to diagnose in small biopsy specimens, particularly in patients, usually infants, with diffusely enlarged liver that may present with bone marrow fibrosis and without circulating blasts (77,144). Other systemic malignancies that may infiltrate the liver in children include *Langerhans-cell histiocytosis* (LCH) (145), characteristically displaying CD1a, langerin, and S100 positive LCH cells, and that may present with either cystic dilatation or biliary sclerosis and fibrosis. *Familial hemophagocytic lymphohistiocytosis* may also involve the liver, demonstrating Kupffer-cell hypertrophy and portal macrophages with erythrophagocytosis, and lymphohistiocytic infiltration of the portal tracts. Perforin and MUNC13–4 staining are useful to establish this diagnosis (146).

Transplant pathology

Evaluation of rejection in the pediatric live transplant population follows the same criteria used for adults (Table 3.6). Briefly, the histopathological diagnosis of acute rejection is based on three main histopathological features, including the presence of mixed, but predominantly mononuclear, portal inflammation containing blastic or activated lymphocytes, neutrophils, and eosinophils; subendothelial inflammation of portal and/or terminal hepatic veins; and bile duct inflammation and damage. The minimal findings needed to establish the diagnosis of acute rejection are at least two of the above histopathological features, along with biochemical evidence of liver damage (147,148).

Late cellular rejection is characterized by centrilobular inflammation, necrosis and central vein endothelialitis. The long-term outcome of patients with isolated centrilobular injury seems to be similar to that of patients with centrilobular changes associated with portal-based rejection (149). Chronic rejection is defined by small (< 60 μm) bile duct loss in more than 50% of the portal tracts and obliterative arteriopathy (150).

Biliary atresia is the most common indication for liver transplant in children comprising 60–70% of all candidates. Other frequent causes include intrahepatic cholestatic diseases, metabolic diseases, acute liver failure of unknown cause, and non-resectable malignant tumors, of which the most common is hepatoblastoma (151). Less-common indications include seronegative non-A non-B hepatitis, drug-induced acute liver failure, and autoimmune hepatitis (151).

The most common recurrent diseases in liver transplantation are primary biliary cirrhosis, primary sclerosing cholangitis, and autoimmune hepatitis (152). *De novo* autoimmune hepatitis, consisting of histological chronic hepatitis associated with autoantibody formation and allograft dysfunction, is increasingly recognized as an important complication of liver transplantation, particularly in the pediatric population (153).

Liver steatosis in children

Hepatic steatosis in children should raise the differential diagnosis of inborn errors of metabolism, viral hepatitides, chemotoxicity, and non-alcoholic fatty liver disease (NAFLD). This section will discuss mainly non-alcoholic fatty liver disease.

Non-alcoholic fatty liver disease is increasingly prevalent in children and has become the most common pediatric chronic liver disease in industrialized countries. The recent rise in the prevalence rates of overweight and obesity likely explains the NAFLD epidemic worldwide. This is a multifactorial condition that encompasses a spectrum of histological damage ranging from simple steatosis, non-alcoholic steatohepatitis (NASH), and fibrosis, with potential eventual progression to cirrhosis (154) requiring liver transplantation, which has been well-documented in children (155).

Table 3.6 Grading of acute liver allograft rejection

Grading of acute liver allograft rejection

Indeterminate	Portal inflammatory infiltrate that fails to meet the criteria for the diagnosis of acute rejection
Mild	Rejection infiltrate in a minority of the triads, that is generally mild, and confined within the portal spaces
Moderate	Rejection infiltrate, expanding most or all of the triads
Severe	As above for moderate, with spillover into periportal areas and moderate to severe perivenular inflammation that extends into the hepatic parenchyma and is associated with perivenular hepatocyte necrosis

Rejection activity index (RAI)

Portal inflammation	Mostly lymphocytic inflammation involving, but not noticeably expanding, a minority of the triads	1
	Expansion of most or all of the triads, by a mixed infiltrate containing lymphocytes with occasional blasts, neutrophils and eosinophils	2
	Marked expansion of most or all of the triads by a mixed infiltrate containing numerous blasts and eosinophils with inflammatory spillover into the periportal parenchyma	3
Bile duct inflammation damage	A minority of the ducts are cuffed and infiltrated by inflammatory cells and show only mild reactive changes such as increased nuclear: cytoplasmic ratio of the epithelial cells	1
	Most or all of the ducts infiltrated by inflammatory cells. More than an occasional duct shows degenerative changes such as nuclear pleomorphism, disordered polarity and cytoplasmic vacuolization of the epithelium	2
	As above for 2, with most or all of the ducts showing degenerative changes or focal luminal disruption	3
Venous endothelial inflammation	Subendothelial lymphocytic infiltration involving some, but not a majority of the portal and/or hepatic venules	1
	Subendothelial infiltration involving most or all of the portal and/or hepatic venules	2
	As above for 2, with moderate or severe perivenular inflammation that extends into the perivenular parenchyma and is associated with perivenular hepatocyte necrosis	3

Total RAI Score = _/9; (1–2: undetermined; 3–4: mild; 5–6: moderate; > 6: severe)
(From Banff Schema for Grading Liver Allograft Rejection: An International Consensus Document. *Hepatology* 1997;**25**(3):658–63.)

The pathogenesis of NASH remains unclear, with many aspects unresolved, but it seems that a two-hit hypothesis is the most likely explanation for the histopathological findings (155,156). Macrovesicular steatosis resulting from the discrepancy between synthesis of lipids and their export from the hepatocytes is thought to represent the first hit. Fat accumulation renders the organ more vulnerable to a second hit that leads to inflammation, steatohepatitis, and ultimately, in the event of persisting or recurring damage, to fibrosis and cirrhosis. Microvesicular steatosis as a minor component might be considered a possible precursor of macrovesicular steatosis. However, when predominantly in the liver, it indicates severe hepatocytic damage as a result of defective β-oxidation of fatty acids, and should raise the possibility of drug toxicity (156).

Imaging by ultrasonography or magnetic resonance, liver function tests, serum markers of liver fibrosis, tests for insulin resistance, and hypertransaminasemia despite weight loss, are variably used as surrogate markers of steatosis (157). Pediatric NASH differs from adult, being often clinically suspected merely on grounds of a mild persistent rise in transaminases, with no liver symptoms (154,157). The diagnosis of NAFLD thus emerges from a combination of clinical and histopathological findings (154).

The criteria used for the morphological definition of steatohepatitis are fatty degeneration of liver cells, predominant in zone 3, lobular and/or portal field-dominant inflammatory reaction, direct liver cell damage in the form of ballooned hepatocytes, fibrosis, and possibly accumulation of iron (Table 3.7; 158). These histologic diagnostic criteria for NAFLD may be unevenly distributed in the liver and as a result, diagnosis based on biopsy samples may be associated with considerable sampling error. Indication for liver biopsy include young age, familial history of severe

Table 3.7 Histological criteria for diagnosis of NASH and NAFLD

Grade of fatty degeneration

< 5%	Grade 0
5–33%	Grade 1
34–66%	Grade 2
More than 66%	Grade 3

Grade of lobular inflammation

Absent	Grade 0
Up to two foci per field of view (×200 magnification)	Grade 1
Two to four foci per field of view	Grade 2
More than four foci per field of view	Grade 3

Lipogranulomas are included in the category of inflammation

Microgranulomas	Yes	No
Large lipogranulomas	Yes	No
Portal inflammation	None to minimal	Greater than minimal

Liver cell injury

Ballooning:

Absent	Grade 0		
Few ballooned hepatocytes	Grade 1		
Many ballooned hepatocytes	Grade 2		
Acidophil bodies	None	Rare	Many
Pigmented macrophages	None	Rare	Many
Megamitochondria	None	Rare	Many
Mallory hyaline	None	Rare	Many
Glycogenated nuclei	None	Rare	Many

Fibrosis

Stage 0	None	
Stage 1	Perisinusoidal or periportal	
	1A	Mild delicate, zone 3, perisinusoidal
	1B	Moderate (dense), zone 3 perisinusoidal
	1C	Portal/periportal
Stage 2	Perisinusoidal and portal/periportal	
Stage 3	Bridging fibrosis	
Stage 4	Cirrhosis	

Total grade non-alcoholic steatohepatitis (NAS) activity score; Steatosis grade + Lobular inflammation grade + hepatocyte ballooning =_/8.
Score: 0–2 = non-diagnosis of NAS; 3–4 = non-diagnostic, borderline, or diagnostic; 6–8 = diagnostic of NAS.

disease, inconclusive tests for other pathologies, and suspected advanced fibrosis (157).

Liver fibrosis is the most worrisome histological feature in patients with NAFLD. Early detection of significant fibrosis in children may prevent the development of advanced cirrhosis, its complications, and the need for liver transplantation. Liver biopsy is the gold standard test for the distinction between simple steatosis and NASH, to determine inflammatory activity and stage of fibrosis. Current treatment relies on weight loss, exercise, and changes in lifestyle, although various insulin-sensitizing agents, anti-oxidants, anti-inflammatory, and anti-fibrogenic agents are under evaluation (156,159).

Pathology of the pancreas

Developmental abnormalities

Pancreas agenesis

Pancreatic agenesis is a human disorder caused by defects in pancreas development (160). Complete agenesis is rare and is associated with gallbladder agenesis, diaphragmatic hernia, and growth restriction. More common, although still rare, is the partial pancreatic agenesis of the dorsal pancreas due to embryological failure of the dorsal pancreatic bud to form the body and tail of the pancreas (161). To date, only a few genes have been linked to pancreatic agenesis in humans, with mutations in pancreatic and duodenal homeobox 1 (PDX1) and pancreas-specific transcription factor 1a (*PTF1A*) reported in only five families with described cases (160). Recently, mutations in the *GATA6* gene have been identified in a large percentage of human cases, and a *GATA4* mutant allele has been implicated in a single case (162).

Pancreas ectopia

An ectopic pancreas is abnormally situated pancreatic tissue that possesses its own duct system and vascular supply (163). The most common site for an ectopic pancreas is the gastrointestinal tract (164). Most patients with ectopic pancreas are asymptomatic or exhibit non-specific symptoms. However, there are case reports of diffuse peritonitis associated with perforated gastric ectopic pancreas (164), and ectopic pancreas presenting as a mediastinal cyst (165).

Annular pancreas

Annular pancreas is a rare developmental anomaly that accounts for 1% of neonatal intestinal obstructions (166). It is the condition where the head of the pancreas surrounds the second part of the duodenum like a ring, causing duodenal stenosis. The annular tissue originates from the ventral pancreatic bud and dysregulation of the hedgehog signaling pathway has been shown to be implicated in this anomaly (167). Chromosomal abnormalities are present in one-third of cases of annular pancreas, with trisomy 21 (followed by trisomy 18 and 13) being the most frequently detected anomaly (168). Treatment usually involves surgical correction.

Pancreatic cysts

Congenital pancreatic cysts, particularly solitary cysts, are rare causes of abdominal masses in newborns (168). The etiology of these cysts is unknown and although they have been reported to occur more frequently in the head and body, they can vary in location within the pancreas. Histologically, the cyst is lined by flattened or cuboidal epithelium and the cyst wall shows fibrous tissue, rarely smooth muscle, and nodules of pancreatic tissue (170). The differential diagnosis includes the multiple cysts associated with von Hippel–Lindau syndrome or polycystic kidney disease, and cystic pancreatic tumors (171).

Pancreatic pseudocysts in children are more frequently sequelae of pancreatic trauma or pancreatitis (172). They can cause persistent abdominal pain, nausea, and gastric outlet obstruction (172). The cysts do not have an epithelial lining and consist of a cystic cavity filled with pancreatic secretions and blood (173).

Exocrine pancreas pathology

The mechanism leading to exocrine pancreatic disease in children differs from those encountered in adult patients. Among Caucasian children, cystic fibrosis (CF) is by far the most common inherited disorder associated with abnormal pancreatic function. Examples of rarer, inherited causes of pancreatic dysfunction include Shwachman–Diamond syndrome, Johanson–Blizzard syndrome SDS, Pearson's syndrome, pancreatic agenesis, and isolated enzyme deficiencies. Hereditary pancreatitis and several recently recognized metabolic causes of chronic pancreatitis may also produce severe pancreatic exocrine dysfunction. Table 3.8 displays the main differential diagnosis in abnormalities of the exocrine pancreas.

Table 3.8 Main differential diagnosis in exocrine pancreas abnormalities

Abnormalities of exocrine pancreas	
Predominant pattern/injury type	*Lipomatous atrophy or lipomatous pseudohypertrophy*
Shwachman–Diamond syndrome	Most common cause of pancreatic insufficiency after cystic fibrosis Metaphyseal dysostosis, bone marrow depression, later leukemia AR, SBDS gene; 7q11
Johanson–Blizzard	Congenital aplasia of ala nasi, deafness, dwarfism, absence of permanent teeth UBR1 gene; E3 ubiquitin ligases
Predominant pattern/injury type	*Fibrosis*
Cystic fibrosis	Eosinophilic concretions in acini and ductules CFTR gene
Pearson syndrome	Refractory sideroblastic anemia, vacuolization of bone marrow cells Deletion of mitochondrial DNA
Neonatal hemochromatosis	Acinar deposition of iron

SBDS: Shwachman–Bodian–Diamond syndrome; UBR1: ubiquitin protein ligase E3 component n-recoining 1; CFTR: Cystic fibrosis conductor regulator gene

Cystic fibrosis

Cystic fibrosis is an autosomal recessive disorder, which is caused by a mutation in the cystic fibrosis transmembrane conductance regulator protein, a chloride channel in epithelial cell membranes (174). More than 1500 mutations are known. The incidence is 1/2000–3000 in nations of European origin. The *CFTR* mutation influences the secretion and absorption by epithelium in various organs. The consequences are different, depending on the organ and mutation type, but there is a global tendency for obstruction of secretory glands. The primary organs affected are the respiratory tract, pancreas, gastrointestinal tract, and sweat glands (175).

The disease is most often diagnosed during the first months of life, with a common presentation of salty-tasting sweat, failure to thrive, in the late fetal period or around the time of delivery, with or without obstruction of the intestinal lumen. Morphological changes in the exocrine glands usually develop only after birth and consist of viscous acidophil content in the secretory ducts and acini of the pancreas, leading to complete acinar atrophy, accompanied by fibrosis and lipomatosis (175).

Shwachman–Diamond syndrome

Shwachman–Diamond syndrome (SDS) is an inherited, rare autosomal recessive marrow failure disorder with exocrine pancreatic insufficiency and metaphyseal dysostosis (176). It is the second most common cause of pancreatic insufficiency after cystic fibrosis (177). Pancreatic exocrine and bone marrow dysfunctions, with persistent or intermittent neutropenia in 88–100% of patients, are considered to be universal features of SDS, whereas the associated skeletal dysplasia is variable and not consistently observed (176; see Chapter 10). Patients frequently present failure to thrive, susceptibility to infections, and short stature. Other clinical features include immunologic, hepatic, and cardiac disorders. Few cases have been associated with Hirschsprung's disease and asphyxiating thoracic dystrophy (178).

Mutations in the Shwachman–Bodian–Diamond syndrome (*SBDS*) gene, a highly conserved gene of unknown function residing at 7q11, are found in 90% of patients meeting clinical diagnostic criteria (177). Clonal cytogenetic abnormalities, particularly those involving chromosome 7, such as monosomy 7 or isochromosome 7, may also be found. The patients have a tendency to develop myelodysplasias and later leukemias, usually acute myelogenous leukemia (177).

Histologically, the pancreas reveals exocrine pancreas hypoplasia with lipomatosis (179). There is increased echogenicity of the pancreas by image, described as "white pancreas" (180).

Pearson syndrome

Pearson syndrome is a fatal disorder mostly diagnosed during infancy and caused by mutations of mitochondrial DNA. It usually presents with transfusion-dependent refractory sideroblastic anemia with vacuolization of marrow progenitor cells, exocrine pancreatic dysfunction, and multiorgan involvement, including liver and renal tubular defects (181). It is caused by multiorgan mitochondrial cytopathy that results from defective oxidative phosphorylation owing to mitochondrial DNA deletions. Prognosis is severe and death occurs in infancy or early childhood (182). The pancreas reveals acinar atrophy with fibrosis, but no lipomatosis is identified.

Johanson–Blizzard syndrome

Johanson–Blizzard syndrome is a very rare autosomal recessive disorder caused by mutations in the ubiquitin-protein ligase E3 component N-recognin 1

(*UBR1*) gene (183). The syndrome is characterized by exocrine pancreatic insufficiency and a wide range of additional clinical features, including aplasia or hypoplasia of the alae nasi, oligodontia, sensorineural hearing loss, hypothyroidism, scalp defects, mental retardation, and developmental delay (183). Several other abnormalities in different organs, particularly anorectal, urogenital, and cardiac anomalies, have been reported since the first description of this syndrome four decades ago. Only symptomatic treatment is available.

Pancreatic tumors

Primary pancreatic neoplasms are rare in children and adolescents; thus, our understanding of these tumors is still quite limited (Table 3.9). The most common epithelial neoplasms originating from the exocrine pancreas in children are solid-pseudopapillary tumor, pancreatoblastoma, and acinar cell carcinoma (184–187). Pancreatoblastoma is more common in younger children, whereas solid-pseudopapillary tumor, acinar cell carcinoma, and endocrine tumors are more common in children older than 10 years of age (188). Tumors of endocrine cell origin are divided according to their hormonal production and are considered as a separate category (189; see Chapter 6).

Solid-pseudopapillary tumor

Definition: Solid pseudopapillary tumor (SPN) is an uncommon pancreatic neoplasm of low malignant potential and excellent prognosis, even with distant metastases, and, accounts for 0.13 to 2.7% of pancreatic tumors (186). It occurs predominantly in young women with a median age of 9 to 17 years (186). It is very rare in males and when occurring in older male patients demonstrates a more aggressive behavior (190,191).

Clinical features: SPNs commonly present with abdominal pain and discomfort, and classical features by imaging, as a large, encapsulated, solid, and cystic hemorrhagic mass, located in any section of the pancreas. Patients with SPN have a better overall survival than patients with neuroendocrine tumors or pancreatoblastoma (184). Features associated with more aggressive behavior includes male gender, older age, atypical histopathology (large tumors, diffuse growth, cellular/nuclear atypia, mitotic activity, necrosis, invasion/metastasis), and incomplete resection (185). Surgical resection is dictated by tumor location and remains the treatment of choice (184).

Table 3.9 Main differential diagnoses in pancreatic tumors in children

Exocrine tumors

Solid-pseudopapillary neoplasm	Large, solid, and cystic
Predominant pattern/ injury type	*Papillary, intracytoplasmic PAS positive globules*
Immunohistochemistry	CD56, CD10, nuclear β-catenin, PR
Prognosis	Excellent
Pancreatoblastoma	Large, solitary mass, solid sheets, or acini
Predominant pattern/ injury type	*Squamoid corpuscles*
Immunohistochemistry	Trypsin, chymotrypsin, nuclear β-catenin.
Genetics	APC/β-catenin pathway
Association	Beckwith–Wiedemann syndrome
Acinar cell carcinoma	Large, circumscribed masses
Predominant pattern/ injury type	*Acinar with minimal endocrine and ductal elements*
Immunohistochemistry	Trypsin, chymotrypsin, zymogen granules by EM.
Genetics	APC/β-catenin pathway
Differential	Pancreatoblastoma

Endocrine tumors

Functional	*Hormone-producing tumors: insulinoma, glucagonoma, gastrinoma, VIPoma.*
Insulin	Amyloid
Somatostatin	Psammoma bodies
Non-functional	*CD56, synaptophysin, chromogranin*

Associated syndromes

MEN-type I	Functional adenomas
Zollinger–Ellison	Gastrin-producing adenomas
Carney syndrome	Pheochromocytoma, pancreatic islet cell tumor
Von-Hippel Lindau	Islet cell tumor, cysts, pheochromocytoma

EM: electron microscopy; PR: progesterone receptors; APC: adenomatous polyposis coli

Histology: Grossly, SPNs are usually large, well-circumscribed masses, histologically containing papillary, microcystic, and solid structures, and a uniform population of cells with nuclear grooves and intra-cytoplasmic hyaline globules (Figure 3.8A–D).

Foamy cells and cholesterol clefts can be also identified. A clear-cell variant of SPN of the pancreas has been reported (192). Ultrastructural studies show two cell types, one with large oval nuclei, little-changed mitochondria, and short fragments of granular cytoplasmic reticulum, mainly forming pseudopapillary structures around the vessels. A second cell type is characterized by pronounced nuclear polymorphism with characteristic "coffee bean" morphology (193) and cytoplasm containing large mitochondria with clarified matrix, and often lipofuscin granules. The tumor cells show positive nuclear stain for β-catenin and progesterone receptor, cytoplasmic positivity for CD10, CD56, and vimentin, an intracytoplasmic dot-like immunoreactivity of CD99, and loss of membranous expression of E-cadherin with aberrant nuclear localization of the cytoplasmic domain (194).

Genetics: Solid-pseudopapillary tumors contain few genetic alterations, always including mutations of the CTNNB1/β-catenin gene (Figure 3.8D; 195).

Differential diagnosis: The SPN is the most common cystic neoplasm of the pancreas; however, cystic neuroendocrine neoplasms, cystic degeneration of otherwise solid neoplasms, and exceedingly rare cystic acinar cell neoplasms and lymphoepithelial cysts, should be included in the differential diagnosis (196). Pancreatoblastoma with a cystic component should also be considered when dealing with younger children (185–187).

Pancreatoblastoma

Definition: Pancreatoblastoma (PB) is a very rare childhood tumor originating from the epithelial exocrine cells of the pancreas (189,197,198). Pancreatoblastoma is an embryonal tumor that morphologically resembles the developing embryonic pancreas during the eighth week of development (197). Its incidence is 0.4% among all age groups within the United States (199), but the most common malignant pancreatic tumor in young children under 10 years old (199). Female gender predilection has been demonstrated in some studies, whereas others show no relevant gender-related differences (199). Scarce case reports of PB have been published occurring in the adult population, showing a worse prognosis (200).

Clinical features: The clinical symptomatology includes abdominal pain and discomfort (197). Elevated serum AFP levels are noted in the majority of cases (201). A large, heterogeneous pancreatic mass with calcifications in a young child should always raise

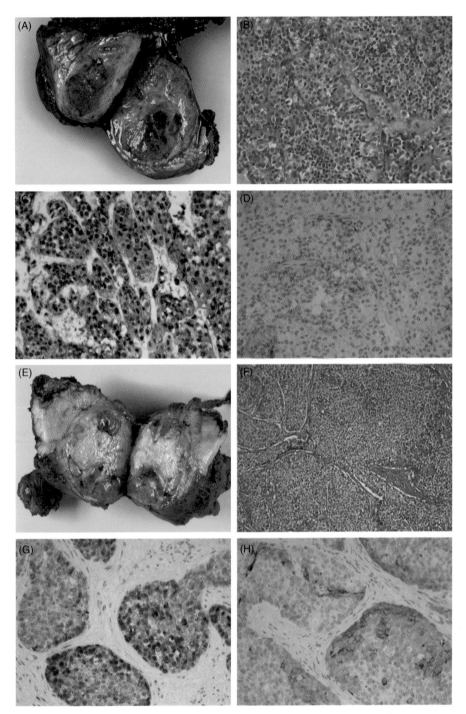

Figure 3.8 Pancreatic tumors seen in children. (A–D) Solid-pseudopapillary tumor. (A) Grossly, the tumor appears as a large solid, with necrotic and hemorrhagic zones. (B) Histologically, the tumor is characterized by solid areas alternating with pseudopapillary structures around the vessel. (C–D) The tumor cells show positive nuclear stain for β-catenin (C) and cytoplasmic positivity for CD56 (D). (E–H) Pancreatoblastoma. (E) The gross appearance shows a well-encapsulated tan to yellow, soft tumor located in the head of the pancreas. (F) Microscopically, the tumor is composed of solid cellular nests separated by dense, stromal bands. The characteristic squamoid corpuscles were not identified in this case. (G) β-catenin is diffusely positive in a nuclear pattern. (H) CEA shows positive membranous stain. Polymerase chain reaction and sequencing of exon 3 of the CTNNB1 gene demonstrate the presence of a codon 33 mutation.

suspicion for PB. Lymph node, liver, lungs, and spleen metastases may be present. Complete surgical resection is the goal of therapy, although many patients are unresectable at diagnosis and require neoadjuvant chemotherapy with good results (188).

Histology: Pancreatoblastoma is most often located in the head or body of the pancreas (201). Grossly, these are well-encapsulated, often large, soft tumors that can extend beyond the pancreatic gland (Figure 3.8E–H). Histology characteristically shows a highly cellular tumor with an epithelial and a mesenchymal component. The epithelial component shows cells arranged in solid sheets and small acini, divided into nodules by a cellular mesenchymal spindle-cell component. The presence of squamoid corpuscles with a morular appearance is the most characteristic feature of this tumor. PBs can also contain both endocrine and exocrine cells, with acinar differentiation being the most prevalent feature (201). Immunohistochemical staining shows a coarsely granular apical cytoplasmic staining for trypsin and chymotrypsin in the acini epithelial component, and zymogen granules by electron microscopy (198,202). The squamoid corpuscles with a morular appearance are positive for cytokeratin, whereas the solid and acinar components of the tumor are negative. Cytokeratin AE1/3 and carcinoembryonic antigen have been shown to be positive in the majority of the cases, and α-fetoprotein can be demonstrated in a few cases. Rarely, positivity for neuron-specific enolase, chromogranin A, and synaptophysin is also seen.

Genetics: Most PB cases are sporadic, but congenital cases have been described in association with Beckwith–Wiedemann syndrome (203), PB often occur with point mutations of the β-catenin gene (Figure 3.8F,G), indicating the relevance of Wnt signaling pathway activation in PB tumorigenesis (204).

Differential diagnosis: The differential diagnosis of PB includes acinar cell carcinoma and neuroendocrine tumors (198,202). Immunohistochemical stains have been useful; however, given the morphological immunophenotypical overlap between PB and acinar cell carcinoma, it may represent a diagnostic challenge in the pediatric population.

Acinar cell carcinoma

Definition: Acinar cell carcinoma (ACC) of the pancreas is the rarest primary epithelial tumor of the pancreas, accounting for 1–2% of all pancreatic tumors (205). These are carcinomas exhibiting evidence of pancreatic enzyme production by neoplastic cells, with endocrine and ductal components not exceeding 25% of the neoplastic cells (206). Because of its rarity, many clinicopathologic characteristics remain to be further elucidated, and prognostic factors are yet to be well established.

Clinical features: Acinar cell carcinomas occur more often in adults between the 5th and 7th decades of life, carrying a better prognosis in children. In a series of children with exocrine pancreatic tumors, the rates of metastases at presentation in the cases with ACCs were around 75% with a median survival time of 32 months (205). Clinical symptoms vary from abdominal discomfort to palpable masses and the serum AFP levels are usually high in all patients (204).

Macroscopic features: The tumors are relatively circumscribed, large and solid with a fleshy cut surface, with occasionally extensive hemorrhage and necrosis. Some tumors show cystic degeneration and a rare case of acinar cell cystoadenoma has been reported (207).

Histology: The tumors are very cellular and characteristically lack a desmoplastic stroma. Acinar, solid, trabecular, and glandular patterns of growth have been identified and individual tumors are usually mixed (204). Nuclei are round to oval, with minimal pleomorphism and single prominent nucleoli. Overall, the cytoplasm is moderately abundant, eosinophilic, and granular, but in solid, highly cellular tumors scarce cytoplasm can be found. Mitotic activity is variable. Features associated with poor prognosis include size, lymph node and distant metastases, and clinical stage (188). In addition, vascular and perineural invasion have been shown to be associated with poor prognosis (205). The tumoral cells are positive for keratins, BCL10, α-fetal protein, and the pancreatic enzymes lipase, chymotrypsin, and trypsin (208). Periodic acid–Schiff is positive in the cytoplasmic granules, which are resistant to treatment with diastases. CAM 5.2 is present in acini cells, however there is no labeling for AE1 antibody, nor with antibodies against cytokeratins 7, 19, and 20. Electron microscopy has demonstrated zymogen granules, as well as isolated dense core granules (209). BCL10 and trypsin have been shown to be more reliable immunohistochemical markers than amylase and lipase (210).

Genetics: Allelic losses on chromosome 11p and mutations in the APC/β-catenin signaling pathway has been demonstrated in ACCs, similarly to that described for pancreatoblastoma (204,211)

117

Differential diagnosis: The morphological, immunohistochemical, and clinical features of ACCs overlap with those of pancreatoblastoma (206,212); however, the presence of squamoid corpuscles favors pancreatoblastoma. Histologically, ACCs can also resemble islet cell tumors, but they differ in their ultrastructural and immunohistochemical features.

Neuroendocrine tumors

Neuroendocrine tumors of the pancreas are rare in children and have a larger histopathological diversity than in adults. They usually occur in the setting of genetic syndromes such as multiple endocrine neoplasia type 1, von Hippel–Lindau disease, and neurofibromatosis 1 (213). Rare cases have been reported in the setting of tuberous-sclerosis.

Clinical features: These tumors can be functional or non-functional. The functional neoplasms are associated with a clinical syndrome caused by the release of the endocrine hormone by the neoplasm and are divided into insulinomas, glucagonomas, gastrinomas, and vasoactive intestinal peptide secreting tumors (VIPomas). They usually occur in younger patients than the non-functional tumors (214). The paucity of cases reported in the literature, in addition to the lack of understanding of biologic behavior, has led to a lack of consensus concerning optimal management strategy. Presentation differs compared to adult counterparts and prognosis is generally better, even when lymph node metastases occur. Prognostic factors include size, large-vessel invasion, spread to lymph nodes, and metastasis (214).

Histology: Histologically, the tumors have a nested or trabecular pattern of growth, with cells showing uniform, salt and pepper nuclei. Amyloid deposition has been associated with insulin-producing neoplasms whereas psammoma bodies are more common in somatostatin-producing tumors (212). Immunohistochemical stains for chromogranin, synaptophysin, and CD56 are usually positive, with variable distribution in the tumor cells. Immunohistochemical stains for specific hormones help in the classification (212,186).

Differential diagnosis: The differential diagnosis is broad and includes solid pseudopapillary tumor, acinar cell carcinoma, and pancreatoblastoma. Nuclear labeling for β-catenin is useful in differentiating pseudopapillary tumor and pancreatoblastoma. The expression of pancreatic enzymes favors acinar cell carcinoma (212).

Pancreatic hamartoma

Pancreatic hamartomas are extremely rare tumors (215), with only few cases reported in the literature. The most common clinical presentation in children is a cystic abdominal mass and elevated pancreatic enzymes (215). Grossly, the tumor is composed of cystic and solid components, and the microscopic findings include numerous variably sized, dilated ducts lined by tall columnar mucinous cells surrounded by a stroma that exhibits foci of cellular condensations resembling primitive pancreatic mesenchyme. Acinar and endocrine cells are often seen budding into the ducts (216). The differential diagnosis includes pancreatoblastoma, pancreatic pseudocyst, and lymphangioma.

Pancreatitis

The most common causes of acute pancreatitis in children include biliary disease, drug-induced pancreatitis, recurrent hereditary pancreatitis, and trauma. Pancreatitis is also seen in children with metabolic and multisystemic disorders (217,218) and is idiopathic in over 30% of cases diagnosed.

Acknowledgement

Some of the artwork in this chapter was prepared by Mr. Michael Todd, Department of Histopathology, Audiovision, St. James University Hospital, Leeds, UK

References

1. Lipp W. The early structural development of the liver parenchyma in man. Z. Mikrosk. Anat. Forsch. 1952;59(1–3):161–86.

2. Shiojiri N. Development and differentiation of bile ducts in the mammalian liver. Microsc. Res. Tech. 1997;39(4):328–35.

3. Ruchelli ED Jr. Russo P, Ruchelli E and Picolli DA, Editors. Pathology of Pediatric Gastrointestinal and Liver Disease, Springer, 2004. 192.

4. Cleveland MH, Sawyer JM, Afelik S, Jensen J, Leach SD. Exocrine ontogenies: on the development of pancreatic acinar, ductal and centroacinar cells. Semin. Cell Dev. Biol. 2012;23(6):711–9.

5. Landsman L, Whitchurch TJ, Vanderlaan RL, *et al.* Pancreatic mesenchyme regulates epithelial organogenesis throughout development. PLoS Biol. 2011; 9(9):e1001143.

6. Rieck S BE, Wright CV. Lineage determinants in early endocrine development. Semin. Cell. Dev. Biol. 2012;23(6):673–84.

7. Rappaport AM, Borowy ZJ, Lougheed WM, Lotto WN. Subdivision of hexagonal liver lobules into a structural and functional unit; role in hepatic physiology and pathology. Anat. Rec. 1954;**119**(1):11–33.

8. Keiding S. Bringing physiology into PET of the liver. J. Nucl. Med. 2012;**53**(3):425–33.

9. Byrne JA, Meara NJ, Rayner AC, Thompson RJ, Knisely AS. Lack of hepatocellular CD10 along bile canaliculi is physiologic in early childhood and persistent in Alagille syndrome. Lab. Invest. 2007;**87**(11):1138–48.

10. Skandalakis LJ RJJ, Gray SW, Skandalakis JE. Surgical embryology and anatomy of the pancreas. Surg. Clin. North Am. 1993;**73**(4):661–97.

11. Sue M CS, Dickson RC, Macalindong C, *et al.* Variation between centers in technique and guidelines for liver biopsy. Liver 1996;**16**(4):267–70.

12. Scoazec JY. Liver biopsy: which role in patient management? Ann. Pathol. 2010;**30**(6):464–9.

13. Lefkowitch JH. Hepatobiliary pathology. Curr. Opin. Gastroenterol. 2006;**22**(3):198–208.

14. Finn LS KA. Recommendations for handling of pediatric liver biopsy specimens. Semin. Diagn. Pathol. 1998;**15**(4):300–5.

15. Turányi E DK, Csomor J, Schaff Z, Paku S, Nagy P. Immunohistochemical classification of ductular reactions in human liver. Histopathology 2010;**57**(4):607–14.

16. Van Den Heuvel MC, Visser L, Muller M, *et al.* Expression of anti-OV6 antibody and anti-N-CAM antibody along the biliary line of normal and diseased human livers. Hepatopathology 2001;**33**(6):1387–93.

17. Yerushalmi B Sr, Narkewicz MR, Smith D, Ashmead JW, Wenger DA. Niemann-pick disease type C in neonatal cholestasis at a North American Center. J. Pediatr. Gastroenterol. Nutr. 2002;**35**(1):44–50.

18. Kurbegov AC, Haas JE, Mierau GW, *et al.* Biliary diversion for progressive familial intrahepatic cholestasis:improved liver morphology and bile acid profile. Gastroenterology 2003;**125**(4):1227–34.

19. Hughes JL BA, Poulos A. Establishment of a normal range of morphometric values for peroxisomes in paediatric liver. Virchows Arch. A Pathol. Anat. Histopathol. 1993;**423**(6):453–7.

20. Asher LV IB, Shrestha MP, Ticehurst J, Baze WB. Virus-like particles in the liver of a patient with fulminant hepatitis and antibody to hepatitis E virus. J. Med. Virol. 1990;**31**(3):229–33.

21. Ishak KG. Inherited metabolic diseases of the liver. Clin. Liver Dis. 2002;**6**(2):455–79.

22. Jevon GP, Dimmick JE. Histopathologic approach to metabolic liver disease: Part 1. Pediatr. Dev. Pathol. 1998;**1**(3):179–99.

23. Jevon GP, Dimmick JE. Histopathologic approach to metabolic liver disease: Part 2. Pediatr. Dev. Pathol. 1998;**1**(4):261–9.

24. Jevon GP, and Dimmick JE. Metabolic diseases in childhood. In: Russo P, Ruchelli E and Picolli DA, Editors, Pathology of Pediatric Gastrointestinal and Liver Disease, Springer 2004. 270–299.

25. de Bie P, Muller P, Wijmenga C, Klomp LW. Molecular pathogenesis of Wilson and Menkes disease: correlation of mutations with molecular defects and disease phenotypes. J. Med. Genet. 2007;**44**(11):673–88.

26. Ludwig J, McDonald GS, Dickson ER, Elveback LR, McCall JT. Copper stains and the syndrome of primary biliary cirrhosis. Evaluation of staining methods and their usefulness for diagnosis and trials of penicillamine treatment. Arch. Pathol. Lab. Med. 1979;**103**(9):467–70.

27. Muller-Hocker J, Meyer U, Wiebecke B, *et al.* Copper storage disease of the liver and chronic dietary copper intoxication in two further German infants mimicking Indian childhood cirrhosis. Pathol. Res. Pract. 1988;**183**(1):39–45.

28. Fairbanks KD, Tavill AS. Liver disease in α 1-antitrypsin deficiency: A review. Am. J. Gastroenterol. 2008;**103**(8):2136–41; quiz:42.

29. Goebel HH, Muller HD. Storage diseases: diagnostic position. Ultrastruct. Pathol. 2013;**37**(1):19–22.

30. de Duve C. Lysosomes revisited. Eur. J. Biochem. 1983;**137**(3):391–7.

31. Rutledge JC. Progressive neonatal liver failure due to type C Niemann–Pick disease. Pediatr. Pathol. 1989;**9**(6):779–84.

32. Bennett MJ, Hale DE, Coates PM, Stanley CA. Postmortem recognition of fatty acid oxidation disorders. Pediatr. Pathol. 1991;**11**(3):365–70.

33. Whitington PF. Neonatal hemochromatosis: A congenital alloimmune hepatitis. Semin. Liver Dis. 2007;**27**(3):243–50.

34. Jorgensen MJ. The ductal plate malformation. Acta Pathol. Microbiol. Scand. Suppl. 1977;(**257**):1–87.

35. Raynaud P, Tate J, Callens C, *et al.* A classification of ductal plate malformations based on distinct pathogenic mechanisms of biliary dysmorphogenesis. Hepatology 2011;**53**(6):1959–66.

36. Gunay-Aygun M. Liver and kidney disease in ciliopathies. Am. J. Med. Genet. C Semin. Med. Genet. 2009;**151C**(4):296–306.

37. Chandok N. Polycystic liver disease: A clinical review. Ann. Hepatol. 2012;**11**(6):819–26.

119

38. Bessho K, Bezerra JA. Biliary atresia: will blocking inflammation tame the disease? Annu. Rev. Med. 2011;**62**:171–85.

39. Jablonska B. Biliary cysts: etiology, diagnosis and management. World J. Gastroenterol. 2012;**18**(35):4801–10.

40. Todani T, Watanabe Y, Narusue M, Tabuchi K, Okajima K. Congenital bile duct cysts: Classification, operative procedures, and review of thirty-seven cases including cancer arising from choledochal cyst. Am. J. Surg. 1977;**134**(2):263–9.

41. Alonso-Lej F, Rever WB, Jr., Pessagno DJ. Congenital choledochal cyst, with a report of 2, and an analysis of 94, cases. Int. Abstr. Surg. 1959;**108**(1):1–30.

42. Debray D, Pariente D, Urvoas E, Hadchouel M, Bernard O. Sclerosing cholangitis in children. J. Pediatr. 1994;**124**(1):49–56.

43. Batres LA, Russo P, Mathews M, et al. Primary sclerosing cholangitis in children: A histologic follow-up study. Pediatr. Dev. Pathol. 2005;**8**(5):568–76.

44. Turnpenny PD, Ellard S. Alagille syndrome: pathogenesis, diagnosis and management. Eur. J. Hum. Genet. 2012;**20**(3):251–7.

45. Knöpfle G AA, Fischer HP. Cholestasis-associated hepatopathies in neonates and infants. Pathologe 2008;**29**(1):61–72.

46. Hadchouel M FM. Histologic diagnosis of neonatal cholestasis. Ann. Pathol. 1995;**15**(5):357–64.

47. Ovchinsky N MR, Lefkowitch JH, Lavine JE. Liver biopsy in modern clinical practice: A pediatric point-of-view. Adv. Anat. Pathol. 2012;**19**(4):250–62.

48. Nightingale S, Day AS, Webber MT, Ward KA, O'Loughlin EV. Chronic hepatitis B and C infection in children in New South Wales. Med. J. Aust. 2009;**190**(12):670–3.

49. Abdel-Hady M BS, Sira J, Brown RM, et al. Chronic hepatitis C in children – review of natural history at a National Centre. J. Viral Hepat. 2011;**18**(10):e535–40.

50. Congly SE SA, Meddings L, Kaplan GG, Myers RP. Amoebic liver abscess in USA: A population-based study of incidence, temporal trends and mortality. Liver Int. 2011;**31**(8):1191–8.

51. CDC Balamuthia mandrillaris transmitted through organ transplantation Mississippi, 2009. MMWR Morb. Mortal. Wkly Rep. 2010;**59**(36):1165–70.

52. Méchaï F, Ficko C, Barruet R, Imbert P, Rapp C. Budd-Chiari syndrome as a vascular complication of amebic liver abscess. Am. J. Trop. Med. Hyg. 2009;**81**(5):768–9.

53. Hakyemez IN AG, Savli H, Küçükbayrak A, Gürel S, Taş T. Fascioliasis Case: A not Rare Cause of Hypereosinophilia in Developing Countries, Present in

Developed too. Mediterr. J. Hematol. Infect. Dis. 2012;**4**(1):e2012029.

54. Treska V SA, Mukensnabl P, Manakova T, et al. Liver abscess in human toxocariasis. Bratisl. Lek. Listy. 2011;**112**(1):644–7.

55. Andrade ZA. Schistosomiasis and liver fibrosis. Parasite Immunol. 2009;**31**(11):656–63.

56. Abath FG, Montenegro CE, Wynn TA, Montenegro SM. Immunopathogenic mechanisms in schistosomiasis: what can be learnt from human studies? Trends Parasitol. 2006;**22**(1):85–91.

57. Yanagisawa S YT, Tanaka T. Clinical diagnosis of Schistosoma japonicum infection complicating infective endocarditis and liver cirrhosis. Intern. Med. 2010;**49**(11):1001–5.

58. Moedy JL, Lerman SJ, White RJ. Fatal disseminated herpes simplex virus infection in a healthy child. Am. J. Dis. Child. 1981;**135**(1):45–7.

59. Barton LL W-WS, Gutierrez JA, Lee DM. Herpes simplex virus hepatitis in a child: case report and review. Pediatr. Infect. Dis. J. 1999;**18**(11):1026–8.

60. Bedel AN, Hemmelgarn TS, Kohli R. Retrospective review of the incidence of cytomegalovirus infection and disease after liver transplantation in pediatric patients: comparison of prophylactic oral ganciclovir and oral valganciclovir. Liver Transpl. **18**(3):347–54.

61. Lautenschlager I HK, Jalanko H, et al. Persistent cytomegalovirus in liver allografts with chronic rejection. Hepatology 1997;**25**(1):190–4.

62. Bobić B NA, Radivojević SK, Klun I, Djurković-Djaković O. Echinococcosis in Serbia: An issue for the 21st century? Foodborne Pathog. Dis. 2012;**9**(11):967–73.

63. Djuricic SM GS, Kafka DI, et al. Cystic echinococcosis in children – the seventeen-year experience of two large medical centers in Serbia. Parasitol. Int. 2010;(**59**):257–61.

64. Hesse AA NA, Hassan HS, Hashish AA. Parasitic infestations requiring surgical interventions. Semin. Pediatr. Surg. 2012;**21**(2):142–50.

65. Oral A, YM, Demirci E, et al. A case of undifferentiated embryonic liver sarcoma mimicking cystic hydatid disease in an endemic region of the world. J. Pediatr. Surg. 2011;**46**(11):e5–9.

66. Mieli-Vergani G VD. Autoimmune hepatitis in children: what is different from adult AIH? Semin. Liver Dis. 2009;**29**(3):297–306.

67. Lefkowitch JH, Honig CL, King ME, Hagstrom JW. Hepatic copper overload and features of Indian childhood cirrhosis in an American sibship. N. Engl. J. Med. 1982;**307**(5):271–7.

68. Scheuer P. Childhood liver disease and metabolic disorders. In Lefkowitch J, editor, *Scheuer's Liver Biopsy Interpretation*, seventh edn. Amsterdam: Elsevier; 2005.

69. Lopez-Terrada D. Hepatoblastoma: new insights into the biology of embryonal tumors of the liver. In Mackinnon AC, editor, *Pediatric Neoplasia: Advances in Molecular Pathology and Translational Medicine, Molecular and Translational Medicine*. Milwaukee, IL: Humana Press; 2012:243–58.

70. Weinberg AG, Finegold MJ. Primary hepatic tumors of childhood. Hum. Pathol. 1983;**14**(6):512–37.

71. Ishak KG, ZD; Stocker JT. Hepatocellular carcinoma. In Ishak KG GZ, Stocker JT, editors, *Atlas of Tumor Pathology: Tumors of the Liver and Intrahepatic Bile Ducts*. Washington DC: Armed Forces Institute of Pathology; 1999:199–230.

72. Finegold MJ. Hepatic tumors in childhood. In Russo P, Ruchelli E, Piccoli DA, editors, *Pathology of Pediatric Gastrointestinal and Liver Disease*. New York: Springer Verlag; 2004.

73. Feusner J, Buckley J, Robison L, Ross J, Van Tornout J. Prematurity and hepatoblastoma: more than just an association? J. Pediatr. 1998;**133**(4):585–6.

74. National Cancer Institute Surveillance, Epidemiology and End Results (database on the Internet). http://seer.cancer.gov/ (accessed May 2014).

75. Stocker JT. *Hepatic Tumors in Children*, second edn, Balistrier W, editor. Philadelphia: Lippincott, Williams and Wilkins; 2001.

76. Lopez-Terrada D, Alaggio R, de Davila MT, *et al.* Towards an international pediatric liver tumor consensus classification: proceedings of the Los Angeles COG liver tumors symposium. Mod. Pathol. 2014;**27**(3):472–91.

77. Haas JE, Muczynski KA, Krailo M, *et al.* Histopathology and prognosis in childhood hepatoblastoma and hepatocarcinoma. Cancer 1989;**64**(5):1082–95.

78. Haas JE, Feusner JH, Finegold MJ. Small cell undifferentiated histology in hepatoblastoma may be unfavorable. Cancer 2001;**92**(12):3130–4.

79. Ortega JA, Douglass EC, Feusner JH, *et al.* Randomized comparison of cisplatin/vincristine/fluorouracil and cisplatin/continuous infusion doxorubicin for treatment of pediatric hepatoblastoma: a report from the Children's Cancer Group and the Pediatric Oncology Group. J. Clin. Oncol. 2000;**18**(14):2665–75.

80. Schneider NR, Cooley LD, Finegold MJ, Douglass EC, Tomlinson GE. The first recurring chromosome translocation in hepatoblastoma: der(4)t(1;4)(q12;q34). Genes Chromosomes Cancer 1997;**19**(4):291–4.

81. Yeh YA, Rao PH, Cigna CT, *et al.* Trisomy 1q, 2, and 20 in a case of hepatoblastoma: possible significance of 2q35-q37 and 1q12-q21 rearrangements. Cancer Genet. Cytogenet. 2000;**123**(2):140–3.

82. Tomlinson GE, Douglass EC, Pollock BH, Finegold MJ, Schneider NR. Cytogenetic evaluation of a large series of hepatoblastomas: numerical abnormalities with recurring aberrations involving 1q12-q21. Genes Chromosomes Cancer 2005;**44**(2):177–84.

83. Cairo S, Armengol C, De Reynies A, *et al.* Hepatic stem-like phenotype and interplay of Wnt/beta-catenin and Myc signaling in aggressive childhood liver cancer. Cancer Cell 2008;**14**(6):471–84.

84. Cairo S, Wang Y, de Reynies A, *et al.* Stem cell-like micro-RNA signature driven by Myc in aggressive liver cancer. Proc. Natl. Acad. Sci. USA 2010;**107**(47):20471–6.

85. Darbari A, Sabin KM, Shapiro CN, Schwarz KB. Epidemiology of primary hepatic malignancies in U.S. children. Hepatology 2003;**38**(3):560–6.

86. Ishak KG, Glunz PR. Hepatoblastoma and hepatocarcinoma in infancy and childhood. Report of 47 cases. Cancer 1967;**20**(3):396–422.

87. Bellani FF, Massimino M. Liver tumors in childhood: epidemiology and clinics. J. Surg. Oncol.. Suppl. 1993;**3**:119–21.

88. Moore SW, Hesseling PB, Wessels G, Schneider JW. Hepatocellular carcinoma in children. Pediatr. *Surg Int.* 1997;**12**(4):266–70.

89. Weinberg AG, Mize CE, Worthen HG. The occurrence of hepatoma in the chronic form of hereditary tyrosinemia. J. Pediatr. 1976;**88**(3):434–8.

90. Demers SI, Russo P, Lettre F, Tanguay RM. Frequent mutation reversion inversely correlates with clinical severity in a genetic liver disease, hereditary tyrosinemia. Hum. Pathol. 2003;**34**(12):1313–20.

91. Coire CI, Qizilbash AH, Castelli MF. Hepatic adenomata in type Ia glycogen storage disease. Arch. Pathol. Lab. Med. 1987;**111**(2):166–9.

92. Bianchi L. Glycogen storage disease I and hepatocellular tumours. Eur. J. Pediatr. 1993;**152** Suppl 1:S63–70.

93. Kingston JE, Draper GJ, Mann JR. Hepatoblastoma and polyposis coli. Lancet 1982;**1**(8269):457.

94. Giardiello FM, Petersen GM, Brensinger JD, *et al.* Hepatoblastoma and APC gene mutation in familial adenomatous polyposis. Gut 1996;**39**(96):867–9.

95. Ettinger LJ, Freeman AI. Hepatoma in a child with neurofibromatosis. Am. J. Dis. Child. 1979;**133**(5):528–31.

96. Weinstein S, Scottolini AG, Loo SY, Caldwell PC, Bhagavan NV. Ataxia telangiectasia with hepatocellular carcinoma in a 15-year-old girl and studies of her kindred. Arch. Pathol. Lab. Med. 1985;**109**(11):1000–4.

97. Geoffroy-Perez B, Janin N, Ossian K, *et al.* Cancer risk in heterozygotes for ataxia-telangiectasia. Int. J. Cancer 2001;**93**(2):288–93.

98. Ucar C, Caliskan U, Toy H, Gunel E. Hepatoblastoma in a child with neurofibromatosis type I. Pediatr. Blood Cancer 2007;**49**(3):357–9.

99. Abbondanzo SL, Manz HJ, Klappenbach RS, Gootenberg JE. Hepatocellular carcinoma in an 11-year-old girl with Fanconi's anemia. Report of a case and review of the literature. Am. J. Pediatr. Hematol. Oncol. 1986;**8**(4):334–7.

100. Vileisis RA, Sorensen K, Gonzalez-Crussi F, Hunt CE. Liver malignancy after parenteral nutrition. J. Pediatr. 1982;**100**(1):88–90.

101. Rabinovitz M, Imperial JC, Schade RR, Van Thiel DH. Hepatocellular carcinoma in Alagille's syndrome: A family study. J. Pediatr. Gastroenterol. Nutr. 1989;**8**(1):26–30.

102. Taat F, Bosman DK, Aronson DC. Hepatoblastoma in a girl with biliary atresia: coincidence or co-incidence. Pediatr. Blood Cancer 2004;**43**(5):603–5.

103. Katzenstein HM, Krailo MD, Malogolowkin MH *et al.* Hepatocellular carcinoma in children and adolescents: results from the Pediatric Oncology Group and the Children's Cancer Group intergroup study. J. Clin. Oncol. 2002;**20**(12):2789–97.

104. Farhi DC, Shikes RH, Murari PJ, Silverberg SG. Hepatocellular carcinoma in young people. Cancer 1983;**52**(8):1516–25.

105. Hirohashi S IK. Tumours of the liver and intrahepatic bile ducts. In Hanmilton Sr AL, editor, *Pathology and Genetics of Tumours of the Digestive System.* Lyon: IARC Press; 2000.

106. Edmondson HA, Steiner PE. Primary carcinoma of the liver: A study of 100 cases among 48,900 necropsies. Cancer 1954;**7**(3):462–503.

107. Torfs CP, Christianson RE. Anomalies in Down syndrome individuals in a large population-based registry. Am. J. Med. Genet. 1998;**77**(5):431–8.

108. El-Serag HB, Davila JA, Petersen NJ, McGlynn KA. The continuing increase in the incidence of hepatocellular carcinoma in the United States: An update. Ann. Intern. Med. 2003;**139**(10):817–23.

109. Katzenstein HM, Krailo MD, Malogolowkin MH, *et al.* Fibrolamellar hepatocellular carcinoma in children and adolescents. Cancer 2003;**97**(8):2006–12.

110. Capurro M, Wanless IR, Sherman M *et al.* Glypican-3: A novel serum and histochemical marker for hepatocellular carcinoma. Gastroenterology 2003;**125**(1):89–97.

111. Wu PC, Fang JW, Lau VK *et al.* Classification of hepatocellular carcinoma according to hepatocellular and biliary differentiation markers. Clinical and biological implications. Am. J. Pathol. 1996;**149**(4):1167–75.

112. Varma V, Cohen C. Immunohistochemical and molecular markers in the diagnosis of hepatocellular carcinoma. Adv. Anat. Pathol. 2004;**11**(5):239–49.

113. Libbrecht L, De Vos R, Cassiman D *et al.* Hepatic progenitor cells in hepatocellular adenomas. Am. J. Surg. Pathol. 2001;**25**(11):1388–96.

114. Gouysse G, Frachon S, Hervieu V *et al.* Endothelial cell differentiation in hepatocellular adenomas: implications for histopathological diagnosis. J. Hepatol. 2004;**41**(2):259–66.

115. Wong N, Lai P, Pang E, *et al.* A comprehensive karyotypic study on human hepatocellular carcinoma by spectral karyotyping. Hepatology 2000;**32**(5):1060–8.

116. Kakar S, Chen X, Ho C, Burgart LJ, *et al.* Chromosomal changes in fibrolamellar hepatocellular carcinoma detected by array comparative genomic hybridization. Mod. Pathol. 2009;**22**(1):134–41.

117. Anders RA, Yerian LM, Tretiakova M, *et al.* cDNA microarray analysis of macroregenerative and dysplastic nodules in end-stage hepatitis C virus-induced cirrhosis. Am. J. Pathol. 2003;**162**(3):991–1000.

118. Lee TH, Tai DI, Cheng CJ, *et al.* Enhanced nuclear factor-kappa B-associated Wnt-1 expression in hepatitis B- and C-related hepatocarcinogenesis: identification by functional proteomics. J. Biomed. Sci. 2006;**13**(1):27–39.

119. Graveel CR, Jatkoe T, Madore SJ, Holt AL, Farnham PJ. Expression profiling and identification of novel genes in hepatocellular carcinomas. Oncogene 2001;**20**(21):2704–12.

120. Okabe H, Satoh S, Kato T, *et al.* Genome-wide analysis of gene expression in human hepatocellular carcinomas using cDNA microarray: identification of genes involved in viral carcinogenesis and tumor progression. Cancer Res. 2001;**61**(5):2129–37.

121. Lee JS, Chu IS, Heo J, *et al.* Classification and prediction of survival in hepatocellular carcinoma by gene expression profiling. Hepatology 2004;**40**(3):667–76.

122. Prokurat A, Kluge P, Kosciesza A, *et al.* Transitional liver cell tumors (TLCT) in older children and adolescents: A novel group of aggressive hepatic tumors expressing beta-catenin. Med. Pediatr. Oncol. 2002;**39**(5):510–8.

123. Bioulac-Sage P, Laumonier H, Couchy G, *et al.* Hepatocellular adenoma management and phenotypic classification: the Bordeaux experience. Hepatology 2009;**50**(2):481–9.

124. Bouyn CI, Leclere J, Raimondo G, *et al.* Hepatic focal nodular hyperplasia in children previously treated for a solid tumor. Incidence, risk factors, and outcome. Cancer 2003;**97**(12):3107–13.

125. Heerema-McKenney A, Leuschner I, Smith N, Sennesh J, Finegold MJ. Nested stromal epithelial tumor of the liver: six cases of a distinctive pediatric neoplasm with frequent calcifications and association with cushing syndrome. Am. J. Surg. Pathol. 2005;**29**(1):10–20.

126. Rod A, Voicu M, Chiche L, *et al.* Cushing's syndrome associated with a nested stromal epithelial tumor of the liver: hormonal, immunohistochemical, and molecular studies. Eur. J. Endocrinol. 2009;**161**(5):805–10.

127. Hill DA, Swanson PE, Anderson K, *et al.* Desmoplastic nested spindle cell tumor of liver: report of four cases of a proposed new entity. Am. J. Surg. Pathol. 2005;**29** (1):1–9.

128. Brodsky SV, Sandoval C, Sharma N, *et al.* Recurrent nested stromal epithelial tumor of the liver with extrahepatic metastasis: case report and review of literature. Pediatr. Dev. Pathol. 2008;**11**(6):469–73.

129. Rajaram V, Knezevich S, Bove KE, Perry A, Pfeifer JD. DNA sequence of the translocation breakpoints in undifferentiated embryonal sarcoma arising in mesenchymal hamartoma of the liver harboring the t (11;19)(q11;q13.4) translocation. Genes Chromosomes Cancer 2007;**46**(5):508–13.

130. Shehata BM, Gupta NA, Katzenstein HM, *et al.* Undifferentiated embryonal sarcoma of the liver is associated with mesenchymal hamartoma and multiple chromosomal abnormalities: A review of eleven cases. Pediatr. Dev. Pathol. 2011;**14**(2):111–6.

131. Lopez-Terrada D, Finegold MJ. Tumors of the liver. In Suchy F, Sokol RJ, Balistreri WF, editors, *Liver Disease in Children*. New York: Cambridge University Press; 2014.

132. Cajaiba MM, Sarita-Reyes C, Zambrano E, Reyes-Mugica M. Mesenchymal hamartoma of the liver associated with features of Beckwith-Wiedemann syndrome and high serum α-fetoprotein levels. Pediatr. Dev. Pathol. 2007;**10**(3):233–8.

133. Dehner LP, Ishak KG. Vascular tumors of the liver in infants and children. A study of 30 cases and review of the literature. Arch. Pathol. 1971;**92**(2):101–11.

134. Walter JW, North PE, Waner M, *et al.* Somatic mutation of vascular endothelial growth factor receptors in juvenile hemangioma. Genes Chromosomes Cancer 2002;**33**(3):295–303.

135. Hadzic N, Finegold MJ. Liver neoplasia in children. Clin. Liver Dis. 2011;**15**(2):443–62.

136. Mo JQ, Dimashkieh HH, Bove KE. GLUT1 endothelial reactivity distinguishes hepatic infantile hemangioma from congenital hepatic vascular malformation with associated capillary proliferation. Hum. Pathol. 2004;**35**(2):200–9.

137. McCarville MB, Kao SC. Imaging recommendations for malignant liver neoplasms in children. Pediatr. Blood Cancer 2006;**46**(1):2–7.

138. Errani C, Zhang L, Panicek DM, Healey JH, Antonescu CR. Epithelioid hemangioma of bone and soft tissue: A reappraisal of a controversial entity. Clin. Orthop. Relat. Res. 2011;**470**(5):1498–506.

139. Bale PP, RE; Stevens, MM. Pathology and behavior of juvenile rhabdomyosarcoma In Finegold M, editor, *Pathology of Neoplasia in Children and Adolescents*. Philadelphia, PA: WB Saunders; 1986:196–222.

140. Russo P, Biegel JA. SMARCB1/INI1 alterations and hepatoblastoma: Another extrarenal rhabdoid tumor revealed? Pediatr. Blood Cancer 2009;**52**(3):312–3.

141. Conrad RJ, Gribbin D, Walker NI, Ong TH. Combined cystic teratoma and hepatoblastoma of the liver. Probable divergent differentiation of an uncommitted hepatic precursor cell. Cancer 1993;**72**(10):2910–3.

142. Barsky SH, Linnoila I, Triche TJ, Costa J. Hepatocellular carcinoma with carcinoid features. Hum. Pathol. 1984;**15**(9):892–4.

143. Ruck P, Harms D, Kaiserling E. Neuroendocrine differentiation in hepatoblastoma. An immunohistochemical investigation. Am. J. Surg. Pathol. 1990;**14**(9):847–55.

144. Mann JR, Kasthuri N, Raafat F, *et al.* Malignant hepatic tumours in children: incidence, clinical features and aetiology. Paediatr. Perinat. Epidemiol. 1990;**4**(3):276–89.

145. Kaplan KJ, Goodman ZD, Ishak KG. Liver involvement in Langerhans' cell histiocytosis: A study of nine cases. Mod. Pathol. 1999;**12**(4):370–8.

146. Filipovich AH. Hemophagocytic lymphohistiocytosis and related disorders. Curr. Opin. Allergy Clin. Immunol. 2006;**6**(6):410–5.

147. Banff schema for grading liver allograft rejection: An international consensus document. Hepatology 1997;**57**(9):2248–66.

148. Rosenthal P EJ, Heyman MB, Snyder J, *et al.* Pathological changes in yearly protocol liver biopsy specimens from healthy pediatric liver recipients. Liver Transpl. Surg. 1997;**3**(6):559–62.

149. Sundaram SS, Melin-Aldana H, Neighbors K, Alonso EM. Histologic characteristics of late cellular rejection, significance of centrilobular injury, and long-term outcome in pediatric liver transplant recipients. Liver Transpl. 2006;**12**(1):58–64.

150. Inomata Y TK. Pathogenesis and treatment of bile duct loss after liver transplantation. J. Hepatobiliary Pancreat. Surg. 2001;**8**(4):316–22.

151. Gotthardt D RC, Weiss KH, Encke J, *et al.* Fulminant hepatic failure: etiology and indications for liver transplantation. Nephrol. Dial. Transplant. 2007;**22**(8):5–8.

152. Faust TW. Recurrent primary biliary cirrhosis, primary sclerosing cholangitis, and autoimmune hepatitis after transplantation. Semin. Liver Dis. 2000;**20**(4):481–95.

153. Czaja AJ. Diagnosis, pathogenesis, and treatment of autoimmune hepatitis after liver transplantation. Dig. Dis. Sci. 2012;**57**(9):2248–66.

154. Alisi A, Feldstein AE, Villani A, Raponi M, Nobili V. Pediatric nonalcoholic fatty liver disease: A multidisciplinary approach. Nat. Rev. Gastroenterol. Hepatol. 2012;**9**(3):152–61.

155. Day CP. Clinical spectrum and therapy of non-alcoholic steatohepatitis. Dig. Dis. 2012;**30** Suppl 1:69–73.

156. Pinzani M. Pathophysiology of non-alcoholic steatohepatitis and basis for treatment. Dig. Dis. 2011;**29**(2):243–8.

157. Alisi A, Carpino G, Nobili V. Paediatric nonalcoholic fatty liver disease. Curr. Opin. Gastroenterol. 2013;**29**(3):279–84.

158 Tannapfel A, Denk H, Dienes HP, *et al.* Histopathological diagnosis of non-alcoholic and alcoholic fatty liver disease. Virchows Arch. 2011;**458**(5):511–23.

159. Nobili V, Svegliati Baroni G, Alisi A, *et al.* A 360-degree overview of paediatric NAFLD: Recent insights. J. Hepatol. 2012;**58**(6):1218–29.

160. Joo YE, Kang HC, Kim HS, *et al.* Agenesis of the dorsal pancreas: A case report and review of the literature. Korean J. Intern. Med. 2006;**21**(4):236–9.

161. Lang K, Lasson A, Muller MF, *et al.* Dorsal agenesis of the pancreas – a rare cause of abdominal pain and insulin-dependent diabetes. Acta Radiol. **53**(1):2–4.

162. Xuan S, Borok MJ, Decker KJ, *et al.* Pancreas-specific deletion of mouse Gata4 and Gata6 causes pancreatic agenesis. J. Clin. Invest. 2012;**122**(10):3516–28.

163. Ginsburg M, Ahmed O, Rana KA, *et al.* Ectopic pancreas presenting with pancreatitis and a mesenteric mass. J. Pediatr. Surg. 2013;**48**(1):e29–32.

164. Fukino N, Oida T, Mimatsu K, *et al.* Diffuse Peritonitis due to Perforated Gastric Ectopic Pancreas. Case Rep. Gastroenterol. 2012;**6**(3):689–94.

165. Szabados S, Lenard L, Tornoczky T, Varady E, Verzar Z. Ectopic pancreas tissue appearing in a mediastinal cyst. J. Cardiothorac. Surg. 7:22.

166. Pansini M, Magerkurth O, Haecker FM, Sesia SB. Annular pancreas associated with duodenal obstruction. BMJ. Case Rep. 2012;2012.

167. Etienne D, John A, Menias CO, *et al.* Annular pancreas: A review of its molecular embryology, genetic basis and clinical considerations. Ann. Anat. 2012;**194**(5):422–8.

168. Antonarakis SE, Lyle R, Dermitzakis ET, Reymond A, Deutsch S. Chromosome 21 and down syndrome: from genomics to pathophysiology. Nat. Rev. Genet. 2004;**5**(10):725–38.

169. Auringer ST, Ulmer JL, Sumner TE, Turner CS. Congenital cyst of the pancreas. J. Pediatr. Surg. 1993;**28**(12):1570–1.

170. Boulanger SC, Borowitz DS, Fisher JF, Brisseau GF. Congenital pancreatic cysts in children. J. Pediatr. Surg. 2003;**38**(7):1080–2.

171. Stringer MD, Davison SM, McClean P, *et al.* Multidisciplinary management of surgical disorders of the pancreas in childhood. J. Pediatr. Gastroenterol. Nutr. 2005;**40**(3):363–7.

172. Cabrera R, Otero H, Blesa E, Jimenez C, Nunez R. (Pancreatic pseudocyst. Review of 22 cases). Cir. Pediatr. 1997;**10**(2):49–53.

173. Houben CH, Ade-Ajayi N, Patel S, *et al.* Traumatic pancreatic duct injury in children: minimally invasive approach to management. J. Pediatr. Surg. 2007;**42**(4):629–35.

174. Edelman A, Saussereau E. (Cystic fibrosis and other channelopathies). Arch. Pediatr. 2012;**19** Suppl 1: S13–6.

175. Wiehe M, Arndt K. Cystic fibrosis: A systems review. AANA J. 2010;**78**(3):246–51.

176. Zairat'iants OV, Miagkova LP, Podymova SD, Mel'nichenko GA, Burmakin IuA. Congenital hypoplasia of the pancreas with lipomatosis and bone marrow dysfunction (Shwachman syndrome). Arkh. Patol. 1991;**53**(7):71–4.

177. Myers KC, Davies SM, Shimamura A. Clinical and molecular pathophysiology of Shwachman-Diamond syndrome: An update. Hematol. Oncol.. Clin. North. Am. 2013;**27**(1):117–28, ix.

178. Michels VV, Donovan GK. Shwachman syndrome: unusual presentation as asphyxiating thoracic dystrophy. Birth Defects Orig. Artic. Ser. 1982;**18**(3B):129–34.

179. Durie PR. Inherited and congenital disorders of the exocrine pancreas. Gastroenterologist 1996;**4**(3):169–87.

180. Schneider K, Harms K, Fendel H. The increased echogenicity of the pancreas in infants and children: the white pancreas. Eur. J. Pediatr. 1987;**146**(5):508–11.

181. Manea EM, Leverger G, Bellmann F, *et al.* Pearson syndrome in the neonatal period: two case reports and review of the literature. J. Pediatr. Hematol. Oncol. 2009;**31**(12):947–51.

182. Williams TB, Daniels M, Puthenveetil G, *et al.* Pearson syndrome: unique endocrine manifestations including neonatal diabetes and adrenal insufficiency. Mol. Genet. Metab. **106**(1):104–7.

183. Rezaei N, Sabbaghian M, Liu Z, Zenker M. Eponym: Johanson–Blizzard syndrome. Eur. J. Pediatr. 2010;**170** (2):179–83.

184. Luttges J. What's new? The 2010 WHO classification for tumours of the pancreas. Pathologe 2011;**32** Suppl 2:332–6.

185. Ansari D, Elebro J, Tingstedt B, *et al.* Single-institution experience with solid pseudopapillary neoplasm of the pancreas. Scand. J. Gastroenterol. 2011;**46**(12):1492–7.

186. Rojas Y, Warneke CL, Dhamne CA, *et al.* Primary malignant pancreatic neoplasms in children and adolescents: A 20 year experience. J. Pediatr. Surg. 2012;**47**(12):2199–204.

187. Sakorafas GH, Smyrniotis V, Reid-Lombardo KM, Sarr MG. Primary pancreatic cystic neoplasms of the pancreas revisited. Part IV: rare cystic neoplasms. Surg. Oncol. 2012;**21**(3):153–63.

188. Perez EA, Gutierrez JC, Koniaris LG, *et al.* Malignant pancreatic tumors: incidence and outcome in 58 pediatric patients. J. Pediatr. Surg. 2009;**44**(1):197–203.

189. Stoica-Mustafa E, Pechianu C, Iorgescu A, *et al.* Pathological characteristics and clinical specifications in gastroenteropancreatic neuroendocrine tumors: A study of 68 cases. Rom. J. Morphol. Embryol. 2012;**53**(2):351–5.

190. Bouassida M, Mighri MM, Bacha D, *et al.* Solid pseudopapillary neoplasm of the pancreas in an old man: Age does not matter. Pan. Afr. Med. J. 2012;**13**:8–.

191. Nasit JG, Jetly D, Shah M. Solid pseudopapillary tumor of pancreas in a male child: a diagnosis by fine needle aspiration cytology. Fetal Pediatr. Pathol. 2013;**32**(4):265–70.

192. Tanino M, Kohsaka S, Kimura T, *et al.* A case of clear cell variant of solid-pseudopapillary tumor of the pancreas in an adult male patient. Ann. Diagn. Pathol. 2012;**16**(2):134–40.

193. Vtyurin BV, Chekmaryova IA, Dubova EA, Podgornova MN, Shchegolev AI. Ultrastructural characteristics of solid pseudopapillary tumors of the pancreas. Bull. Exp. Biol. Med. **151**(2):230–3.

194. Nguyen NQ, Johns AL, Gill AJ, *et al.* Clinical and immunohistochemical features of 34 solid pseudopapillary tumors of the pancreas. J. Gastroenterol. Hepatol. 2011;**26**(2):267–74.

195. Wu J, Jiao Y, Dal Molin M, *et al.* Whole-exome sequencing of neoplastic cysts of the pancreas reveals recurrent mutations in components of ubiquitin-dependent pathways. Proc. Natl. Acad. Sci. USA 2011;**108**(52):21188–93.1

196. Igbinosa O. Pseudopapillary tumor of the pancreas. An algorithmic approach. JOP. 2011;**12**(3):262–5.

197. Defachelles A-S, Rocourt N, Branchereau S, Peuchmaur M. Pancreatoblastoma in children: diagnosis and therapeutic management. Bull. Cancer 2012;**99**(7–8):793–9.

198. Balasundaram C, Luthra M, Chavalitdhamrong D, *et al.* Pancreatoblastoma: A rare tumor still evolving in clinical presentation and histology. JOP 2012;**13**(3):301–3.

199. Bien E, Godzinski J, Dall'igna P, *et al.* Pancreatoblastoma: A report from the European cooperative study group for paediatric rare tumours (EXPeRT). Eur. J. Cancer. 2011;**47**(15):2347–52.

200. Cavallini A, Falconi M, Bortesi L, *et al.* Pancreatoblastoma in adults: A review of the literature. Pancreatology 2009;**9**(1–2):73–80.

201. Xu C, Zhong L, Wang Y, *et al.* Clinical analysis of childhood pancreatoblastoma arising from the tail of the pancreas. J. Pediatr. Hematol. Oncol. 2012;**34** (5):177–81.

202. Sigel CS, Klimstra DS. Cytomorphologic and immunophenotypical features of acinar cell neoplasms of the pancreas. Cancer Cytopathol. 2013.

203. Glick RD, Pashankar FD, Pappo A, Laquaglia MP. Management of pancreatoblastoma in children and young adults. J. Pediatr. Hematol. Oncol. 2012;**34** Suppl 2:S47–50.

204. Park M, Koh KN, Kim BE, *et al.* Pancreatic neoplasms in childhood and adolescence. J. Pediatr. Hematol. Oncol. 2011;**33**(4):295–300.

205. Ellerkamp V, Warmann SW, Vorwerk P, Leuschner I, Fuchs J. Exocrine pancreatic tumors in childhood in Germany. Pediatr. Blood Cancer 2012;**58**(3):366–71.

206. Sipos B, Kloppel G. Acinar cell carcinomas and pancreatoblastomas: related but not the same. Pathologe 2005;**26**(1):37–40.

207. Huang Y, Cao YF, Lin JL, Gao F, Li F. Acinar cell cystadenocarcinoma of the pancreas in a 4-year-old child. Pancreas 2006;**33**(3):311–2.

208. Cingolani N, Shaco-Levy R, Farruggio A, Klimstra DS, Rosai J. A-fetoprotein production by pancreatic tumors exhibiting acinar cell differentiation: study of five cases, one arising in a mediastinal teratoma. Hum. Pathol. 2000;**31**(8):938–44.

209. Ordonez NG, Mackay B. Acinar cell carcinoma of the pancreas. Ultrastruct. Pathol. 2000;**24**(4):227–41.

210. Yantiss RK, Chang H-K, Farraye FA, Compton CC, Odze RD. Prevalence and prognostic significance of acinar cell differentiation in pancreatic endocrine tumors. Am. J. Surg. Pathol. 2002;**26**(7):893–901.

211. Abraham SC, Wu T-T, Hruban RH, *et al.* Genetic and immunohistochemical analysis of pancreatic acinar cell carcinoma: frequent allelic loss on chromosome 11p and alterations in the APC/beta-catenin pathway. Am. J. Pathol. 2002;**160**(3):953–62.

212. Tapia B, Ahrens W, Kenney B, Touloukian R, Reyes-Mugica M. Acinar cell carcinoma vs. solid pseudopapillary tumor of the pancreas in children: A comparison of two rare and overlapping entities with review of the literature. Pediatr. Dev. Pathol. 2008;**11**(5):384–90.

213. Arva NC, Pappas JG, Bhatla T, *et al.* Well-differentiated pancreatic neuroendocrine carcinoma in tuberous sclerosis: case report and review of the literature. Am. J. Surg. Pathol. 2012;**36**(1):149–53.

214. Kuiper P, Verspaget HW, van Slooten H-J, *et al.* Pathological incidence of duodenopancreatic neuroendocrine tumors in the Netherlands: A Pathologisch Anatomisch Landelijk Geautomatiseerd Archief study. Pancreas 2010;**39**(8):1134–9.

215. Sueyoshi R, Okazaki T, Lane GJ, *et al.* Multicystic adenomatoid pancreatic hamartoma in a child: Case report and literature review. Int. J. Surg. Case Rep. 2013;**4**(1):98–9100.

216. Thrall M, Jessurun J, Stelow EB, *et al.* Multicystic adenomatoid hamartoma of the pancreas: A hitherto undescribed pancreatic tumor occurring in a 3-year-old boy. Pediatr. Dev. Pathol. 2008;**11**(4):314–20.

217. Mekitarian Filho E, Carvalho WB, Silva FD. Acute pancreatitis in pediatrics: A systematic review of the literature. J. Pediatr. (Rio J). 2012;**88**(2):101–14.

218. Suchi M. The pancreas. In Stocker JT, Dehner LP, Hussain AN, editors, *Stocker and Dehner's Pediatric Pathology*, third edn. Philadelphia, PA: Wolters Kluwer/Lippincott, Williams and Wilkins; 2011.

Head and neck

Jo McPartland, Alena Skálová, Rajeev Shukla, and Roman Kodet

Introduction

The head and neck region in childhood presents the pathologist with a wide range of lesions, some similar to those encountered in adults, others unique to childhood.

The majority of pediatric surgical samples from this region are of inflammatory and developmental conditions. Many developmental anomalies and syndromes affect the head and neck region, but this chapter will concentrate on those lesions that are commonly removed and present as surgical pathology specimens.

For ease of reference, this chapter is divided according to anatomic site, although some conditions can occur in more than one region.

The ear

External ear

Pediatric surgical samples from the external ear are rare. Benign lesions are mostly limited to pre-auricular developmental anomalies, described below, with branchial arch anomalies, and keloid scarring of the ear lobe, associated with ear piercing. Malignant tumors can rarely present in the external ear canal in childhood, and are almost exclusively rhabdomyosarcomas.

Rhabdomyosarcoma

A primitive malignant tumor with phenotypic and biological features of embryonic skeletal muscle.

Clinical features: Rhabdomyosarcoma is rare in any part of the body. Rhabdomyosarcoma and its variants are discussed in greater detail in the section on salivary gland pathology (below), and in Chapter 11. There is a distinct group arising in the head and neck of children,

often very young, with a predilection for the palate, middle ear, and orbit. This section focuses on its occurrence as a primary tumor in the external ear canal. Most of these tumors arise in the middle ear with extension into the external canal as an "aural polyp." Embryonal rhabdomyosarcoma should be excluded in any child presenting with a polyp in the external ear canal.

Macroscopy: Usually polypoid specimens with myxoid appearance.

Histology: The majority of rhabomyosarcomas at this site are of embryonal subtype (1,2). Many of these have characteristics of botryoid tumors (see Chapter 11).

Differential diagnosis: Inflammatory aural polyps with lymphoid infiltrates and other small round cell tumors (see Chapter 11) are the main differential diagnoses. It is important to maintain a high index of suspicion to make a diagnosis of rhabdomyosarcoma (3).

Yolk sac tumor has been described as a polypoid tumor presenting in the external ear canal. However, this is histologically distinct, being composed of small round blue cells arranged in a vacuolated pattern with formation of Schiller–Duval bodies and expressing α-fetoprotein (4).

Middle ear

Middle-ear pathology is more common in children due to their narrow eustachian tubes and increased risk of eustachian tube dysfunction.

Otitis media

Otitis media is any inflammation of the middle ear, and is one of the most common diseases in young children. Most cases are managed medically, with only a minority requiring surgical intervention and yielding tissue for histopathological diagnosis. The

Essentials of Surgical Pediatric Pathology, ed. Marta C. Cohen and Irene Scheimberg. Published by Cambridge University Press.
© Cambridge University Press 2014.

clinical diagnoses of acute and chronic otitis media have pathological correlates, but there is significant histological overlap.

Clinical presentation: Acute otitis media (AOM) usually presents with otalgia, fever, or otorrhoea, with abnormal otoscopic findings of the tympanic membrane. AOM is a recurrent disease. More than one-third of children experience six or more episodes of AOM by the age of seven years.

Otitis media with effusion (OME), or "glue ear," formerly termed serous OM or secretory OM, is a middle-ear effusion of any duration that lacks the associated signs and symptoms of infection (e.g., fever, otalgia, and irritability). OME usually follows an episode of AOM.

Chronic suppurative OM is a chronic inflammation of the middle ear that persists for at least six weeks and is associated with otorrhoea through a perforated tympanic membrane.

Histology: Chronic otitis media causes mucinous metaplasia of the middle ear mucosa, with associated inflammatory cell infiltration composed of lymphocytes, plasma cells, and macrophages. There may be associated granulation tissue, fibrosis, cholesterol granuloma, cholesteatoma, inflammatory aural polyp, ossicular erosion, or new bone formation.

Cholesteatoma

Abnormal collections of squamous epithelium and keratinous debris that usually involve the middle ear and mastoid. The term cholesteatoma is actually a misnomer, as the lesion is not a neoplasm and does not contain cholesterol. Cholesteatomas may cause progressive bone erosion of ossicles and surrounding bone, but are not neoplastic (5).

Clinical presentation: Cholesteatomas are either congenital or acquired, the latter occurring far more frequently.

Congenital cholesteatomas present as a white mass behind an intact eardrum in a child with no previous history of ear surgery, perforation, or tympanic membrane retraction (6). They can occur anywhere in the temporal bone, but have a predilection for the anterosuperior quadrant of the middle ear, just above the eustachian-tube opening (7).

Acquired cholesteatomas form after birth, usually as a result of chronic middle-ear disease. They form in three ways: (i) from focal retractions of the tympanic membrane (retraction-pocket cholesteatomas); (ii) superficial epithelium enters the middle ear through a perforation of the tympanic membrane along a temporal-bone fracture line; and (iii) squamous epithelium is introduced into the middle ear after surgery, as a complication of tympanoplasty, or by creeping in alongside a retained tympanostomy tube (secondary acquired cholesteatoma).

Cholesteatomas usually present with unremitting or recurrent painless otorrhoea, often with hearing loss. Dizziness or symptoms of central nervous system (CNS) complications such as sigmoid sinus thrombosis, epidural abscess, or meningitis are rare (8).

Genetics: There is no known association with genetic abnormalities, even in congenital cholesteatoma (9).

Macroscopy: The specimen usually submitted for histology consists of yellow-white waxy material. Rarely in congenital cholesteatoma, an intact small cyst is submitted.

Histology: Histologically similar to an epidermal inclusion cyst at any other site, these are cystic formations lined by keratinizing, stratified squamous epithelium, the so-called matrix, lying on top of dense connective tissue of varied thickness, the perimatrix. As many of these specimens are curettings, intact cysts are rarely seen. Most of the specimens show keratin lamellae and/or strips of keratinizing squamous epithelium. There may be a lympho-plasmacytic infiltrate and/or granulation tissue and a foreign-body type of reaction if the perimatrix is included. Papillary hyperplasia and koilocytosis may be predictors of aggressiveness (10). We have not seen viral cytopathic changes in our material and are not convinced that there is any established histological feature of prognostic significance.

Differential diagnosis: Rarely, dermoid cysts can occur at these sites, distinguished by the presence of skin adnexal structures in the cyst wall, or hair shafts in the cyst content (11). Cholesterol granulomas and cholesteatomas can also occur together (12–14). In these cases, it is possible that the original lesion was a cholesteatoma that progressed, causing obstruction of the air-space network in the bone, leading to concomitant growth of a cholesterol granuloma (14). It is important to make the distinction between cholesterol granuloma and cholesteatoma because of treatment differences. Cholesterol granulomas will resolve after internal drainage into the mastoid cavity or middle ear, relieving the obstruction, and restoring the normal pneumatization of the bone (14). Cholesteatomas require complete surgical removal, have a recurrence rate of up to 50%, and often result in hearing loss (15).

Heterotopic brain tissue has been found in the middle ear in association with cholesteatomas, and may occur due to brain herniation (16).

Cholesterol granuloma

Descriptive term used for a granulomatous reaction to blood breakdown products, primarily cholesterol in pneumatized skull bones.

Clinical features: Occur most commonly in the pneumatized petrous apex of the temporal bone, but also may be seen in other pneumatized portions of the temporal bone, including mastoid air cells and middle ear space (17). They are thought to arise secondarily following disease states where normally ventilated air-containing bony spaces are obstructed, such as in chronic or acute otitis media, cholesteatoma, or mastoiditis (18). Cholesterol granulomas generally grow silently, with clinical presentation after the lesion has caused bony destruction and compression of cranial nerves V–VIII, structures within the inner ear, or the brainstem (15). Symptoms can include headache, diplopia, vertigo, dizziness, hearing loss, and facial paralysis (17).

Macroscopy: Usually cystic lesions with a thin brown-yellow fibrous capsule and luminal contents consisting of watery chocolate-colored fluid (14).

Histology: Extensive granulomatous response with cholesterol clefts surrounded by multinucleated giant cells, hemosiderin-laden and foamy macrophages, lymphocytes, plasma cells, and abnormal blood vessels (12). In severe cases, there may be evidence of bone destruction (17).

Differential diagnosis: There may be overlapping histological features with inflammatory aural polyp (see below).

Inflammatory aural polyp

Growth in the external ear canal that may be attached to the tympanic membrane, or may grow from the middle ear space.

Clinical features: Aural polyps usually present with chronic otorrhoea or with hearing loss, aural bleeding, otalgia, and vertigo. Typically, polyps arc unilateral, protruding through the tympanic membrane from the middle ear cleft and completely occluding the external auditory canal. Chronic otitis media and cholesteatoma are the most frequent underlying etiology of polyps, with rare systemic inflammatory infections and lymphoproliferative processes as alternative causes (19).

Macroscopy: Polypoidal, soft to rubbery, tan white to pink.

Histology: Polyps show a chronic inflammatory cell infiltrate, including lymphocytes, plasma cells, histiocytes, and eosinophils. The stroma includes granulation tissue varying in appearance from edematous and richly vascularized to fibrous with decreased vascularity. Multinucleate giant cells, cholesterol granulomata, keratin flakes, and calcific debris (tympanosclerosis) may be seen (20). The surface of the polyp may be ulcerated or there may be pseudostratified columnar or cuboidal epithelium or metaplastic squamous epithelium. The finding of a combination of raw granulation tissue, with keratin flakes or as a mass, makes the presence of an underlying cholesteatoma highly likely (21).

Differential diagnosis: In general, the presence of a mixed inflammatory cell infiltrate indicates that the polyp is benign. However, the inflammatory component may obscure an underlying neoplastic process like rhabdomyosarcoma or Langerhans-cell histiocytosis (LCH), which are known to present as aural polyps in children (19).

Salivary gland choristoma

Heterotopic, non-growing normal salivary gland tissue that can occur in different locations in the head and neck, where it is not usually found, most commonly in the middle ear.

Clinical features: Very rare developmental anomaly of the second branchial arch that presents in the first and second decades, usually with unilateral conductive hearing loss, sometimes with co-existent glue ear (22,23).

Macroscopy: The choristoma is often a lobulated mass, attached posteriorly in the region of the oval window, with absent or malformed ossicles (23). It may appear as a pearly white mass and mimic a cholesteatoma.

Histology: Composed of histologically normal salivary gland tissue, usually of mixed mucous and serous elements (24).

Inner ear

There are numerous malformations of the inner ear; this topic is beyond the scope of this compact text, but is excellently reviewed elsewhere (25).

The nose, paranasal sinuses, and nasopharynx

The nasal cavity, paranasal sinuses, and nasopharynx are host to a wide variety of neoplastic and non-neoplastic conditions. There are some differences in the normal histology between children and adults. At birth, the nasopharynx is lined by respiratory-type epithelium, but this is mostly replaced by stratified squamous epithelium by later childhood. Mucosal lymphoid tissue in the anterior nasopharynx (adenoids) is particularly prominent in childhood.

Inflammatory lesions

Viral and bacterial inflammatory lesions are very common in this region, but fortunately histological examination is required only in the small proportion of cases that are destructive, involve a large area of mucosa, or result in a mass.

Fungal infection

Fungal infections are often destructive and at times may present as mass lesions. A variety of fungi affect the nose and sinuses, *Mucor* and *Aspergillus* being the most common. Angioinvasion may result in necrosis and hemorrhage. The inflammation may range from minimal to a neutrophilic abscess or granulation tissue.

Fungal balls of *Aspergillus* hyphae may grow in the sinuses with a variable inflammatory response. Invasive *Aspergillus*, although more common in the immunocompromised, can occur in immunocompetent individuals (26).

Allergic non-invasive rhinosinusitis is considered to be an allergic response to *Aspergillus* similar to allergic bronchopulmonary aspergillosis. Biopsies in these cases show tenacious mucin, large numbers of eosinophils and Charcot–Leyden crystals – so-called "allergic mucin" (27), and fungal hyphae are not always seen.

Granulomatous conditions

Mycobacterial infection

Leprosy affects the nasal mucosa in 95% of cases and sometimes is an initial manifestation (28). Pathology is similar to cutaneous leprosy. The tuberculoid end of the spectrum with well-formed granulomata is rare. *Tuberculosis* of the sinonasal mucosa is an uncommon manifestation of hematogenous spread.

Rhinosporidiosis is a chronic granulomatous infection of the mucous membranes that usually manifests as vascular friable polyps that arise from the nasal mucosa or external structures of the eye; it usually affects persons in or from southern India and Sri Lanka. Histologically, characteristic sporangia of *R. seeberi* are seen in the subepithelium, with mixed active chronic inflammation.

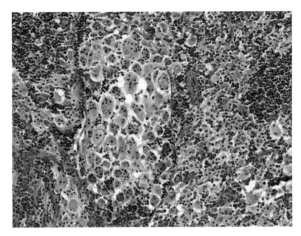

Figure 4.1 Rosai–Dorfman disease showing prominent emperipolesis (H&E × 400).

Sporangia are thick walled and contain up to several thousand spores (29).

Rhinoscleroma is a chronic granulomatous condition of the nose and other structures of the upper respiratory tract, caused by infection with *Klebsiella rhinoscleromatis*. Rhinoscleroma is endemic to areas of Africa, South-East Asia, Central and South America, and Central and Eastern Europe, with an increased incidence in Spain, possibly due to immigration. Histologically, Rhinoscleroma is characterized by sheets of foamy histiocytes and variable numbers of plasma cells. The main differential diagnosis is lepromatous leprosy and extranodal forms of Rosai–Dorfman disease. Lepromatous leprosy cases are strongly positive for acid-fast bacilli (multibacillary), whereas *K. rhinoscleromatis* are gram-negative rods. *Rosai–Dorfman disease* cases characteristically show large S100-positive histiocytes, exhibiting phagocytosis of leucocytes (emperipolesis) (Figure 4.1; 30).

Midline destructive disease (lethal midline granuloma/midfacial necrotizing lesions)

A heterogenous group of disorders presenting with one or more infiltrative and destructive mucosal lesions of the upper aerodigestive tract, excluding those caused by trauma, toxic agents, or infections. The differential diagnosis for midline destructive diseases includes Wegener's granulomatosis (WG), Sinonasal NK/T cell lymphoma, idiopathic midline destructive disease, polyarteritis nodosa, allergic granulomatosis, and foreign body granuloma. Superficial biopsies are usually inadequate for diagnosis because of the associated necrosis. The best results are achieved if the superficial scab is removed and a generous biopsy is performed.

Histology: The classical triad of histological findings in WG includes necrosis, granulomatous inflammation and vasculitis affecting arterioles, small arteries, and veins (31). Granulomata are rarely well formed and are often seen as loose, ill-defined aggregates of histiocytes with nuclear debris. Scattered giant cells and foci of coagulative necrosis of the connective tissue are often seen. Variable numbers of plasma cells and eosinophils are present. Nasal biopsy is diagnostic only in 20–40% of cases (32,33). Diagnostic criteria have been proposed for the diagnosis of WG on head and neck biopsies (32).

Sino-nasal NK/T cell lymphoma is sometimes seen in children (31). Clinically and histologically it may resemble WG with necrosis and inflammation (34). The presence of atypical lymphocytes defines this condition. These atypical cells tend to be angiocentric, mimicking vasculitis. These cells are usually CD56+, CD3+, EBV+. Those which are negative for CD56 are required to show expression of CD3, EBV, and cytotoxic proteins (granzyme B, TIA1 and perforins).

Idiopathic midline destructive granuloma (IMDD) is characterized by the absence of atypical lymphocytes and typical vasculitis (35). Clinically there is lack of renal or pulmonary involvement.

Nasal polyps

Broadly defined, any benign or malignant tumor may present as a polyp. Discussion in this section is limited to polyps of the nasal and paranasal sinuses due to non-neoplastic proliferation of stromal and epithelial elements, of which there are two clinicopathologically distinct subtypes: (i) inflammatory polyps and (ii) antro-choanal polyps.

Inflammatory polyps

Clinical features: Inflammatory polyps are typically bilateral and multiple, and involve the nasal cavity and the paranasal sinuses. The majority of inflammatory polyps in children occur in a setting of cystic fibrosis (CF). They are seen in nearly 20% of children with CF and may be the first manifestation of the disease. Adult-type polyps can be seen in older children where there is an association with asthma or chronic rhinitis.

Macroscopy: These are multiple translucent polyps with a broad base. The cut surface is edematous.

Histology: These lesions represent a localized outgrowth of the lamina propria due to the accumulation of edema-like fluid, with varying degrees of inflammation and fibroblastic proliferation. The surface may show squamous metaplasia in long-standing lesions. The stroma contains mucous glands in variable numbers. Typically they are less numerous than in normal mucosa (36). The stroma is edematous in most cases, but may become fibrotic in long-standing cases. Stromal cell atypia may be seen. Inflammation is variable and may show a predominance of neutrophils, eosinophils, or plasma cells. Thickened basement membranes and eosinophil predominance does not necessarily indicate an allergic etiology (37). In CF, nasal polyps usually lack basement membrane thickening and submucosal hyalinization, show fewer eosinophils, and the mucous glands and cysts contain predominantly acidic Alcian-blue-positive mucin, in contrast to neutral mucin in non-CF-associated inflammatory polyps. Goblet cells in both conditions contain acidic mucin (38).

Antrochoanal polyps

Benign lesions originating from the maxillary sinus mucosa, growing through the accessory ostium into the middle meatus and, thereafter, protruding posteriorly to the choana and nasopharynx.

Clinical features: Patients usually present with unilateral nasal obstruction and nasal discharge. Some cases present with headache (mostly unilateral), epistaxis, or sleep apnea. Occasionally, larger masses may prolapse posteriorly and hang down from the nasopharynx, becoming visible from the mouth.

Macroscopy: Large, solitary, gray-white, smooth polyp with a stalk of variable length, usually with a firm and fibrous body.

Histology: Similar to inflammatory nasal polyp with minor differences. These polyps usually lack basement membrane thickening. The stroma is variable, but is often less edematous and more fibrous, as compared to a typical nasal polyp, with fewer glandular elements. Stromal inflammation is patchy and eosinophil prominence is seen in only 20% of cases (39).

Many sino-nasal polyps show scattered, mildly atypical stromal cells. Occasionally, a significant population of pleomorphic or overtly bizarre stromal cells is present, raising the possibility of sarcoma (Figure 4.2; 40). These changes are more often seen in younger patients and in

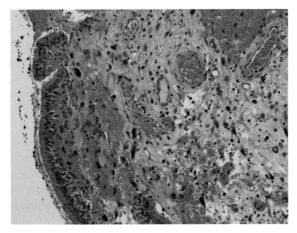

Figure 4.2 Nasal polyp featuring atypical stromal cells (H&E × 200).

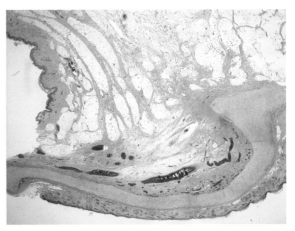

Figure 4.3 Congenital hairy polyp (H&E × 100) featuring surface squamous epithelium with skin adnexal structures overlying a core containing adipose tissue and cartilage.

polyps with pronounced stromal fibrosis, and are more common in antrochoanal polyps than in nasal polyps. The atypical cells tend to concentrate in perivascular or submucosal regions. They are spindled cells with variably enlarged, angulated dark nuclei and abundant eosinophilic cytoplasm, so that the nuclear to cytoplasmic ratio is maintained. Mitoses are rare or absent, and there is no increase in cellularity or vascularity. Based on these features, it is usually possible to exclude malignancy, but in some cases immunohistochemistry may be required to exclude rhabdomyosarcoma. These atypical cells are negative for Myo D1 and myogenin and show smooth-muscle actin (SMA), vimentin, and actin positivity, indicating a myofibroblastic phenotype.

Congenital hairy polyps

Congenital hairy polyps are the most common congenital nasopharyngeal mass (41).

There are many differing views in the literature regarding the origin and embryology of hairy polyps; 10% of cases occur with first or second branchial arch malformations (41), and one theory is that hairy polyps are forms of accessory auricles, being embryonic displacements of first or second branchial arch tissue (42). However, this does not account for hairy polyps occurring outside of the distribution of the first and second branchial arches, or the absence of cartilage in some hairy polyps.

Clinical presentation: Presentation is often soon after birth with respiratory compromise or feeding difficulties, but clinical features vary with the site of the mass. The female:male ratio is 6:1 (43); 60% of cases occur in the nasopharynx or superior velum; other sites include the oropharynx, tonsillar area,

eustachian tube, or middle ear (41,44). In 10% of cases there is secondary development of a cleft palate, as the hairy polyp prevents fusion of the secondary palatal shelves during embryogenesis (45). One case report details the co-existence of a nasopharyngeal hairy polyp with multiple synchronous similar "bigerminal teratomas" in the neck (46).

Macroscopy: The polyps are usually pedunculated and vary in size from 0.5 to 6 cm (47).

Histology: Hairy polyps characteristically contain only ectodermal and mesodermal components, with skin, including dermis and skin appendages, overlying mature adipose tissue, with cartilage in some cases (Figure 4.3).

Differential diagnosis: Distinguished from dermoid cysts, which contain only tissue of ectodermal origin. Hairy polyps have no malignant potential, unlike teratomas.

Congenital pleomorphic adenoma (salivary gland anlage tumor)

Salivary gland anlage tumor (SGAT) is a nasopharyngeal pedunculated polypoid lesion that presents with respiratory distress at birth or within the first few weeks of life (48,49).

Clinical presentation: Usually presents as a polypoid mass in the nasopharynx (48–51). There may be involvement of the posterior nasal septum (52). The polypoid nasopharyngeal lesion may be attached to the mucosa by a thin delicate pedicle. Obstruction of the upper respiratory tract, with progressive respiratory distress is the most common presenting feature.

Bleeding from the nose and mouth of the newborn may be seen (49). Among seven cases with follow-up information, six were disease-free at 1–6 years after treatment (49).

Macroscopic features: Polypoid pedunculated mass measuring between 1.3 and 3.0 cm with a bosselated surface. The tumor is attached by a thick stalk to the nasopharynx, is soft in consistency, and white to pink in color. The mucosal surface is intact in most cases (49,50).

Histology: Salivary gland anlage tumor is characterized by solid cords and branching duct-like structures that appear to originate from the surface mucosa. Some of the duct-like structures have focal squamous lining resembling sialometaplasia. The tumor is divided by variously thick septa into nodules composed of fascicles of spindle-shaped and ovoid cells with indistinctive borders, eosinophilic cytoplasm, and bland nuclei. Within these nodules, the cells focally form glands, cystic spaces, and squamous cell nests (Figure 4.4). In one case, widespread necrotic foci, partially lined by squamous epithelium with necrotic debris and erythrocytes in the centre, were noted (51). The epithelial structures exhibit immunoreactivity for cytokeratins and epithelial membrane antigen (EMA), while solid stromal-like nodules co-express vimentin, SMA, and cytokeratin.

Differential diagnosis: Salivary gland anlage tumor is a benign lesion characterized by non-recurring clinical behavior. The biphasic multinodular growth pattern and solid nodules composed of mesenchyme-like

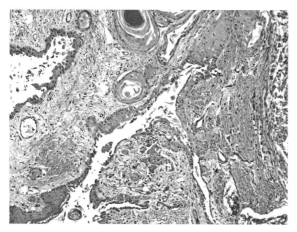

Figure 4.4 Salivary anlage tumor (congenital pleomorphic adenoma): SGAT is characterized by solid cords and branching duct-like structures that appear to originate from the surface mucosa. Some of the duct-like structures have focal squamous lining resembling sialometaplasia (H&E).

spindle-shaped cells mimic synovial sarcoma. The presence of budding epithelium from the surface mucosa in SGAT, its actin positivity and lack of numerous mitoses are major distinguishing features from synovial sarcoma. Low-grade mucoepidermoid carcinoma can be distinguished because of the presence of spindled actin-positive stromal cells and keratinizing squamous epithelium in SGAT. Another tumor composed of cystic-squamous, glandular, and spindle-shaped cell formations is ectopic hamartomatous thymoma (53), which is actin negative, not congenital, and does not occur in the nasopharynx.

Midline nasopharyngeal cysts

Midline nasopharyngeal cysts may be deep or superficial. Deep cysts originate from the median embryonal pharyngeal recess, posterior to Rathke's pouch. Superficial cysts may arise from the midline pharyngeal recess during nasopharyngeal tonsillar development. Superficial cysts may also arise from obstruction of a seromucinous gland duct. Superficial cysts may be incidentally removed during adenoidectomy, but the deep cysts are too deeply situated (52).

Histology: Cysts may be lined by squamous or columnar epithelium, or both.

Differential diagnosis: Cysts lined by squamous or columnar lining in the *lateral* wall of the nasopharynx with lymphoid tissue in the wall are most likely branchial pouch derivatives (52).

Nasolabial cyst

Non-odontogenic developmental cyst, located behind the ala nasi, extending beneath the nasal floor and anteriorly into the upper labio-gingival sulcus.

Clinical presentation: Although developmental in origin, presentation is usually in adulthood with a painless mass beneath one ala.

Histology: Cyst lined by ciliated columnar or cuboidal epithelium with mucous glands (54).

Heterotopic central nervous system tissue

Mass composed of mature brain tissue isolated from the cranial cavity or spinal canal (55). It is also known as *nasal glioma* or *nasal glial heterotopia*. It is a congenital malformation in which there is anterior displacement of mature cerebral tissue that has lost connection with the intracranial contents.

Clinical features: Most patients present at birth, and 90% of cases are diagnosed by the age of two. There is

133

no gender predilection. The lesion is situated externally, on or near the bridge of the nose in 60% of cases, and within the nasal cavity in 30% of cases. Extranasal lesions present as a mass over the dorsum of the nose. The intranasal lesions usually present with nasal obstruction or nasal deformity. Heterotopic CNS tissue can also occur in the scalp (56), orbit (57), pterygopalatine fossa (58), pharynx (59,60), palate (61), lips (62), tongue (63), and middle ear (55). One-third of pharyngeal heterotopic CNS tissues are associated with cleft palate or choanal stenosis. Incomplete excision can be accompanied by recurrence in 15–30% of cases, but there is no local aggressive behavior or malignant potential.

Macroscopy: The lesion appears as a polypoid, smooth, soft, gray-tan, non-translucent mass, usually measuring 1–3 cm.

Histology: Non-encapsulated lesion, composed of large or small islands of glial tissue and interlacing bands of vascularized fibrous connective tissue. The glial tissue merges with the collagen of the stroma or dermis, and fibrosis tends to be greater with longer-standing lesions. Gemistocytic astrocytes are commonly seen. Mitoses are absent. Neurons are rare or absent. Rarely, choroid plexus, ependyma-lined clefts and pigmented retinal epithelium are seen, especially in the palate and nasopharynx (Figure 4.5). The glial tissue can be confirmed by immunohistochemistry for glial fibrillary acidic protein (GFAP) or S100 protein.

Differential diagnosis: The histologic differential diagnoses include nasal encephalocele, a fibrosed nasal polyp, or teratoma. Histologically, heterotopia may be indistinguishable from encephalocele and appropriate imaging is necessary to exclude this possibility. It is suggested that encephaloceles have readily identifiable neurons, whereas they are rare to find in nasal neuroglial heterotopia. Fibrosis may obscure glial elements in long-standing cases and be mistaken for a fibrosed nasal polyp (64). The subtle glial component on routine microscopy can be accentuated with a trichrome stain or by GFAP/S100 staining. Teratoma with mature glial elements can usually be distinguished by the presence of other components.

Ectopic meningioma

Benign neoplasms of meningothelial cells occurring at extracranial sites.

Clinical presentation: Primary ectopic meningiomas of the sinonasal tract are rare, comprising <0.5% of non-epithelial neoplasms (65). They should be distinguished from intracranial meningiomas with extracranial/extraspinal extension (65,66). Any age can be affected, and there is a slight female predilection. Symptoms include a mass (often polypoid), nasal obstruction, epistaxis, sinusitis, pain, headache, seizure, exophthalmos, periorbital edema, visual disturbance, ptosis, and facial deformity (65,66). Primary ectopic meningiomas have not been reported to metastasize.

Macroscopy: The tumors range up to 8 cm, with a mean of about 3 cm. They may infiltrate bone and rarely ulcerate the mucosa. The cut surface is gray-white, tan, or pink, gritty, and firm to rubbery. Calcifications and fragments of bone are frequently visible.

Histology: Sinonasal meningiomas can exhibit a variety of histological patterns, most commonly meningotheliomatous, characterized by lobules of cells with a whorl formation, indistinct cell borders, and bland nuclei with delicate chromatin (66). Intranuclear pseudoinclusions and psammoma bodies are common. Other variants can also occur in the sinonasal tract. Meningiomas are immunoreactive for EMA and vimentin. Cytokeratin is usually negative, or rarely focally and weakly positive; 50% are positive for progesterone receptor and 25% for estrogen receptor. Glial fibrillary acidic protein and SMA are negative.

Differential diagnosis: The differential diagnoses include carcinoma, melanoma, aggressive psammomatoid ossifying fibroma, and follicular dendritic cell sarcoma/tumor (65,67).

Craniopharyngioma

Exceptionally, craniopharyngioma can arise in the nasopharynx or can involve the nasopharynx through

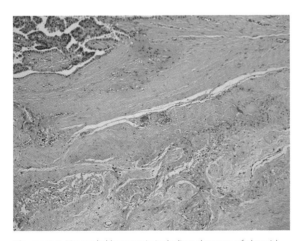

Figure 4.5 Neuroglial heterotpia including elements of choroid plexus (H&E × 200).

downward invasion from a suprasellar location. The morphological features are identical to the suprasellar counterpart (68,69).

Nasal chondromesenchymal hamartoma

Nasal chondromesenchymal hamartoma (NCMH) is a rare benign lesion of the nasal cavity and/or paranasal sinuses with characteristic histology featuring stromal and chondroid tissue in various proportions.

Clinical features: NCMHs occur predominantly in infants under one year of age, but are well described in older children and adults (70–74). The clinical manifestations include respiratory and feeding difficulties, rhinorrhoea, epistaxis, visual disturbances, and otitis media. Occasionally, orbital involvement leads to ophthalmoplegia, proptosis, ptosis, hypotropia, or enophthalmos (72,74–77). Intracranial extension can result in neurological signs such as hydrocephalus and oculomotor disturbances (4). On imaging, it may appear aggressive with bony erosion, thinning, and displacement, and can raise suspicion of malignancy. Intracranial extension through the cribriform plate is not infrequent (72,74). There have been no reported cases of malignant transformation.

Histology: NCMH is characterized by a variety of mesenchymal components with a focally lobular architecture. The most prominent components are irregular islands of mature and immature hyaline cartilage with occasional binucleated chondrocytes. The islands of cartilage are well demarcated from the surrounding stromal tissues, which have a myxoid background and consist of a relatively bland and compact spindle-cell population with variable cellularity, but without nuclear atypia or atypical mitoses (Figure 4.6; 72,74). Reactive bone, small thick-walled vessels, cystic formation, and erythrocyte-filled spaces may be seen (72,74). Smooth muscle actin, S-100, vimentin, KP-1, and Leu-7 are positive, while cytokeratin, EMA, and desmin are negative (74,75).

Genetics: The pathogenesis of NCMH is still unknown. Although called hamartoma, it most likely represents a neoplastic process. It has been described in association with pleuropulmonary blastoma (PBP) (76) and the translocation t(12;17)(q24.1; q21) (8). It is suggested that NCMH is part of the familial disease complex associated with PPB, and patients affected with NCMH may have a familial predisposition to childhood malignant and dysplastic disease.

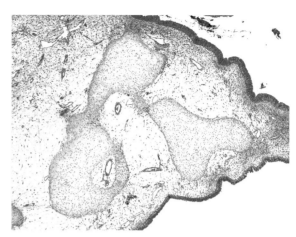

Figure 4.6 Chondromesenchymal hamartoma featuring lobules of cartilage set in a myxoid stroma containing spindled cells (H&E × 10).

Nasopharyngeal angiofibroma

A tumor composed of variable fibrous and vascular elements, seen almost exclusively in young males.

Clinical features: Nasopharyngeal angiofibroma represents <1% of all nasopharyngeal tumors and <0.5% of all head and neck tumors (78,79). It is almost exclusively seen in boys and adolescent-to-young men with a peak in the second decade of life. If a female is affected, testicular feminization has to be excluded.

The tumor arises in the postero-lateral nasal wall of the nasopharynx, usually in the region of the superior margin of the sphenopalatine foramen and the posterior aspect of the middle turbinate. The tumor displaces and distorts, rather than invades, adjacent structures, with pressure necrosis causing tissue destruction. Depending on the site of involvement, patients may present with nasal obstruction and/or recurrent epistaxis, nasal discharge, facial deformity, proptosis, diplopia, exophthalmos, sinusitis, otitis media, tinnitus, rhinorrhea, deafness, headaches, dyspnoea, and, rarely, anosmia or pain (78,80,81). The diagnosis is generally made on clinical findings and imaging. Angiography allows for identification of the feeding vessel(s) and presurgical embolization.

Macroscopy: Angiofibromas are polypoid with a rounded or multinodular contour, with nodularity increasing with age. They have well-defined margins, but are not encapsulated. The cut-surface is reticulated, and whorled to spongy in appearance. A whorled appearance correlates with a dominant fibrous element on histology, while a spongy appearance correlates with marked vascularity.

135

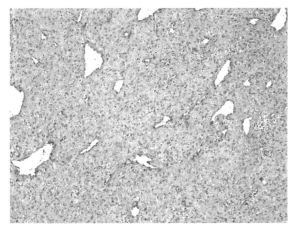

Figure 4.7 Nasopharyngeal angiofibroma composed of small vessels set in fibrous stroma. This example includes a few lymphocytes in the stroma (H&E × 100).

Histology: There are of two main components, stroma and vessels. Younger lesions are more vascular, whereas collagenous stroma predominates in long-standing tumors. Within a lesion there is regional variability with peripheral areas showing more vascularity, and central areas showing stromal predominance. The overlying mucosa may show squamous metaplasia. The vessels are mostly thin-walled, slit-like ("stag horn"), or dilated, with calibers ranging from capillary size to large, patulous vessels. The muscular layer can be absent, focal and pad-like, or circumferential. In addition to the abnormal muscle, these vessels also lack elastic fibers. Lack of normal constriction of these vessels can lead to uncontrolled bleeding. The fibrous stroma consists of plump, spindled, round, angular, or stellate-shaped cells and a varying amount of fine and coarse collagen fibers (Figure 4.7). Background myxoid degeneration is common, especially in embolized specimens. The stromal cell nuclei are generally bland, but they may be multinucleated or show some degree of pleomorphism in the more cellular areas. Mast cells may be seen, but other inflammatory elements are usually absent, unless there is surface ulceration (82). Preoperative embolization may lead to infarction and the presence of Gelfoam or other iatrogenic embolic material in the sections.

There are no definite histological prognostic markers. Microvessel density using CD105 has been shown to be of some prognostic significance (83). Sarcomatous transformation is rare, usually following radiation therapy (84).

The stromal cells are immunoreactive with vimentin only, except in areas of increased fibrosis, where

focal SMA may be identified. Stromal and endothelial cells are variably reactive with androgen and estrogen/progesterone receptors. CD34 and CD31 highlight the endothelium. The stromal cells are negative for S-100 protein. Nuclear β-catenin positivity in stromal cells is seen in a large majority of cases.

Genetics: Many genetic abnormalities have been identified, including activating β-catenin gene alterations and p53 loss (85).

Differential diagnosis: The differential diagnosis includes lobular capillary hemangioma (pyogenic granuloma), nasal inflammatory polyps with fibrosis, or atypical stromal cells, antrochoanal polyps, and peripheral nerve sheath tumor.

Nasopharyngeal carcinoma

Carcinoma arising in the nasopharyngeal mucosa that shows light microscopic or ultrastructural evidence of squamous differentiation.

Clinical features: Nasopharyngeal carcinoma (NPC) is rare in children, accounting for 1–3% of all pediatric malignancies and 20–50% of all nasopharyngeal tumors in this age group (86,87). Nasopharyngeal carcinoma is highly prevalent in southern China, South-East Asia, and the Middle East (88). There is a strong etiological association with Epstein–Barr virus (EBV) (89). Nasopharyngeal carcinoma usually originates in the lateral wall of the nasopharynx, but can then extend to the skull base or the palate, nasal cavity, or oropharynx. Distant metastases may also occur. Cervical lymphadenopathy is the initial presentation in many patients, or there may be local symptoms related to the primary tumor, including pain, nasal obstruction or bleeding, otitis media, hearing loss, and cranial nerve palsies.

Macroscopic features: The tumor can appear as a smooth bulge in the mucosa, a discrete raised nodule, with or without surface ulceration, or a frankly infiltrative fungating mass.

Histology: Nasopharyngeal carcinoma is divided into two groups: (i) squamous cell carcinoma (keratinizing squamous cell carcinoma), and (ii) non-keratinizing carcinoma (including differentiated and undifferentiated carcinoma). Nasopharyngeal carcinoma in childhood and adolescence is almost exclusively of non-keratinizing type, the majority showing undifferentiated morphology (90). Keratinizing squamous cell carcinomas will not be discussed further as they are very rare in the pediatric population.

The *non-keratinizing undifferentiated* subtype is characterized by syncytial-appearing large tumor cells

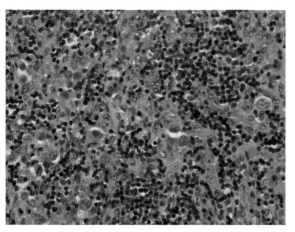

Figure 4.8 Non-keratinizing nasopharyngeal carcinoma showing Schminke-type pattern, with epithelial cells mingling with lymphoid cells (H&E × 400).

with indistinct cell borders, scanty cytoplasm, round-to-oval vesicular nuclei, and large central nucleoli. The cells often appear crowded or even overlapping. There can be small foci of primitive squamous differentiation. A typical feature is the presence of a variable lymphoid infiltrate, ranging from rare inflammatory cells to a dense infiltrate that obscures the epithelial nature of the tumor, giving rise to the term "lymphoepithelial carcinoma." Two histological patterns may occur: Regaud type, with a well-defined collection of epithelial cells surrounded by lymphocytes and connective tissue, and Schmincke type, in which the tumor cells are distributed diffusely and intermingle with the inflammatory cells (Figure 4.8). Coagulative necrosis, epithelioid granulomata, and eosinophils may be present (91,92).

The majority of tumor cells show strong staining for pan-cytokeratin (AE1/AE3). Cytokeratins 7 and 20 are negative (93). Immunoreactivity for EMA is often only focal (94). Lymphoid cells are a mixture of T-cells and B-cells, usually with T-cells predominating.

Non-keratinizing nasopharyngeal carcinoma is associated with EBV in virtually 100% of cases, with *in situ* hybridization for EBV-encoded early RNA (EBER) being the most reliable method to demonstrate infection. Epstein–Barr virus latent membrane protein-1 (LMP1) is positive in only 30–40% of cases, and immunostaining is often patchy and weak (86,95).

Genetics: Several associations have been described between the frequency of human leukocyte antigen (HLA) Class I genes in certain populations and the risk of developing NPC (96).

Differential diagnosis: In small biopsies, the epithelial nature of the tumor may be missed in cases with dense lymphoid infiltrate. Conversely, clusters of germinal center cells, a tangentially sectioned crypt with reactive changes, lymphoid hyperplasia, featuring increased numbers of immunoblasts, and lymphoid tissue-associated high endothelial venules can be mistaken for NPC (97). Immunohistochemistry for cytokeratin, CD45, CD34, and fresh tissue fluorescence in-situ hybridization (FISH) for EBER will help, depending on the differential diagnosis. Negative FISH for EBER would render a diagnosis of nasopharyngeal carcinoma most unlikely (97). Nasopharyngeal carcinoma can mimic large-cell lymphoma or Hodgkin's lymphoma. NPC with marked cellular spindling can mimic a high-grade sarcoma. In most cases, the diagnosis can be reached by identifying a component of typical NPC, with further confirmation by cytokeratin immunoreactivity.

Esthesioneuroblastoma (ENB)

Esthesioneuroblastoma or olfactory neuroblastoma is a rare, aggressive tumor of the sinonasal region originating from olfactory neuroepithelium. It is clinico-pathologically distinct from neuroblastoma elsewhere in the body, and is more closely related to neuroendocrine carcinoma (NEC) of the sino-nasal region.

Clinical presentation: Esthesioneuroblastoma can occur at any age, with peak incidence in the second and fifth decades of life (98,99). Up to 15 years of age, the estimated incidence is 0.1/100 000, but it is the most common cancer of the nasal cavity (99).

ENB generally presents with nasal symptoms, including obstruction, epistaxis, discharge, unilateral polyps, or anosmia. The initial symptoms tend to be subtle, with clinical diagnosis of rhinosinusitis or nasal polyps (100), the tumoral nature often being an unexpected pathological finding.

Macroscopy: Generally mucosa-covered, soft, polypoid, often highly vascular masses varying from less than 1 cm to a large mass filling the nasal cavity and extending into the paranasal sinuses, orbit, and/or cranial cavity.

Histology: Characteristically composed of circumscribed lobules or nests separated by a richly vascularized fibrous stroma. Less often, the tumor shows a diffuse growth pattern. The neoplastic cells have uniform, small, round nuclei with scant cytoplasm, dispersed ("salt and pepper") coarse-to-fine nuclear chromatin, and inconspicuous nucleoli. Nuclear pleomorphism, mitoses, and necrosis are usually absent, but higher-grade tumors show all three. The cells have indistinct borders and are surrounded by a neurofibrillary matrix. Perivascular pseudorosettes, Homer–Wright-type pseudorosettes and less commonly Flexner–Wintersteiner type (true neural rosettes) are seen. Occasional divergent differentiation with glandular, squamous, teratomatous, or rhabdomyoblastic elements may be seen (101).

Hyam's histologic grading scheme reportedly provides prognostic information, with grade I patients having a uniformly good outcome and grade IV patients all dying of disease (102,103).

The majority of cases express neuron-specific enolase (NSE), synaptophysin, neurofilament protein (NFP), class III β-tubulin, and microtubule-associated protein. S100 protein is limited to the sustentacular cells in the periphery of the neoplastic lobules, which may be sparse in higher-grade tumors. Immunoreactivity may be seen for chromogranin, GFAP, and Leu-7. Epithelial markers, CD45, HMB-45, desmin, and CD99 are absent. Proliferation marker studies using Ki-67 and MIB-1 have shown correlation with tumor grade.

Differential diagnosis: The differential diagnosis includes other small, round cell tumors that can occur in the sinonasal tract, i.e. sinonasal undifferentiated carcinoma, lymphoma, rhabdomyosarcoma, mucosal malignant melanoma, and neuroendocrine carcinomas.

Tumors of bone and cartilage

These lesions are covered in Chapter 12. Of note, the craniofacial bones are a common site of origin for osteoma, juvenile active ossifying fibroma, benign fibro-osseus lesions (ossifying fibroma and fibrous dysplasia), and LCH (104).

Oral lesions

Jaw cysts

Jaw cysts can be divided into *odontogenic cysts* that derive from odontogenic epithelium, and have either developmental or inflammatory etiology, and *non-odontogenic cysts* derived from other epithelial structures (105).

Inflammatory odontogenic cysts

Radicular cyst

Radicular cysts occur at the roots of non-vital teeth, in which the dental pulp is necrotic, usually due to tooth decay. There is periapical granulation tissue, and the inflammation stimulates the growth of the rests of

Malassez in the periodontal ligament. Subsequent central liquefactive necrosis leads to cyst formation (105,106).

Clinical presentation: Lesions most commonly occur in young adults and are rare in deciduous teeth (107). The anterior maxilla is the most common site, around the lateral incisors, although the mandible is more commonly affected when deciduous teeth are involved (106).

Radiographically, the lesion presents as a radiolucent region of bone destruction at the root apex. Cysts may also occur at the lateral side of the tooth, known as a *lateral radicular cyst.*

Macroscopy: The lesion is often friable and received piecemeal, with the structure of the cyst not evident. Intact cysts may show a thickened wall, and the lumen may contain altered blood or cholesterol crystals (106).

Histology: The cyst is lined by spongiotic and inflamed non-keratinizing stratified squamous epithelium. Eosinophilic, hyaline Rushton bodies may be seen within the epithelium, and up to 40% of cases show mucous cells, with rare ciliated cells in some (105,106). The surrounding wall is of fibrous connective tissue showing an inflammatory cell infiltrate. Collections of lipid-laden macrophages may be seen. Other inflamed odontogenic and non-odontogenic cysts can appear histologically identical. The association of the cyst with a decayed tooth is therefore vital to the diagnosis. If a radicular cyst remains in the jaw after the associated tooth has been extracted, it is termed a *residual cyst.*

Paradental cyst

Inflammatory odontogenic cysts occurring at the lateral side of the tooth, at the junction of the enamel cap and the root. In contrast to the lateral radicular cyst, they occur in association with a vital tooth, which may be partially or fully erupted.

Clinical presentation: The majority are located in the mandible, with more than 60% in association with the third molar, usually presenting in early adulthood, while cysts in association with the lower first and second molars present at a mean age of 8.7 and 17.4 years, respectively (108). Apart from the vitality of the associated tooth, macroscopic and microscopic features are similar to the radicular cyst.

Developmental odontogenic cysts

Dentigerous cyst

Dentigerous cysts arise when fluid accumulates between the crown of a tooth and the reduced enamel epithelium that remains after enamel formation is complete.

Clinical presentation: They always occur in association with an unerupted tooth, most commonly the third mandibular molars, followed by maxillary third molars, maxillary canines, and premolars of the maxilla and mandible, and very rarely the incisors (109). They can rarely occur around an unerupted deciduous tooth, and have also been reported in association with supernumerary teeth (110). Presentation is usually in adolescents and young adults.

Radiographically, there is a unilocular radiolucent cyst surrounding the crown of the tooth only in the *central* variety, while *lateral* cysts only partially surround the crown, as they develop laterally along the tooth root, and the *circumferential* variety surrounds the crown and extends along the root (106).

Dentigerous cysts are usually successfully treated by enucleation with removal of the associated tooth.

Histology: The cyst is lined by a thin layer of non-keratinizing stratified squamous epithelium without rete ridges. Mucous cells, ciliated cells, eosinophilic cuboidal cells, and intraepithelial pseudomicrocysts may be seen, mimicking the rare glandular odontogenic cyst (111). If the cyst becomes inflamed, the epithelium becomes hyperplastic, with rete ridges developing, and can appear identical to a radicular cyst (105).

Differential diagnosis: Keratocystic odontogenic tumor and cystic ameloblastoma, which have a propensity to recur (112), and dental follicles.

Dental follicles

The dental follicle is a sac that surrounds a developing tooth.

Clinical presentation: A dental follicle can be visualized radiographically around impacted teeth as a pericoronal radiolucency. An enlarged dental follicle can appear radiologically identical to a small dentigerous cyst, the cut-off point between the two usually taken as a pericoronal lucency in excess of around 3 mm (106,113). Specimens may be sent for histopathological analysis with the question of whether they represent a dentigerous cyst or a dental follicle.

Histology: The dental follicle should be lined by reduced enamel epithelium. However, some may be lined by stratified squamous epithelium, even when pericoronal lucency is less than 2.5 mm and appear histologically identical to a dentigerous cyst. Therefore,

identification of a cystic cavity at the time of surgery may be the only way to distinguish between the two (113).

Lateral periodontal cysts

These cysts are thought to arise from rests of Malassez, remnants of dental lamina epithelium, and lie lateral to the roots close to the tooth crown (105).

Clinical presentation: These cysts are very rare in childhood, usually affecting older adults, most often in the premolar-canine-incisor region of the mandible, but also in the anterior maxilla (105,106). When the cyst is multilocular, it is known as the *Botryoid odontogenic cyst*.

Histology: The cyst is lined by thin non-keratinizing squamous or cuboidal epithelium with focal thickenings that contain numerous clear cells with glycogen-rich cytoplasm, and sometimes show a swirled architecture (105). Recurrence is unusual after enucleation, but is more common in the multicystic botryoid variants (114).

Glandular odontogenic cyst

Definition: This is a rare odontogenic cyst that usually presents in older adults, although rare cases have been seen in teenagers (115); 80% occur in the mandible, and 60% in the anterior jaws (111).

Radiographically it presents as a well-defined unilocular or multilocular radiolucency involving the periapical area of multiple teeth. Rare cases have been associated with an unerupted tooth, mimicking a dentigerous cyst, and lateral periodontal relationship is also rarely seen (111). Cysts can vary from 1 cm in size to extensive destructive lesions within the jaw (106).

Histology: The cyst is lined partly by non-keratinizing stratified squamous epithelium and partly by cuboidal or columnar epithelium, with surface eosinophilic hobnailed cells required for the diagnosis. Other features include apocrine snouting, intraepithelial microcysts, clear cells, mucous goblet cells, ciliated cells, papillary projections, and focal epithelial thickenings similar to the thickened plaques of the lateral periodontal cyst, in addition to swirled areas. Multicystic spaces are common (111,115).

Differential diagnosis: Diagnoses to consider are the lateral periodontal and botryoid odontogenic cysts, and cystic intraosseus mucoepidermoid carcinoma, although the latter would be exceptionally rare in childhood. Metaplastic change in a dentigerous cyst is a possibility for those in association with an uner-upted tooth (111). After excision, 30 to 50% of cysts recur, in some cases multiply (111,115).

Keratocystic odontogenic tumors

Keratocystic odontogenic tumors (KCOT) were for-merly known as odontogenic keratocysts. They are benign cystic intraosseus tumors with potentially aggressive and infiltrative behavior (112).

Clinical presentation: KCOTs present over a wide age range from the first to the ninth decades, with a peak in the second and third decades. The mandible is involved in 65–83% of cases, often at the angle (112).

Radiographically, KCOTs are often small unilocu-lar radiolucencies, with larger cysts more likely to be multilocular.

Genetics: Multiple cysts, which may be metachro-nous or synchronous, are usually part of nevoid basal cell carcinoma syndrome (NBCCS), and present at a younger age than sporadic KCOTs (116). This syndrome is caused by PTCH gene mutation, which has also been shown to be involved in sporadic KCOTs (112).

Macroscopy: Lesions may be unilocular or multi-locular, with a thin, often collapsed cyst lining, and keratinous cyst content may be present.

Histology: KCOTs are lined by parakeratotic strati-fied squamous epithelium approximately four to eight layers thick, without rete ridges. There is a prominent and often palisaded basal layer of columnar or cuboi-dal cells, often showing nuclear hyperchromatism. Suprabasilar mitoses are common. The layer of para-keratin is often corrugated, and may be subtle in some cases, causing diagnostic difficulty (Figure 4.9). There

is no granular cell layer. The cyst wall may contain smaller daughter cysts and solid epithelial nests, more common with NBCCS (116). KCOTs tend to recur after enucleation, and partial jaw resection may be required in some cases. Follow-up is essential due to the common presence of daughter cysts and multiple lesions (112).

Orthokeratinized odontogenic cysts

Clinical presentation: They most often occur in males from the second to fifth decades, usually presenting in the posterior mandible in association with an unerup-ted tooth (117).

Radiographically, they most often present as a uni-locular radiolucency up to 7 cm, with rare multilocular variants (106).

Histology: Histologically, the cyst lining is of orthokeratinized stratified squamous epithelium with a granular cell layer. The basal layer is composed of flattened cuboidal cells without palisading. Recurrence is very rare.

Non-odontogenic cysts

Palatal cysts

Around two thirds of babies are born with two to three small yellow-white palatal cysts around 1 mm in diam-eter. They are usually found in the midline at the junc-tion of the soft and hard palates, and are thought to develop from persistent islands of epithelial cells at the site of palatal shelf fusion (118). Similar cysts are found on the gums of 25–53% babies, known as *gingival cysts of the newborn*, or *dental lamina cysts* (118,119), derived from remnants of the dental lamina. Lesions are less common in premature babies, increasing in incidence towards term (120). Both types of lesion spontaneously resolve in the weeks or months after birth, and so are rarely seen by the histopathologist, but show a lining of stratified squamous epithelium with keratotic or para-keratotic content (121).

Nasopalatine duct cyst

Nasopalatine duct cysts (NPDCs) also known as incisive canal cysts, are the most common non-odontogenic maxillary cyst, affecting 1% of the population (122). Nasopalatine duct cysts are thought to arise from epi-thelial remnants of the nasopalatine duct, which is the fetal connection between the nasal cavity and developing maxilla. As the anterior palate fuses, the connection narrows, forming the incisive canals that carry nerves, vessels, and epithelial rests of the degenerated nasopala-tine duct (123).

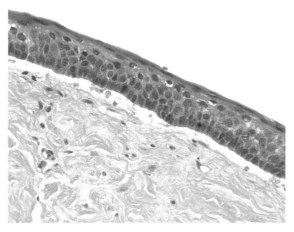

Figure 4.9 Keratocystic odontogenic tumor (H&E × 400), with basal palisading and subtle parakeratosis.

Clinical presentation: Around 30% of cases are asymptomatic, being incidentally identified on routine radiographs. Presentation is rare in childhood, with most presenting in the fourth to sixth decades.

Radiographically, a well-defined radiolucency is present in the anterior mandible, with average size of 17 mm (122).

Histology: Nasopalatine duct cysts may be lined by a combination of stratified squamous epithelium, pseudostratified columnar epithelium, with or without cilia and goblet cells, simple columnar, and simple cuboidal epithelium (123). The fibrovascular wall may contain minor salivary gland tissue and cartilage, and secondary inflammatory changes may be seen.

Congenital granular cell tumor (CGCT)

Congenital granular cell tumor also known as congenital epulis, is a rare tumor that originates from anterior alveolar ridge mucosa, most often in the maxilla, with rare cases affecting the tongue (124). Histogenesis is not clear, but ultrastructural studies support a mesenchymal origin (125).

Clinical presentation: The lesions are usually present at birth, or develop shortly after. There is a strong female predominance, 9:1; in 10% of cases, lesions are multiple. Large lesions may cause feeding problems or respiratory compromise. Spontaneous regression has been reported (126).

Macroscopy: Pedunculated, sometimes lobulated nodules, usually 0.5–2 cm in size, but up to 9 cm in some cases (127).

Histology: The core is composed of tightly packed, large, histiocyte-like polygonal cells with granular eosinophilic cytoplasm and small dark nuclei, with virtually no discernible stroma. The overlying epithelium is atrophic. Odontogenic epithelial rests may be seen (127). In contrast to granular cell myoblastomas, which may appear histologically similar, CGCT are negative for S100 and NSE. Vimentin, PGP 9.5, and CD68 are positive (128).

Orofacial granulomatosis

This is a generic term including granulomatous inflammation affecting the mouth or oropharynx submucosa, for which there is a wide differential diagnosis, including Crohn's disease, granulomatous cheilitis of Miescher or of Melkersson–Rosenthal syndrome, sarcoidosis, WG, granulomatous gingivitis, cholesterol granuloma, foreign-body granuloma, and infections such as tuberculosis, syphilis, fungi, or *Salmonella* (127).

Clinical presentation: This varies with the underlying condition. Some granulomata may be lobulated nodules or papules, some may cluster together to give a cobblestoned mucosa in conditions such as Crohn's disease, while some patients may present with lip swelling.

Macroscopy: The pathologist usually receives an incisional biopsy of labial mucosa, or biopsies of other intraoral sites. Ulceration may be present in some cases.

Histology: Histological appearances and the presence of micro-organisms or necrosis will vary according to the underlying cause. Excluding particular infective causes and WG, granulomata are usually small, well-defined, and non-caseating, composed of epithelioid histiocytes, including multinucleated giant cells, with or without surrounding chronic inflammation. Multiple levels of a labial biopsy may be required to reveal the granulomata.

Differential diagnosis: Surgeons may interpret *orofacial granulomatosis* as being synonymous with Crohn's disease; pathologists should ensure that their report reflects the range of possible differential diagnoses from the above list, depending on the particular histological features of the case.

Central giant-cell granuloma (CGCG)

Central giant-cell granuloma occurs in the jaws and craniofacial skeleton, and is thought to be a reactive process, rather than a true neoplasm. This lesion is discussed in Chapter 12.

Melanotic neuroectodermal tumor of infancy (MNTI)

Melanotic neuroectodermal tumor of infancy is a very rare tumor of neural crest origin, with a predilection for the head and neck region. It is probably a dysembryogenetic neoplasm that recapitulates the early embryonic retina (129).

Clinical presentation: Melanotic neuroectodermal tumor of infancy predominantly affects the anterior maxilla of infants in the first year of life, but other sites include the mandible, skull, meninges, brain, soft tissues of the head and neck region and extremities, long bones, and the paratesticular region, including the epididymis (130). It presents as a rapidly growing mass, which often destroys underlying bone and may displace teeth. Based on published cases, 7% of cases have been associated with metastatic disease, with 36% resulting in local recurrence (130). Elevated plasma and urinary catecholamines may be present.

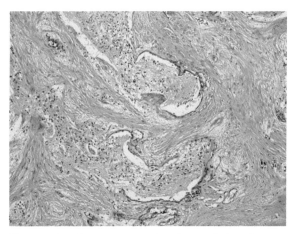

Figure 4.10 Melanotic neuroectodermal tumor of infancy featuring a dual population of neuroblastic cells and pigmented epithelioid cells, with fibroblastic stroma (H&E × 100).

Macroscopy: Usually 2–4 cm in diameter, up to 10 cm in some cases; may be a lobulated, firm mass with white, blue, or black discoloration on cut surface.

Histology: The tumor shows a biphasic pattern. Large polygonal epithelioid cells, with open vesicular nuclei and intracellular melanin granules, are arranged in alveolar and tubular structures. The second intermixed population is of smaller neuroblastic cells, with a background fibrovascular stroma that may contain neurofibrillary or glial elements (Figure 4.10). Most MNTIs show cytological atypia, but mitoses are usually low at < 2/10 hpf (131). Although very rare cases may show more severe atypia or abundant mitoses, in most cases, histological features cannot distinguish malignant from benign behavior (132). Large cells are positive with HMB-45, NSE, cytokeratin, and vimentin, and are variably positive for EMA. Small cells are positive for CD56 and NSE, with variable positivity with Leu7, synaptophysin, GFAP, and S100 (130). Focal positivity with desmin and chromogranin has been described (129). NB84a and neurofilament are negative (129,130). CD99 positivity has been reported in a single case of a highly mitotically active tumor that behaved aggressively, and had a Ki67 fraction of 25% (132).

Electronmicroscopy reveals cells with melanosomes at various stages of maturation, and cells with neuroblastic features, including neurosecretory granules and cytoplasmic processes (129).

Differential diagnosis: Other melanin-containing tumors, pigmented ectomesenchymoma and pigmented intraosseous odontogenic carcinoma of the maxilla.

Larynx

Laryngocele

Air or fluid-filled dilatation of the laryngeal saccule. While internal laryngoceles are confined to the larynx, combined internal–external and external laryngoceles can present as a neck mass adjacent to the thyro-hyoid membrane.

Laryngeal hemangioma

The are benign vascular tumors similar to those found elsewhere in the body (see Chapter 1).

Clinical features: Presentation is usually in the neonatal period or in the first six months of life, often with progressive or intermittent stridor. There is female predominance (133). Lesions may be associated with simultaneous cutaneous hemangiomas, and some may be associated with the PHACES syndrome (Posterior fossa malformations–hemangiomas–arterial anomalies–cardiac defects–eye abnormalities–sternal cleft, and supraumbilical raphe syndrome) (134). As with other infantile hemangiomas, lesions show a tendency to regress after an initial period of growth.

Macroscopy: These are usually subglottic tumors that may be sessile growths of variable color, or may be circumferential in nature.

Histology: Similar to hemangiomas of infancy seen elsewhere. Although small studies have revealed GLUT-1 negativity in some lesions (135), and there are other case reports of pyogenic granulomas in the larynx (136), a recent larger series revealed GLUT-1 positivity in all 18 cases tested, indicating that the majority of such lesions are hemangiomas of infancy (133). GLUT-1 staining should be carried out on all cases to allow correct designation.

Respiratory papilloma/papillomatosis

A rare disease in which solitary, or more commonly, multiple, exophytic squamous wart-like lesions occur within the respiratory tract (137). The papillomata can occur anywhere in the aerodigestive tract, but are most frequent in the larynx, and tend to be recurrent, leading to the term *recurrent respiratory papillomatosis* (RRP).

Clinical features: Recurrent respiratory papillomatosis is caused by human papilloma virus (HPV) with subtypes 6 and 11 accounting for more than 90% cases (138). Human papilloma virus infection in children is related to maternal genital infection

(139). Presentation is with dysphonia and stridor, less commonly with chronic cough, recurrent pneumonia, dyspnea, and acute life-threatening events (139–141). Delayed diagnosis may result in an acute presentation with respiratory distress, requiring urgent tracheotomy.

Squamous papillomata in children and adults follow diverse clinical courses. Extensive growth with rapid recurrences is more common in children, and the relatively small airway in children predisposes to airway obstruction. Disease progression is more frequent in the juvenile form, usually associated with subglottic papillomata and prior tracheotomy (142).

Cases of RRP occur mainly at sites where ciliated and squamous epithelia are juxtaposed. It primarily involves the larynx, especially the vocal cords, but extralaryngeal extension has been identified in 30% of children and in 16% of adult patients (140). The most frequent extralaryngeal sites are, in descending order: oral cavity, trachea, bronchi, lung parenchyma, and esophagus (143). Tracheotomy is associated with more frequent extension into the tracheobronchial tree. Any injury to ciliated mucosa after surgical procedures may result in squamous metaplasia, creating an iatrogenic squamous–ciliary junction, and a new potential site for further tumors (143).

The clinical course is highly variable, from spontaneously remitting to aggressive and recurrent disease (139). The overall mortality rate of patients with RRP ranges from 4–14% (140), often due to asphyxia, infection, and pulmonary complications (140,141).

Malignant change in children has been described, but is extremely rare in the absence of a history of irradiation, or other promoters (144,145). The overall incidence of cancer development for irradiated patients is 14%, and 2% for the non-irradiated (145). Malignancies occur preferentially in the tracheobronchial tree in children, and in the larynx in adults (144,145).

Macroscopy: When papillomata are microscopic and spread, they give the mucosa a velvety appearance, and when macroscopic or exophytic, they appear as cauliflower-like projections. These lesions may be sessile or pedunculated and typically appear pinkish to white (146).

Histology: Squamous papillomata are composed of finger-like or frond-like projections of squamous mucosa, containing thin fibrovascular cores. Arborization with secondary or tertiary branching of papillae may be present. Frequently, there is basal and parabasal cell hyperplasia, usually extending up to the mid-portion. Mitoses may be prominent within this area. Scattered koilocytes may be seen in the superficial part of the epithelium (147). Mild-to-moderate nuclear atypia with hyperchromasia, increased nuclear cytoplasmic ratio, and increased mitoses may be seen. Some authors have suggested that these features may predict an aggressive clinical course. However, no definite histological prognosticators of local recurrence and malignant transformation have been identified (148).

Differential diagnosis: Verrucous carcinoma and papillary squamous cell carcinoma may have morphological overlap with respiratory papillomatosis, but are not seen in children, so there is no genuine morphological differential diagnosis.

Cervical developmental anomalies

The differential diagnosis of head and neck masses in children includes a variety of congenital cysts, sinuses, and fistulae that are the results of defective embryonic development. Thyroglossal duct anomalies are the most common of this group, followed by branchial cleft and arch anomalies, dermoid cysts, and median cervical clefts (149).

Thyroglossal duct anomalies

The thyroid gland begins to develop from a midline endodermal thickening in the floor of the primordial pharynx, at around 24 days postfertilization. The thickening then forms a hollow thyroid diverticulum (primordium) within the tongue. With embryonic growth, the diverticulum descends into the neck, ventral to the developing hyoid bone and laryngeal cartilages, while still connected to the tongue via the thyroglossal duct. The thyroid diverticulum becomes solid and divides into the left and right lobes of the thyroid gland, divided by the isthmus. The lumen of the thyroglossal duct should obliterate by week 7. A proximal remnant, the foramen cecum, persists at the base of the tongue, and in about 50% of people, a distal remnant remains, the pyramidal lobe of the thyroid (150). If the thyroglossal duct does not obliterate before formation of the mesodermal anlage of the hyoid bone, it will persist clinically as a cyst (151).

Clinical presentation: Most thyroglossal duct anomalies are diagnosed before five years of age, but can occur in adulthood (151). They most often present as a painless midline cystic neck mass. Although 60% are located adjacent to the hyoid bone, they can be located anywhere along the path of embryonic descent of the thyroid, with 24% between the base of tongue and hyoid bone, 13% between the hyoid bone and the pyramidal lobe, and 3% within the tongue in one series (152), with rarer reports of intrathyroid cysts (153–155). About 10–25% may be lateral, occurring more often on the left, and raise the differential diagnosis of a branchial cleft anomaly (156). Cysts may become infected and spontaneously rupture, fistulating to the skin, or discharge into the mouth via the foramen cecum. This risk of infection is the main indication for surgical removal (151). There are rare cases of respiratory compromise or sudden infant death due to airway obstruction from lesions at the base of the tongue (157,158).

In median ectopic thyroid, all of the thyroid tissue can be located in a thyroglossal duct cyst (149), rendering the patient hypothyroid after surgical removal. Carcinoma can occur within thyroglossal duct remnants, with a reported incidence of between less than 1% and 6.5% (159,160). Most cases occur in adults, but it is reported in children as young as six (161). Papillary thyroid carcinomas are the most common carcinoma to occur, but follicular lesions can also develop.

Macroscopic: Cysts are usually 2–3 cm in diameter, but can be as large as 10 cm. A long duct-like structure is often submitted for examination, usually with a portion of the hyoid bone. Multiple transverse sections and serial sections or deeper levels may be required to demonstrate the diagnostic features of the duct.

Histology: A thyroglossal duct cyst (TDC) may be lined by respiratory or squamous epithelium, or a combination of both. However, the epithelial lining may be replaced by inflammatory granulation tissue and fibrosis in cases where infection has occurred. Thyroid tissue is found in the wall in up to 40% of cases, if serial sections are performed (162), but its presence is not required to make the diagnosis (Figure 4.11). Histological examination of the hyoid bone sometimes reveals the tract extending into the bone; decalcification and sampling of the hyoid bone should be done in all cases.

Differential diagnosis: As the epithelial lining of a TDC can be identical to that of a branchial cleft cyst, and lymphoid tissue can also be found in the wall of a thyroglossal duct cyst, these two cyst types may appear histologically identical. In such cases, clinico-pathological correlation concerning the site of the cyst and the relationship to the hyoid bone, or the

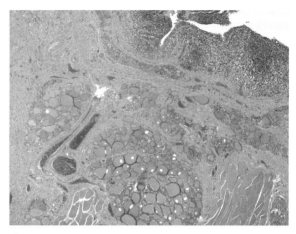

Figure 4.11 Thyroglossal duct cyst (H&E × 40) featuring lining of respiratory-type epithelium, with lymphoid and thyroid tissue in the wall.

path of descent of the thyroid, may be crucial. Rare cysts have been reported with features of both thyroglossal duct and branchial cleft anomalies, and even bronchogenic cysts (155,163). However, it should be remembered that as ectopic thyroid tissue can be present anywhere along the path of embryonic descent, it may be present incidentally within the walls of other cyst types. We have seen several otherwise typical dermoid cysts with thyroid tissue in the wall.

Branchial arch anomalies

Four pairs of branchial arches (more correctly known as pharyngeal arches) develop during the fourth week of development. The arches are separated on the external, ectodermal surface by clefts called pharyngeal grooves, and by pharyngeal pouches internally on the endodermal surface (150). In humans, the pharyngeal clefts and pouches are obliterated during normal development by the invasion of surrounding mesenchyme, and the arches develop into the structures of the head and neck (164).

Clinical presentation: Branchial anomalies occur if there is incomplete obliteration of the clefts and pouches, and can present as cysts, fistulae, and sinuses. Patients can present from infancy through to adulthood, with equal sex incidence; 2–10% of cases are bilateral. The site of the lesion depends on which branchial cleft the anomaly is derived from.

Macroscopy: Variable, depending on whether the specimen is a cyst, sinus or fistula. Cysts are usually

2–6 cm in diameter and may contain keratinous material, and there may be superimposed inflammatory and fibrotic changes.

Genetics: Rare cases may be inherited as part of branchio-oculo-facial syndrome, an autosomal dominant craniofacial disorder with variable expression, featuring branchial anomalies, hearing loss, and renal anomalies (165).

First branchial cleft anomalies

These account for between 8 and 18% of branchial anomalies (166, 167). The first (mandibular) arch forms the mandible, part of the maxillary process and parts of the inner ear. The first cleft and pouch form the external auditory canal, the eustachian tube, the middle ear cavity, and the mastoid air cells.

Clinical presentation: They are more common in girls, and can present at any age from infancy to the elderly (166). They present with purulent drainage from the ear, periauricular swelling in the parotid region, or as a fistula or abscess in the neck, above the horizontal plane of the hyoid bone (168). Infection is common; they are often misdiagnosed, and frequently recur if resection is incomplete (169). In the largest series of 39 cases reported, 28% were fistulae, 51% sinuses, and 21% cysts (168). In 10% of cases, there is an asymptomatic membranous attachment between the floor of the external auditory canal and the tympanic membrane (168).

Subclassification: Defects are divided into two types (169,170). *Type I* defects are embryological duplication anomalies of the membranous external auditory canal. They are usually located medial, inferior, or posterior to the concha and pinna, and pass lateral to the facial nerve. *Type II* defects are derived from the first branchial cleft *and* the first and second branchial arches; they are associated with defects of the membranous external auditory canal and cartilaginous elements, and are thought to be embryological duplication anomalies of both the external auditory canal *and* pinna. They present as preauricular, infraauricular, or postauricular swellings just below the angle of the mandible, anterior to the sternocleidomastoid muscle (168). Fistulous tracts extend through the parotid gland, pass medial to the facial nerve, and may extend into the external auditory canal, although connection with the middle ear is very rare.

Histology: Type I defects are derived only from ectodermal elements of the first branchial cleft, so they are lined by keratinizing stratified squamous

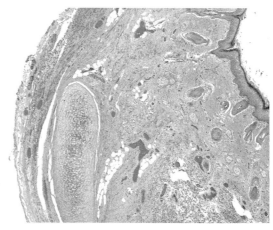

Figure 4.12 Type II first branchial arch anomaly (H&E × 40), featuring ectodermal and mesodermal elements, with stratified squamous epithelium with skin adnexal structures and cartilage.

epithelium only, with no adnexal structures or cartilage. Lymphoid tissue is common. As type II defects are derived from ectodermal and mesodermal elements, they show keratinizing stratified squamous epithelium with skin adnexae and bars of hyaline cartilage (Figure 4.12). It may not be possible to distinguish type I from type II lesions, especially in the presence of infection, but the lesions may be classified simply as either cysts, sinuses, or fistulae (166).

Differential diagnosis: A type I first branchial arch anomaly can mimic an epidermoid cyst. The differential diagnoses of type II defects are dermoid cysts and the rare cystic sebaceous lymphadenoma of the parotid gland (171).

Second branchial cleft anomalies

These account for from 69 to 95% of branchial anomalies (164,167). The second (hyoid) arch forms the hyoid bone and the adjacent neck region, while the second pouch develops into the tonsillar and supratonsillar fossae.

Clinical presentation: They usually present as a fistula or cyst in the lower anterolateral neck, anterior to the sternocleidomastoid muscle. Cysts are more common, and usually present in adults aged 20–40 (149). Fistulae usually present in infancy, draining along the anterior border of the sternocleidomastoid muscle in the lower third of the neck (164). Fistulous tracts follow the carotid sheath, passing over the hypoglossal nerve, between the internal and external carotid arteries, terminating in the tonsillar fossa.

Subclassification: Second-arch anomalies are classified into four types, depending on their location

(149,172). *Type I* lesions lie anterior to the sternocleidomastoid muscle and do not contact the carotid sheath. The most common are *type II* lesions, which pass deep to the sternocleidomastoid muscle, and may be anterior or posterior to the carotid sheath. *Type III* lesions pass between the internal and external carotid arteries and lie adjacent to the pharynx. *Type IV* lesions lie medial to the carotid sheath, close to the pharynx, and adjacent to the tonsillar fossa.

Histology: Of these lesions, 90% are lined by squamous epithelium, 8% by respiratory-type epithelium, and 2% by both (173). Cyst content may be keratinous, mucoid, or serous, and may contain cholesterol crystals or purulent material; 97% contain lymphoid tissue within the wall. This can be nodular or diffuse in arrangement, and may contain germinal centers and show features of nodal architecture, with subcapsular and medullary sinuses (173). Sebaceous glands and salivary gland tissue may be seen, and xanthogranulomatous inflammation, mimicking a malignancy, has been reported (174). Respiratory epithelium is more common in sinuses and fistulae (164), and in cases where infection has occurred, the epithelium may be replaced by granulation tissue and fibrosis. Rarely, squamous cell carcinoma arises within branchial cleft anomalies in adults, and such cases require careful assessment to distinguish primary branchogenic carcinoma from a cystic metastasis (175).

Third and fourth branchial cleft anomalies

These are rare, accounting for between 3 and 10% of branchial anomalies (176,177). They are thought to derive from persistence of the thymopharyngeal duct of the third branchial pouch, often passing through or adjacent to the thyroid, usually on the left side (178).

Clinical presentation: Generally as a neck abscess or suppurative thyroiditis, or tracheal compression and stridor in neonates (179–181); patients can present at any age. Third-cleft anomalies present at the lower anterior border of the sternocleidomastoid muscle, level with the superior pole of the thyroid, with 89% on the left (149,180). Fourth branchial arch anomalies present as lateral cysts in the lower third of the neck, with 94% occurring on the left side (179).

Histology: Third and fourth anomalies are lined by stratified squamous epithelium or ciliated respiratory-type epithelium and often contain thymic tissue (149,182). Rarely, parathyroid tissue may be present

(183). Distinction from cysts arising from thymic or parathyroid rests is made by the connection of branchial anomalies to the piriform sinus.

Congenital midline cervical cleft

A rare congenital anomaly, most likely caused by a failure of midline fusion of the first and second branchial arches during development.

Clinical presentation: It presents at birth with a midline defect of the anterior neck skin, a superior overhanging skin tag, a sinus tract passing inferiorly from the skin defect, and usually a subcutaneous fibrous cord (184). It is usually an isolated defect, but rare cases have been associated with midline clefts of the tongue, lower lip, mandible, and sternum (149). The subcutaneous cord can prevent full extension of the neck and lead to micrognathia and torticollis (184).

Preauricular lesions

Preauricular skin pits or tags occur in 0.3–5% of the population (185). Some preauricular sinuses and cysts are remnants of the first pharyngeal groove, but others are ectodermal folds sequestered during formation of the auricle (150).

Genetics: Some preauricular lesions may be part of a syndrome such as Treacher–Collins, Goldenhar, or branchio-oculo-facial syndromes. Hearing testing and renal ultrasound should be considered when other anomalies are present (186).

Histology: Histologically, sinus tracts may show features of infection. Preauricular tags typically consist of a central bar of elastic cartilage surrounded by subcutaneous fat with a covering of skin.

Cervical chondrocutaneous remnants

Similar to preauricular skin tags, but located in the lateral neck, usually anterior to the sternocleidomastoid muscle. They consist of skin covering a central bar of elastic cartilage, are rarely bilateral, and are commonly associated with other anomalies involving the auditory, respiratory, gastrointestinal, genitourinary, cardiovascular, musculoskeletal, or visual systems, with some part of branchio-oculo-facial syndrome (165,187,188). These remnants are thought to derive from second branchial arch structures (187). Differential diagnosis is of skin tags associated with a thyroglossal duct remnant.

Cervical thymic remnants, thymic cysts, and thymopharyngeal duct cysts

The thymus develops from the third pharyngeal pouch. Bilateral thymic primordia descend along the paired thymopharyngeal ducts, coming together in the midline to form the thymus, before continuing to migrate inferiorly into the superior mediastinum (150). Embryonic remnants of the thymus may therefore be found anywhere along the path of descent, from the mandible to the sternal notch.

Clinical presentation: A large pediatric autopsy study found abnormally positioned thymic tissue in 1% of children, most often in the anterior neck near the thyroid gland, but with one case at the left base of skull (189). Of these children, 71% had features consistent with DiGeorge syndrome, and of those who did not, half had no mediastinal thymic tissue present (189).

Cervical thymic remnants and cysts are usually asymptomatic, but they can present with dysphagia or dyspnoea, and rarely as an emergency with airway obstruction (190–192). *Ectopic solid thymic tissue* usually presents as an asymptomatic neck mass in infancy, with the majority of children under three years of age (193–195).

Thymic cysts are more common, and usually present between 2 and 10 years, during the period of prepubertal thymic enlargement, with the remainder in early adulthood (196). Although all thymic cysts are strictly speaking remnants of the thymopharyngeal duct, the term *thymopharyngeal duct cyst* is used when the cyst maintains a connection to the pharynx at the piriform sinus (197–199). Thymopharyngeal duct cysts are the rarest of the thymic embryonic remnants. With cervical thymic cysts, 50% can extend into the mediastinum (196,200), presenting different surgical challenges, and care should be taken to ensure that ectopic cervical thymic tissue is not the only thymic tissue present, to avoid total thymectomy on resection.

Macroscopy: Average size is around 7 cm, but cysts can measure up to 11 cm in diameter (191).

Histology: The cyst lining may be stratified squamous, columnar, or cuboidal epithelium, and may show secondary changes, with granulation tissue, fibrosis, and cholesterol clefts. Thymic tissue is present in the wall, with lymphoid tissue and squamous components with Hassall's corpuscles. Even a small amount of thymic tissue designates the cyst as a thymic cyst,

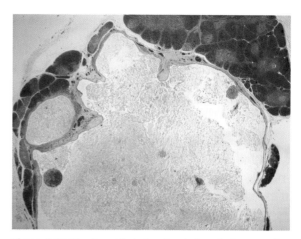

Figure 4.13 Thymic cyst including thymic tissue in the cyst wall (H&E × 10).

and thorough sampling and sectioning may be required to demonstrate this (Figure 4.13). Due to their common origin in the third pharyngeal pouch, parathyroid tissue may be found embedded within normally sited thymus glands, and may also be found with ectopic thymic tissue (201) and in the wall of thymic cysts (202). However, such cysts, including both thymus and parathyroid gland tissue, are probably better designated as *third pharyngeal pouch cysts*.

Parathyroid cysts

Parathyroid cysts are rare neck masses that most often present in adults, but with rare reports of cases occurring in the first and second decades (203–205), and one report in infancy (206). Some cysts may derive from embryonic remnants of the third and fourth pharyngeal pouches, while others may represent cystic degeneration in an abnormal gland (see also Chapter 6).

Clinical presentation: Presentation is usually with an anterior neck mass below the thyroid gland, with 65% occurring in association with the inferior parathyroid glands, but cysts can occur anywhere in the anterior neck, within the thyroid gland itself, or even posterior to the thyroid (207,208). The majority of cysts are non-functioning; functioning cysts are associated with hyperparathyroidism and hypercalcaemia, and are more likely to be due to cystic degeneration in a hyperplastic or adenomatous gland (207).

Macroscopy: Cysts range from 1 to 10 cm in diameter and are thin-walled and unilocular (209).

Histology: A cyst lined by cuboidal or cubo-columnar epithelium with chief cells or oxyphil cells within the wall. Even if diagnostic parathyroid tissue is absent, the diagnosis can be made by parathyroid hormone levels in the cyst fluid (207).

Differential diagnosis: Parathyroid gland tissue may be present as part of a branchial cleft cyst, which would show a stratified squamous epithelial lining (183).

Dermoid cysts

The soft tissues of the face form from the merging of the frontal, maxillary, and mandibular facial processes. Ectodermal elements can be trapped along lines of embryonic fusion, later forming dermoid cysts. They comprise ectodermal and endodermal elements only; if mesodermal components are found, the lesion should be designated a teratoma.

Clinical presentation: A large series of pediatric head and neck dermoid cysts from the Mayo Clinic revealed 61% to be periorbital, and 18% cervical, with 4% showing intracranial extension (210). The most common congenital midline nasal masses are dermoid cysts (211), which may also present in the floor of the mouth (212). A third of cases are congenital in presentation, with most presenting by age six (213).

Macroscopy: Average size is around 1 cm (210), although a giant variant mimicking a cystic hygroma has been reported (214).

Histology: The cyst is lined by keratinizing stratified squamous epithelium with skin adnexal structures in the wall. Cysts arising near to the median canthus of the eye may show lacrimal gland tissue in the wall, and this should be included in the histology report, to alert the surgeon to the possibility of damage to the lacrimal gland apparatus (215).

Differential diagnosis: Branchial cleft cyst, discussed above.

Foregut duplication cysts

These arise from the division of the embryonic foregut, and include bronchogenic cysts and duplication cysts of the gut.

Clinical presentation: Foregut duplication cysts of the head and neck are uncommon, and may arise in the oral cavity, including the tongue, oropharynx, supraglottis, intra- or extralaryngeal, anterior midline, anterolateral neck, or even paraspinally (216–218).

Macroscopy: Cysts feature a thin cyst wall, are often tubular in shape, and may contain either serous or mucoid fluid (219).

Histology: Cysts may be lined by stratified squamous, pseudostratified ciliated columnar or gastric-type epithelium, or sometimes a combination of these. Those cysts lined by respiratory-type epithelium with seromucinous glands *or* cartilage, *or* both, in the wall are classified as bronchogenic cysts. A smooth muscle layer is also usually present. Cartilage is found less often in cervical bronchogenic cysts than in mediastinal or thoracic variants (219) (see Chapter 5). In infected cases, squamous epithelium may be present, and scanty lymphoid tissue may also be present, making surgical identification of location important in the distinction from branchial cleft cysts.

Tumors of the neck with thymic or related branchial pouch differentiation

A classification for this rare group of tumors occurring in the thyroid and soft tissues of the neck with four groups has been suggested: ectopic hamartomatous thymoma, ectopic cervical thymomas, spindle epithelial tumor with thymus-like differentiation (SETTLE), and carcinoma showing thymus-like differentiation (CASTLE). The most common in the pediatric setting is SETTLE, a rare tumor of the thyroid and perithyroid tissues that most often occurs in children and adolescents (220).

Teratoma

These are neoplasms derived from totipotential cells that typically contain elements from all three germ cell layers, with tissues foreign to the site of origin. However, some monodermal or bidermal tumors are now also classified as teratomas.

Clinical presentation: Teratomas of the head and neck comprise around 5% of teratomas in infancy and childhood (221). They are most often diagnosed shortly after birth. The most common site is the anterior or lateral neck, where the thyroid may be involved (cervico-thyroidal teratoma), followed by the face, oropharynx or nasopharynx, where the tumor may protrude from the mouth, and orbit (221). Respiratory compromise leading to death may be caused by large cervical or oro/nasopharyngeal masses. Some cases may be diagnosed antenatally, and *ex utero* intrapartum surgical intervention can be used to establish an airway in such cases (222).

Macroscopy: Teratomas vary markedly in size, with one large pediatric head and neck series reporting sizes from 3 to 11 cm (221). Tumors are typically well circumscribed, and the cut surface may vary from solid to cystic, depending on the component tissue types, and may include bone and cartilage.

Histology: Tumors show a mixture of mature and immature tissues from all three germ-cell layers, which may include CNS tissue, retinal tissue, skin and skin adnexal structures, smooth muscle, adipose tissue, glandular epithelium, tooth formation, cartilage, and bone. Although immature elements may be present, congenital and infantile tumors of the head and neck usually behave in a benign fashion, although rare metastases have been reported (223). The presence of a yolk sac tumor or embryonal carcinoma is rare in head and neck tumors, but thorough sampling is important to detect such components.

Differential diagnosis: Sinonasal teratocarcinoma (combination of malignant teratoma and carcinosarcoma) with a triphasic growth pattern including epithelial, mesenchymal, and primitive neuroectodermal components is exceptionally rare in childhood (224). Salivary gland anlage tumor, a hamartoma of the midline nasopharynx usually occurring in neonates, can be mistaken for a teratoma, and is discussed later in the chapter (224). Nasopharyngeal teratomas with an intracranial component may contain neuroglial tissue, and need to be distinguished from an encephalocele.

Vascular lesions

Vascular lesions and tumors are covered in detail in Chapters 1 and 11, and specific sections on infantile hemangiomas are covered in the laryngeal and salivary gland sections of this chapter.

Lymphatic malformations

These are rare congenital lymphatic system malformations that occur throughout the body with greater frequency in the cervicofacial area. Traditionally, lymphatic malformations were described as lymphangioma, cystic hygroma, lymphangioma circumscriptum, and lymphangiomatosis (225). These lesions are now classified as simple (slow-flow) malformations, rather than neoplasms, and the terminology of lymphatic malformation is preferred (226). Lymphatic malformations can be simple when composed of only lymphatic vessels, or be part of compound lesions when other vascular elements, i.e, capillaries, arteries, and veins are present (see Chapter 1).

Clinical features: The majority present antenatally or within the first two years of life. The incidence ranges from 1.2 to 2.8 per 1000 newborns, with a slight male predilection (227). Symptoms are related to the size of malformation and compression of adjacent structures. Rapid enlargement due to inflammation, infection, or hemorrhage into the mass may bring a subclinical lesion to medical attention. The clinical course is variable with stable to erratic growth, or even spontaneous regression. A subgroup of larger lesions in the neck present as cystic hygroma. These are painless non-pulsatile masses in the neck with a rubbery consistency that are covered by normal colored skin. Lymphatic VMs are the most common bases for macrocheilia, macroglossia, macrotia, and macromelia (228).

Genetics: Several theories have been proposed to explain the origin of this abnormality (229). Macrocystic LMs can be associated with several congenital disorders, including Down syndrome and other trisomy disorders, Turner syndrome, hydrops fetalis, Noonan syndrome, and several others. No evidence for inheritance exists, suggesting that the possible genetic causes are compatible with life only as somatic mutations in a restricted area of the lymphatic network (230,231).

Macroscopy: Typical lesions are multilocular cysts filled with clear or yellow lymph fluid.

Histology: See Chapter 1.

Cranial fasciitis

This is a benign fibroblastic tumor of the skull (232).

Clinical features: It occurs almost exclusively in children under the age of six years, with median age of presentation of approximately 21 months. There are rare case reports in adults (233). The male:female ratio is 2:1 (232). Prior trauma to the affected area is a possible etiological factor (232,234–237). A familial predisposition has also been suggested (237). The lesions are characteristically rapidly growing, firm, and non-tender. Parieto-temporal regions are most commonly affected (232). In most cases, the lesion arises from the deep fascia of the scalp and erodes into the underlying calvaria, but one case of purely intracranial cranial fasciitis has been reported (236). The lesions are usually single. Imaging reveals a single lytic skull lesion. Erosion of the outer table of the skull is most common, although extension through the

149

inner table and involvement of the dura has been seen in approximately one-third of reported cases.

Macroscopy: The lesion is usually tan to gray-white, and may appear myxoid. The median size at presentation is around 2.5 cm, although they may attain a size as large as 15 cm (238).

Histology: Cranial fasciitis is considered as a variant of nodular fasciitis (see Chapter 11).The tumor cells are positive for vimentin and SMA, but negative for S100, desmin, Alk, CD34, MyoD1 and myogenin. A small proportion of these tumors may show nuclear β-catenin positivity (239).

Genetics: A subset of cases are associated with molecular alterations leading to aberrant persistence and nuclear localization of β-catenin. It is suggested that this subset has clinical and molecular features similar to desmoid fibromatosis and Gardner fibroma, in that some cases occur in association with FAP and show loss-of-function APC mutations, whereas other cases occur sporadically and show either gain-of-function CTNNB1 mutations or other yet-unidentified mutations (239). In view of this association with FAP, immunohistochemistry for β-catenin should be performed in all cases with the clinico-pathological features of cranial fasciitis. This will alert the clinician to the possibility of future occurrence of colonic adenomas and adenocarcinomas in this small subgroup.

Salivary glands

Introduction

Salivary gland tumors are rare in children and adolescents. Pediatric salivary-gland tumors account for 2.5–5% of the total number of salivary- gland tumors (240–242). Several features distinguish salivary-gland tumors in the pediatric age group, compared to those in adults, in particular a much greater frequency of non-epithelial benign tumors, a higher proportion of malignant tumors, when non-epithelial ones are excluded, and a different incidence of various salivary-gland types (243). Monomorphic adenomas are virtually absent in children, and benign epithelial tumors are less common than in adults. The most common benign tumors are pleomorphic adenoma and hemangioma; together they account for about 90% of benign salivary-gland tumors in children (242). The incidence of mucoepidermoid and acinic-cell carcinoma is remarkable, they account for almost 60% of malignant epithelial salivary-gland

tumors in children (241). Less than 0.25% of all salivary-gland tumors are found in children under 10 years of age (240), and perinatal (congenital and neonatal) epithelial salivary tumors are considered exceedingly rare (244).

Congenital malformations of salivary glands

Salivary polycystic dysgenetic disease

This is a very rare condition resembling morphologically cystic anomalies of other organs, such as the kidney, liver, and pancreas.

Clinical presentation: Polycystic dysgenetic disease of the parotid gland is a very rare inherited or familial developmental disorder, not associated with polycystic disease of other organs. Most patients present with bilateral parotid gland swelling in childhood. However, some lesions are not recognized until adulthood. The disorder occurs almost exclusively in females. Polycystic dysgenetic disease only affects the parotid glands, usually bilaterally. It is a non-neoplastic developmental lesion of the parotid gland without risk of malignant transformation.

Genetics: No association with polycystic disease of other organs has been documented.

Macroscopy: Bilateral irregular swelling of parotid glands with prominent nodularity, reflecting multiple parenchymal cysts of salivary-gland tissue. The cut surface displays a multicystic spongy appearance.

Histology: Salivary-gland lobules are enlarged by multifocal and diffuse cystic dilatations of intercalated ducts. The parotid glands maintain their lobular architecture, and some lobules are affected more severely than others. The glands have honeycomb or latticework-like patterns (Figure 4.14). The cysts are irregularly sized (up to a few mm) and lined by flat, cuboidal-to-low-columnar epithelium, sometimes with apocrine-like appearances. The lumina of cystic spaces contain eosinophilic proteinaceous material with spherical microliths. No dysplasia has been documented. Remnants of salivary acini are seen between the cysts, and thick fibrous interlobular septa are often prominent (245,246).

Differential diagnosis: Cystic salivary-gland neoplasms, such as mucoepidermoid carcinoma, cystadenoma, and low-grade cystadenocarcinoma. These tumors are unilateral and they do not maintain the lobular architecture of sclerosing dysgenetic disease.

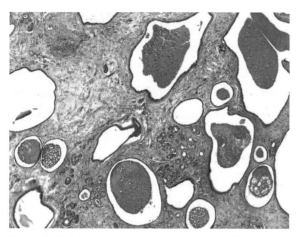

Figure 4.14 Salivary polycystic disease: salivary gland lobules are enlarged by multifocal and diffuse cystic dilatation of intercalated ducts. The glands have honeycomb or latticework-like patterns (H&E × 10).

Non-neoplastic lesions

Cysts: mucocele

Two types of mucocele are recognized – *extravasation* and *retention*, the former being ten-times commoner than the latter. An extravasation mucocele is defined as pooling of mucus in the connective tissue in a cavity not lined by epithelium, while a mucus retention cyst is defined as pooling of mucus in a cystic cavity.

Clinical presentation: Most patients with *extravasation* mucocele are under 30 years of age, and the minor glands are most often affected. The incidence by site is lower lip 65%, palate 4%, buccal mucosa 10%, and (in the major glands) parotid 0.6%, submandibular 1.2%, and sublingual 1.1%. The pathogenesis is traumatic severance of a duct, leading to mucus pooling. *Retention* cysts can occur at any age, and the mucus pool is within an epithelial-lined cavity, likely to be a dilated excretory duct.

Macroscopy: An extravasation mucocele presents in the lip as a raised, often blue, dome-shaped swelling of the mucosa, usually 2–10 mm in diameter, but it is generally larger in the sublingual gland in the floor of the mouth where it is known as a ranula.

Histology shows a rounded pool of mucus in fibrous tissue with inflammation, particularly macrophages.

Differential diagnosis: Mucus retention cysts must be distinguished from cystic neoplasms of minor salivary glands, such as low-grade mucoepidermoid carcinoma (MEC), cystadenoma, and inverted ductal papilloma. The presence of mucus cells in a benign cyst can make differential diagnosis from MEC difficult. Distinction is based on evidence of proliferative activity in MEC, such as increased cell stratification, multicystic structure, and invasive growth.

Ranula

A ranula is a cystic extravasation mucocele that arises from the sublingual salivary gland, most often from a ruptured main duct (247) or from acini that have ruptured secondary to obstruction (248). The extravasated mucin induces a macrophage response, and granulation tissue formation with subsequent fibrosis. The sublingual glands are spontaneous continuous secretors, explaining their propensity to develop ranulas.

Clinical presentation: Ranulas can occur at any age, and may be congenital and diagnosed antenatally (249), but are most frequent in the second decade (250). There is an association with HIV infection, which should be borne in mind in geographic areas of high prevalence (251).

Simple *intraoral* ranulas do not extend beyond the oral cavity, while *plunging* or *cervical* ranulas extend through the mylohyoid muscle in the floor of the mouth (which is discontinuous in one third of individuals) (252), or extend into the neck posteriorly. Plunging ranulas usually present with a painless neck mass in the submental or submandibular region, and may be misdiagnosed as thyroglossal duct cysts or lymphatic malformations (253,254). A rare presentation with acute respiratory distress in a child has been reported (255). Many cases do not show a co-existent intraoral ranula on clinical examination, although mucin extrasation is usually evident radiologically or histologically. Large lesions may extend deeply into the neck, and even into the anterior mediastinum and skull base.

Macroscopy: Usually cystic in appearance, can be of variable size, with mucinous content evident, sometimes entering the surrounding tissues.

Histology: Pseudocysts with no epithelial lining. Extravasated mucus is usually surrounded by mucin-laden macrophages surrounding the pseudocyst, with fibrosis predominating over time.

Benign tumors

Pleomorphic adenoma (PA)

Pleomorphic adenoma is characterized by architectural rather than cellular pleomorphism. Epithelial and

151

modified myoepithelial cells are intermingled with tissues of myxoid, mucoid, and chondroid appearance.

Clinical presentation: Pleomorphic adenoma is the most common benign epithelial tumor of minor and major salivary glands both in adults and children. They account for up to 40% of all primary salivary-gland tumors in children (243). Although most often found in young to middle-aged women, they can occur in either sex and at any age.

Genetics: Pleomorphic adenoma is characterized by recurrent rearrangement involving transcription factors PLAG1 on chromosome 8q12 and HMGA2 on chromosome 12q15 (256).

Macroscopy: Grossly, PAs are solitary, firm, and well-circumscribed tumors, some of them even appear encapsulated. Many other cases, however, lack encapsulation and can be multifocal. On cut section, the tumors have a glistening pale homogenous or vaguely bosselated surface.

Histology: Biphasic cellular proliferation composed of variable proportions of epithelial, myoepithelial, and mesenchymal-like areas, characterized by chondroid, hyaline, and myxoid stroma. Ducts are lined by flat, cuboidal, or columnar epithelial cells, with little or no atypia. The ducts are usually small tubules, but can be cystically dilated and also arranged in a cribriform pattern. Proliferation rate and MIB1 index is low.

The luminal layer cells are positive for cytokeratins and EMA, while the myoepithelial cells co-express cytokeratin CK 14, GFAP, p63 protein, calponin, CD10, and muscle-specific actin.

Differential diagnosis. Includes benign tumors, such as myoepithelioma and basal-cell adenoma, and malignant tumors, such as adenoid cystic carcinoma (AdCCa) and polymorphous low-grade adenocarcinoma (PLGA) of minor glands. Pleomorphic adenoma with a predominance of myoepithelial cells differs from myoepithelioma and basal-cell adenoma by the presence of chondromyxoid stroma and ductal tubular structures. Adenoid cystic carcinoma (AdCCa) and PLGA can be distinguished by their infiltrative growth pattern. Juvenile PA may contain embryonal immature structures and must be distinguished from other congenital salivary-gland tumors, in particular congenital basal-cell adenoma, hybrid basal-cell adenoma/adenoid cystic carcinoma, sialoblastoma, and salivary-gland anlage tumor (257).

Myoepithelioma

This is a benign neoplasm composed almost exclusively of myoepithelial cells. It represents the end spectrum of benign salivary-gland tumors, which also includes pleomorphic adenoma and basal-cell adenoma.

Clinical presentation: The incidence of myoepithelioma depends on how strict criteria are applied for diagnosis. It accounts for 0.3 to 1.5% of all salivary-gland tumors, and for 2.2 to 5.7% of all major and minor benign salivary-gland tumors, respectively (258). The age of patients ranges between 9 and 95 and the average age is 47 years. The most common sites include the parotid gland (48%), and the hard and soft palates (35%), but all salivary glands may be affected.

Macroscopy: Grossly, myoepitheliomas are well-circumscribed, encapsulated, and have yellow-tan color and glistening cut surface.

Histology: There are solid, myxoid, and reticular growth patterns. A variety of cell morphologies has been recognized, including spindle, plasmacytoid or hyaline, epithelioid, and clear (259). Most tumors are composed of a single predominant cell type. Spindle-cell myoepithelioma is composed of interlacing fascicles of spindle-shaped myoepithelial cells. These tumors are often very cellular, with little intervening stroma, and may be multinodular. Rarely, spindle-shaped myoepithelioma may show lipomatous metaplasia (260). Myoepitheliomas of minor glands tend to be composed of plasmacytoid (hyaline) cells, while parotid gland myoepitheliomas are mostly composed of epithelioid or spindle-shaped cells. The clear-cell variant occurs in both major and minor salivary glands, but it is rare. It is composed predominantly of clear polygonal cells with abundant optically clear cytoplasm containing large amounts of glycogen, but devoid of mucin and fat (261). The unusual reticular variant is characterized by net-like arrangements of interconnected cell cords within abundant loose myxoid, richly vascularized stroma. Oncocytic change in myoepithelial cells is uncommon and can occur in both benign pleomorphic adenomas and myoepitheliomas (262). Nuclear polymorphism is generally minimal in benign myoepitheliomas; however, a mild-to-moderate nuclear atypia can be seen in oncocytic metaplasia with no increase in proliferative activity (262). Collagenous crystalloids can be observed in myoepitheliomas of both minor and major salivary glands (263). Immunohistochemically, there may be considerable variability in staining within the same tumor and between different tumors. However, almost all tumors express S100 protein and broad-spectrum cytokeratins (AE1–AE3) and some cytokeratin subtypes, mostly CK14 and CK 5/6. α-Smooth-muscle actin and muscle-specific actin are expressed in spindle-shaped myoepithelial cells, but they are usually absent from epithelioid and plasmacytoid cells. Staining for CD10, calponin, smooth-muscle heavy chain, and maspin, is inconsistent in neoplastic myoepithelial cells. The nuclear transcription factor p63, vimentin, and GFAP are positive in most benign myoepitheliomas.

Differential diagnosis: Spindle-cell myoepithelioma should be distinguished from schwannoma, fibrous histiocytoma, synovial sarcoma, and solitary fibrous tumor. The clear-cell variant must be distinguished from other clear-cell tumors of salivary glands, both primary and secondary, in particular from metastatic renal-cell carcinoma. Immunohistochemistry is valuable in demonstration of the myoepithelial phenotype in these tumors. Myoepithelial carcinoma, in contrast to benign myoepithelioma, shows invasive growth, necrosis, and high proliferative index (MIB1). Pleomorphic adenoma with predominance of myoepithelial cells differs from myoepithelioma by the presence of chondromyxoid stroma and ductal tubular structures.

Cystadenoma

Rare, benign neoplasm composed of multicystic growth pattern often with intraluminal papillary projections. The epithelial lining may be oncocytic, apocrine, epidermoid, or mucous.

Clinical presentation: Represents 0.7 to 8.1% of all benign salivary tumors, but it is probably underestimated, as some cases of cystadenoma are classified as non-descriptive monomorphic adenomas (264). The average age of patients is about 50 years of age (range from 8 to 89). The tumors are unlikely to recur, but rare cases of mucinous cystadenomas with malignant transformation have been reported (265). There are two major variants, papillary oncocytic type and mucous cell type (264).

Macroscopy: The cut section reveals multiple small cystic spaces of variable sizes with intraluminal proliferations. The tumors are well circumscribed and encapsulated.

Histology: Composed of numerous cystic spaces lined by variable epithelium with focal intraluminal papillary proliferations. The individual cystic spaces are separated by dense fibrous stroma or may be devoid of any intervening stroma with cystic spaces arranged in a "back-to-back" pattern. The cysts' lining

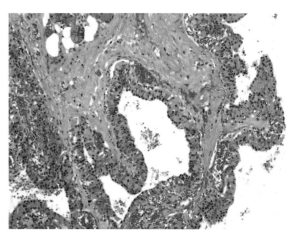

Figure 4.15 Cystadenomas are composed of numerous cystic spaces lined by variable epithelium with focal intraluminal papillary proliferations (H&E × 20).

epithelium is mostly columnar and cuboidal. Oncocytic, mucous, and apocrine cells are sometimes present focally or may predominate. Rarely, the cysts may be lined exclusively by mucous cells; such tumors are called cystadenoma, mucous cell type (Figure 4.15). An oncocytic variant of papillary cystadenoma is composed of oncocytes present in unilayered or bilayered papillary structures. The lumina often contain eosinophilic material with scattered epithelial, foamy, or inflammatory cells. Rarely, psammoma bodies and crystalloids have been described within the luminal secretion (266).

Differential diagnosis: Simple cyst, duct ectasia, polycystic dysgenetic disease, intraductal papilloma, low-grade mucoepidermoid carcinoma, and the recently described striated duct adenoma (267). Both duct ectasia and simple cysts have simple epithelial linings without papillary intraluminal projections. In addition, duct ectasia, in contrast to cystadenoma, is often associated with fibrosis and chronic inflammatory infiltration. Polycystic dysgenetic disease is extremely rare and involves the whole gland (245). Intraductal papilloma has overlapping histological features with papillary cystadenoma; however, intraductal papilloma is a unicystic lesion with prominent intracystic papillary proliferation, while cystadenomas are multicystic tumors. Low-grade mucoepidermoid carcinoma shares some histological features with the mucous cell variant of cystadenoma. Solid islands composed of intermediate cells are characteristic of mucoepidermoid carcinoma; moreover cystadenoma is well circumscribed without invasive growth. Striated duct adenoma is a

153

rare salivary-gland neoplasm composed of unilayered ducts resembling striated ducts of a normal gland, but without a myoepithelial layer, and with minimal intervening stroma and variable cystic ductal spaces (267). Striated duct adenoma is composed mostly of closely packed ductal structures. In contrast, cystadenoma is always composed of prevailing cystic formations.

Sclerosing polycystic adenosis (SPA)

Sclerosing polycystic adenosis is a rare salivary-gland lesion (268) characterized by a resemblance to epithelial proliferative lesions of the breast, such as fibrocystic disease and sclerosing breast adenosis. Less than 50 cases have been reported in the world literature so far.

Clinical presentation: Patients typically present with a slow-growing mass, some of which have pain or sensation. Sclerosing polycystic adenosis occurs within a broad age range from children to elderly, with a mean of 40 years (range from 9 to 84 years of age). Recurrence is possible in about on-third of cases, usually related to incomplete excision and possible multifocal disease. To date, none of the patients have developed metastases or died secondary to disease (269,270).

Macroscopy: Grossly, most tumors are firm or rubbery, well circumscribed, and surrounded by normal salivary-gland tissue. The tumors range in size from 0.3–7 cm. The cut surface is pale and glistening with multiple tiny visible cystic spaces ranging from 1–3 mm in diameter.

Histology: The tumors have a very variable appearance with a well-circumscribed, partly encapsulated mass and preservation of the lobular architecture, and a variable amount of inflammatory infiltrate in a sclerotic stroma. Multiple dilated ducts are often lined by a flattened bilayered epithelium. The ductal cells comprise a spectrum of vacuolated, foamy, apocrine, and mucous appearances, and focal squamous metaplasia may also be present. The hallmark of the tumors is a presence of large acinar cells with numerous coarse eosinophilic PAS-positive cytoplasmic granules (Figure 4.16). Some ducts contain solid and cribriform epithelial proliferations with vacuolated foamy cells having a sebaceous-like appearance. In all cases, there is focal intraluminal epithelial proliferation, giving rise to solid, microcystic, and cribriform structures. There is mild-to-severe nuclear polymorphism, even amounting to low-grade ductal carcinoma *in situ* (269,270). In places, tiny cell aggregates and small ducts embedded in sclerotic

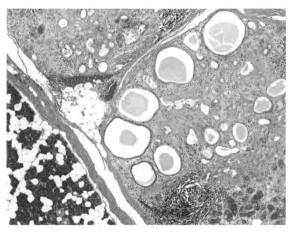

Figure 4.16 Sclerosing polycystic adenosis: multiple dilated ducts are often lined by a flattened bilayered epithelium. The ductal cells comprise a spectrum of vacuolated, foamy, apocrine, and mucous appearances, and focal squamous metaplasia may be also present. The hallmark of the tumors is a presence of large acinar cells with numerous coarse eosinophilic PAS-positive cytoplasmic granules (H&E × 20).

stroma reminiscent of stromal invasion can also be present (271).

The ductal and acinar cells are positive for cytokeratin (AE1–3 and CAM5.2), variably positive for EMA, S100, anti-mitochondrial antibody, and are negative for CEA, p53, and HER-2/neu. Acinar cells with coarse eosinophilic cytoplasm are positive for GCDFP-15. In all cases, about 15 to 20% of the epithelial cells express progesterone receptors. Estrogen receptors were detected, at least focally, in about 5% of ductal cells in the dysplastic and hyperplastic foci. Ducts filled with hyperplastic and dysplastic epithelium were surrounded by an intact myoepithelial layer, positive for SMA, p63, and calponin.

Differential diagnosis: Most cases of SPA are initially misdiagnosed as tumors, such as mucoepidermoid and acinic cell carcinomas, cystadenocarcinoma, and pleomorphic adenoma. Major microscopic clues to a correct diagnosis include maintenance of the lobular architecture of the gland, ductal ectasia, scar-like hyalinized fibrous sclerosis, and a spectrum of foam, apocrine, granular, and mucous cells, in addition to the presence of tubuloacinar structures composed of large acinar cells with prominent, brightly eosinophilic granules. Intraductal hyperplasia, particularly if associated with dysplasia, may lead one to suspect a neoplastic process, but clues to the benign nature of SPA are that it is well circumscribed, lacks an invasive growth pattern, and that mitotic/proliferative activity is low. Major differential diagnoses include PA and chronic sclerosing sialadenitis. The definitive lobular growth pattern and large Paneth-cell-like acinic cells of SPA are not seen in pleomorphic adenomas. In contrast, SPA lacks a prominent myoepithelial cell component and chondromyxoid stroma typical of PA. Chronic sclerosing sialadenitis lacks the nodular pattern and typical structural heterogeneity of SPA, though both lesions share prominent fibrosis. Moreover, large acinic cells with coarse PAS-positive zymogen-like cytoplasmic granules are not seen in chronic sclerosing sialadenitis.

Benign mesenchymal tumors

Mesenchymal tumors of the salivary glands are less common than epithelial neoplasms, in general. However, in childhood non-epithelial tumors contribute about two-thirds of salivary-gland tumors (243). In early childhood, hemangiomas markedly predominate over epithelial neoplasms and they account for approximately 90% of all salivary-gland neoplasms in infancy. In total, hemangiomas contribute to about 60% of all neoplasms in the salivary glands in childhood, followed by lymphangiomas (about 30%) (272).

Hemangioma

Most hemangiomas involving the salivary glands are usually immature and cellular, and are classified under the category of infantile (juvenile) hemangioma – hemangioma of infancy. In older children, cavernous hemangiomas may be encountered.

Clinical presentation: Infantile hemangiomas of the salivary glands are diagnosed mostly in newborns and infants. At this age group they are the most common neoplasms of the salivary glands. The female to male ratio is 2.3:1 (273). The tumor develops usually in the parotid gland and presents as a unilateral soft mass causing facial asymmetry. The overlying skin may have a bluish or red discoloration. Infantile hemangioma may also involve the submandibular gland or it may appear as a multifocal process. Rarely, especially if large, hemangiomas may be a cause of Kasabach–Merritt syndrome (274), but this is more common with kaposiform hemangioendothelioma (see Chapter 13).

Macroscopy: The size of the tumor varies from 2 to 8 cm. On the cut section the tumor is poorly defined without a capsule, and has a lobulated pattern and a dark red color.

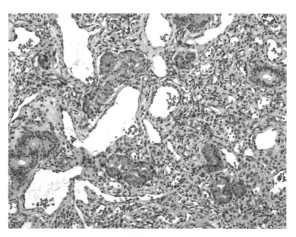

Figure 4.17 Infantile (juvenile) hemangioma: the tumor infiltrates the parotid gland. Individual acini and ducts are widely separated by a mass of newly formed capillaries. They are of a variable size and shape with opened lumina in this microscopical field (H&E × 20).

Histology: Infantile hemangiomas form multilobulated clusters of variously maturing capillaries, usually of a similar size. The tumor infiltrates salivary-gland tissue and, typically, it is not encapsulated, so that residual acini and ducts of the salivary-gland tissue are easily identified (Figure 4.17). In the parotid gland, hemangiomas may also involve the facial nerve. Early diagnosed lesions tend to be immature, with plump endothelial cells; the vascular lumina are poorly developed or almost indiscernible. Although mitotic figures are frequent, atypical mitoses are not found. There is an admixture of mast cells. At later stages the capillaries are better defined with opened lumina and flattened endothelium. This feature is best seen at the tumor periphery. The hemangioma may regress with a loss of cellularity and stromal fibrosis. Due to frequent spontaneous regression of the tumor, conservative follow-up or treatment with steroids or interferon is currently preferred to surgical resection, so biopsy specimens are less frequent (275). A progression of a residual congenital hemangioma with features closer to cavernous hemangioma than to the juvenile form, and with some solid spindled and epithelioid foci, to epithelioid angiosarcoma has been reported (276). Cavernous hemangiomas are much less frequent and they do not differ from cavernous hemangiomas involving other organs. They are diagnosed in older children and the parotid gland is most frequently affected. Cavernous hemangiomas do not show a tendency to regress like the infantile (juvenile) types. Secondary changes such as thrombosis may be found in cavernous hemangiomas. Vascular markers are useful for identification of endothelial cells, such as FVIII,

CD31, and CD34. Likewise, anti-smooth-muscle actin maps the pericytes. GLUT1 is useful in differentiating infantile (juvenile) hemangioma from other vascular lesions such as vascular malformations and pyogenic granulomas (277,278). Its role in discriminating other soft-tissue lesions is limited as positivity has been described in a wide spectrum of both benign and malignant soft tissue and bone tumors, including Ewing's sarcoma/primitive neuroectodermal tumor (PNET) (279).

Differential diagnosis: Infantile (juvenile) hemangiomas may occasionally resemble a malignancy due to their immaturity and infiltrative growth, occasionally involving the facial nerve. Simple silver impregnation and/or immunohistochemical investigations reveal the cellular components and lead to the appropriate diagnosis.

Lymphatic malformations

Lymphatic malformations, as described above, may be a primary tumor of the salivary glands, but more frequently the glands are involved by lymphatic malformations affecting soft tissues of the head and neck region. Primary lymphatic malformations, similar to hemangiomas, commonly affect the parotid gland (243,280–282).

Other benign mesenchymal neoplasms are rare in childhood. They include schwannoma, plexiform neurofibroma, lipoma, nodular fasciitis, solitary fibrous tumor, and myofibromatosis (see Chapter 13; 272,283–285).

Malignant tumors

Mucoepidermoid carcinoma (MEC)

Mucoepidermoid carcinoma is a malignant glandular epithelial neoplasm characterized by mucous, intermediate, and epidermoid cells with columnar, clear-cell, and onocytic features. The vast majority of MEC in children are of a low grade.

Clinical presentation: Mucoepidermoid carcinoma is the most common primary salivary-gland malignancy in children. Symptoms can include pain, paraesthesia, bleeding, mucosal ulcerations, and facial nerve palsy. Several systems have been proposed for the grading of MEC, based on the proportion of the cystic component, neural invasion, necrosis, number of mitoses, anaplasia, and MIB1 index (286,287).

Genetics: The recurrent translocations t(11;19) and t(11;15) resulting in *CRTC1-MAML2* or *CRTC3-*

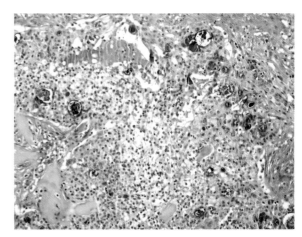

Figure 4.18 Mucoepidermoid carcinoma is characterized by mixture of epidermoid, mucus-producing, and intermediate cells in variable proportions (mucicarmine staining × 20).

MAML2 fusion oncogenes, respectively, are identified in a large proportion of low-grade MEC of the salivary gland and have an impact on prognosis (288,289).

Macroscopy. Firm, often cystic tumors with well-defined or infiltrative margins.

Microscopy: Characterized by a mixture of epidermoid, mucus-producing, and intermediate cells in variable proportions (Figure 4.18), the tumors are usually multicystic with a variable solid component. Cystic spaces are lined by mucus-producing and intermediate cells; solid areas are composed of epidermoid and intermediate cells, but true keratinization is absent. Clear- and oncocytic-cell differentiation may be present focally or may predominate. Epidermoid cells of MEC co-express p63 and high-molecular-weight cytokeratins (CK 14 and CK 5/6), while myoepithelial markers and S100 protein are negative.

Differential diagnosis: This includes benign necrotizing sialometaplasia (NSM), hyalinizing clear-cell carcinoma, and mammary analog secretory carcinoma (MASC) (290). NSM can rarely simulate low-grade MEC in children; however, NSM retains the lobular architecture of the normal gland and lacks cystic spaces. Hyalinizing clear-cell carcinoma may mimic the clear-cell variant of MEC, but is devoid of mucus-producing cells. Recently recognized MASC is characterized by microcystic spaces, within which there is abundant PAS-positive secretory material (Figure 4.19), and by a t(12;15) translocation encoding *ETV6-NTRK3* gene fusion. The distinction can be made by the lack of a cobblestone-like appearance with intercellular bridges, true squamoid areas, or basal-like intermediate cells in MASC. In addition,

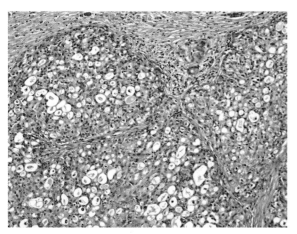

Figure 4.19 Mammary analog secretory carcinoma (MASC) is characterized by microcystic spaces within which there is abundant PAS-positive secretory material (H&E × 20).

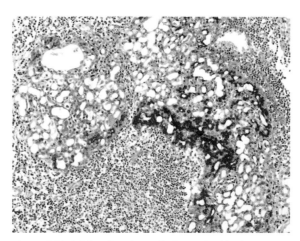

Figure 4.20 Acinic-cell carcinoma is characterized by the presence of well-differentiated serous acinar cells with abundant cytoplasmic PAS-positive zymogen granules, resistant to diastase digestion (periodic acid–Schiff–diastase staining × 20).

MASC lacks p63 staining and shows diffuse S100 positivity in most cases, which would be distinctly unusual in MEC.

Acinic-cell carcinoma (AciCCa)

Acinic-cell carcinoma is a malignant salivary-gland tumor in which at least some of the neoplastic cells demonstrate serous acinar cell differentiation.

Clinical presentation: Acinic-cell carcinoma represents the second most common salivary malignancy in children. Together with mucoepidermoid carcinoma, they account for almost 60% of malignant salivary-gland tumors in children (291). Only 4% of patients with AciCCa are under 20 years old (292).

Macroscopy: Most tumors are well circumscribed, but not encapsulated. The cut surface is multilobular, and tan to red in color. They vary from firm to soft, and solid to cystic.

Histology: By definition, AciCCa is characterized by the presence of well-differentiated serous acinar cells with abundant cytoplasmic PAS-positive zymogen granules, resistant to diastase digestion (Figure 4.20). However, several other cell types, such as intercalated ductal, vacuolated, clear, and non-specific glandular cells are recognized. Solid/lobular and microcystic growth patterns are most commonly seen in AciCCa, but macrocystic, follicular (thyroid gland-like), papillary cystic patterns are also recognized. The immunoprofile is not specific. A new potentially useful marker DOG1 shows intense apical membranous staining around lumina as well as complete membranous and variable cytoplasmic staining in AciCCa (293).

Differential diagnosis: The most common tumor entity in salivary-gland pathology that mimics AciCCa is a recently described entity, called mammary analog secretory carcinoma, MASC (281). The MASC neoplastic cells resemble intercalated duct cells, and they have low-grade nuclei with distinctive nuclear membranes and centrally located nucleoli. However, the large serous acinar cells with cytoplasmic PAS-positive zymogen-like granules typical of AciCCa are completely absent in MASC. In contrast to MASC, classic AciCCa shows an intact ETV6 gene, and is usually S100 protein negative. Consistently strong DOG1 staining in AciCCa can be utilized to support the diagnosis. In equivocal cases, demonstration of the *ETV6-NTRK3* translocation is diagnostic of MASC and is absent in conventional AciCCa.

Adenoid cystic carcinoma (AdCC)

Adenoid cystic carcinoma is a basaloid biphasic salivary-gland tumor consisting of epithelial and myoepithelial cells in cribriform, solid (basaloid), and tubular structures in variable proportions.

Clinical presentation: The third most common malignant salivary gland tumor in childhood, AdCC is a common tumor that occurs in both minor and major salivary glands, but most often in the submandibular or minor salivary glands, particularly the palate. The tumor often has a relentless clinical course that includes late recurrences and distant metastatic disease. Despite apparently slow growth, outcome over the long term is poor. There is no particular age or sex predilection. A system of three grades, based on the presence of tubular,

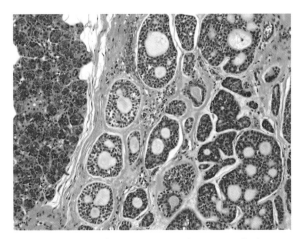

Figure 4.21 Adenoid cystic carcinomas characteristically show multiple cribriform structures, composed of epithelial and basal/myoepithelial cells. The nuclei are usually dark, hyperchromatic, and angulated (H&E × 20).

cribriform, and solid patterns has shown that outcome is better in tubular AdCC, while the worst prognosis is seen in solid AdCC. Nevertheless, the clinical stage appears to be a better predictor than grade.

Genetics: Recently, the translocation between chromosomes 6 and 9 was described in AdCC of both breast and salivary glands. This translocation fuses the *MYB* gene and the *NFIB* gene, which leads to a characteristic chimeric transcript (294). The MYB/NFIB fusion transcript, present in at least one-third of AdCCs, has emerged as a potential therapeutic target (295).

Macroscopy: Adenoid cystic carcinoma are infiltrative without encapsulation, but may be well circumscribed, and are firm in consistency.

Histology: Adenoid cystic carcinoma is a generally solid tumor in which the cribriform pattern is easily recognised (Figure 4.21); however, tubular and solid structures can also be present. The commonest growth patterns are:

Cribriform: Multiple cribriform structures composed of epithelial and basal/myoepithelial cells. The nuclei are usually dark, hyperchromatic, and angulated. Mitoses are easy to find and may be abundant. The contents of the spaces can be loose and basophilic, or dense and eosinophilic.

Tubular: Composed of small tubules lined by one or two cell types, luminal and abluminal without significant cytological atypia. Because of this bland cytological appearance it may be mistaken for basal cell adenoma, except for the presence of infiltration.

Solid (basaloid): Large solid sheets of tumor cells, sometimes with comedo-like central necrosis. Within the solid masses of tumor cells, there are small duct-like spaces surrounded by a definite layer of epithelial cells.

Differential diagnosis: Cribriform and pseudocystic spaces are characteristic of AdCC, but many other tumor types can show the same structures, in particular, pleomorphic adenoma, basal-cell adenoma, epithelial-myoepithelial carcinoma, and low-grade salivary-duct carcinoma (low-grade cribriform cystadenocarcinoma). The most important histological differential diagnosis is between AdCC and polymorphous low-grade adenocarcinoma (PLGA). The distinction is based on cytologic features. While the cells of PLGA are uniform, cuboidal with vesicular low-grade nuclei, the cells of AdCC display basaloid features, they have mitotic activity, high MIB1 index, and nuclei are angulated (296).

Sialoblastoma

This is a low-grade malignant neoplasm usually present at birth or shortly thereafter, composed of epithelial basaloid and myoepithelial cells that recapitulate the primitive salivary-gland anlage. Sialoblastoma was initially referred to as embryoma (297); since that time, approximately 40 tumors that fit into a definition of sialoblastoma have been reported under different names (298).

Clinical presentation: Sialoblastoma arises almost exclusively in the perinatal period, with rare cases presenting after two years of age (299).

Macroscopy: Grossly, the tumors range up to 15 cm, are well circumscribed, and even partly encapsulated. In other cases, they may be locally invasive with extension to adjacent soft tissues and bone.

Histology: Recapitulates the embryonic development of major salivary glands (300). The tumors have variable histological patterns, composed of variably sized nests and solid sheets of basaloid cells with focal ductal differentiation, and cystic and microcystic change. The tumor cells are fairly uniform with minimal cytoplasm and round-to-oval nuclei with only slight polymorphism. Mitoses are frequent and may be numerous; atypical mitoses are not present. Neural and occasionally vascular invasion may be found (Figure 4.22). Anti-cytokeratin and EMA antibodies stain ductal elements and occasional basaloid epithelial cells in the solid nests. Luminal cells express S100 protein and actin.

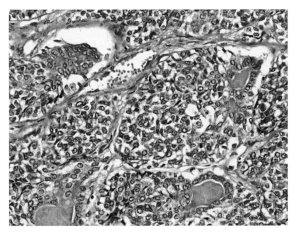

Figure 4.22 Sialoblastoma: the tumor cells and fairly uniform with minimal cytoplasm and round to oval nuclei with only slight polymorphism. Mitoses are frequently found and may be numerous, atypical mitoses are not present. Neural and occasionally vascular invasion may be found (H&E × 20).

Differential diagnosis: Pleomorphic adenoma is exceedingly rare in the neonatal age group and is distinguished by chondromyxoid stroma and combination of epithelial and myoepithelial cells with duct formation and metaplastic changes. Basal-cell adenoma is very rare in the neonatal population, and it consists of uniform basaloid cells without mitoses and polymorphism. Adenoid cystic carcinoma is also exceedingly rare in the neonatal age group and it is characterized by invasive growth and formation of abundant extracellular matrix presenting with cribriform and pseudocystic patterns.

Endodermal sinus tumor (yolk sac)

Endodermal sac tumors (EST) are aggressive malignant germ-cell-derived neoplasms characterized by the presence of Schiller–Duval bodies admixed with papillae, tubules, microcysts,and sheets of primitive cells within a myxoid extracellular background.

Clinical presentation: Very aggressive malignant tumors with short survival time, ESTs are documented in adults and children. Within the head and neck, these tumors occur mostly in the sinonasal tract and in the nasopharynx. Only two cases of EST of the parotid gland in children have been reported so far (301,302).

Histology (see also Chapter 9): The tumor often shows a reticular pattern characterized by anastomosing small glandular spaces. In other places, it may be composed of microcystic, solid, and papillary structures lined by irregular neoplastic cells. Periodic acid–Schiff stain-positive diastase-resistant intracellular and extracellular globules are present. Tumor cells are positive for α-fetoprotein.

Differential diagnosis: Immature teratoma, sialoblastoma, and poorly differentiated adenocarcinoma should be considered. Endodermal sinus tumor is characterized by Schiller–Duval bodies and positive staining for α-fetoprotein. Particularly immature teratomas with papillary areas may be reminiscent of EST, but must be distinguished because their prognosis in children is favorable after complete resection. In contrast, ESTs in children are very aggressive neoplasms which require adjuvant cisplatin-based chemotherapy.

Rhabdomyosarcoma

Rhabdomyosarcomas represent a group of immature mesenchymal neoplasms with a variously expressed potential to skeletal muscle differentiation. Two major subtypes are known to occur in childhood, embryonal and alveolar rhabdomyosarcomas (303). In salivary glands the embryonal subtype has been described by several authors (304,305), the alveolar being exceptional. The alveolar subtype may affect older children or young adults (272,306,307). Rhabdomyosarcomas contribute to about 7% of all malignant tumors of the salivary glands in children and adolescents up to 18 years of age (272).

Clinical presentation: Generally a mass and swelling of the facial region (304). As the parotid gland or soft tissues around it are affected, most commonly the symptomatology also depends on the extent of the tumor at the time of diagnosis. Less commonly the tumor may cause tenderness or pain and facial nerve paralysis. At late stages tumor invasion into the surrounding soft tissues, nasopharynx, fossa pterygopalatina, and base of the skull may be found, and it may also involve other cranial nerves than the facial nerve. Advanced lesions with a local invasion are grouped as so-called parameningeal rhabdomyosarcomas, having an unfavorable prognosis.

Macroscopy: Most affect the parotid gland. The size of the tumor varies from 3 to 5 cm, and it may become larger as the tumors spread into the surrounding compartments. If the tumor reaches beyond the margins of the salivary-gland tissue, it may be difficult to assign the primary site to the salivary glands.

Histology: Embryonal rhabdomyosarcoma may present under various morphological appearances. It may present in its classical form of a solid mass without any structural characteristics, being cytologically variant from a spindle-cell component to myxoid areas

159

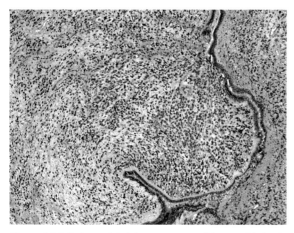

Figure 4.23 Embryonal rhabdomyosarcoma of the parotid gland. The tumor is close to Stenon's duct. It is formed by poorly differentiated polygonal cells with features of atypia (H&E × 20).

and polygonal cell sheets. It may, though very rarely, appear in the form of sarcoma botryoides growing into the Stensen's duct (Figure 4.23). The tumor forms polypoid masses protruding into the major salivary duct or protruding from the Stensen's duct caruncle (305). Under the salivary-duct epithelium there is a typical cambium layer. The remaning parts of the polyps are typically less cellular, with a predominant extracellular myxoid matrix and scattered tumor cells. Tissue deeper in the parotid gland may be involved in the tumor, composed of cellular tissue with predom inantly undifferentiated cells and scattered rhabdo-myoblasts (see Chapter 11). Some rhabdomyoblasts may appear vacuolated due to accumulation of intra-cytoplasmatic glycogen. Sarcoma botroides of the major salivary ducts should be regarded as primary to the salivary glands. See Chapter 11 for further histology and immunocytochemistry.

Differential diagnosis. A typical embryonal rhab-domyosarcoma with sarcoma botryoides features is recognized due to its characteristic growth pattern and a rhabdomyoblastic differentiation. Occasionally, rhabdomyosarcomas may be immature.To rule out the Ewing's/PNET tumor, CD99 and FLI-1 proteins may be added to the spectrum of antibodies used, as well as NB84 to help distinguish metastatic neuroblas-toma (284). Leukocyte common antigen (LCA) and other lymphoid markers may be useful to rule out a lymphoma under some circumstances. A desmoplastic small round-cell tumor was described affecting a young adult female and this tumor should be kept in the differential diagnostic list, along with the other

small round-cell tumors in childhood (308). In cases of alveolar rhabdomyosarcoma and Ewing's/PNET tumors, fluorescence *in situ* hybridization demon-strates typical chromosomal breaks (at the sites of genes FOXO1(FKHR) and EWS, respectively), or adding the translocation probes demonstrates the most common translocations t(2;13), in the case of alveolar rhabdomyosarcoma and t(11;22) in the case of Ewing's/PNET. If adequate isolates of mRNA are available, PCR is now routinely engaged. Other malignant mesenchymal neoplasms of the salivary glands may occur, but are rare diseases even in adults – liposarcoma, leiomyosarcoma, synovial sar-coma, desmoplastic small round-cell tumor, and Ewing's/PNET 274). In children, aggressive fibroma-tosis has been reported, and due to an unfavorable site of origin it may progress with life-threatening complications (272,309).

References

1. Abbas A, Awan S. Rhabdomyosarcoma of the middle ear and mastoid:a case report and review of the literature. Ear Nose Throat J. 2005;**84**:780,782,784.

2. Durve DV, Kanegaonkar RG, Albert D, Levitt G. Paediatric rhabdomyosarcoma of the ear and temporal bone. Clin. Otolaryngol Allied Sci. 2004;**29**:32–7.

3. Schwartz RH, Movassaghi N, Marion ED. Rhabdomyosarcoma of the middle ear:a wolf in sheep's clothing. Pediatrics. 1980;**65**:1131–3.

4. Fukunaga M, Miyazawa Y, Harada T, Ushigome S, Ishikawa E. Yolk sac tumour of the ear. Histopathology 1995;**27**:563–567.

5. Isaacson G. Diagnosis of pediatric cholesteatoma. Pediatrics 2007;**120**:603–608.

6. Levenson MJ, Parisier SC, Chute P, *et al.* A review of twenty congenital cholesteatomas of the middle ear in children. Otolaryngol. Head Neck Surg. 1986;**94**:560–567.

7. Koltai PJ, Nelson M, Castellon RJ, *et al.* The natural history of congenital cholesteatoma. Arch. Otolaryngol. Head Neck Surg. 2002;**128**:804–809.

8. Manolidis S, Kutz JW Jr. Diagnosis and management of lateral sinus thrombosis. Otol. Neurotol. 2005;**26**:1045–51.

9. Albino AP, Kimmelman CP, Parisier SC. Cholesteatoma:a molecular and cellular puzzle. Am. J. Otol. 1998;**19**:7–19.

10. Ferekidis E, Nikolopoulos TP, Yiotakis J, *et al.* Correlation of clinical and surgical findings to histological features (koilocytosis, papillary hyperplasia) suggesting papillomavirus involvement in

the pathogenesis of cholesteatoma. Int. Med. Sci. Monit. 2006;**12**:368–71.

11. Johnston DR, Whittemore K, Poe D, Robson CD, Perez-Atayde AR. Diagnostic and surgical challenge: middle ear dermoid cyst in 12 month old with branchio-oto-renal syndrome and multiple middle-ear congenital anomalies. J. Pediatr. Otorhinolaryngol. 2011;**75**:1341–5.

12. Ferlito A, Devaney KO, Rinaldo A, *et al.* Clinicopathological consultation: Ear cholesteatoma vs. cholesterol granuloma. Ann. Otol. Rhinol. Laryngol. 1997;**106**:79–85.

13. Ferlito A. A review of the definition, terminology and pathology of aural cholesteatoma. J. Laryngol. Otol. 1993;**107**:483–8.

14. Martin N, Sterkers O, Mompoint D, Julien N, Nahum H. Cholesterol granulomas of the middle ear cavities: MR imaging. Radiology 1989;**172**:521–5.

15. Chang P, Fagan PA, Atlas MD, Roche J. Imaging destructive lesions of the petrous apex. Laryngoscope 1998;**108**:599–604.

16. Mcgregor DH, Cherian R, Kepes JJ, *et al.* Case reports: heterotopic brain tissue of the middle ear associated with cholesteatoma. Am. J. Med. Sci. 1994;**308**:180–183.

17. Lustig LR, Cheung SW, Jackler RK. Subcochlear petrous cholesterol granuloma involving the infratemporal fossa. Otolaryngol. Head Neck Surg. 1998;**119**:685–9.

18. House JL, Brackmann DE. Cholesterol granuloma of the cerebellopontine angle. Arch. Otolaryngol. 1982;**108**:504–6.

19. Gliklich RE, Cunningham MJ, Eavey RD. The cause of aural polyps in children. Arch. Otolaryngol. Head Neck Surg. 1993;**119**:669–71.

20. Gaafar H, Maher A, Al-Ghazzawi E. Aural polypi: A histopathological and histochemical study. ORL J. Otorhinolaryngol. Relat. Spec. 1982;**44**(2):108–15.

21. Milroy CM, Slack RWT, Maw AR, Bradfield JWB. Aural polyps as predictors of underlying cholesteatoma. J. Clin. Pathol. 1989;**42**:460–465.

22. Supiyaphun P, Snidvongs K, Shuangshoti S. Salivary gland choristoma of the middle ear:case treated with KTP laser. J. Laryngol. Otol. 2000;**114** :528–32.

23. Hinni ML, Beattie CW. Salivary gland choristoma of the middle ear:a case report and review of the literature. Ear Nose Throat J. 1196;**75**:422–4.

24. Michaels LM, Hellquist HB. Neoplasma and similar lesions of the middle ear. In Michaels LM, Hellquist HB, editors, *Ear, Nose and Throat Histopathology*, second edn. London: Springer-Verlag; 2001:66–76.

25. Michaels LM, Hellquist HB. Malformations of the middle and inner ear. In Michaels LM, Hellquist HB,

editors, *Ear, Nose and Throat Histopathology*, second edn. London: Springer-Verlag; 2001:77–91.

26. Webb BJ, Vikram HR. Chronic invasive sinus aspergillosis in immunocompetent hosts:a geographic comparison. Mycopathologia 2010;**170**:403–10.

27. Katzenstein AL, Sale SR, Greenberger PA. Pathologic findings in allergic aspergillus sinusitis. A newly recognized form of sinusitis. Am. J. Surg. Pathol. 1983;**7**:439–43.

28. Pollack JD, Pincus RL, Lucente FE. Leprosy of the head and neck. Otolaryngol. Head Neck Surg. 1987;**97**:93–6.

29. Das S, Kashyap B, Barua M, *et al.* Nasal rhinosporidiosis in humans:new interpretations and a review of the literature of this enigmatic disease. Med. Mycol. 2011;**49**:311–5.

30. Ramadass T, P. Thulasi Das, Geetha N, *et al.* Extranodal Manifestation of Rosai Dorfman Disease of the Nasopharynx. Indian J. Otolaryngol. Head Neck Surg. 2007;**59**:178–81.

31. Zagolski O, Dwivedi RC, Subramanian S, Kazi R. Non-Hodgkin's lymphoma of the sino-nasal tract in children. J. Can. Res. Ther. 2010;**6**:5–10.

32. Devaney KO, Travis WD, Hoffman G, *et al.* Interpretation of head and neck biopsies in Wegener's granulomatosis. A pathologic study of 126 biopsies in 70 patients. Am. J. Surg. Pathol. 1990;**14**:555–64.

33. Del Buono EA, Flint A. Diagnostic usefulness of nasal biopsy in Wegener's granulomatosis. Hum. Pathol. 1991;**22**:107–10.

34. Metgud RS, Doshi JJ, Gaurkhede S, Dongre R, Karle R. Extranodal NK/T-cell lymphoma, nasal type (angiocentric T-cell lymphoma): A review about the terminology. J. Oral Maxillofac. Pathol. 2011;**15**:96–100.

35. Borges A, Fink J, Villablanca P, Eversole R, Lufkin R. Midline destructive lesions of the sinonasal tract: simplified terminology based on histopathologic criteria. Am. J. Neuroradiol. 2000;**21**:331–6.

36. Tos M, Mogensen C. Mucous glands in nasal polyps. Arch. Otolaryngol. 1977;**103**:407–13.

37. Saitoh T, Kusunoki T, Yao T, *et al.* Relationship between epithelial damage or basement membrane thickness and eosinophilic infiltration in nasal polyps with chronic rhinosinusitis. Rhinology 2009;**47**:275–9.

38. Oppenheimer EH, Rosenstein BJ. Differential pathology of nasal polyps in cystic fibrosis and atopy. Lab. Invest. 1979;**40**:445–9.

39. Min YG, Chung JW, Shin JS, Chi JG. Histologic structure of antrochoanal polyps. Acta Oto-Laryngologica 1995;**115**:543–7.

40. Batsakis JG. Stromal cell atypia in sinonasal polyposis. Ann. Otol. Rhinol. Laryngol. 1986;**95** (3 Pt 1):321–2.

41. Burns BV, Axon PR, Pahade A. "Hairy polyp" of the pharynx in association with an ipsilateral branchial sinus: evidence that the "hairy polyp" is a second branchial arch malformation. J. Laryngol. Otol. 2001;**115**:145–8.

42. Heffner DK, Thompson LDR, Schall DG, *et al*. Pharyngeal dermoids ("hairy polyps") as accessory auricles. Ann. Otol. Rhinol. Laryngol. 1996;**10**:819–824.

43. Foxwell PB, Kellham BH. Teratoid tumours of the nasopharynx. J. Laryngol. Otol. 1958;**72**:647–657.

44. Eichel BS, Hallberg OE. Hamartoma of the middle ear and eustachian tube: Report of a case. Laryngoscope 1966;**76**:1810–5.

45. Haddad J Jr, Senders CW, Leach CS, Stool SE. Congenital hairy polyp of the nasopharynx associated with cleft palate:report of two cases. Int. J. Pediatr. Otorhinolaryngol. 1990;**20**(2):127–35.

46. Delides A, Sharifi F, Karagianni E, *et al*. Multifocal bigerminal mature teratomas of the head and neck. J. Laryngol. Otol. 2006;**120**:967–969.

47. Nicklaus P, Forte V, Thorner P. Hairy polyp of the Eustachian tube. J. Otolaryngol. 1991;**20**:254–257.

48. Har-El G, Zirkin HY, Tovi F, Sidi J. Congenital pleomorphic adenoma of the nasopharynx. J. Laryngol. Otol. 1985;**99**:1281–1287.

49. Dehner LP, Valbuena L, Perez-Atayde A, *et al*. Salivary gland anlage tumor ("congenital pleomorphic adenoma"): A clinicopathologic, immunohistochemical and ultrastrucutural study of nine cases. Am. J. Surg. Pathol. 1994;**18**:25–36.

50. Buchino JJ. Salivary gland anlage tumor: A newly recognized clinicopatohlogic entity of uncertain histogenesis. Adv. Anatom. Pathol. 1995;**2**:94–98.

51. Michal M, Sokol L, Mukenšnabl P. Salivary gland anlage tumor. A case with widespread necrosis and large cyst formation. Pathology 1996;**28**:128–130.

52. Michaels LM, Hellquist HB. The nasopharynx: normal anatomy and histology; adenoids; infections. In Michaels LM, Hellquist HB, editors, *Ear, Nose and Throat Histopathology*, second edn. London: Springer-Verlag; 2001:259–63.

53. Rosai J. Limas S, Husband EM. Ectopic hamartomatous thymoma. A distinctive benign lesion of lower neck. Am. J. Surg. Pathol. 1984;**8**:501–513.

54. Michaels LM, Hellquist HB. The nose and paranasal sinuses: Miscellaneous conditions. In Michaels LM, Hellquist HB, editors, *Ear, Nose and Throat Histopathology*, second edn. London: Springer-Verlag; 2001:247–56.

55. Gyure KA, Thompson LDR, Morrison AL. A clinicopathological study of 15 patients with neuroglial heterotopias and encephaloceles of the middle ear and mastoid region. Laryngoscope 2000;**110**:1731–5.

56. Zook EG, Nickey WM, Pribaz JJ. Heterotopic brain tissue in the scalp. Plast. Reconstr. Surg. 1984;**73**:660–3.

57. Elder JE, Chow CM, Holmes AD. Heterotopic brain tissue in the orbit: case report. Br. J. Ophthalmol. 1989;**73**:928–31.

58. Kallman JE, Loevner LA, Yousem DM, *et al*. Heterotopic brain in the pterygopalatine fossa. AJNR Am. J. Neuroradiol. 1997;**18**:176–9.

59. Okulski EG, Biemer JJ, Alonso WA. Heterotopic pharyngeal brain. Arch. Otolaryngol. 1981;**107**:385–6.

60. Cohen AH, Abt AB. An unusual case of neonatal respiratory obstruction:heterotopic pharyngeal brain tissue. J. Pediatr. 1970;**76**:119–22.

61. Fuse T, Aoyagi M, Ota N, *et al*. Heterotopic brain tissue of the soft palate. ORL J. Otorhinolaryngol. Relat. Spec. 1992;**54**:54–6.

62. Pasyk KA, Agenta LC, Marks MW, Friedman RJ. Heterotopic brain presenting as a lip lesion. Cleft Palate J. 1988;**25**:48–52.

63. Knox R, Pratt M, Garvin AJ, White B. Heterotopic lingual brain in the newborn. Arch. Otolaryngol. Head Neck Surg. 1989;**115**:630–2.

64. Kamerer DB, Love GL, Riehl PA. Intranasal encephalocele masking as nasal polyp in an adult patient. Arch. Otolaryngol. 1983;**109**:420–1.

65. Thompson LD, Gyure KA. Extracranial sinonasal tract meningiomas:a clinicopathologic study of 30 cases with a review of the literature. Am. J. Surg. Pathol. 2000;**24**:640–50.

66. Friedman CD, Costantino PD, Teitelbaum B, Berktold RE, Sisson GA. Primary extracranial meningiomas of the head and neck. Laryngoscope 1990;**100**:41–4.

67. Wenig BM, Vinh TN, Smirniotopoulos JG, *et al*. Aggressive psammomatoid ossifying fibromas of the sinonasal region: A clinicopathologic study of a distinct group of fibro-osseous lesions. Cancer 1995;**76**:1155–65.

68. Maier HC. Craniopharyngioma with erosion and drainage into the nasopharynx. An autobiographical case report. J. Neurosurg. 1985;**62**:132–4.

69. Maiuri F, Corriero G, Elefante R, Cirillo S, Giamundo A. Craniopharyngioma of the cranial base and nasopharynx. Surg. Neurol. 1987;**27**:191–4.

70. McDermott MB, Ponder TB, Dehner LP. Nasal chondromesenchymal hamartoma: An upper respiratory tract analogue of the chest wall mesenchymal hamartoma. Am. J. Surg. Pathol. 1998;**22**:425–33.

71. Alrawi M, McDermott M, Orr D, Russell J. Nasal chondromesenchymal hamartoma presenting in an adolescent. Int. J. Pediatr. Otorhinolaryngol. 2003;**67**:669–72.

72. Norman ES, Bergman S, Trupiano JK. Nasal chondromesenchymal hamartoma:report of a case and review of the literature. Pediatr. Dev. Pathol. 2004;**7**:517–20.

73. Ozolek JA, Carrau R, Barnes EL, Hunt JL. Nasal chondromesenchymal hamartoma in older children and adults: series and immunohistochemical analysis. Arch. Pathol. Lab. Med. 2005;**129**:1444–50.

74. Johnson C, Nagaraj U, Esguerra J, *et al.* Nasal chondromesenchymal hamartoma: radiographic and histopathologic analysis of a rare pediatric tumor. Pediatr. Radiol. 2007;**37**:101–4.

75. Kim DW, Low W, Billman G, Wickersham J, Kearns D. Chondroid hamartoma presenting as a neonatal nasal mass. Int. J. Pediatr. Otorhinolaryngol. 1999;**47**:253–9.

76. Priest JR, Williams GM, Mize WA, *et al.* Nasal chondromesenchymal hamartoma in children with pleuropulmonary blastoma: A report from the International Pleuropulmonary Blastoma Registry. Int. J. Pediatr. Otorhinolaryngol. 2010;**74**:1240–4.

77. Behery RAE, Bedrnicek J, Lazenby A, *et al.* Translocation t(12;17)(q24.1;q21) as the sole anomaly in a nasal chondromesenchymal hamartoma arising in a patient with pleuropulmonary blastoma. Pediatr. Dev. Pathol. 2012;**15**:249–53.

78. Beham A, Fletcher CD, Kainz J, *et al.* Nasopharyngeal angiofibroma: An immunohistochemical study of 32 cases. Virchows Arch. A Pathol. Anat. Histopathol. 1993;**423**:281–5.

79. Lund VJ, Stammberger H, Nicolai P, Castelnuovo P, *et al.* European position paper on endoscopic management of tumours of the nose, paranasal sinuses and skull base. Rhinology Supplement. 2010;**22**:1–143.

80. Bremer JW, Bryan NH, De Sando LW, Ljones GC. Angiofibroma: treatment trends in 150 patients during 40 years. Laryngoscope 1986;**96** 1321–9.

81. Lasjaunias P, Picard L, Manelfe C, Moret J, Doyon D. Angiofibroma of the nasopharynx. A review of 53 cases treated by embolisation. The role of pretherapeutic angiography. Pathophysiological hypotheses. J. Neuroradiol. 1980;**7**:73–95.

82. Andrade NA, Andrade JSC, Silva PDM, *et al.* Nasopharyngeal Angiofibroma:Review of the Genetic and Molecular Aspects. Int. Arch. Otorhinolaryngol. 2008;**12**:442–9.

83. Wang, J-J., Sun, X-C., Hu, L., *et al.* Endoglin (CD105) expression on microvessel endothelial cells in juvenile nasopharyngeal angiofibroma: Tissue microarray analysis and association with prognostic significance. Head Neck 2013;**35**:1719–25.

84. Spagnolo DV, Papadimitriou JM, Archer M. Post irradiation malignant fibrous histiocytoma arising in juvenile nasopharyngeal angiofibroma and producing α-1-antitrypsin. Histopathology 1984;**8**:339–52.

85. Coutinho-Camillo CM, Brentani MM, Nagai MA. Genetic alterations in juvenile nasopharyngeal angiofibromas. Head Neck 2008;**30** :390–400.

86. Ayan I, Nasopharyngeal carcinoma in children: retrospective review of 50 patients. Int. J. Radiation Oncol.. Biol. Phys. 1996;**35**:485–92.

87. Ingersoll L, Shiao Y. Donaldson WS, Giesler J, *et al.* Nasopharyngeal carcinoma in the young: A combined M.D. Anderson and Stanford experience. Int. J. Radiation Oncol.. Biol. Phys. 1990;**19** :881–7.

88. Yu MC, Yuan JM. Epidemiology of nasopharyngeal carcinoma. Semin. Cancer Biol. 2002;**12**:421–9.

89. Raab-Traub N. Epstein-Barr virus in the pathogenesis of NPC. Semin. Cancer Biol. 2002;**12**:431–41.

90. Ong YK, Tan HK. I. Nasopharyngeal carcinoma in children. Int. J. Pediatr. Otorhinolaryngol. 2000;**55**:149–54.

91. Leighton SE, Teo JG, Leung SF, *et al.* Prevalence and prognostic significance of tumor-associated tissue eosinophilia in nasopharyngeal carcinoma. Cancer 1996;**77**:436–40.

92. Looi L. Tumor-associated tissue eosinophilia in nasopharyngeal carcinoma. A pathologic study of 422 primary and 138 metastatic tumors. Cancer 1987;**59**:466–70.

93. Franchi A, Moroni M, Massi D, *et al.* Sinonasal undifferentiated carcinoma, nasopharyngeal-type undifferentiated carcinoma, and keratinizing and nonkeratinizing squamous cell carcinoma express different cytokeratin patterns. Am. J. Surg. Pathol. 2002;**26**:1597–604.

94. Friedrich RE, Bartel-Friedrich S, Lobeck H, Niedobitek G, Arps H. Epstein-Barr virus DNA, intermediate filaments and epithelial membrane antigen in nasopharyngeal carcinoma. Anticancer Res. 2000;**20**:4909–16.

95. Pathmanathan R, Prasad U, Chandrika G, *et al.* Undifferentiated, nonkeratinizing, and squamous cell carcinoma of the nasopharynx. Variants of Epstein-Barr virus-infected neoplasia. Am. J. Pathol. 1995;**146**:1355–67.

96. Li X, Fasano R, Wang E, Yao KT, Marincola FM. HLA Associations with Nasopharyngeal Carcinoma. Curr. Mol. Med. 2009;**9**(6):751–65.

97. Carbone A, Micheau C. Pitfalls in microscopic diagnosis of undifferentiated carcinoma of nasopharyngeal type (lymphoepithelioma). Cancer 1982;**50**:1344–51.

98. Bisogno G, Soloni P, Conte M, *et al.* Esthesioneuroblastoma in pediatric and adolescent age.

A report from the TREP project in cooperation with the Italian Neuroblastoma and Soft Tissue Sarcoma Committees. BMC Cancer 2012 ;**12**:117.

99. Benoit MM, Bhattacharyya N, Faquin W, Cunningham M. Cancer of the nasal cavity in the pediatric population. Pediatrics 2008;**121**:141–5.

100. Zhang M, Zhou L, Wang DH, Huang WT, Wang SY. Diagnosis and management of esthesioneuroblastoma. J. Otorhinolaryngol. Relat. Spec. 2010;**72**:113–8.

101. Faragalla H, Weinreb, I. Olfactory Neuroblastoma: A Review and Update Advances in Anatom. Pathol. 2009;**16**:322–31.

102. Hyams VJ. Tumors of the upper respiratory tract and ear. In Hyams VJ, Batsakis JG, Michaels L, editors, *Atlas of Tumor Pathology*, 2nd series, Fascile 25. Washington, DC: Armed Forces Institute of Pathology; 1988:240–8.

103. Miyamoto R C, Lyon L. Gleich, Paul W. *et al.* Esthesioneuroblastoma and sinonasal undifferentiated carcinoma: Impact of histological grading and clinical staging on survival and prognosis. Laryngoscope. 2000;**11**:1262–5.

104. Michaels LM, Hellquist HB. Neoplasms of cartilage and bone. In Michaels LM, Hellquist HB, editors, *Ear, Nose and Throat Histopathology*, second edn. London: Springer-Verlag; 2001:236–46.

105. Slootweg PJ. Lesions of the jaws. Histopathology 2009;**54**:401–18.

106. Neville BW, Damm DD, Allen CM. Odonotgenic Cysts and Tumors. In Gnepp DR, editors, *Diagnostic Surgical Pathology of the Head and Neck*. Philadelphia, PA: Saunders; 2001:605–49.

107. Mass E, Kaplan I, Hirshberg A. A clinical and histopathological study of radicular cysts associated with primary molars. J. Oral. Pathol. Med. 1995;**24**:458–61.

108. Philipsen HP, Reichart PA, Ogawa I, Suei Y, Takata T. The inflammatory paradental cyst: A critical review of 342 cases from a literature survey, including 17 new cases from the author's files. J. Oral. Pathol. Med. 2004;**33**:147–55.

109. Naclério H, Simões WA, Zindel D, *et al.* Dentigerous cyst associated with an upper permanent central incisor: case report and literature review. J. Clin. Pediatr. Dent. 2002;**26**:187–92.

110. Vucicevic Boras V, Mohamad Zaini Z, Savage NW. Supernumerary tooth with associated dentigerous cyst in an infant. A case report and review of differential diagnosis. Aust. Dent. J. 2007;**52**(2):150–3.

111. Fowler CB, Brannon RB, Kessler HP, Castle JT, Kahn MA. Glandular odontogenic cyst: Analysis of 46 cases with special emphasis on microscopic criteria for diagnosis. Head Neck Pathol. 2011;**5**:364–75.

112. Barnes L, Eveson JW, Reichart P, *et al. World Health Organization Classification of Tumors: Pathology and Genetics of Head and Neck Tumors.* Lyon: IARC Press;2005.

113. Daley TD, Wysocki GP. The small dentigerous cyst A diagnostic dilemma. Oral Surg. Oral Med. Oral Pathol. Oral Radiol. Endod. 1995;**79**:77–81.

114. Greer RO Jr, Johnson M. Botryoid odontogenic cyst: clinicopathologic analysis of ten cases with three recurrences. J. Oral Maxillofac. Surg. 1988;**46**:574–9.

115. Kaplan I, Anavi Y, Hirshberg A. Glandular odontogenic cyst: A challenge in diagnosis and treatment. Oral Dis. 2008;**14**:575–81.

116. Woolgar JA, Rippin JW, Browne RM. The odontogenic keratocyst and its occurrence in the nevoid basal cell carcinoma syndrome. Oral Surg. Oral Med. Oral Pathol. 1987;**64**:727–30.

117. Wright JM. The odontogenic keratocyst: orthokeratinized variant. Oral Surg. Oral Med. Oral Pathol. 1981;**51**:609–18.

118. Jorgenson RJ, Shapiro SD, Salinas CF, Levin LS. Intraoral findings and anomalies in neonates. Pediatrics 1982;**69** :577–82.

119. Friend GW, Harris EF, Mincer HH, *et al.* Oral anomalies in neonate, by race and gender, in urban setting. Pediatr. Dent. 1990;**12**:157–61.

120. Donley CL, Nelson LP. Comparison of palatal and alveolar cysts of the newborn in premature and full-term infants. Pediatr. Dent. 2000;**22**:321–4.

121. Fromm A. Epstein's pearls, Bohn's nodules and inclusion-cysts of the oral cavity. J. Dent. Child. 1967;**34**:275–87.

122. Swanson KS, Kaugars GE, Gunsolley JC. Nasopalatine duct cyst:an analysis of 334 cases. J. Oral Maxillofac. Surg. 1991;**49**:268–71.

123. Nelson BL, Linfesty RL. Nasopalatine duct cyst. Head and Neck Pathol. 2010;**4**:121–122.

124. Loyola AM, Gatti AF, Pinto DS Jr, Mesquita RA. Alveolar and extra-alveolar granular cell lesions of the newborn:report of case and review of literature. Oral Surg. Oral Med. Oral Pathol. Oral Radiol. Endod. 1997;**84**:668–71.

125. Tucker MC, Rusnock EJ, Azumi N, Hoy GR, Lack EE. Gingival granular cell tumors of the newborn. An ultrastructural and immunohistochemical study. Arch. Pathol. Lab. Med. 1990;**114**:895–8.

126. Jenkins HR, Hill CM. Spontaneous regression of congenital epulis of the newborn. Arch. Dis. Child. 1989;**64**:145–7.

127. Bouquot JE, Nikai Hiromasa. Lesions of the oral cavity. In Gnepp DR, editor, *Diagnostic Surgical Pathology of*

the Head and Neck. Ed. Philadelphia, PA: Saunders, 2001;141–238.

128. Vered M, Dobriyan A, Buchner A. Congenital granular cell epulis presents an immunohistochemical profile that distinguishes it from the granular cell tumor of the adult. Virchows Arch. 2009;**454**:303–10.

129. Pettinato G, Manivel JC, d'Amore ES, *et al.* Melanotic neuroectodermal tumor of infancy. A reexamination of a histogenetic problem based on immunohistochemical, flow cytometric, and ultrastructural study of 10 cases. Am. J. Surg. Pathol. 1991;**15**:233–45.

130. Fowler DJ, Chisholm J, Roebuck D, *et al.* Melanotic neuroectodermal tumor of infancy:clinical, radiological, and pathological features. Fetal Pediatr. Pathol. 2006;**25**:59–72.

131. Kapadia SB, Frisman DM, Hitchcock CL, *et al.* Melanotic neuroectodermal tumor of infancy. Clinicopathological, immunohistochemical, and flow cytometric study. Am. J. Surg. Pathol. 1993;**17**:566–573.

132. Barrett AW, Morgan M, Ramsay AD, *et al.* A clinicopathologic and immunohistochemical analysis of melanotic neuroectodermal tumor of infancy. Oral Surg. Oral Med. Oral Pathol. Oral Radiol. Endod. 2002;**93**:688–98.

133. Badi AN, Kerschner JE, North PE, *et al.* Histopathologic and immunophenotypic profile of subglottic hemangioma:multicenter study. Int. J. Pediatr. Otorhinolaryngol. 2009;**73**:1187–91.

134. Mahadi S, Malpas T, O'Donnell A, Roman K, Jephson C. PHACES syndrome. Arch. Dis. Child Fetal Neonatal Ed. 2012;**97**:F209–10.

135. Roehm CE, Chelius DC, Larrier D, *et al.* Postcricoid vascular lesions:histopathological and immunohistochemical diagnosis. Laryngoscope 2011;**121**:397–403.

136. Walner DL, Parker NP, Kim OS, Angeles RM, Stich DD. Lobular capillary hemangioma of the neonatal larynx. Arch. Otolaryngol. Head Neck Surg. 2008;**134**:272–7.

137. Goon P, Sonnex C, Jani P, Stanley M, Sudhoff H. Recurrent respiratory papillomatosis:an overview of current thinking and treatment. Eur. Arch. Otorhinolaryngol. 2008;**265**:147–51.

138. Donne AJ, Hampson L, Homer JJ, Hampson IN. The role of HPV type in recurrent respiratory papillomatosis. Int. J. Pediatr. Otorhinolaryngol. 2010;**74**:7–14.

139. Bauman NM, Smith RJ. Recurrent respiratory papillomatosis. Pediatr. Clin. North Am. 1996;**43**:1385–401.

140. Boston M, Derkay CS. Recurrent respiratory papillomatosis. Clin. Pulm. Med. 2003;**10**:10–16.

141. Derkay CS, Darrow DH. Recurrent respiratory papillomatosis of the larynx: current diagnosis and treatment. Otolaryngol. Clin. North Am. 2000;**33**:1127–42.

142. Weiss MD, Kashima HK. Tracheal involvement in laryngeal papillomatosis. Laryngoscope 1983;**93**:45–8.

143. Kashima H, Mounts P, Leventhal B, Hruban RH. Sites of predilection in recurrent respiratory papillomatosis. Ann. Otol. Rhinol. Laryngol. 1993;**102**:580–3.

144. Rady PL, Schnadig VJ, Weiss RL, Hughes TK, Tyring SK. Malignant transformation of recurrent respiratory papillomatosis associated with integrated human papillomavirus type 11 DNA and mutation of p53. Laryngoscope 1998;**108**:735–40.

145. Solomon D, Smith RR, Kashima HK, Leventhal BG. Malignant transformation in non-irradiated recurrent respiratory papillomatosis. Laryngoscope 1985;**95**:900–4.

146. Derkay CS, Wiatrak B. Recurrent Respiratory Papillomatosis: A Review, Laryngoscope 2008;**118**;1236–47.

147. Poljak M, Seme K, Gale N. Detection of human papillomaviruses in tissue specimens. Adv. Anat. Pathol. 1998;**5**:216–34.

148. Quick CA, Foucar E, Dehner LP. Frequency and significance of epithelial atypia in laryngeal papillomatosis. Laryngoscope 1979;**89**:550–60.

149. Acierno SP, Waldhausen JHT. Congenital cervical cysts, sinuses and fistulae. Otolaryngol. Clin. North Am. 2007;**40**:161–76.

150. Moore KL, Persaud V. The Pharyngeal Apparatus. In Moore KL, Persaud V, editors, *Before We Are Born: Essentials of Embryology and Birth Defects*, sixth edn. Philadelphia, PA: Saunders, 2003:151–188.

151. Foley DS, Fallat ME. Thyroglossal duct and other congenital midline cervical anomalies. Semin. Pediatr. Surg. 2006;**15**:70–5.

152. Allard RH. The thyroglossal cyst. Head Neck Surg. 1982;**5**:134–46.

153. Pérez-Martínez A, Bento-Bravo L, Martínez-Bermejo MA, *et al.* An intra-thyroid thyroglossal duct cyst. Eur. J. Pediatr. Surg. 2005;**15**:428–30.

154. North JH Jr, Foley AM, Hamill RL. Intrathyroid cysts of thyroglossal duct origin. Am. Surg. 1998;**64**:886–8.

155. Sonnino RE, Spigland N, Laberge JM, Desjardins J, Guttman FM. Unusual patterns of congenital neck masses in children. J. Pediatr. Surg. 1989;**24**:966–9.

156. Shifrin A, Vernick J. A thyroglossal duct cyst presenting as a thyroid nodule in the lateral neck. Thyroid 2008;**18**:263–5.

157. Diaz MC, Stormorken A, Christopher NC. A thyroglossal duct cyst causing apnea and cyanosis in a neonate. Pediatr. Emerg. Care. 2005;**21**:35–7.

158. Byard RW, Bourne AJ, Silver MM. The association of lingual thyroglossal duct remnants with sudden death in infancy. Int. J. Pediatr. Otorhinolaryngol. 1990;**20**:107–12.

159. Doshi SV, Cruz RM, Hilsinger RL Jr. Thyroglossal duct carcinoma: A large case series. Ann. Otol. Rhinol. Laryngol. 2001;**110**:734–8.

160. Forest VI, Murali R, Clark JR. Thyroglossal duct cyst carcinoma:case series. J. Otolaryngol. Head Neck Surg. 2011;**40**:151–6.

161. Peretz A, Leiberman E, Kapelushnik J, Hershkovitz E. Thyroglossal duct carcinoma in children:case presentation and review of the literature. Thyroid 2004;**14**:777–85.

162. Solomon JR, Rangecroft L. Thyroglossal duct lesions in children. J. Pediatr. Surg. 1984;**19**:555–61.

163. Tyson RW, Groff DB. An unusual lateral neck cyst with the combined features of a bronchogenic, thyroglossal, and branchial cleft origin. Pediatr. Pathol. 1993;**13**:567–72.

164. Waldhausen JH. Branchial cleft and arch anomalies in children. Semin. Pediatr. Surg. 2006;**15**:64–9.

165. Milunsky JM, Maher TM, Zhao G, Wang Z, *et al*. Genotype-phenotype analysis of the branchio-oculo-facial syndrome. Am. J. Med. Genet. A. 2011;**155A**:22–32.

166. Olsen KD, Maragos NE, Weiland LH. First branchial cleft anomalies. Laryngoscope 1980;**90**:423–36.

167. Schroeder JW Jr, Mohyuddin N, Maddalozzo J. Branchial anomalies in the pediatric population. Otolaryngol. Head Neck Surg. 2007;**137**:289–95.

168. Triglia JM, Nicollas R, Ducroz V, *et al*. First branchial cleft anomalies:a study of 39 cases and a review of the literature. Arch. Otolaryngol. Head Neck Surg. 1998;**124**:291–5.

169. Aronsohn RS, Batsakis JG, Rice DH, Work WP. Anomalies of the first branchial cleft. Arch. Otolaryngol. 1976;**102**:737–40.

170. Work WP. Newer concepts of first branchial cleft defects. Laryngoscope 1972;**82**:1581–93.

171. Chandrasekar T, Ramani P, Anuja N, *et al*. Unilocular cystic sebaceous lymphadenoma:a rare tumour. Ann. R. Coll. Surg. Engl. 2007;**89**:1–3.

172. Mukherji SK, Fatterpekar G, Castillo M, Stone JA, Chung CJ. Imaging of congenital anomalies of the branchial apparatus. Neuroimag. Clin. N. Am. 2000;**10**:75–93, viii.

173. Bhaksar SN, Bernei JL. Histogenesis of branchial cysts: A report of 468 cases. Am. J. Pathol. 1959;**35**:407–23.

174. Sarioglu S, Unlu M, Adali Y, Erdag TK, Men S. Branchial cleft cyst with xanthogranulomatous inflammation. Head Neck Pathol. 2012;**6**:146–9.

175. Khafif RA, Prichep R, Minkowitz S. Primary branchiogenic carcinoma. Head Neck. 1989;**11**:153–63.

176. Choi SS, Zalzal GH. Branchial anomalies:a review of 52 cases. Laryngoscope 1995;**105**:909–13.

177. Ford GR, Balakrishnan A, Evans JN, *et al*. Branchial cleft and pouch anomalies. J. Laryngol. Otol. 1992;**106**:137–43.

178. James A, Stewart C, Warrick P, *et al*. Branchial sinus of the piriform fossa:reappraisal of third and fourth branchial anomalies. Laryngoscope 2007;**117**:1920–24.

179. Nicoucar K, Giger R, Pope HG Jr, Jaecklin T, Dulguerov P. Management of congenital fourth branchial arch anomalies: A review and analysis of published cases. J. Pediatr. Surg. 2009;**44**:1432–9.

180. Nicoucar K, Giger R, Jaecklin T, Pope HG Jr, Dulguerov P. Management of congenital third branchial arch anomalies:a systematic review. Otolaryngol. Head Neck Surg. 2010;**142**:21–8.

181. Nicollas R, Ducroz V, Garabédian EN, Triglia JM. Fourth branchial pouch anomalies:a study of six cases and review of the literature. Int. J. Pediatr. Otorhinolaryngol. 1998;**44**:5–10.

182. Thomas B, Shroff M, Forte V, *et al*. Revisiting imaging features and the embryologic basis of third and fourth branchial anomalies. AJNR Am. J. Neuroradiol. 2010;**31**:755–60.

183. Redleaf MI, Walker WP, Alt LP. Parathyroid adenoma associated with a branchial cleft cyst. Arch. Otolaryngol. Head Neck Surg. 1995 ;**121**:113–5.

184. McInnes CW, Benson AD, Verchere CG, Ludemann JP, Arneja JS. Management of congenital midline cervical cleft. J. Craniofac. Surg. 2012 ;**23**:e36–8.

185. Roth DA, Hildesheimer M, Bardenstein S, *et al*. Preauricular skin tags and ear pits are associated with permanent hearing impairment in newborns. Pediatrics 2008;**122**:e884–90.

186. Scheinfeld NS, Silverberg NB, Weinberg JM, Nozad V. The preauricular sinus:a review of its clinical presentation, treatment,and associations. Pediatr. Dermatol. 2004;**21**:191–6.

187. Atlan G, Egerszegi EP, Brochu P, *et al*. Cervical chrondrocutaneous branchial remnants. Plast. Reconstr. Surg. 1997;**100**:32–9.

188. Nasser HA, Iskandarani F, Berjaoui T, Fleifel S. A case report of bilateral cervical chondrocutaneous remnants with review of the literature. J. Pediatr. Surg. 2011;**46**:998–1000.

189. Bale PM, Sotelo-Avila C. Maldescent of the thymus: 34 necropsy and 10 surgical cases, including 7 thymuses

medial to the mandible. Pediatr. Pathol. 1993;**13**:181–190.

190. Shah SS, Lai SY, Ruchelli E, *et al.* Retropharyngeal aberrant thymus. Pediatrics 2001;**108**(5):E94.

191. Sturm-O'Brien AK, Salazar JD, Byrd RH, *et al.* Cervical thymic anomalies–the Texas Children's Hospital experience. Laryngoscope 2009;**119**:1988–93.

192. Jones JE, Hession B. Cervical thymic cysts. Ear Nose Throat J. 1996;**75**(10):678–80.

193. Khariwala SS, Nicollas R, Triglia JM, *et al.* Cervical presentations of thymic anomalies in children. Int. J. Pediatr. Otorhinolaryngol. 2004;**68**:909–14.

194. Statham MM, Mehta D, Willging JP. Cervical thymic remnants in children. Int. J. Pediatr. Otorhinolaryngol. 2008;**72**):1807–13.

195. Scott KJ, Schroeder AA, Greinwald JH Jr. Ectopic cervical thymus:an uncommon diagnosis in the evaluation of pediatric neck masses. Arch. Otolaryngol. Head Neck Surg. 2002;**128**:714–7.

196. De Caluwé D, Ahmed M, Puri P. Cervical thymic cysts. Pediatr. Surg Int. 2002;**18**:477–9.

197. Kuperan AB, Quraishi HA, Shah AJ, Mirani N. Thymopharyngeal duct cyst:a case presentation and literature review. Laryngoscope 2010;**120** Suppl 4:S226.

198. Kaufman MR, Smith S, Rothschild MA, Som P. Thymopharyngeal duct cyst:an unusual variant of cervical thymic anomalies. Arch. Otolaryngol. Head Neck Surg. 2001;**127**:1357–60.

199. Burton EM, Mercado-Deane MG, Howell CG, *et al.* Cervical thymic cysts: CT appearance of two cases including a persistent thymopharyngeal duct cyst. Pediatr. Radiol. 1995;**25**:363–5.

200. Kelley DJ, Gerber ME, Willging JP. Cervicomediastinal thymic cysts. Int. J. Pediatr. Otorhinolaryngol. 1997;**39**:139–46.

201. Daneshbod Y, Banani A, Kumar PV. Aberrant thymus and parathyroid gland presenting as a recurrent lateral neck mass: A case report. Ear Nose Throat J. 2006 Jul;**85**:452–3.

202. Berenos-Riley L, Manni JJ, Coronel C, De Wilde PC. Thymic cyst in the neck. Acta Otolaryngol. 2005;**125**:108–12.

203. Entwistle JW, Pierce CV, Johnson DE, *et al.* Parathyroid cysts: report of the sixth and youngest pediatric case. J. Pediatr. Surg. 1994;**29**:1528–9.

204. Turner A, Lampe HB, Cramer H. Parathyroid cysts. J. Otolaryngol. 1989;**18**:311–3.

205. Sánchez A, Carretto H. Treatment of a nonfunctioning parathyroid cyst with tetracycline injection. Head Neck. 1993;**15**:263–5.

206. Wu W. (The diagnosis and surgical management of parathyroid cysts). Zhonghua Wai Ke Za Zhi. 1995;**33**:673–4.

207. Clark OH. Parathyroid cysts. Am. J. Surg. 1978;**135**:395–402.

208. Atwan M, Chetty R. An unusual "thyroid cyst": intrathyroidal parathyroid cyst. Endocr. Pathol. 2011;**22**:108–11.

209. Calandra DB, Shah KH, Prinz RA, *et al.* Parathyroid cysts: A report of eleven cases including two associated with hyperparathyroid crisis. Surgery 1983;**94**:887–92.

210. Pryor SG, Lewis JE, Weaver AL, Orvidas LJ. Pediatric dermoid cysts of the head and neck. Otolaryngol. Head Neck Surg. 2005;**132**:938–42.

211. Hanikeri M, Waterhouse N, Kirkpatrick N, *et al.* The management of midline transcranial nasal dermoid sinus cysts. Br. J. Plast. Surg. 2005;**58**:1043–50.

212. Bloom D, Carvalho D, Edmonds J, Magit A. Neonatal dermoid cyst of the floor of the mouth extending to the midline neck. Arch. Otolaryngol. Head Neck Surg. 2002;**128**:68–70.

213. McAvoy JM, Zuckerbraun L. Dermoid cysts of the head and neck in children. Arch. Otolaryngol. 1976;**102**:529–31.

214. Ro EY, Thomas RM, Isaacson GC. Giant dermoid cyst of the neck can mimic a cystic hygroma:using MRI to differentiate cystic neck lesions. Int. J. Pediatr. Otorhinolaryngol. 2007;**71**:653–8.

215. Kim NJ, Choung HK, Khwarg SI. Management of dermoid tumor in the medial canthal area. Korean J. Ophthalmol. 2009;**23**:204–6.

216. Kieran SM, Robson CD, Nosé V, Rahbar R. Foregut duplication cysts in the head and neck: presentation, diagnosis, and management. Arch. Otolaryngol. Head Neck Surg. 2010;**136**:778–82.

217. Teissier N, Elmaleh-Bergès M, Ferkdadji L, *et al.* Cervical bronchogenic cysts:usual and unusual clinical presentations. Arch. Otolaryngol. Head Neck Surg. 2008;**134**:1165–9.

218. Eaton D, Billings K, Timmons C, *et al.* Congenital foregut duplication cysts of the anterior tongue. Arch. Otolaryngol. Head Neck Surg. 2001;**127**:1484–7.

219. Luna MA and Pfaltz M. Cyst of the neck, unknown primary tumor, and neck dissection. In Gnepp DR, editor, *Diagnostic Surgical Pathology of the Head and Neck*. Philadelphia, PA: Saunders; 2001:650–80.

220. Chan JK, Rosai J. Tumors of the neck showing thymic or related branchial pouch differentiation:a unifying concept. Hum. Pathol. 1991;**22**:349–67.

221. Tapper D, Lack EE. Teratomas in infancy and childhood. A 54-year experience at the Children's Hospital Medical Center. Ann. Surg. 1983;**198**:398–409.

222. Lazar DA, Olutoye OO, Moise KJ Jr, *et al.* Ex-utero intrapartum treatment procedure for giant neck masses-fetal and maternal outcomes. J. Pediatr. Surg. 2011;**46**:817–22.

223. Rothschild MA, Catalano P, Urken M, *et al.* Evaluation and management of congenital cervical teratoma. Arch. Otolaryngol. Head Neck Surg. 1994;**120**:444–8.

224. Rotenberg B, El-Hakim H, Lodha A, *et al.* Nasopharyngeal teratocarcinosarcoma. Int. J. Pediatr. Otorhinolaryngol. 2002 Feb 1;**62**:159–64.

225. Levine C. Primary disorders of the lymphatic vessels. A unified concept. J. Pediatr. Surg. 1989;**24**:233.

226. Waner M, Suen JY. A classification of congenital vascular lesions. In Waner M, Suen JY, editors, *Hemangiomas and Vascular Malformations of the Head And Neck*. New York:Wiley-Liss;1999:1–12.

227. Review Hemangiomas, cystic hygromas, and teratomas of the head and neck. Filston HC Semin. Pediatr. Surg. 1994;**3**:147–59.

228. Mulliken JB. Vascular anomalies. In Aston SJ, Beasley RW, Thorne CHM, editors, *Grabb and Smith Plastic Surgery*, fifth edn. New York: Lippincott Raven Publishers;1997.

229. Kennedy TL. Cystic hygroma-lymphangioma:a rare and still unclear entity. Laryngoscope 1989;**99**:1–10.

230. Chervenak FA, Isaacson G, Blakemore KJ, *et al.* Fetal cystic hygroma. Cause and natural history. N. Engl. J. Med. 1983;**309**:822–5.

231. Kalof AN, Cooper K. D2–40 immunohistochemistry – so far! Adv. Anat. Pathol. 2009;**16**:62–4.

232. Lauer DH, Enziger FM. Cranial fasciitis of childhood. Cancer 1980;**45**:401–6.

233. Marciano S, Vanel D, Mathieu MC. Cranial fasciitis in an adult: CT and MR imaging findings. Eur. Radiol. 1999;**9**:1650–2.

234. Ringsted J, Ladefoged C, Bjerre P. Cranial fasciitis of childhood. Acta Neuropathol. 1985;**66**:337–9.

235. Sato Y, Kitamura T, Suganuma Y, *et al.* Cranial fasciitis of childhood: A case report. Eur. J. Pediatr. Surg. 1993;**3**:107–9.

236. Pagenstecher A, Emmerich B, van Velthoven V, *et al.* Exclusively intracranial cranial fasciitis in a child: case report. J. Neurosurg. 1995;**83**:744–7.

237. Adler R, Wong CA. Cranial fasciitis simulating histiocytosis. J. Pediatr. 1986;**109**:85–8.

238. Govender PV, Jithoo R, Chrystal V, *et al.* Cranial fasciitis:case illustration. J. Neurosurg. 2001;**94**:681.

239. Rakheja D, Cunningham JC, Mitui M, *et al.* A subset of cranial fasciitis is associated with dysregulation of the Wnt/β-catenin pathway. Mod. Pathology. 2008;**21**:1330–1336.

240. Seifert G, Okabe H, Caselitz J. Epithelial salivary gland tumors in children and adolescents. Analysis of 80 cases (Salivary gland register 1965–1984). Otorhinolaryngol. Rel. Spec. 1986;**48**:137–49.

241. Batsakis JG, Luna MA, El-Naggar AK. Salivary gland tumors in children. Otol. Rhinol. Laryngol. 1991;**100**:869–71.

242. Krolls SO, Trodahl JN, Boyers RC. Salivary gland lesions in children. Cancer 1972;**30**:459–69.

243. Lack EE, Upton MP. Histopathologic review of salivary gland tumors in childhood. Arch. Otolaryngol. Head Neck Surg. 1988;**114**:898–906.

244. Batsakis JG, Mackay B, Ryka F, Seifert RW. Perinatal salivary gland tumors (Embryomas). J. Laryngol. Otol. 1988;**102**:1007–11.

245. Seifert G, *et al.* Bilateral dysgenetic polycystic parotid glands. Morphological analysis and differential diagnosis of this rare disease of salivary glands. Virchows Arch. A Pathol. Anat. Histol. 1981;**390**:273–88.

246. Dobson CM, *et al.* Polycystic disease of the parotid glands:case report of a rare entity and review of the literature. Histopathology 1987;**11**:953–61.

247. McGurk M, Eyeson J, Thomas B, Harrison JD. Conservative treatment of oral ranula by excision with minimal excision of the sublingual gland:histological support for a traumatic etiology. J. Oral Maxillofac. Surg. 2008;**66**:2050–7.

248. Harrison JD. Modern management and pathophysiology of ranula:literature review. Head Neck. 2010 ;**32**:1310–20.

249. Onderoglu L, Saygan-Karamürsel B, Deren O, *et al.* Prenatal diagnosis of ranula at 21 weeks of gestation. Ultrasound Obstet. Gynecol. 2003;**22**:399–401.

250. Zhao YF, Jia Y, Chen XM, Zhang WF. Clinical review of 580 ranulas. Oral Surg. Oral Med. Oral Pathol. Oral Radiol. Endod. 2004;**98**:281–7.

251. Syebele K, Bütow KW. Oral mucoceles and ranulas may be part of initial manifestations of HIV infection. AIDS Res. Hum. Retrovir. 2010;**26**:1075–8.

252. Langlois NE, Kolhe P. Plunging ranula:a case report and a literature review. Hum. Pathol. 1992;**23**:1306–8.

253. Jain R, Morton RP, Ahmad Z. Diagnostic difficulties of plunging ranula:case series. J. Laryngol. Otol. 2012;**126**:506–10.

254. Osborne TE, Haller JA, Levin LS, *et al.*, Submandibular cystic hygroma resembling a plunging ranula in a neonate. Review and report of a case. Oral Surg. Oral Med. Oral Pathol. 1991;**71**:16–20.

255. Effat KG. Acute presentation of a plunging ranula causing respiratory distress:case report. J. Laryngol. Otol. 2012;**126**:861–3.

256. Voz ML, Agten NS, Van de Ven WJ, Kas K. PLAG1, the main translocation target in pleomorphic adenoma of the salivary glands, is a positive regulator of IGF-II. Cancer Res. 2000;**60**:106–13.

257. Seifert G, Donath K. Juvenile pleomorphic parotid adenoma of embryonal structures. Pathologe 1998;**19**:286–91.

258. Gnepp DR, Henley JD, Simpson RHW, Eveson J. Salivary and lacrimal glands. In Gnepp DR, editor, *Diagnostic Surgical Pathology of the Head and Neck*. Philadelphia, PA: Saunders, 2009:449–51.

259. Sciubba JJ, Brannon RB. Myoepithelioma of salivary glands:report of 23 case. Cancer 1982;**49**:562–72.

260. Stárek I, Skálová A, Simpson RHW, *et al*. Spindle cell myoepithelial tumors of parotid gland with extensive lipomatous metaplasia. Virchows Arch. 2001;**439**:762–7.

261. Dardick I, Thomas MJ, van Nostrand AW. Myoepithelioma-new concepts of histology and classification:a light and electron microscopic study. Ultrastruct. Pathol. 1989;**13**:187–224.

262. Skalova A, Michal M, Ryška A, *et al*. Oncocytic myoepithelioma and pleomorphic adenoma. Virchows Arch. 1999;**434**:537–46.

263. Skálová A, Michal M, Leivo I, *et al*. Analysis of collagen isotypes in crystalloid structures of salivary gland tumors. Hum. Pathol. 1992;**23**:748–55.

264. Skálová A, Michal M. Cystadenoma: Tumours of the salivary glands In Barnes EL, Eveson JW, Reichart P. Sidransky D, editors, *World Health Organization Classification of Tumours: Pathology and Genetics of Head and Neck Tumours*. Lyon, France:IARC Press; 2005: 273–4.

265. Michal M, Skalova A, Mukensnabl P. Micropapillary carcinoma arising in mucinous cystadenoma. Virchows Arch. 2000;**437**:465–8.

266. Skálová A, Leivo I, Wolf H, Fakan F. Oncocytic cystadenoma of the parotid gland with tyrosine-rich crystals. Path. Res. Pract. 2000;**196**:849–51.

267. Weinreb I, Simpson RHW, Skalova A, *et al*. Ductal adenomas of salivary gland showing features of striated duct differentiation ('striated duct adenoma'): A report of six cases. Histopathology 2010;**57**:707–15.

268. Smith BC, Ellis GL, Slater LJ, *et al*. Sclerosing polycystic adenosis of major salivary glands:A clinicopathologic analysis of nine cases. Am. J. Surg. Pathol. 1996;**20**:161–70.

269. Skalova A, Michal M, Simpson RHW, *et al*. Sclerosing polycystic adenosis of parotid gland with dysplasia and ductal carcinoma in situ: Report of three cases with immunohistochemical and ultrastructural examination. Virchows Arch. 2002;**440**:29–35.

270. Skalova A, Gnepp DR, Simpson RHW, *et al*. Clonal nature of sclerosing polycystic adenosis of salivary glands demonstrated by using the polymorphism of the human androgen receptor locus (HUMARA) as a marker. Am. J. Surg. Pathol. 2006;**30**:939–944.

271. Petersson F, Tan PH, Hwang JSG. Sclerosing polycystic adenosis of parotid gland: report of a bifocal, paucicystic variant with ductal carcinoma in situ and pronounced stromal distortion mimicking stromal invasion. Head Neck Pathol. 2011;**5**:188–92.

272. Bentz BG, Hughes CA, Ludemann JP, Maddalozzo J. Masses of the salivary gland region in children. Arch. Otolaryngol. Head Neck Surg. 2000;**126**:1435–9.

273. Weiss I, Lipari BA, Meyer L, *et al*. Current treatment of parotid hemangiomas. Laryngoscope 2011;**121**:1642–50.

274. Takato T, Komuro Y, Yonehara Y. Giant hemangioma of the parotid gland associated with Kasabach-Merritt syndrome:a case report. J. Oral Maxillofac. Surg. 1993:**51**:425–8.

275. Sinno H, Thibaudeau S, Coughlin R, Chitte S, Williams B. Management of infantile parotid gland hemangiomas: A 40-year experience. Plast. Reconstr. Surg. 2010:**125**:265–273.

276. Damiani S, Corti B, Neri F, Collina G, Bertoni F. Primary angiosarcoma of the parotid gland arising from benign congenital hemangioma. Oral Surg. Oral Med. Oral Pathol. Oral Radiol. Endod. 2003;**96**:66–9.

277. Leon-Villapalos J, Wolfe K, Kangesu L. GLUT-1: An extra diagnostic tool to differentiate between haemangiomas and vascular malformations. Br. J. Plast. Surg. 2005:**58**:348–52.

278. Johann AC, Salla JT, Gomez RS, de Aguiar MC, Gontijo B, Mesquita RA. GLUT-1 in oral benign vascular lesions. Oral Dis. 2007;**13**:51–5.

279. Ahrens WA, Ridenour RV, 3rd, Caron BL, Miller DV, Folpe AL. GLUT-1 expression in mesenchymal tumors: An immunohistochemical study of 247 soft tissue and bone neoplasms. Hum. Pathol. 2008;**39**:1519–26.

280. Kennedy T, Briant TD. Parotid lymphangioma. J. Otolaryngol. 1977;**6**:23–7.

281. Schroeder BA, Czarnecki DJ, Wells RG, Sty JR. Salivary gland scintigraphy. Cystic hygroma of the parotid. Clin. Nucl. Med. 1987;**12**:485–6.

282. Taylor BG, Cohn I, Jr. Tumors of the salivary glands. Curr. Probl. Cancer 1978;**3**:1–43.

283. Cho KJ, Ro JY, Choi J, *et al*. Mesenchymal neoplasms of the major salivary glands: clinicopathological features of 18 cases. Eur. Arch. Otorhinolaryngol. 2008;**265** Suppl 1:S47–56.

284. Jaryszak EM, Shah RK, Bauman NM, *et al*. Unexpected pathologies in pediatric parotid lesions:management

paradigms revisited. Int. J. Pediatr. Otorhinolaryngol. 2011;**75**:558–63.

285. Carr MM, Fraser RB, Clarke KD. Nodular fasciitis in the parotid region of a child. Head Neck 1998;**20**:645–648.

286. Goode RK, El-Naggar AK. Mucoepidermoid carcinoma: Tumours of the salivary glands. In Barnes EL, Eveson JW, Reichart P. Sidransky D, editors, *World Health Organization Classification of Tumours: Pathology and Genetics of Head and Neck Tumours.* Lyon, France: IARC Press; 2005:219–20.

287. Skálová A, Lehtonen H, Boguslawsky K, Leivo I: Prognostic significance of cell proliferation in mucoepidermoid carcinomas of salivary gland. Clinicopathological study using MIB 1 antibody in paraffin sections. Hum. Pathol. 1994;**25**:929–35.

288. Okabe M, Miyabe S, Nagatsuka H, *et al.* MECT1-MAML2 fusion transcript defines a favorable subset of mucoepidermoid carcinoma. Clin. Cancer Res. 2006;**12**:3902–7.

289. Nakayama T, Miyabe S, Okabe M, *et al.* Clinicopathological significance of the CRTC3-MAML2 fusion transcript in mucoepidermoid carcinoma. Mod. Pathol. 2009;**22**:1575–81.

290. Skalova A, Vanecek T, Sima R, *et al.* Mammary analogue secretory carcinoma of salivary glands, containing the ETV6-NTRK3 fusion gene: A hitherto undescribed salivary gland tumor entity. Am. J. Surg. Pathol. 2010;**34**:599–608.

291. Luna MA, Batsakis JG, El-Naggar AK. Pathology consultation. Salivary gland tumors in children. Ann. Otol. Rhinol. Laryngol. 1991;**100**:869–71.

292. Ellis G, Simpson RHW. Acinic cell carcinoma: Tumours of the salivary glands. In Barnes EL, Eveson JW, Reichart P. Sidransky D, editors, *World Health Organization Classification of Tumours:Pathology and Genetics of Head and Neck Tumours.* Lyon, France: IARC Press; 2005:216–8.

293. Chenevert J, Duvvuri U, Chiosea S, *et al.* DOG1: A novel marker of salivary acinar and intercalated duct differentiation. Mod. Pathol. 2012;**25**:919–29.

294. Nordkvist A, Mark J, Gustaffson H, *et al.* Non-random chromosome rearrangenments in adenoid cystic carcinoma of salivary glands. Genes Chromosomes Cancer 1994;**10**:115–21.

295. Persson M, Andrén Y, Mark J, *et al.* Recurrent fusion of MYB and NFIB transcription factor genes in carcinoma of the breast and head and neck. Proc. Natl. Acad. Sci. USA 2009;**106**:18740–4.

296. Skálová A, Simpson RHW, Lehtonnen H, Leivo I. Assessment of proliferative activity using the MIB1 antibody helps to distinguish polymorphous low grade adenocarcinoma from adenoid cystic carcinoma of salivary glands. Path. Res. Pract. 1997;**193**:695–703.

297. Vawter GF, Tefft M. Congenital tumors of parotid gland. Arch. Pathol. 1966;**82**:242–5.

298. Taylor GP. Congenital epithelial tumor of the parotid-sialoblastoma. Pediatr. Pathol. 1988;**88**:447–52.

299. Adkins GF. Low grade basaloid adenocarcinoma of the salivary gland in childhood: the so called hybrid basal cell adenoma-adenoid cystic carcinoma. Pathology 1990;**22**:187–90.

300. Brandwein M, Al-Naeif NS, Manwani D, *et al.* Sialoblastoma. Clinicopathological/ immunohistochemical study. Am. J. Surg. Pathol. 1999;**23**:342–348.

301. Viva E, Zorzi F, Annibale G, *et al.* Endodermal sinus (yolk sac) tumor of the parotid gland:a case report. Int. J. Pediatr. Otorhinolaryngol. 1992;**24**:269–74.

302. Sredni ST, da Cunha IW, de Carvalho Filho NP, *et al.* Endodermal sinus tumor of the parotid gland in a child. Pediatr. Dev. Pathol. 2004;**7**:77–80.

303. Newton WA, Jr., Gehan EA, Webber BL, *et al.* Classification of rhabdomyosarcomas and related sarcomas. Pathologic aspects and proposal for a new classification – an Intergroup Rhabdomyosarcoma Study. Cancer 1995;**76**:1073–85.

304. Salomao DR, Sigman JD, Greenebaum E, Cohen MB. Rhabdomyosarcoma presenting as a parotid gland mass in pediatric patients:fine-needle aspiration biopsy findings. Cancer 1998;**84**:245–51.

305. Kapadia SB, Dhir R, Fujii H, *et al.* Botryoid embryonal rhabdomyosarcoma of Stensen's duct. Am. J. Otolaryngol. 1996;**17**:127–32.

306. Valencerina Gopez E, Dauterman J, Layfield LJ. Fine-needle aspiration biopsy of alveolar rhabdomyosarcoma of the parotid: A case report and review of the literature. Diagn. Cytopathol. 2001;**24**:249–52.

307. Walterhouse DO, Pappo AS, Baker KS, *et al.* Rhabdomyosarcoma of the parotid region occurring in childhood and adolescence. A report from the Intergroup Rhabdomyosarcoma Study Group. Cancer 2001;**92**:3135–46.

308. Yin WH, Guo SP, Yang HY, Chan JK. Desmoplastic small round-cell tumor of the submandibular gland–a rare but distinctive primary salivary gland neoplasm. Hum. Pathol. 2010;**41**:438–42.

309. Pulec JL. Aggressive fibromatosis (fibrosarcoma) of the facial nerve. Ear Nose Throat J. 1993;**72**:460–7, 470–2.

Respiratory system

Gail Deutsch and Erin R. Rudzinski

Introduction

Pediatric lung disorders, particularly non-neoplastic, comprise entities and histologic patterns that differ significantly from that described in the adult literature. Areas of dissimilarity are particularly apparent within neonates and young children, who are likely to present early in life with a congenital lung malformation, primary disorder of lung development, lung growth abnormality, or genetic abnormality in surfactant production and homeostasis. There is high variability in morbidity and mortality associated with infant lung disorders, highlighting the critical need for accurate diagnosis (1). A multidisciplinary approach to these disorders is necessary, with appropriate clinical, radiographic, pathologic, and frequent molecular evaluations required to result in a specific diagnosis. As such, proper processing of the tissue is critical to provide a comprehensive diagnostic evaluation, including tissue for culture, light microscopy, immunohistochemistry, electron microscopy, and genetic studies (2).

This chapter will highlight several disorders that are characteristic of the pediatric age group, particularly those that present in infancy and within the first few years of life.

Congenital lung malformations

With the routine practice of fetal ultrasonography, congenital lung abnormalities are increasingly being recognized antenatally, often resulting in resection of these lesions well before they manifest with respiratory compromise. While there is no consistent nomenclature system to describe the variety of congenital lung abnormalities, they frequently share common modes of pathogenesis and histologic features (3–5). For example, congenital cystic pulmonary airway malformations, intralobar sequestration, pulmonary hyperplasia, and congenital lobar overinflation are thought to be related to airway obstruction with or without secondary dysplastic changes, while bronchogenic cysts and extralobar sequestration are manifestations of aberrant foregut budding and differentiation.

Bronchogenic cyst

Bronchogenic or bronchial cysts are unilocular cysts that recapitulate the bronchial structure, without connection to the lung. They arise from anomalous foregut budding during development.

Clinical presentation: Most commonly occur in the mid-mediastinum or subcarinal area, but may be intralobar, subdiaphragmatic or even cutaneous (6,7). The time of clinical presentation is variable and related to compression of adjacent structures (e.g., trachea, bronchi, esophagus), infection, or rupture. Patients typically present later in life with recurrent coughing, wheezing, dysphagia, or pneumonia, but neonatal presentation or incidental detection on chest radiographs taken for unrelated reasons is not unusual. On imaging, bronchogenic cysts appear as round water-density masses with sharp margins that may have air-fluid levels. Management consists of surgical resection.

Macroscopy: Cysts are unilocular and, if intraparenchymal, do not connect with the normal tracheobronchial tree. They are filled with clear serous fluid, unless infected, in which case the fluid may be turbid.

Histology: The cysts are lined by ciliated columnar bronchial epithelium with frequent inflammation, ulceration, and squamous metaplasia. The wall recapitulates that of the normal bronchus, containing smooth muscle, submucosal glands, and plates of

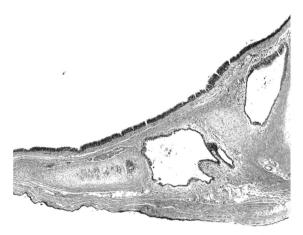

Figure 5.1 Incidental posterior mediastinal mass discovered in a 9-year-old imaged for abdominal trauma.

cartilage. Multiple sections may be required to demonstrate cartilage, the presence of which is diagnostic of this lesion (Figure 5.1).

Differential diagnosis: When inflamed and intraparenchymal, bronchogenic cysts need to be distinguished from a lung abscess or a large cyst (Stocker Type I congenital pulmonary airway malformation (CPAM)). Unlike a bronchogenic cyst, both of these have multiple bronchial lumina and typically communicate with the normal tracheobronchial tree, although in CPAM this connection is not normal and the bronchus may be atretic. Other foregut-derived cysts should also be excluded, including enteric cysts, which are lined by gastric or intestinal epithelium. Cystic teratomas also occur in the mediastinum, but are multilocular and contain ectodermal, mesodermal, and endodermal derivatives other than bronchial epithelium.

Congenital pulmonary airway malformation

Congenital pulmonary airway malformation (CPAM), previously known as congenital cystic adenomatoid malformation (CCAM), is the most common lung malformation of the lower respiratory tract. Under the Stocker classification, it has been categorized into five separate subtypes, based upon the size of the cysts and their resemblance to the tracheobronchial tree (tracheal, bronchial, bronchiolar, or alveolar) (8), but the pathogenesis and terminology of all the types is debated (3). For example, Type 0 CPAM is also known as acinar dysplasia, Type 3 CPAM resembles

pulmonary hyperplasia, and Type 4 CPAM is thought to represent a form of type I pleuropulmonary blastoma. Type 1 CPAM is typically a large cystic lesion lined by ciliated bronchial epithelium (large cyst type) and Type 2 CPAM (small cyst type) comprises bronchiolar spaces and is commonly associated with lobar sequestrations and bronchial atresia.

Clinical presentation: The presentation of CPAMs is variable; patients may present with respiratory distress in the newborn period or remain asymptomatic until later in life. Most cases are now detected by routine prenatal ultrasound. Large lesions typically cause symptoms by compromising alveolar growth during development. Mediastinal shift with subsequent development of polyhydramnios and hydrops may develop in rapidly enlarging lesions (9). Congenital pulmonary airway malformations are sporadic lesions that can arise in any lobe; infrequently they involve multiple lung lobes (10). A large-cyst CPAM is the most common type, and by imaging presents as a lung mass with cysts measuring greater than 2 cm. A small-cyst CPAM is comprised of multiple small cysts, which may be heterogeneous on imaging, based on the presence of cystic and solid components. Small-cyst CPAMs may be associated with other congenital anomalies, including cardiovascular, renal, and diaphragmatic hernia (11). Mechanisms resulting in CPAM formation are debated, but they are thought to arise from *in utero* bronchial obstruction during development (4,5). Recurrent pulmonary infection is a common complication of CPAM, which may lead to clinical presentation. Surgical resection is the treatment of choice. There are rare case reports of malignancy arising in CPAM, particularly bronchioalveolar carcinoma (12,13).

Macroscopy: A large-cyst CPAM is defined as having cysts greater than 2 cm in diameter, but often they are larger. It may be unilocular or multilocular and septated, replacing the normal lung parenchyma. Small-cyst CPAM is a localized lesion within a lung lobe comprising multiple irregular cysts (< 2 cm) (Figure 5.2a). Dissection of the proximal airways is required to assess for bronchial obstruction, which is frequently seen (Figure 5.2b).

Histology: Large-cyst CPAM is lined by columnar respiratory epithelium with smooth muscle in the wall. Clusters of mucigenic cells may be present, and rarely cartilage (Figure 5.2b). Small-cyst CPAM is composed of increased bronchiolar-like profiles lined by cuboidal to ciliated respiratory epithelium. Unlike normal bronchioles, they are not accompanied by arteries.

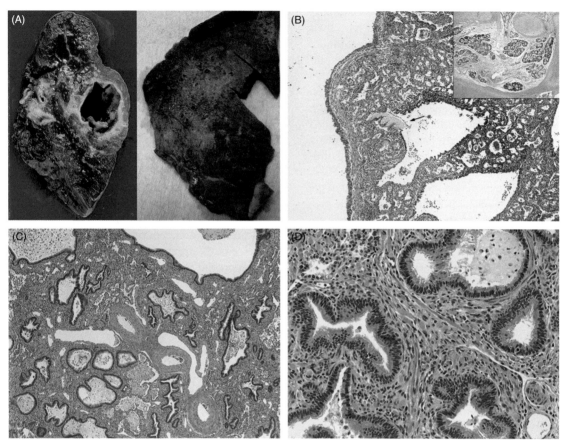

Figure 5.2 (a) Congenital pulmonary airway malformation. Gross appearance of a large cyst type CPAM (left panel) and small cyst type CPAM (right panel). The large-cyst CPAM is often unilocular while the small-cyst CPAM is a mixture of relatively solid regions interspersed with small cysts. (b) Congenital pulmonary airway malformation, large cyst type (Stocker type 1). These large cysts are lined by respiratory epithelium with smooth muscle in the wall; focal mucigenic epithelium resembling gastric foveolar epithelium may be seen (arrow). (H&E × 4). Luminal occlusion (bronchial atresia) was present in a lobar bronchus (inset). (c–d) Extralobar sequestration (ELS) with congenital pulmonary airway malformation, small-cyst type (Stocker type 2). (c) Many ELS show features of small-cyst CPAM with back-to-back bronchiolar structures that are frequently filled with mucin and muciphages, evidence of bronchial obstruction. Thick-walled arteries reflect systemic vascular supply (H&E × 10). (d) Rhabdomyomatous differentiation may be prominent in small-cyst CPAM (H&E ×20).

The adjacent and intervening alveoli are simplified in appearance. Rhabdomyomatous differentiation with small bundles of skeletal muscle may be present around the cysts.

Differential diagnosis: The most consequential entity that may be confused with a CPAM is a type I pleuropulmonary blastoma (PPB). Cystic PPB has nests of primitive spindle cells that condense beneath the lining of the cysts, which is largely alveolar in appearance, vs. respiratory. Atypical nodules of cartilage are frequently present in PPB. A large-cyst CPAM should be distinguished from an intrapulmonary bronchogenic cyst or pneumatocele. A bronchogenic cyst is unilocular and self-contained without connection to adjacent lung. A pneumatocele is composed of thin-walled, air-filled cysts in the lung, which may be a sequela to pneumonia or positive-pressure ventilation. The cysts of a pneumatocele are not lined by respiratory epithelium. An abnormal systemic arterial supply can be seen in large-cyst CPAM, making it challenging to differentiate from an intrapulmonary sequestration (3); the diagnosis of a hybrid lesion is rendered in such cases.

Pulmonary sequestrations

Pulmonary sequestrations are masses of non-functioning lung that do not connect to the normal tracheobronchial tree and have a systemic arterial blood supply, usually from the thoracic or abdominal aorta (14). They are classified as intralobar when they occur within the visceral pleural lining of a lung lobe, and extralobar when they are separate from the lung and have their own pleural lining. They are the second most common lung lesion detected antenatally, after congenital pulmonary airway malformations/CPAM.

Clinical presentation: Although intralobar sequestration (ILS) and extralobar sequestration (ELS) both commonly occur on the left side, and are supplied by anomalous systemic arteries, they are distinctly different in clinical presentation and presumed pathogenesis (15).

Extralobar sequestration more commonly presents in the fetal and neonatal period, and has a male predominance (8). Similar to bronchogenic cysts they are believed to arise from a foregut-derived supernumerary lung bud, but contain distal lung parenchyma. There is frequent association with other anomalies, especially congenital diaphragmatic hernia, cardiac abnormalities, and other duplications. Extralobar sequestration may present as an intrathoracic, subdiaphragmatic, or retroperitoneal mass.

In contrast to ELS, ILS equally affects males and females, and is rarely associated with other congenital malformations. If not detected by routine prenatal ultrasound, they typically present in childhood or adolescence with cough and recurrent pulmonary infections. In some cases the lesion is detected as an incidental finding on a chest radiograph. Radiographically, ILS typically appears as a dense mass within the pulmonary parenchyma; infection can lead to cystic change with fluid levels. Most ILS is located in the lower lobes and are fed by systemic arteries from the thoracic or abdominal aorta. There is generally vascular drainage to the pulmonary venous system of the affected lobe, but systemic venous drainage may occur. The abnormal vascular supply is defined by angiography prior to surgical resection, which is curative. There is debate whether ILS is a congenital or an acquired lesion, the latter supported by the late age of presentation and history of recurrent infection. Some authors have proposed that ILS represents systemic arterial supply to an otherwise developmentally normal lung that became infected, or lung involved by bronchial atresia and/or CPAM, which are frequently present (16).

Macroscopy: Extralobar sequestration resembles an accessory lobe of lung with its own pleura. It contains a vascular pedicle with a systemic artery and draining vein. In contrast, ILS is contained within a lung lobe. On cut section, ILS is usually well demarcated from the adjacent normal lung. It is often altered by prolonged infection and inflammation. Thick-walled feeding systemic arteries may be apparent, distinct from the normal bronchovascular structures. The lesion may resemble a CPAM with cystic spaces, including dilated airways filled with mucus. In both ELS and ILS, an atretic bronchus may be found in the proximal portion of the lesion. The bronchus is often dilated and filled with mucus, similar to that seen in bronchial atresia.

Histology: ELS have absent or reduced numbers of cartilaginous bronchi and variably mature alveolar spaces. The vessels are large and thick-walled, reflecting systemic vascular supply. Depending on the presence of proximal airway obstruction, there may be mucus accumulation. Features of small-cyst CPAM (Stocker, type 2), with back-to-back bronchiolar structures, are present in approximately 50% of cases (17). As in typical small-cyst CPAM, there may be striated muscle fibers present. Although similar histologically to ELS, ILS has more consistent findings of proximal airway obstruction, including dilated bronchi filled with mucus and alveolar filling by foamy macrophages. Depending upon the age of presentation and presence of concurrent infection, inflammation and dense fibrosis may be present.

Differential diagnosis: Due to the histologic overlap, ILS can be difficult to distinguish from a CPAM or isolated bronchial atresia without knowledge of a systemic arterial supply. When infected, it may be confused with a chronic pneumonia, although the latter has a normal bronchial connection to the involved lung.

Pulmonary hyperplasia and congenital lobar overinflation

Pulmonary hyperplasia or excessive growth of the parenchyma is the result of airway obstruction during development, which blocks the outflow of fetal fluid leading to increased alveolar growth. Pulmonary hyperplasia has also been referred to as type 3 cystic adenomatoid malformation in the Stocker classification (8). The pathogenesis and clinical characteristics of congenital lobar overinflation/emphysema are similar, in that intrinsic or extrinsic compression of an airway results in overexpansion of a lobe, albeit due to alveolar distension by air, and not increased alveolar growth. In congenital lobar overinflation (CLO) the compressed airway acts as a one-way valve, resulting in air trapping postnatally.

Clinical presentation: Like many of the congenital cystic lesions, pulmonary hyperplasia is most frequently seen in the setting of airway obstruction. Upper airway obstruction, such as tracheal or laryngeal atresia affects all lung lobes, while bronchial atresia and stenosis results in focal hyperplasia. Extrinsic airway compression from a bronchogenic cyst or anomalous vessel could result in a hyperplastic or overinflated lung lobe. Weak or absent bronchial cartilage resulting in airway collapse is a common intrinsic etiology of CLO. Pulmonary hyperplasia may manifest *in utero* with polyhydramnios or fetal hydrops, from compression of the venous return to the heart. In both pulmonary hyperplasia and CLO, newborns usually present with dyspnea in early life. Chest radiographs demonstrate progressive hyperinflation or hyperlucency of a lobe. Marked overinflation may lead to compression of the adjacent lung and mediastinal shift.

Macroscopy: In both pulmonary hyperplasia and CLO the involved lung lobes are enlarged, bulky, and often pale.

Histology: Pulmonary hyperplasia, diffuse or focal, is characterized by a striking increase in alveoli in relation to airways, which can be confirmed by the radial alveolar count. Alveoli are often abnormally enlarged and simplified, and there may be a decrease or absence of interlobular septa. Cystic maldevelopment (CPAM, small-cyst type) may be seen. In CLO there is airspace enlargement without alveolar wall disruption or maldevelopment.

Differential diagnosis: Pulmonary hyperplasia is differentiated from CLO in that the volume increase is due to absolute increase in alveoli vs. alveolar enlargement. Radial alveolar counts can be helpful in this circumstance. In a full-term infant the radial alveolar count should average five alveolar spaces, which increases to approximately 8–10 by one year of life (18,19). While CLO may be referred to as congenital lobar emphysema, the term "emphysema" is inaccurate, as alveolar wall destruction does not accompany alveolar expansion.

Primary disorders of lung development (diffuse developmental)

Acinar dysplasia

Acinar dysplasia is a rare disorder representing the most extreme form of lung developmental arrest, with formation of little or no acinar structures and no alveoli. It is conjectured that a signaling defect between the bronchial bud and adjacent lung mesenchyme results in failure of acinar structures to form, resembling the pseudoglandular stage of lung development. It has also been referred to as acinar aplasia or cystic adenomatoid malformation type 0 (8).

Clinical presentation: Infants are generally term and have immediate onset of severe respiratory compromise refractory to resuscitative measures. Survival is rare beyond a few hours and only with maximum support. The majority of affected infants are female. Rarely, malformations have been identified in other organs (20). As the disorder is incompatible with life the diagnosis may be made only at autopsy.

Hereditary/genetic features: Although extremely rare, a few familial cases have been reported (21,22). Investigational studies in an individual case has demonstrated a reduction in transforming growth factor-β signaling (23), but no genetic etiology for the disorder has been defined.

Macroscopy: The lungs are small, often with thickened interlobular septa.

Histology: Lungs show striking growth arrest with predominantly only bronchi and bronchioles present. Acinar structures are essentially absent, with no significant formation of saccules and no alveoli (Figure 5.3a). The interlobular septa are frequently thickened. Cartilage and airway smooth muscle may be prominent. Although there are no type II cells, the airway epithelium shows normal differentiation with ciliated cells and expression of Clara-cell secretory protein (23).

Differential diagnosis: Acinar dysplasia should be distinguished from severe pulmonary hypoplasia. Clinical history and the absence of other anomalies limiting lung growth should distinguish between the two.

Congenital alveolar dysplasia

Congenital alveolar dysplasia is a developmental disorder in which maturational arrest occurs in the late canalicular or early saccular stage of lung development. There have been very few reported cases in the literature with variable terminology including "alveolar capillary dysplasia without misalignment of pulmonary veins" (24).

Clinical presentation: Infants are born at term and present early in life with respiratory distress, which may be complicated by pulmonary hypertension and

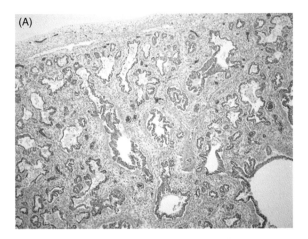

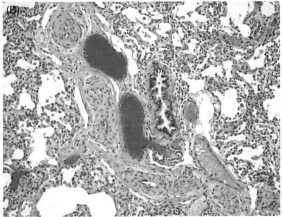

Figure 5.3 (a) Acinar dysplasia. This primary disorder of lung development shows only proximal airway development composed of bronchial and bronchiolar structures (H&E × 4). (b) Alveolar capillary dysplasia with misalignment of pulmonary veins. Pulmonary veins, which are normally in the interlobular septa, are malpositioned adjacent to pulmonary arteries and bronchioles. Small arteries show marked hypertensive changes and veins are dilated and congested (H&E × 10).

cardiac failure. They may survive weeks with intensive support, including mechanical ventilation and ECMO (extracorporeal membrane oxygenation), but succumb after being weaned off. Diagnosis is frequently made at autopsy.

Macroscopy: Lung weight is normal, but may be increased due to congestion.

Histology: The lung structure is immature with no well-formed alveoli present. Acini are simplified and frequently have abundant intervening loose mesenchyme, which should be distinguished from fibrosis. Depending on the stage of growth arrest there may be saccular spaces with early alveolar septation. There may be a reduction of capillaries within alveolar walls.

Differential diagnosis: Although they may share similar lobular maldevelopment, congenital alveolar dysplasia can be differentiated from alveolar capillary dysplasia with misalignment of the pulmonary veins, as the veins are appropriately positioned in the interlobular septa. Congenital alveolar dysplasia may be difficult to separate from reparative lung injury in infants who have been on ventilatory support. Lung immaturity should be uniform without diffuse superimposed acute injury, such as reactive type II cells and fibrosis. The diagnosis of congenital alveolar dysplasia cannot be made with certainty in premature infants due to similar lung immaturity.

Alveolar capillary dysplasia with misalignment of pulmonary veins

Alveolar capillary dysplasia with misalignment of pulmonary veins (ACDMPV), variably termed alveolar capillary dysplasia (ACD) and congenital alveolar capillary dysplasia, is a rare uniformly lethal developmental disorder of the lung. It is named based on distinctive abnormalities of the pulmonary vasculature, as well as the alveolar structures. Although the disorder may be suspected clinically, currently the diagnosis can only be established by lung biopsy or autopsy, although genetic testing may play a greater role in the future.

Clinical presentation: Affected infants are term or near-term and typically develop respiratory distress and severe pulmonary hypertension within a few hours or days after birth. They demonstrate no sustained response to extensive therapeutic interventions, including inhaled nitric oxide and ECMO, and usually die within the first few weeks of life. A few cases of delayed presentation to weeks or months with longer survival have rarely been described (25–28). Lung transplantation has rarely been attempted. The majority (around 80%) of infants with ACDMPV have additional congenital malformations, with cardiac (commonly hypoplastic left heart), gastrointestinal (intestinal malrotation and atresias), and renal abnormalities the most frequent (29–31).

Hereditary/genetic features: Inactivating point mutations in *FOXF1* or overlapping microdeletions encompassing the *FOX* transcription factor gene cluster on chromosome 16q24.1 have been found in a subset of patients with ACDMPV and concurrent anomalies (32,33). Based on the phenotype of patients with microdeletions vs. point mutations, it is theorized that ACDMPV results from haploinsufficiency of *FOXF1*, while the frequent associated cardiac and gastrointestinal anomalies are due to haploinsufficiency for the neighboring *FOXC2* and *FOXL1* genes (32). *FOXF1* is a transcription factor expressed in embryonic foregut mesenchyme and is essential for cell migration during murine vasculogenesis and lung development (34,35). Of the known cases of ACDMPV, approximately 10% have a familial association, usually with an affected sibling (30,36–38). A recent case examining a family with five of six children affected with ACDMPV suggests *FOXF1* is paternally imprinted (39).

Macroscopy: The lungs at autopsy are often deeply congested, with normal to increased lung weight.

Histology: Alveolar capillary dysplasia with misalignment of pulmonary veins is defined by a characteristic constellation of histologic features, of which anomalously situated pulmonary veins accompanying bronchioles and small pulmonary arteries in the same adventitial sheath is essential (Figure 5.3b). Normally, pulmonary veins are in the interlobular septa, arising from small veins, which drain pulmonary lobules. In conjunction with the abnormally positioned veins, there is frequently a decrease in veins within the interlobular septa, although larger veins, including those adjacent to proximal airways, are usually present. Small pulmonary arteries show marked medial hypertrophy and there is muscularization of intra-acinar vessels. There is often abnormal lobular architecture with reduced and enlarged alveoli. The capillary density within the alveolar walls is decreased compared to normal lung, with dilatation and poor approximation of capillaries to the alveolar space. Lymphangiectasia is present in a subset of cases.

D2-40 immunostaining may be helpful in distinguishing the abnormally positioned veins from lymphatic spaces within bronchovascular bundles. An endothelial marker such as CD31 highlights the reduced capillaries within alveolar walls.

Differential diagnosis: Histologically, ACDMPV should be distinguished from other disorders that demonstrate a similar arrest in lung development, including congenital alveolar dysplasia and advanced pulmonary hypoplasia. While these disorders also demonstrate lobular simplification and frequently vascular changes, they do not have malpositioned veins. The characteristic constellation of findings may be subtle, particularly when the lung sample is limited, with few bronchovascular bundles for evaluation and there is regional variation in venous congestion. In autopsy material there is often superimposed reactive changes related to the terminal course, which may obscure findings. Patchy distribution of malpositioned veins has rarely been reported (40) and multiple lung sections may be required for confirmation.

Lung growth abnormalities and related processes

Lung growth abnormalities

Lung growth abnormalities reflect impaired alveolarization of prenatal or postnatal onset. Unlike primary disorders of lung development (diffuse developmental disorders), lung growth abnormalities are largely secondary to another process and may be seen in a variety of settings. These pulmonary disorders are the leading cause of morbidity and mortality in the preterm neonate, whose lungs are often morphologically and functionally immature.

Clinical presentation: Deficient lung growth is a common finding in infants who undergo lung biopsy to determine the etiology of respiratory dysfunction felt to be out of proportion to their known clinical condition and co-morbidities (1,41). While impaired lung growth is traditionally considered to occur in the context of prenatal onset pulmonary hypoplasia and prematurity, it also occurs in infants with congenital heart disease as well as those with chromosomal disorders (Table 5.1).

The majority of cases with pulmonary hypoplasia are secondary to congenital anomalies or pregnancy complications that inhibit lung development. As distension of the lung with amniotic fluid and fetal respiratory movements is required for prenatal lung growth, any mechanism that interferes with these processes can result in pulmonary hypoplasia (Figure 5.4a). The severity of the lung growth abnormality depends on the mechanism of hypoplasia and the timing of the insult. Conditions that occur early in pregnancy (diaphragmatic hernia, renal anomalies) may interfere with airway branching as well as alveolar development, while later events (premature rupture of membranes, central nervous system lesions), will only impact alveolar formation.

As lung maturation continues well into the postnatal period, with most alveolarization occurring within the first year of life (18), postnatal events can impact lung growth as well. Postnatal growth abnormalities predominate in infants with chronic lung disease of prematurity (also known as

Table 5.1 Lung growth abnormalities

Pulmonary hypoplasia (restriction of prenatal lung growth)

- Oligohydramnios
  - Prolonged rupture of membranes
  - Renal dysfunction (bladder outlet obstruction, cystic kidneys)
- Restriction of thoracic volume
  - Diaphragmatic hernia
  - Pleural effusions (including hydrops fetalis)
  - Thoracic deformity due to skeletal dysplasia
  - Space-occupying lesions (CPAMs, sequestrations, lymphatic malformation)
- Central nervous system lesions, neuromuscular disorders, and other agents resulting in decreased fetal breathing

Chronic lung disease related to prematurity (clinical bronchopulmonary dysplasia)

Congenital heart disease

- Disorders with reduced pulmonary blood flow
  - Tetralogy of Fallot
  - Pulmonary artery stenosis/atresia
  - Hypoplastic right heart
- Cyanotic heart disease impairing postnatal alveolarization

Chromosomal abnormalities

- Trisomy 21 with poor postnatal alveolarization (often manifests with subpleural cysts)
- Other chromosomal defects

chronic neonatal lung disease and clinically bronchopulmonary dysplasia/BPD). Chronic neonatal lung disease (CNLD), which encompasses BPD, is a disorder of lung injury and repair. It usually follows some form of acute injury or disorder that requires treatment with high concentrations of oxygen and mechanical ventilation. This acute lung injury may be hyaline membrane disease (see below) or lung injury as a result of pneumonia, sepsis, or meconium aspiration. Multiple factors likely lead to deficient alveolarization in infants with congenital heart disease and chromosomal disorders, including hypoxia and abnormal pulmonary blood flow (42,43).

The incidence of CNLD is increasing as the survival of extremely premature infants improves, but its clinical presentation is milder with current therapeutic practices. Radiographic findings are variable, based on etiology, age of the infant, and severity of the growth abnormality. Subpleural cysts may be present, and are frequently seen in deficient lung growth associated with Down syndrome (43).

Macroscopy: Grossly, the ratio of lung weight to body weight (LW/BW) is the most reliable parameter of lung growth (44). In a large autopsy series, the tenth percentile of LW/BW in normal preterm lungs (< 37 weeks) varied between 2.48% and 2.59%, and in term infants 1.2%; values less than these would suggest pulmonary hypoplasia (44,45). Similar to the radiographic appearance, severe lung growth abnormalities may manifest with cysts in the lung, most prominent in the subpleural space.

Histology: Lung growth abnormalities demonstrate lobular simplification with enlarged alveolar spaces, which lack complexity. Classic CNLD/BPD is typified by variable inflation of the lung, with a combination of dilated alveoli and interstitial fibrosis. Bronchiolar stenosis and bronchiolectasis, representative of small airway injury, accompany these changes, and account for alternating areas of hyperexpansion and atelectasis (46). Following the widespread use of surfactant replacement and improved ventilatory and other therapies, the histology of "new BPD"/chronic neonatal lung disease is characterized by more uniform inflation without significant fibrosis or airway injury (47). However, alveoli remain simplified and enlarged, often accentuated in the subpleural space, reflecting disruption of postnatal alveolarization (Figure 5.4b). In prenatal-onset pulmonary hypoplasia, there is a diffuse reduction and simplification of alveolar spaces, which is often accompanied by prominence of the bronchovascular structures and a widened interstitium. Hypertensive changes of the pulmonary arteries are commonly seen and are especially prominent in infants with severe lung growth abnormality or Down syndrome, the latter with or without associated cardiac abnormalities (48; Figure 5.4c). As discussed below, pulmonary interstitial glycogenosis (PIG) is a frequent histologic finding in lungs demonstrating impaired growth.

Differential diagnosis: Due to the presence of alveolar enlargement and simplification, a lung growth abnormality is often misinterpreted as emphysematous change or a consequence of lung remodeling after injury. However, unlike in these processes, in lung growth abnormality there is no evidence of a destructive process, including inflammation, type II cell hyperplasia, or significant fibrosis. When severe, a deficient lung growth is easily recognized, but more subtle cases may be difficult to distinguish without comparison to an age-matched control. Radial alveolar count, which is the number of alveoli transected by a perpendicular line drawn from the center of a respiratory bronchiole to the nearest septal division

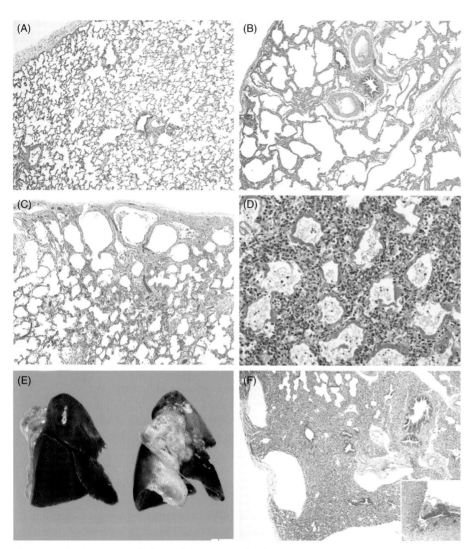

Figure 5.4 (a–c) Lung-growth abnormalities. Compared with an age-matched lung at the same magnification (a), the lung biopsy from an 8-month-old former term infant in which the pregnancy was complicated by oligohydramnios (H&E × 4) (b) demonstrates impaired alveolarization, with reduced and markedly enlarged airspaces. Hypertensive changes of the pulmonary arteries are seen, which frequently accompany severe lung-growth disorders. In postnatal onset lung-growth disorders (H&E × 4) (c), deficient alveolarization is often most prominent in the subpleural space with cystic dilatation of alveoli (H&E ×10). (d) Hyaline membrane disease. Hyaline membrane disease of 48 hours' duration in an infant born at 30 weeks. Eosinophilic membranes line alveolar ducts and there is septal widening from congested capillaries, inflammatory cells, and early collagen deposition. (H&E × 20). (e–f) Pulmonary interstitial emphysema. (e) Marked pulmonary interstitial emphysema with bubbly cysts superimposed on hyaline membrane disease in a premature infant with respiratory distress syndrome. (f) Angulated cystic spaces from dissected air are in the subpleural space and around bronchovascular bundles, often accompanied by histiocytes and multinucleated giant cells (inset) (H&E × 10).

or pleural margin, may be helpful in determining decreased lung growth. The radial alveolar count in a full-term infant should average five alveolar spaces, and increases to approximately 8–10 by one year of life (18,19). Unfortunately, radial alveolar count is a method that requires standardized inflation of the lung as the radial alveolar count is substantially reduced in uninflated lungs.

Hyaline membrane disease

Hyaline membrane disease (HMD), the pathologic correlate of respiratory distress of the newborn (RDS), is a form of acute lung injury caused by an inadequate amount of pulmonary surfactant (49). Surfactant is necessary to maintain adequate surface tension in the alveolus during expiration. Insufficient surfactant leads to atelectasis and decreased gas exchange, resulting in severe hypoxia and acidosis.

Clinical presentation: Cases of classic HMD and subsequent development of chronic neonatal lung disease of prematurity/BPD have become infrequent due to improvement in therapies, including antenatal administration of corticosteroids to mothers delivering prematurely, surfactant replacement, and advances in mechanical ventilation and oxygen treatment (47). HMD usually occurs in very premature neonates, whose lungs are deficient in endogenous surfactant due to relative immaturity of type II pneumocytes. However, HMD may arise in any condition resulting in type II cell injury, including fetal/perinatal asphyxia, meconium aspiration, and sepsis (50). In addition to prematurity, risk factors for HMD include male sex, white race, cesarean delivery without preceding labor, multiple gestation, and maternal diabetes (51). HMD is a common cause of respiratory distress in the first day of life, and despite supportive measures, remains a significant cause of infant morbidity and mortality (52). Infants present within the first few hours of birth, with tachypnea, retractions, expiratory grunting, and progressive cyanosis. The typical radiographic appearance in infants with RDS is decreased expansion, with diffuse reticulogranular opacification of the lungs and air bronchograms.

Macroscopy: The lungs are dark red, firm, and diffusely congested, resembling liver. On cut surface they are markedly atelectatic.

Histology: Hyaline membranes may appear as early as 3–4 hours after the development of symptoms and are well formed by 12–24 hours. The pathology of HMD, including the reparative process, is analogous to that of diffuse alveolar damage in older patients. Hyaline membranes consist of cellular debris, fibrin, and plasma transudate, forming homogeneous eosinophilic material adherent to the alveolar surface (Figure 5.4d). They may be bright yellow if the infant has unconjugated hyperbilirubinemia. The lung also shows alveolar collapse, congestion, hemorrhage, desquamation of epithelial cells, and lymphatic dilatation. As most infants are premature, there is lung immaturity, which correlates with gestational age. If the process does not resolve, progression to more classic CNLD/BPD with airway and interstitial fibrosis, may be seen as early as 36 hours after birth.

Differential diagnosis: Hyaline membranes are essentially a by-product, not the cause, of neonatal respiratory failure, and careful attention should be given to elucidating the mechanism of type II cell injury. In a term or post-term infant with RDS, meconium aspiration, acute infection, and pulmonary hemorrhage may be the etiology of HMD. The early stages of chronic neonatal lung disease and those related to therapeutic intervention cannot be easily separated from HMD. It is important to distinguish HMD from an inherited disorder of surfactant metabolism (e.g., SP-B or ABCA3 deficiency), which may have a similar clinical presentation. Hereditary disorders of surfactant production typically show alveolar filling from proteinaceous material, diffuse type II cell hyperplasia, and variable accumulation of macrophages.

Pulmonary interstitial emphysema

Pulmonary interstitial emphysema (PIE) is an acquired condition that may complicate any pulmonary disorder in which there is airway overdistension, often due to mechanical ventilation. Air gains access to the lung via rupture of small bronchioles or alveoli, dissecting along connective tissue sheaths of the bronchovascular bundles, interlobular septa and pleura.

Clinical presentation: Pulmonary interstitial emphysema occurs most frequently in conjunction with respiratory distress of the newborn, in which there is reduced lung compliance and positive pressure ventilation is being employed (53). By compressing adjacent functional lung tissue and vascular structures, PIE can further compromise an already critically ill neonate by impeding oxygenation, ventilation, and blood flow. Subpleural blebs may rupture into the pleural space, resulting in a pneumothorax. Migration of interstitial air may produce pneumomediastinum or pneumopericardium. The radiographic appearance of PIE is tubular and cystic lucencies that may coalesce in the subpleural space to form pseudocysts.

Macroscopy: The extent of PIE can vary, with single or numerous cysts, involving both lungs diffusely or localized to one or multiple lobes. The air-filled cysts are frequently subpleural (Figure 5.4e).

Histology: Round or elongated empty spaces of variable size are present beneath the pleura and along bronchovascular bundles and interlobular septa (Figure 5.4f). In persistent disease, the prolonged presence of air elicits a foreign-body response with multinucleated giant cells lining the cystic spaces; eosinophils are also frequently seen.

Differential diagnosis: The air-filled spaces in PIE may resemble a lung growth disorder or even a cystic lung malformation. However, the spaces in PIE are limited to the interstitial tissues without alveolar involvement, although associated atelectasis is often present. Primary or secondary pulmonary lymphangiectasia may also resemble PIE; immunostains to label the endothelium or lymphatics (e.g., CD31, D2-40) can be helpful in these circumstances.

Pulmonary interstitial glycogenosis

Pulmonary interstitial glycogenosis (PIG), previously referred to as cellular interstitial pneumonitis (54), is an idiopathic neonatal lung disorder characterized by expansion of the interstitium by glycogen-laden mesenchymal cells.

Clinical presentation: Pulmonary interstitial glycogenosis is a disorder that is unique to neonates and young infants, with the preponderance of cases observed in children less than six months of age. Most infants are symptomatic in the first few days to weeks of life, often after an initial period of well being (1,55). The clinical presentation can be variable, ranging from indolent tachypnea and hypoxemia to refractory pulmonary hypertension and acute respiratory failure requiring nitric oxide and mechanical ventilation. No common imaging appearance has been identified, but case series have reported diffuse infiltrates or hazy opacities on chest radiographs (56–58). Pulmonary interstitial glycogenosis can occur in either term or preterm infants, and may be an isolated disorder or a component of another congenital or neonatal condition. PIG commonly occurs in the setting of deficient lung growth (see above), such as chronic neonatal lung of prematurity and pulmonary hypoplasia (1), but has also been observed in infants with congenital heart disease, pulmonary hypertension, meconium aspiration, and lung malformations, including congenital lobar emphysema and CPAM. There is clinical and pathologic evidence to support that PIG is often a self-limited disorder, which may respond to high-dose pulse corticosteroids, as well as spontaneously resolving over time (55,57,59). Ultimately, however, the prognosis is related to the presence of co-morbidities, particularly a lung growth abnormality or congenital heart disease (1). Patients may remain symptomatic for months and require supplemental oxygen.

Hereditary/genetic features: Although there are rare reports of PIG occurring in siblings (56), there is no evidence to support a genetic etiology. That PIG is often associated with conditions related to lung

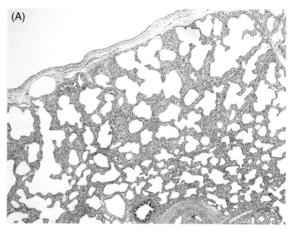

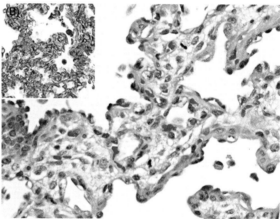

Figure 5.5 Pulmonary interstitial glycogenosis. (a) Interstitial widening and cellularity in this condition can be diffuse or patchy, and is typically associated with a concurrent lung-growth abnormality (H&E ×4). (b) The cells are spindled with vacuolated cytoplasm and indistinct cell borders. Mitotic activity is frequently seen (H&E ×40). These mesenchymal cells exhibit strong vimentin immunoreactivity (inset).

development and injury has led some authors to suggest that the accumulation of mesenchymal cells is a non-specific reactive feature of the neonatal lung (60).

Histology: The term PIG was coined by Canakis *et al.* based on the histologic finding of increased glycogen-laden mesenchymal cells in the alveolar interstitium (55). There is patchy or diffuse expansion of the alveolar walls by bland oval cells with vacuolated cytoplasm and indistinct cell borders (Figure 5.5a–b). A patchy distribution is frequent when PIG occurs in the setting of a lung growth abnormality (1). Associated inflammation or fibrosis in the interstitium is absent. Periodic acid–Schiff (PAS) stain may demonstrate PAS-positive diastase labile material within the cytoplasm of the cells. As the preservation of glycogen is influenced by the use of aqueous fixatives (i.e., 10% formalin) the presence of PAS positivity may be difficult to demonstrate on routine sections. Electron microscopy is considered the best approach to reveal the accumulation of monoparticulate glycogen in these mesenchymal cells. Treating ultrathin sections with tannic acid enhances visualization of glycogen (55). As PIG commonly occurs in the setting of another pulmonary process, particularly deficient lung growth, it is critical to fully assess the lung architecture for other abnormalities. The cells are strongly immunopositive for vimentin, and focally for smooth-muscle actin. In normal conditions, vimentin-positive cells are present around airways and vessels, but not in the alveolar septa. They are negative for other muscle and inflammatory markers, including desmin, leukocyte common antigen, CD68, and lysozyme.

Differential diagnosis: As PIG generally has a favorable prognosis, it is essential to distinguish it from other neonatal pulmonary disorders that have a similar clinical presentation, but high morbidity and mortality, including ACDMPV and a surfactant dysfunction disorder. Pulmonary interstitial glycogenosis/chronic interstitial pneumonitis has sometimes been confused with chronic pneumonitis of infancy, the latter frequently associated with mutations in surfactant protein C (*SFTPC*). Dissimilar to PIG, surfactant dysfunction disorders have uniform type II cell hyperplasia and some degree of PAS-positive proteinaceous material within alveoli, as well as within macrophages. Likewise, pulmonary involvement in metabolic disorders (e.g., glycogen storage disease, Gaucher disease, Niemann–Pick disease) does rarely manifest with stored material within the airspaces and interstitium, but in contrast to PIG the accumulating cells are histiocytes and should stain for macrophage markers.

Neuroendocrine cell hyperplasia of infancy

Neuroendocrine cell hyperplasia of infancy (NEHI) is a disorder of unclear etiology that occurs in infants and young children. Characteristic clinical presentation and imaging appearance by high-resolution CT (HRCT) often obviates the need for lung biopsy. Pathologic diagnosis of NEHI rests on finding an increased proportion of neuroendocrine cells within the airways, in the absence of other significant abnormalities in the lung.

Clinical presentation: NEHI occurs in otherwise healthy term or near-term infants who present with tachypnea and retractions, generally of insidious onset, in the first few months to year of life (61). Crackles and hypoxemia are common and many patients develop failure to thrive. Symptom exacerbation frequently occurs with upper respiratory infections. HRCT findings are characteristic with segmental ground-glass opacities centrally and in the right middle lobe and lingual (62). Infant pulmonary function testing in NEHI patients demonstrates profound physiologic small airway obstruction with air-trapping (63,64). The majority of patients gradually improve over time, although they may remain symptomatic with exercise intolerance and require supplemental oxygen long term. There have been no deaths reported and no patients have required lung transplantation (1,61,64).

Hereditary/genetic features: While the etiology of NEHI is unknown, familial cases with affected siblings have been identified, suggesting there may be a genetic predisposition (65). The stimulus for increased neuroendocrine cells is unclear and whether pulmonary neuroendocrine cells are simply a marker of NEHI or are directly involved in the pathogenesis of the disorder has yet to be defined. Investigators have demonstrated a correlation between neuroendocrine cell number and the severity of small airway obstruction by infant pulmonary function testing, suggesting a potential causal role (64). As pulmonary neuroendocrine cells are important in oxygen sensing and release bioactive products that affect airway and arterial tone, it has been hypothesized that increased neuroendocrine cells can cause ventilation/perfusion mismatch within the lung (61).

Histology: Lung biopsies in NEHI are characteristic in their lack of significant inflammation or architectural abnormalities, and may be interpreted as normal (Figure 5.6a). Mild airway smooth-muscle hyperplasia and increased alveolar macrophages are frequently present and prominent neuroepithelial bodies (NEBs) may be seen around alveolar ducts. Patchy mild peri-airway lymphocytic inflammation and fibrosis are commonly seen, especially following an illness or with a history of aspiration, but are not diffuse or severe enough to support an etiology for the patient's clinical hypoxemia (64). Interstitial inflammation, fibrosis, or an alveolar filling processing (pneumonia, proteinosis) should be absent. Diagnosis of NEHI rests on finding an increased proportion of neuroendocrine cells

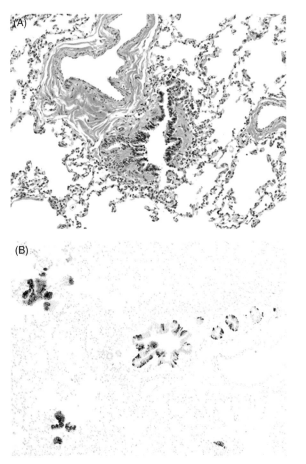

Figure 5.6 Neuroendocrine cell hyperplasia of infancy (NEHI). (a) Lung biopsy from an 8-month-old former term infant with chronic tachypnea, retractions, hypoxemia, and failure to thrive shows mild findings, including hyperplasia of airway smooth muscle and accumulation of alveolar macrophages (H&E × 10). (b) Bombesin immunostaining highlights the increased neuroendocrine cells within bronchioles and prominent neuroepithelial bodies around alveolar ducts (× 40).

within bronchioles, best seen by bombesin and serotonin immunohistochemistry (61). Neuron-specific enolase, calcitonin, synaptophysin, and chromogranin have been shown to be less reliable in demonstrating this increase in neuroendocrine cell number. Immunohistochemical assessment of NEHI requires an adequate biopsy with at least 8–10 airways for evaluation. More than one biopsy site is recommended, as wide intra- and intersubject variability in neuroendocrine cell number has been reported, which does not relate to the imaging appearance of the regions biopsied (64).

Currently, formal criteria for defining neuroendocrine cell excess in NEHI are lacking, and outside the

setting of a pathologist experienced with the disorder, morphometric quantification of bombesin staining may be required (64). Bombesin-immunopositive cells are seen in greater than 75% of the non-cartilaginous airways, most evident in the distal respiratory bronchioles. One or more individual airways with greater than 10% bombesin-immunopositive area or cell number of the airway epithelium are frequently present, as well as clusters of neuroendocrine cells (neuroepithelial bodies) around alveolar ducts (Figure 5.6b).

Differential diagnosis: An increased number of neuroendocrine cells have been associated with a variety of other pulmonary conditions, including BPD, sudden infant death syndrome, pulmonary hypertension, and cystic fibrosis (66–71). The lung biopsy in NEHI should be free of diagnostic abnormalities characteristic of a known pulmonary process such as architectural disruption (as seen in lung growth abnormalities), diffuse/advanced airway injury (bronchiectasis, obliterative bronchiolitis), and significant hypertensive changes of the pulmonary vasculature. Correlation of the histology with the clinical presentation and radiographic findings is essential.

Surfactant dysfunction disorders

Surfactant dysfunction disorders comprise genetic abnormalities that disrupt normal surfactant metabolism, including genes for surfactant protein B (*SFTPB*), surfactant protein C (*SFTPC*), ATP-binding cassette transporter A3 (*ABCA3*), and thyroid transcription factor gene *NKX2.1* (TTF-1) (72–75). Surfactant is necessary to reduce surface tension at the air–liquid interface and prevent collapse of the lung at the end of expiration. These disorders cause significant mortality and morbidity, including lethal respiratory failure in term neonates, and interstitial lung disease in older infants, children, and adults (76,77). As there is considerable overlap in the clinical features and lung pathology findings associated with these disorders, genetic testing is essential for establishing a specific diagnosis in patients with suspected surfactant disorders (Table 5.2).

Clinical presentation: Surfactant dysfunction disorders are becoming a frequent cause of unexplained respiratory compromise in the otherwise normal full-term newborn. Infants with surfactant protein B (SP-B) deficiency generally develop respiratory distress shortly after birth that is rapidly fatal without transplant. Partial SP-B deficiency can be associated with milder symptoms which worsen over time

Table 5.2 Surfactant dysfunction disorders

	SFTPB	ABCA3	SFTPC	NKX2.1
Mechanism	Surfactant dysfunction	Surfactant dysfunction	Aggregation of misfolded proSP-C	Surfactant dysfunction; growth arrest
Inheritance	Recessive	Recessive	Dominant or sporadic	Dominant or sporadic
Age of onset	Newborn	Newborn to adolescent	Newborn to adult	Newborn to child
Clinical findings	RDS	RDS; ILD	RDS; ILD	RDS; ILD hypothyroid, hypotonia, chorea
Outcome	Fatal	Variable	Variable	Variable
Pathology	PAP, DIP	PAP, DIP, NSIP, UIP	CPI, PAP, DIP, NSIP, UIP	Growth, PAP, DIP, NSIP, minimal
Ultrastructure of lamellar bodies	No normal forms; multivesicular bodies	Normal to small with dense inclusions	Normal with variable abnormal forms	Normal with variable abnormal forms

Table adapted from 90. RDS, respiratory distress syndrome; ILD, interstitial lung disease, PAP, pulmonary alveolar proteinosis; DIP, desquamative interstitial pneumonitis; CPI, chronic pneumonitis of infancy; NSIP, nonspecific interstitial pneumonitis; UIP, usual interstitial pneumonitis

(78,79). Infants with deficiency of ABCA3 may have a similar phenotype to SP-B deficiency with fatal disease in infancy, but may also present with interstitial lung disease in older children with varying degrees of clinical manifestation. Cough, tachypnea, hypoxemia, and failure to thrive are frequently reported. Patients with surfactant protein C (SP-C) mutations have even more variable age of onset of symptoms, from months after birth to adult life. Patients generally have milder disease with a prolonged survival. *SFTPC* mutations are a recognized cause of idiopathic and familial pulmonary fibrosis in older children and adults. Haploinsufficiency of *NKX2.1* results in "Brain–Thyroid–Lung" syndrome, with affected individuals having a variable degree of pulmonary disease, thyroid dysfunction, and neurological abnormalities (e.g., hypotonia, chorea, seizures). Affected patients may present with RDS in infancy, but other patients develop a more chronic lung disease, including recurrent infections (75). Evidence of chronic diffuse lung disease (digital clubbing, failure to thrive, ground glass infiltrates on HRCT, and peripheral lung cysts) should increase suspicion for any of these surfactant mutations.

Hereditary/genetic features: Hereditary SP-B and ABCA3 deficiency are autosomal recessive disorders, while cases of SP-C and *NKX2.1* dysfunction are autosomal dominant or sporadic. Most disease-causing mutations in *SFTPB* result in a complete lack of mature SP-B protein necessary for normal surfactant function, resulting in lethal neonatal disease.

Mutations in *ABCA3* appear to be the most common of genetic surfactant dysfunction disorders, with loss or reduced function of the ABCA3 protein (80,81). ABCA3 is a transmembrane protein found on the limiting plate of lamellar bodies in which surfactant is stored prior to secretion. The variability of disease caused by ABCA3 mutations is thought to depend upon the degree of ABCA3 dysfunction, with no functional surfactant in the neonatal form. Disease-causing *SFTPC* mutations result in production of abnormal proSP-C, which is thought to fold incorrectly. It is not currently known how these mutations produce disease. *NKX2.1* plays an important role in SP-B, SP-C, and ABCA3 expression, and reduced amounts of one or more of these proteins due to haploinsufficiency of *NKX2.1* is the presumed etiology for lung disease. The variable clinical outcome of these disorders, even in families with the same mutations, suggests the contribution of other genetic, epigenetic, or environmental factors (82,83). Genetic testing for diagnosis is not 100% sensitive as the current approach in clinical laboratories is to look at mutations in exons, while functionally significant variants in untranslated regions will be missed.

Histology: Different histologic patterns in infants and young children with these genetic abnormalities have been reported, including pulmonary alveolar proteinosis (PAP), chronic pneumonitis of infancy (CPI), desquamative interstitial pneumonia (DIP), and non-specific interstitial pneumonia (NSIP) (84). Proteinosis (PAP) with accumulation of granular

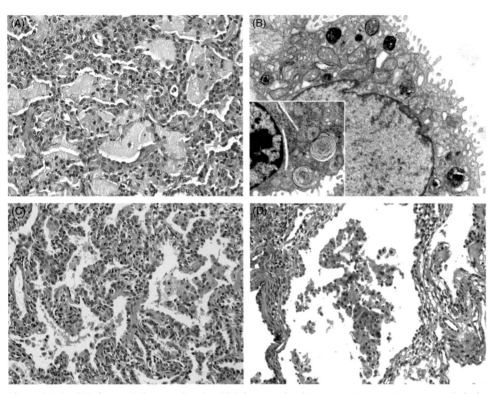

Figure 5.7 (a–d) Surfactant dysfunction disorders. (a) Pulmonary alveolar proteinosis pattern is more typical of infants with mutations in surfactant protein B gene and ABCA3 gene (H&E × 20). (b) Lamellar bodies are markedly abnormal in surfactant protein B mutations (normal comparison, inset). (c) Chronic pneumonitis of infancy pattern in an infant with a surfactant protein C mutation, with lobular remodeling, prominent type II cells, macrophage accumulation, and some proteinosis (H&E × 20). (d) Lung biopsy from an older child with a surfactant protein C mutation is less cellular with more interstitial fibrosis; scant proteinaceous material with cholesterol clefts and foamy macrophages is focally seen (H&E × 20).

eosinophilic, PAS-positive material is more likely to be associated with *SFTPB* and *ABCA3* mutations, while accumulation of intra-alveolar macrophages with cholesterol clefts and an interstitial infiltrate (CPI pattern) is more typical in patients with a *SFTPC* mutation (1; Figure 5.7a,c). DIP can be seen in both *ABCA3* and *SFTPC* mutations. With the exception of *NKX2.1*, surfactant dysfunction mutations that present in infancy show diffuse hyperplasia of alveolar type II cells, variable accumulation of foamy macrophages, and some degree of PAS-positive diastase-resistant proteinaceous material in distal airspaces (1). A degree of abnormal lung growth is frequently present. Lung from older children and adults with *ABCA3* and *SFTPC* mutations tends to show the histologic pattern of NSIP or even UIP (usual interstitial pneumonitis), although a small amount of proteinosis is usually present (88,85; Figure 5.7d).

In individuals with *NKX2.1* mutations the pulmonary histology is quite heterogeneous, and may even

be normal (75). While the predominant histological feature of altered surfactant metabolism is usually pneumocyte hyperplasia, alveolar proteinosis, and accumulation of macrophages, other cases have demonstrated deficient lung growth or NSIP as the principal defect (75,86).

Electron microscopy can be helpful, as both *SFTPB* and *ABCA3* mutations have characteristic ultrastructural findings (74,87). In *SFTPB*, there is absence of normal lamellar bodies with large disorganized multivesicular bodies (Figure 5.7b). In *ABCA3* mutations electron microscopy often demonstrates distinctive changes in lamellar bodies, which are small and contain more densely packed membranes with electron-dense inclusion bodies (74). These abnormal lamellar bodies are often interspersed with normal lamellar bodies and may be infrequent (88). Currently no distinctive ultrastructural abnormalities have been described in association with *SFTPC* and *NKX2.1* mutations, although irregular or disorganized lamellar bodies are often seen among normal forms, including ones resembling that of *ABCA3* mutations (89).

Although stains for surfactant proteins are available, they typically do not assist with the diagnosis (90). The most helpful immunostaining pattern is in the setting of a genetic SP-B deficiency, in which there is absence of mature SP-B expression and aberrant staining for proSP-C in the alveolar lumen (91). The staining pattern in the other surfactant dysfunction disorders is less predictable. Mature SP-B may be absent in *ABCA3* mutations (80) and variable expression for SP-A, SP-B, proSP-C, ABCA3, and TTF-1 have been described in patients with *NKX2.1* mutations (86,89,92,93), consistent with the known role of this gene in regulating surfactant gene expression.

Differential diagnosis: While many cases with the characteristic clinical and histologic findings do not have a mutation, given the complexity of surfactant metabolism it is certain other genetic disorders have yet to be identified. The PAP pattern is also characteristic of patients with antibodies to GM-CSF (granulocyte macrophage colony stimulating factor) (94) or secondary proteinosis in patients with congenital or acquired immunodeficiency. These patients are typically older and do not have the type II cell hyperplasia seen in neonates with surfactant dysfunction mutations; in secondary forms the proteinosis is typically patchy. Pulmonary alveolar proteinosis and cholesterol granulomas have been described in patients with lysinuric protein intolerance, a multisystem disorder caused by mutations in the amino acid transporter gene *SCL7A7* (95). Presentation is variable, with frequent failure to thrive, hepatomegaly, osteopenia, and immune defects.

Cystic fibrosis

Cystic fibrosis, due to mutations in the gene encoding the cystic fibrosis transmembrane conductance regulator (CFTR), is the most common life-shortening inherited disorder in Caucasians. There is prominent involvement of the respiratory tract, as well as other organ systems. Chronic lung disease is the result of increased chloride concentration in secretions, leading to thick tenacious mucus and recurrent infections.

Clinical presentation: The effect of the cystic fibrosis is highly variable between individuals, but typically results in progressive decline in respiratory function in early childhood due to airway obstruction from secretions, recurrent infection, and bronchiectasis. Milder forms may not present until adulthood or

be misdiagnosed as asthma. Patients often have a persistent, productive cough, hyperinflation on radiographs, and pulmonary function tests consistent with obstructive airway disease. *CFTR* mutations increase chloride concentration in exocrine gland secretions, leading to dysfunction of many organ systems, including pancreatic insufficiency (diabetes and fat malabsorption), meconium ileus in the infant, biliary cirrhosis, and male infertility. Inspissated airway mucus causes chronic airway-centered infection. Bacterial colonization (particularly with *Pseudomonas aeruginosa*, *Burkholderia cepacia*, *Staphylococcus aureus*, and *Haemophilus influenzae*) is a constant feature, but the airways may also be colonized by yeast and fungal organisms (especially *Candida* and *Aspergillus*). Patients with cystic fibrosis are at significantly greater risk of contracting non-tuberculous mycobacterial infections, with an estimated disease prevalence of approximately 13% (96). Improvements in the management of cystic fibrosis have resulted in a marked increase in survival. Cystic fibrosis accounts for the highest proportion of lung transplants performed in the pediatric age group.

Hereditary/genetic features: Cystic fibrosis is an autosomal recessive disease caused by homozygous or compound heterozygous mutations in the *CFTR* gene on chromosome 7 (97). The *CFTR* gene encodes an epithelial cyclic adenosine monophosphate-regulated anion channel responsible for bidirectional chloride transport (98). Impaired removal of chloride ions results in decreased sodium and water content in mucus, leading to thick secretions in the airways. Genetic testing for the common mutations in *CFTR* is widely available, but the sweat test remains a common screening tool.

Macroscopy: Bronchiectasis with thickened and fibrotic airways and mucopurulent secretions is characteristic of the disorder (Figure 5.8). Areas of less affected lung may show hyperinflation due to air-trapping. Pleural adhesions and subpleural blebs may be present.

Histology: The histologic features are dependent on the longevity of the pulmonary complications. The large airways may show submucosal gland hypertrophy with mucous plugging. There is acute and chronic bronchiolitis with bronchial wall thickening and mucopurulent secretions in small airways. Purulent material frequently contains colonies of bacteria. Interstitial changes may include foci of organizing pneumonia, interstitial inflammation/fibrosis, and emphysematous change. Colonization by *Aspergillus* may manifest as allergic bronchopulmonary fungal disease.

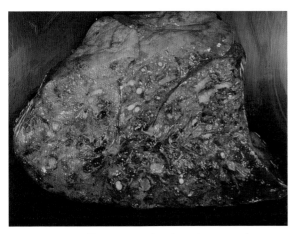

Figure 5.8 Cystic fibrosis. Lungs show bronchiectasis with mucopurulent secretions.

Differential diagnosis: In the absence of genetic confirmation, other entities resulting in bronchiectasis should be considered, including primary ciliary dyskinesia (PCD), immunodeficiencies, and disorders causing tracheobronchomalacia, both congenital and acquired. Primary ciliary dyskinesia is a genetically heterogeneous autosomal recessive disorder affecting ciliary structure and function (99). It is associated with chronic oto-sino-pulmonary disease (sinusitis, bronchiectasis) and organ laterality defects in approximately 50% of patients. Genetic testing for PCD is warranted if clinically suspected, as many PCD patients (around 30%) have normal cilia ultrastructure; conversely, chronic inflammatory disorders can lead to secondary ciliary dysfunction. Patients with immunodeficiencies, both congenital and acquired, are susceptible to infection from a wide range of organisms and may not show the normal inflammatory response expected in immunologically intact individuals.

Williams–Campbell syndrome is a rare congenital disorder characterized by absent or deficient cartilage in the bronchial tree, causing dilatation and collapse of segmental and subsegmental bronchi (100).

Vascular disorders

Persistent pulmonary hypertension of the newborn

Persistent pulmonary hypertension of the newborn (PPHN), also referred to as "persistent fetal circulation" is a clinical syndrome defined by severe hypoxemia and pulmonary hypertension from failure of the normal fetal to neonatal circulatory transition (101). *In utero*, pulmonary blood flow is low due to high pulmonary vascular resistance and shunts (foramen ovale, ductus arteriosus), which permit blood to bypass the pulmonary vascular bed. At birth, pulmonary vascular resistance falls dramatically due to lung inflation and oxygenation. In PPHN this normal transition fails and pulmonary vascular resistance remains high, which results in right-to-left shunting at the foramen ovale, diminished pulmonary blood flow, and hypoxemia.

Clinical presentation: Affected infants are typically late preterm or full term and present with cyanosis and respiratory distress at or shortly after birth. They have evidence of a right-to-left shunt with elevated pulmonary artery pressure. Infants frequently require supplemental oxygen and mechanical ventilation and even may go on ECMO. There are many known etiologies of PPHN, which may be classified as primary or secondary (102). Primary PPHN is related to a decrease in the cross-sectional area of the pulmonary vasculature, as in the case of alveolar capillary dysplasia with misalignment of the pulmonary veins or pulmonary hypoplasia. Secondary PPHN commonly occurs in the setting of congenital heart disease or severe acquired pulmonary disease (i.e., meconium aspiration, neonatal pneumonia), resulting in clinically significant pulmonary vasoconstriction. Persistent pulmonary hypertension of the newborn may also result from decreased *in utero* perfusion/oxygenation or intrapartum asphyxia. It has a high risk of mortality.

Histology: Vascular remodeling is a prominent feature in PPHN that is characterized by increased muscularization of the small pulmonary arteries and abnormal extension of smooth muscle into normally non-muscularized intraacinar vessels (103; Figure 5.9a). In normal infants, the arterial medial thickness decreases rapidly in the first two weeks of life, and resembles the adult by approximately 3–4 months of life (104) Extension of arterial smooth muscle into intraacinar vessels is normally a postnatal phenomenon that does not begin until six months of age and is completed in late adolescence (105). The intima is also infiltrated with fibroblasts and there is often a prominent adventitial sheath around vessels, with increased deposition of collagen and elastin, thought to be a response to local hypoxia (106). The net result of these changes is thickening of the blood vessel wall with increased pulmonary vascular resistance and reduced compliance.

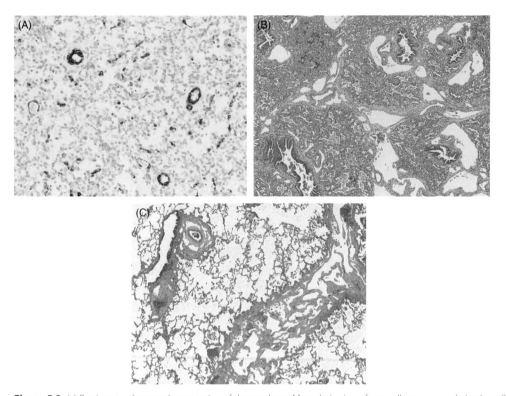

Figure 5.9 (a) Persistent pulmonary hypertension of the newborn. Muscularization of normally non-muscularized small vessels in the alveolar parenchyma is evident by smooth-muscle actin immunostaining (× 20). (b) Lymphangiectasia. A three-month-old infant with total anomalous pulmonary venous return has prominent dilatation of the lymphatic spaces in the bronchovascular spaces and interlobular septa, with associated fibrosis (trichrome stain ×10). (c) Lymphangiomatosis. Lymphatic channels within the interlobular septa are markedly increased, forming complex anastomosing channels (H&E × 10).

Smooth-muscle actin and trichrome stain can help delineate the abnormally muscularized intra-acinar vessels (Figure 5.9a).

Differential diagnosis: As PPHN is a component of many hypoxic neonatal lung diseases, including diffuse developmental disorders of the lung, deficient lung growth, PIG, and congenital abnormalities of surfactant metabolism, it is important to define pathologically, as well as clinically, the potential underlying etiology of vascular remodeling.

Lymphatic disorders

Lymphangiectasia (primary or secondary) and lymphangiomatosis are rare, but still the most common disorders of the pulmonary lymphatic system that present in children (107). Pulmonary lymphangiectasia is characterized by massive dilatation of normal lymphatic vessels due to disordered drainage of lymph in the lungs, while pulmonary lymphangiomatosis is an abnormal proliferation of lymphatic channels in normal locations. Both of these disorders may be isolated to the lung or associated with involvement of other organs.

Clinical presentation: Lymphangiectasia may be primary/congenital or secondary to conditions that increase lymph production or impair lymph drainage. Primary lymphangiectasia may be sporadic or a component of a chromosomal (Down syndrome, Turner syndrome) or genetic disorder (Noonan syndrome, Ehlers–Danlos syndrome). It is hypothesized to be due to a failure of regression of pulmonary interstitial connective tissues in the second trimester of fetal life. Primary lymphangiectasia is usually fatal early in life and may present with stillbirth and fetal hydrops (108,109). It should be suspected in newborns that present at birth with severe respiratory distress and chylous pleural effusions. Imaging findings may be highly suggestive, with pleural effusions and diffuse thickening of the interstitium and interlobular septa (Kerley-B lines). Secondary lymphangiectasia occurs if there is obstruction to lymphatic drainage (surgery, radiation, infection) or increased lymphatic circulation, the latter predominantly in children with congenital heart disease (e.g., total anomalous pulmonary venous return, hypoplastic left heart, congenital mitral stenosis). Depending on the etiology there are localized or diffuse pulmonary interstitial infiltrates and cystic lesions on chest radiograph and MRI. Prognosis depends on the underlying condition.

In contrast to lymphangiectasia, which largely affects neonates, patients with pulmonary lymphangiomatosis typically present in late childhood, although patients ranging from birth to young adults have been reported (110,111). The presentation usually includes recurrent cough, wheeze, and reoccurring chylous pleural effusions, which progress with advancing age. A CT scan of the thorax reveals thickening of the interlobular septa and often extensive involvement of the mediastinum and perihilar regions. Pulmonary lymphangiomatosis frequently involves many other sites, most commonly the mediastinum, bone, and soft tissue. The co-existence of lytic bone lesions and chylothorax is highly suspicious for the diagnosis. The prognosis depends on sites of involvement, but is usually poor with pulmonary and intra-abdominal disease (111). Dietary modifications and sclerotherapy are the main treatment options.

Hereditary/genetic features: Although usually sporadic, several cases of primary congenital pulmonary lymphangiectasia have been reported in siblings, suggesting a genetic etiology (112,113).

Macroscopy: In both entities the dilatation of the subpleural and septal lymphatics give the pleural surface a cobblestone appearance.

Histology: Lymphatics are located adjacent to blood vessels in the bronchovascular spaces and the connective tissue of interlobular septa and the pleura. In pulmonary lymphangiectasia these pre-existing lymphatic channels are diffusely dilated and appear tortuous (Figure 5.9b). If longstanding, there may be widening of the interlobular septa and pleura by dense fibrosis. Compared to lymphangiectasia, lymphangiomatosis has a proliferation of lymphatic spaces in the interlobular septa and pleura, which are accompanied by collagen and fascicles of smooth muscle cells (Figure 5.9c; 70).

Differential diagnosis: Diffuse pulmonary lymphangiectasia may be confused with pulmonary interstitial emphysema (PIE), as the interstitial air-filled spaces may be misinterpreted as dilated lymphatics. Negative immunostaining for a vascular marker (e.g., CD31,

D2-40) and the presence of foreign-body giant cells would support the diagnosis of PIE. As well as PIE and lymphangiectasia, lymphangiomatosis should be distinguished from lymphangioleiomyomatosis (LAM), which affects women of reproductive age. LAM is characterized histologically by cystic spaces and a proliferation of spindle cells that are immunoreactive for HMB-45, as well as smooth-muscle markers (smooth-muscle actin, desmin). The smooth-muscle cells in lymphangiomatosis do not express HMB-45. In addition, LAM disrupts the adjacent lung parenchyma, while lymphangiectasia and lymphangiomatosis do not.

Neoplasms of the airways and lung

Respiratory papillomatosis

Multiple, recurrent squamous papillomas typically involve the larynx, but may extend to the trachea, bronchi, and even pulmonary parenchyma.

Clinical presentation: Juvenile respiratory papillomatosis most often arises in the commissure and anterior third of the vocal cords within the larynx (114,115). Approximately 10% of patients have tracheal or lower airway involvement, with bronchial or pulmonary parenchymal involvement occurring in 2–5% of patients. Patients usually present by 7–10 years of age with hoarseness, stridor, or, rarely, difficulty breathing secondary to airway obstruction. Children with lower airway papillomatosis present at an earlier age (1–2 years vs. 3–4 years of age) and require more surgical procedures. Whether this is due to more extensive spread of papillomatosis or secondary to scarring from multiple surgeries is unclear, however, as lower airway dissemination typically occurs following tracheotomy or intubation performed for tracheal stenosis. Spontaneous regression of laryngeal papillomatosis may occur at puberty, but the mortality from pulmonary and lower airway papillomatosis is high.

Hereditary/genetic features: Papillomatosis is associated with human papillomavirus, particularly types 6 and 11, and is generally thought to be transmitted vertically from mother to child. There is a 200–400-fold increased risk of papillomatosis in infants of mothers with a history of genital warts, as compared to infants of mothers without condylomata. Human papilloma virus-11 infection is associated with more aggressive disease.

Macroscopy: Endoscopically, papillomatosis appears as multiple exophytic, sessile papillary masses.

Histology: Respiratory papillomas have thickened, non-keratinizing squamous epithelium overlying fibrovascular stroma with varying amounts of inflammation. The epithelium may show koilocytic atypia, but high-grade squamous dysplasia or carcinoma are uncommon in children.

Differential diagnosis: Children with lower airway papillomatosis almost always have a history of laryngeal papillomatosis. In rare cases where a history of laryngeal papillomatosis is not obtained, radiographic detection of an intraluminal mass in the airway could raise the possibility of other pediatric bronchial lesions, such as a carcinoid tumor or mucoepidermoid carcinoma. Routine histologic examination easily resolves the diagnosis, however.

Inflammatory myofibroblastic tumor

As the name suggests, inflammatory myofibroblastic tumors (IMTs) are composed of spindled myofibroblastic cells accompanied by an inflammatory infiltrate including plasma cells, lymphocytes, and eosinophils.

Clinical presentation: Most often affecting children and young adults (mean age = 10 years), the lung is a common site of involvement for IMT (116,117). Pulmonary IMT may present with chest pain or dyspnea, or may be entirely asymptomatic. Fever and weight loss occur in some patients, and, rarely, patients develop a clinical syndrome including anemia, thrombocytosis, hypergammaglobulinemia, and an elevated erythrocyte sedimentation rate or C-reactive protein, which disappears upon resection and may reappear with tumor recurrence. On imaging studies, the mass is lobulated, heterogeneous, and may show calcifications.

Macroscopy: Inflammatory myofibroblastic tumor is well circumscribed or multinodular. The cut surface is firm, but may appear whorled or myxoid. Hemorrhage or necrosis can be seen. Tumor size ranges from 1–17 cm, with a mean diameter of 6 cm.

Histology: A reactive pattern of IMT is characterized by loosely arranged myofibroblasts with an edematous, myxoid background, and abundant blood vessels. There is a prominent inflammatory infiltrate of plasma cells, lymphocytes, and eosinophils, which may resemble granulation tissue. Neutrophils may be seen more often with this histologic pattern as well. A more compact, fibrous pattern is characterized by fascicles of spindle cells with a myxoid to collagenous background. The inflammatory component may be diffuse or arranged in small aggregates of plasma cells or true lymphoid nodules. Both of these histologic

patterns may contain large ganglion-like or Reed–Sternberg-like myofibroblasts. The third pattern of IMT shows dense collagen and lacks a prominent inflammatory component, resulting in a scar-like appearance. Rarely, a round-cell histiocytoid pattern characterizes more aggressive tumors. Tumor size, cellularity, and histologic features are not reliable prognostic indicators, however.

Inflammatory myofibroblastic tumors are uniformly immunoreactive for vimentin with variable expression of smooth-muscle actin, muscle-specific actin, and desmin. Focal cytokeratin expression may be seen, but the spindled cells are negative for myogenin, myoglobin, and S100. Inflammatory myofibroblastic tumor is also typically negative for CD117. Anaplastic lymphoma kinase (ALK) staining characterizes approximately 50% of IMT, although ALK rearrangements may be less common in children (118).

Hereditary/genetic features: Anaplastic lymphoma kinase (ALK) immunoreactivity correlates with the presence of a rearrangement involving the *ALK* gene on chromosome 2p23. Fusion partners include *TPM3*, *TPM4*, *CLTC*, and *ATIC*. The fusion partner *RANBP2* may be associated with worse prognosis and is characterized by epithelioid/histiocytoid morphology and a nuclear membrane pattern of ALK staining.

Differential diagnosis: The differential diagnosis varies with the histologic pattern. The loose pattern of IMT can mimic granulation tissue or a reactive process, while the fascicular pattern may resemble a fibrous histiocytoma or a smooth-muscle neoplasm. The collagenous scar-like pattern mimics a desmoid-type fibromatosis.

Fetal lung interstitial tumor (FLIT)

Fetal lung interstitial tumor (FLIT) is a recently named entity described as a lobar-based solid to microcystic mass characterized by immature airspaces with widened septa containing immature interstitial cells.

Clinical presentation: All reported cases presented prenatally or by three months of age (119,120). Most affected infants have some degree of respiratory distress or feeding difficulties, but the mass may be noted incidentally on chest X-ray. Imaging studies demonstrate a well-circumscribed, solid, or partially cystic mass involving the periphery of one lobe. Treatment has primarily consisted of lobectomy or wedge resection, with only one infant receiving postoperative chemotherapy. No local recurrence or metastatic disease is reported to date.

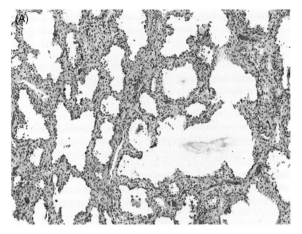

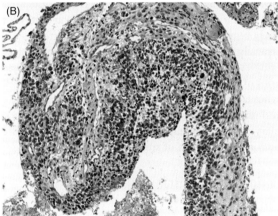

Figure 5.10 (a) Fetal lung interstitial tumor. This focal lesion is composed of alveolar-like cystic spaces with expanded septa containing immature mesenchymal cells (H&E ×20). (b) Pleuropulmonary blastoma. This type I pleuropulmonary blastoma has a condensation of small primitive cells in the cyst walls (H&E ×20).

Macroscopy: Grossly, FLIT is well circumscribed and ranges from 2.0–6.6 cm in diameter. The cut surface of most lesions is described as spongy and pale tan to dark red. There may be focal hemorrhage.

Histology: The mass is microscopically well circumscribed, with a fibrous border and abrupt interface with normal lung parenchyma. The tumor shows immature appearing airspace-like structures with variably widened septa (Figure 5.10a). The interstitium contains a monotonous population of immature round to ovoid cells with glycogenated cytoplasm. The septa lack any condensation of mesenchymal cells beneath the epithelium. Nuclear hyperchromasia, mitotic activity and atypical mitotic figures are absent. The airspace-like structures are lined by a flattened-to-cuboidal non-ciliated epithelium. Occasionally, a spindle-cell component resembling a myofibroblastic tumor may be seen focally.

The interstitial cells of the tumor are diffusely positive for vimentin, with variable expression of desmin and smooth-muscle actin. The interstitial cells are consistently negative for myogenin, however. The epithelial lining of the cystic spaces express cytokeratin and epithelial membrane antigen, as well as thyroid transforming factor-1 (TTF-1).

Hereditary/genetic features: In the few cases examined, a routine karyotype was normal, although one case showed trisomy 8 by fresh tissue, fluorescence *in-situ* hybridization (FISH) . Controversy exists over the relationship between FLIT and PPB, and it is unclear whether FLIT represents a maldevelopment or a potentially malignant neoplasm (119,120). Both FLIT and PPB arise from interstitial mesenchymal cells, but they appear to have very different outcomes.

Differential diagnosis: The differential diagnosis of FLIT includes CPAMs, particularly type 3. Both of these entities demonstrate dilated airspaces and lack cartilage or mucogenic epithelium. Congenital pulmonary airway malformations are typically less well circumscribed than FLIT, however, and their more variably sized cysts are lined by ciliated respiratory epithelium. Type 3 CPAM often involves an entire lobe and is composed of small gland-like spaces lined by ciliated cuboidal epithelium resembling terminal bronchioles.

Both FLIT and PPB are well-circumscribed masses, but types 2 and 3 PPB do not present a diagnostic dilemma as they very rarely present in this age group and characteristically have overtly malignant features in the solid component. The differentiation of FLIT from type 1 cystic PPB relies on the more delicate, multicystic structure of type 1 PPB, the condensation of primitive small cells (many with rhabdomyoblastic differentiation) beneath the epithelial surface in PPB, and the presence of small nodules of primitive cartilage (although not present in all cases of PPB).

Pleuropulmonary blastoma

Pleuropulmonary blastoma (PPB) is a primitive embryonal tumor of the lung characterized by cysts with primitive mesenchymal cells beneath an intact, benign-appearing epithelium. Mesenchymal overgrowth results in an increasingly solid component and correlates with worsening outcomes.

Clinical presentation: The clinical presentation of PPB varies with the natural history of the tumor. Type 1 cystic PPB almost always presents before 30 months of age and may be detected prenatally (121). Affected

191

infants often have respiratory symptoms, including cough and chest pain, and many present with pneumothorax. Up to one-half of cases may be multifocal, and one-third are bilateral. Types 2 and 3 PPB present in slightly older children (mean age = 38 months), but a lung cyst may have been previously identified in some patients. Radiographically, type 1 PPB is a well-circumscribed multilocular cyst, while types 2 and 3 PPB show a mixed solid and cystic, or solid mass, respectively.

Hereditary/genetic features: Approximately 25% of patients with PPB have a hereditary tumor predisposition syndrome in which family members are at increased risk of lung "cysts," cystic nephroma, and other embryonal tumors, such as Wilms tumor or rhabdomyosarcoma. Recent studies mapped the PPB locus to chromosome 14q and implicated *DICER1* in the development of familial PPB (122). DICER1 is a key component in the generation of small RNAs (miRNAs and siRNAs), which regulate gene expression and are critical for stem-cell maintenance, organogenesis, cell-cycle progression, and oncogenesis.

Macroscopy: Type I PPB is well circumscribed and multilocular without solid nodules or plaque-like thickening of the cyst walls. Type 2 PPB is, by definition, a mixed solid and cystic mass, while type 3 PPB is entirely solid. The mass is usually located at the periphery of the lung, and tumor resections may include overlying pleura.

Histology: Type 1 PPB shows cysts lined by flattened-to-cuboidal, non-ciliated epithelial cells. The cyst walls contain continuous to exquisitely focal nests of primitive mesenchymal cells. In many cases these malignant cells condense beneath the epithelial lining, resulting in a well-formed cambium layer (Figure 5.10b). Definitive skeletal muscle differentiation may be seen. In some cases nodules of primitive "blastema"-like cells may be seen, as well as foci of immature cartilage. Occasionally, nodules of spindle cells resembling mature fibroblasts may be the only tumor component differentiating PPB from other lung cysts.

Sarcomatous overgrowth in the tumor septa indicates transition to type 2 PPB. Types 2 and 3 PPB show frankly malignant features, including bizarre pleomorphic giant cells. The tumors are heterogeneous, typically with multiple mesenchymal components including rhabdomyoblastic, chondroid, fibrohistiocytic, and lipoblastic differentiation. Interstitial tumor cells with skeletal muscle differentiation are desmin positive. Myogenin and MyoD1 staining in these cells show a pattern similar to that seen in embryonal rhabdomyosarcoma, with scattered positive cells.

Differential diagnosis: The differential diagnosis varies with the type of PPB. As mentioned previously, type 1 PPB must be differentiated from congenital cystic adenomatoid malformation and FLIT (123). The presence of a cambium layer, at least focally, is most useful in this distinction. The other microscopic features of these entities are described above. With increasingly solid components in type 2 and type 3 PPB, the differential diagnosis shifts to include other sarcomas. Rhabdomyoblastic differentiation is common, and small biopsies of PPB may reveal only embryonal rhabdomyosarcoma-like regions. Reports of rhabdomyosarcomas arising from a lung cyst most likely represent PPB. Pleuropulmonary blastomas are typically very heterogeneous, however, and larger samples reveal varying morphologies, with multiple lines of differentiation. Finally, although uncommon, synovial sarcoma may present with pneumothorax and an underlying primary cystic lung lesion. A primary cystic synovial sarcoma typically has a more uniform population of spindle cells, however (124).

Peripheral primitive neuroectodermal tumor

Primitive neuroectodermal tumors (PNETs)/Ewing's sarcomas arising in the chest wall are eponymously named Askin tumors, and resemble PNETs at other sites (125).

Clinical presentation: Patients may present with fever, chest pain, or a palpable mass. Imaging shows a solid soft-tissue or pleural-based mass, with or without bony invasion.

Hereditary/genetic features: As with Ewing's sarcoma family tumors at other sites, thoracopulmonary PNETs are characterized by rearrangement of the *EWS* gene on chromosome 22 (126).

Macroscopy: Because of the location in the chest wall, these tumors are often diagnosed by incisional or needle biopsies. Resection of Ewing's sarcoma family tumors typically follows neoadjuvant chemotherapy, and gross examination reveals variable necrosis and fibrosis in these treated tumors.

Histology: Thoracopulmonary PNETs demonstrate sheets of small round cells with scant cytoplasm. Alternating light and dark cells, and focal rosette formation may be a clue to the diagnosis of a PNET in these otherwise undifferentiated neoplasms. Strong, diffuse membrane staining for CD99 supports the diagnosis of PNET. The novel marker NKX2.2, a direct target of the EWS-FLI1 fusion protein, is also reportedly more commonly expressed in Ewing's sarcoma family tumors than in other small round-cell tumors (127).

Differential diagnosis: As noted elsewhere, CD99 expression in small round-cell tumors is not specific and lymphoblastic lymphoma, as well as other neoplasms, should be excluded. Monophasic synovial sarcoma occurs in older children and adolescents and can show membranous CD99 expression (128). Confirmation of the appropriate chromosomal translocation or fusion protein, i.e., *EWS* rearrangement in Ewing's/PNET or t (X;18)(*SYT-SSX*) in synovial sarcoma, is useful in difficult cases. Rhabdomyosarcoma may uncommonly involve the chest wall in young children, but myogenin or MyoD1, in addition to CD99, help with this distinction.

References

1. Deutsch GH, Young LR, Deterding RR, *et al.* Diffuse lung disease in young children: Application of a novel classification scheme. Am. J. Respir. Crit. Care Med. 2007;**176**:1120–8.

2. Langston C, Patterson K, Dishop MK, *et al.* A protocol for the handling of tissue obtained by operative lung biopsy: recommendations of the chILD pathology co-operative group. Pediatr. Dev. Pathol. 2006;**9**:173–80.

3. Langston C. New concepts in the pathology of congenital lung malformations. Semin. Pediatr. Surg. 2003;**12**:17–37.

4. Kunisaki SM, Fauza DO, Nemes LP, *et al.* Bronchial atresia: the hidden pathology within a spectrum of prenatally diagnosed lung masses. J. Pediatr. Surg. 2006;**41**:61–5.

5. Riedlinger WF, Vargas SO, Jennings RW, *et al.* Bronchial atresia is common to extralobar sequestration, intralobar sequestration, congenital cystic adenomatoid malformation, and lobar emphysema. Pediatr. Dev. Pathol. 2006;**9**:361–73.

6. Nobuhara KK, Gorski YC, La Quaglia MP, Shamberger RC. Bronchogenic cysts and esophageal duplications: common origins and treatment. J. Pediatr. Surg. 1997;**32**:1408–13.

7. Zvulunov A, Amichai B, Grunwald MH, Avinoach I, Halevy S. Cutaneous bronchogenic cyst: delineation of a poorly recognized lesion. Pediatr. Dermatol. 1998;**15**:277–81.

8. Stocker JT, Drake RM, Madewell JE. Cystic and congenital lung disease in the newborn. Perspect. Pediatr. Pathol. 1978;**4**:93–154.

9. Crombleholme TM, Coleman B, Hedrick H, *et al.* Cystic adenomatoid malformation volume ratio predicts outcome in prenatally diagnosed cystic adenomatoid malformation of the lung. J. Pediatr. Surg. 2002;**37**:331–8.

10. De Santis M, Masini L, Noia G, Cavaliere AF, Oliva N, Caruso A. Congenital cystic adenomatoid malformation of the lung: Antenatal ultrasound findings and fetal-neonatal outcome. Fifteen years of experience. Fetal Diagn. Ther. 2000;**15**:246–50.

11. Stocker JT, Madewell JE, Drake RM. Congenital cystic adenomatoid malformation of the lung. Classification and morphologic spectrum. Hum. Pathol. 1977;**8**:155–71.

12. Granata C, Gambini C, Balducci T, *et al.* Bronchioloalveolar carcinoma arising in congenital cystic adenomatoid malformation in a child: A case report and review on malignancies originating in congenital cystic adenomatoid malformation. Pediatr. Pulmonol. 1998;**25**:62–6.

13. West D, Nicholson AG, Colquhoun I, Pollock J. Bronchioloalveolar carcinoma in congenital cystic adenomatoid malformation of lung. Ann. Thorac. Surg. 2007;**83**:687–9.

14. Landing BH, Dixon LG. Congenital malformations and genetic disorders of the respiratory tract (larynx, trachea, bronchi, and lungs). Am. Rev. Respir. Dis. 1979;**120**:151–85.

15. DeParedes CG, Pierce WS, Johnson DG, Waldhausen JA. Pulmonary sequestration in infants and children: A 20-year experience and review of the literature. J. Pediatr. Surg. 1970;**5**:136–47.

16. Holder PD, Langston C. Intralobar pulmonary sequestration (a nonentity?). Pediatr. Pulmonol. 1986;**2**:147–53.

17. Conran RM, Stocker JT. Extralobar sequestration with frequently associated congenital cystic adenomatoid malformation, type 2: report of 50 cases. Pediatr. Dev. Pathol. 1999;**2**:454–63.

18. Cooney TP, Thurlbeck WM. The radial alveolar count method of Emery and Mithal: A reappraisal 2–intrauterine and early postnatal lung growth. Thorax 1982;**37**:580–3.

19. Cooney TP, Thurlbeck WM. The radial alveolar count method of Emery and Mithal: A reappraisal 1–postnatal lung growth. Thorax 1982;**37**:572–9.

20. Gillespie LM, Fenton AC, Wright C. Acinar dysplasia: A rare cause of neonatal respiratory failure. Acta Paediatr. 2004;**93**:712–3.

193

21. Moerman P, Vanhole C, Devlieger H, Fryns JP. Severe primary pulmonary hypoplasia ("acinar dysplasia") in sibs: A genetically determined mesodermal defect? J. Med. Genet. 1998;**35**:964–5.

22. Deboer EM, Keene S, Winkler AM, Shehata BM. Identical twins with lethal congenital pulmonary airway malformation type 0 (acinar dysplasia): further evidence of familial tendency. Fetal Pediatr. Pathol. 2012;**31**:217–24.

23. Chen MF, Gray KD, Prentice MA, Mariano JM, Jakowlew SB. Human pulmonary acinar aplasia: reduction of transforming growth factor-beta ligands and receptors. Pediatr. Res. 1999;**46**:61–70.

24. Garola RE, Thibeault DW. Alveolar capillary dysplasia, with and without misalignment of pulmonary veins: An association of congenital anomalies. Am. J. Perinatol. 1998;**15**:103–7.

25. Licht C, Schickendantz S, Sreeram N, *et al.* Prolonged survival in alveolar capillary dysplasia syndrome. Eur. J. Pediatr. 2004;**163**:181–2.

26. Shankar V, Haque A, Johnson J, Pietsch J. Late presentation of alveolar capillary dysplasia in an infant. Pediatr. Crit. Care Med. 2006;**7**:177–9.

27. Ahmed S, Ackerman V, Faught P, Langston C. Profound hypoxemia and pulmonary hypertension in a 7-month-old infant: late presentation of alveolar capillary dysplasia. Pediatr. Crit. Care Med. 2008;**9**:e43–6.

28. Al-Hathlol K, Phillips S, Seshia MK, *et al.* Alveolar capillary dysplasia. Report of a case of prolonged life without extracorporeal membrane oxygenation (ECMO) and review of the literature. Early Hum. Dev. 2000;**57**:85–94.

29. Rabah R, Poulik JM. Congenital alveolar capillary dysplasia with misalignment of pulmonary veins associated with hypoplastic left heart syndrome. Pediatr. Dev. Pathol. 2001;**4**:167–74.

30. Sen P, Thakur N, Stockton DW, Langston C, Bejjani BA. Expanding the phenotype of alveolar capillary dysplasia (ACD). J. Pediatr. 2004;**145**:646–51.

31. Antao B, Samuel M, Kiely E, Spitz L, Malone M. Congenital alveolar capillary dysplasia and associated gastrointestinal anomalies. Fetal Pediatr. Pathol. 2006;**25**:137–45.

32. Stankiewicz P, Sen P, Bhatt SS *et al.* Genomic and genic deletions of the FOX gene cluster on 16q24.1 and inactivating mutations of *FOXF1* cause alveolar capillary dysplasia and other malformations. Am. J. Hum. Genet. 2009;**84**:780–91.

33. Yu S, Shao L, Kilbride H, Zwick DL. Haploinsufficiencies of FOXF1 and FOXC2 genes associated with lethal alveolar capillary dysplasia and congenital heart disease. Am. J. Med. Genet. A;**152A**:1257–62.

34. Mahlapuu M, Enerback S, Carlsson P. Haploinsufficiency of the forkhead gene Foxf1, a target for sonic hedgehog signaling, causes lung and foregut malformations. Development. 2001;**128**:2397–406.

35. Astorga J, Carlsson P. Hedgehog induction of murine vasculogenesis is mediated by Foxf1 and Bmp4. Development 2007;**134**:3753–61.

36. Manouvrier-Hanu S, Devisme L, Farre I *et al.* Pulmonary hypertension of the newborn and urogenital anomalies in two male siblings: A new family with misalignment of pulmonary vessels. GenetCouns. 1996;**7**:249–55.

37. Boggs S, Harris MC, Hoffman DJ, *et al.* Misalignment of pulmonary veins with alveolar capillary dysplasia: Affected siblings and variable phenotypic expression. J. Pediatr. 1994;**124**:125–8.

38. Gutierrez C, Rodriguez A, Palenzuela S, Forteza C, Rossello JL. Congenital misalignment of pulmonary veins with alveolar capillary dysplasia causing persistent neonatal pulmonary hypertension: report of two affected siblings. Pediatr. Dev. Pathol. 2000;**3**:271–6.

39. Sen P, Gerychova R, Janku P, *et al.* A familial case of alveolar capillary dysplasia with misalignment of pulmonary veins supports paternal imprinting of *FOXF1* in human. Eur. J. Hum. Genet. 2012;**21**:474–7.

40. Abdallah HI, Karmazin N, Marks LA. Late presentation of misalignment of lung vessels with alveolar capillary dysplasia. Crit. Care Med. 1993;**21**:628 30.

41. Langston C, Dishop MK. Diffuse lung disease in infancy: A proposed classification applied to 259 diagnostic biopsies. Pediatr. Dev. Pathol. 2009;**12**:421–37.

42. Sherer DM, Davis JM, Woods JR, Jr. Pulmonary hypoplasia: A review. Obstet. Gynecol. Surv. 1990;**45**:792–803.

43. Cooney TP, Thurlbeck WM. Pulmonary hypoplasia in Down's syndrome. N. Engl. J. Med. 1982;**307**:1170–3.

44. Wigglesworth JS, Desai R, Guerrini P. Fetal lung hypoplasia: biochemical and structural variations and their possible significance. Arch. Dis. Child. 1981;**56**:606–15.

45. De Paepe ME, Friedman RM, Gundogan F, Pinar H. Postmortem lung weight/body weight standards for term and preterm infants. Pediatr. Pulmonol. 2005;**40**:445–8.

46. Bonikos DS, Bensch KG, Northway WH, Jr., Edwards DK. Bronchopulmonary dysplasia: the pulmonary pathologic sequel of necrotizing bronchiolitis and pulmonary fibrosis. Hum. Pathol. 1976;**7**:643–66.

47. Husain AN, Siddiqui NH, Stocker JT. Pathology of arrested acinar development in postsurfactant bronchopulmonary dysplasia. Hum. Pathol. 1998;**29**:710–7.

48. Chi TPL, Krovetz J. The pulmonary vascular bed in children with Down syndrome. J. Pediatr. 1975;**86**:533–8.

49. Farrell PM, Avery ME. Hyaline membrane disease. Am. Rev. Respir. Dis. 1975;**111**:657–88.

50. Pfenninger J, Tschaeppeler H, Wagner BP, Weber J, Zimmerman A. The paradox of adult respiratory distress syndrome in neonates. Pediatr. Pulmonol. 1991;**10**:18–24.

51. Farrell PM, Wood RE. Epidemiology of hyaline membrane disease in the United States: Analysis of national mortality statistics. Pediatrics 1976;**58**:167–76.

52. Greenough A. Factors adversely affecting lung growth. Paediatr. Respir. Rev. 2000;**1**:314–20.

53. Stocker JT, Madewell JE. Persistent interstitial pulmonary emphysema: Another complication of the respiratory distress syndrome. Pediatrics 1977;**59**:847–57.

54. Schroeder SA, Shannon DC, Mark EJ. Cellular interstitial pneumonitis in infants. A clinicopathologic study. Chest 1992;**101**:1065–9.

55. Canakis AM, Cutz E, Manson D, O'Brodovich H. Pulmonary interstitial glycogenosis: A new variant of neonatal interstitial lung disease. Am. J. Respir. Crit. Care Med. 2002;**165**:1557–65.

56. Onland W, Molenaar JJ, Leguit RJ, et al. Pulmonary interstitial glycogenosis in identical twins. Pediatr. Pulmonol. 2005;**40**:362–6.

57. Lanfranchi M, Allbery SM, Wheelock L, Perry D. Pulmonary interstitial glycogenosis. Pediatr. Radiol. 2002;**40**:361–5.

58. Castillo M, Vade A, Lim-Dunham JE, Masuda E, Massarani-Wafai R. Pulmonary interstitial glycogenosis in the setting of lung growth abnormality: radiographic and pathologic correlation. Pediatr. Radiol. 2010;**40**:1562–5.

59. Deutsch GH, Young LR. Histologic resolution of pulmonary interstitial glycogenosis. Pediatr. Dev. Pathol. 2009;**12**:475–80.

60. Deutsch GH, Young LR. Pulmonary interstitial glycogenosis: words of caution. Pediatr. Radiol. 2010;**40**:1471–5.

61. Deterding RR, Pye C, Fan LL, Langston C. Persistent tachypnea of infancy is associated with neuroendocrine cell hyperplasia. Pediatr. Pulmonol. 2005;**40**:157–65.

62. Brody AS, Guillerman RP, Hay TC, et al. Neuroendocrine cell hyperplasia of infancy: diagnosis with high-resolution CT. AJR Am. J. Roentgenol. 2010;**194**:238–44.

63. Kerby GS, Kopecky C, Wilcox SL, et al. Infant pulmonary function testing in children with neuroendocrine cell hyperplasia with and without lung biopsy. Proc. Am. Thorac. Soc. 2009:A5287.

64. Young LR, Brody AS, Inge TH, et al. Neuroendocrine cell distribution and frequency distinguish neuroendocrine cell hyperplasia of infancy from other pulmonary disorders. Chest 2010.

65. Popler J, Gower W, Mogayzel P, et al. Familial neuroendocrine cell hyperplasia of infancy. Pediatr. Pulmonol. 2010.

66. Perrin DG, McDonald TJ, Cutz E. Hyperplasia of bombesin-immunoreactive pulmonary neuroendocrine cells and neuroepithelial bodies in sudden infant death syndrome. Pediatr. Pathol. 1991;**11**:431–47.

67. Johnson DE, Lock JE, Elde RP, Thompson TR. Pulmonary neuroendocrine cells in hyaline membrane disease and bronchopulmonary dysplasia. Pediatr. Res. 1982;**16**:446–54.

68. Sunday ME, Kaplan LM, Motoyama E, Chin WW, Spindel ER. Gastrin-releasing peptide (mammalian bombesin) gene expression in health and disease. Lab. Invest. 1988;**59**:5–24.

69. Schindler MB, Bohn DJ, Bryan AC, Cutz E, Rabinovitch M. Increased respiratory system resistance and bronchial smooth muscle hypertrophy in children with acute postoperative pulmonary hypertension. Am. J. Respir. Crit. Care Med. 1995;**152**:1347–52.

70. Johnson DE, Wobken JD, Landrum BG. Changes in bombesin, calcitonin, and serotonin immunoreactive pulmonary neuroendocrine cells in cystic fibrosis and after prolonged mechanical ventilation. Am. Rev. Respir. Dis. 1988;**137**:123–31.

71. Scher H, Miller YE, Aguayo SM, et al. Urinary bombesin-like peptide levels in infants and children with bronchopulmonary dysplasia and cystic fibrosis. Pediatr. Pulmonol. 1998;**26**:326–31.

72. Nogee LM, de Mello DE, Dehner LP, Colten HR. Brief report: deficiency of pulmonary surfactant protein B in congenital alveolar proteinosis. N. Engl. J. Med. 1993;**328**:406–10.

73. Nogee LM, Dunbar AE, 3rd, Wert SE, Askin F, Hamvas A, Whitsett JA. A mutation in the surfactant protein C gene associated with familial interstitial lung disease. N. Engl. J. Med. 2001;**344**:573–9.

74. Shulenin S, Nogee LM, Annilo T, Wert SE, Whitsett JA, Dean M. ABCA3 gene mutations in newborns with fatal surfactant deficiency. N. Engl. J. Med. 2004;**350**:1296–303.

195

75. Hamvas A, Deterding RR, Wert SE, *et al*. Heterogeneous pulmonary phenotypes associated with mutations in the thyroid transcription factor gene NKX2–1. Chest 2013;**144**:794–804.

76. Hartl D, Griese M. Interstitial lung disease in children – genetic background and associated phenotypes. Respir. Res. 2005;**6**:32.

77. Bullard JE, Wert SE, Nogee LM. ABCA3 deficiency: neonatal respiratory failure and interstitial lung disease. Semin. Perinatol. 2006;**30**:327–34.

78. Ballard PL, Nogee LM, Beers MF *et al*. Partial deficiency of surfactant protein B in an infant with chronic lung disease. Pediatrics 1995;**96**:1046–52.

79. Dunbar AE, 3rd, Wert SE, Ikegami M *et al*. Prolonged survival in hereditary surfactant protein B (SP-B) deficiency associated with a novel splicing mutation. Pediatr. Res. 2000;**48**:275–82.

80. Brasch F, Schimanski S, Muhlfeld C, *et al*. Alteration of the pulmonary surfactant system in full-term infants with hereditary ABCA3 deficiency. Am. J. Respir. Crit. Care Med. 2006;**174**:571–80.

81. Cheong N, Madesh M, Gonzales LW, *et al*. Functional and trafficking defects in ATP binding cassette A3 mutants associated with respiratory distress syndrome. J. Biol. Chem. 2006;**281**:9791–800.

82. Hallik M, Annilo T, Ilmoja ML. Different course of lung disease in two siblings with novel ABCA3 mutations. Eur. J. Pediatr. 2013 (Epub ahead of print).

83. Thavagnanam S, Cutz E, Manson D, Nogee LM, Dell SD. Variable clinical outcome of ABCA3 deficiency in two siblings. Pediatr. Pulmonol. 2013;**48**:1035–8.

84. Chibbar R, Shih F, Baga M, *et al*. Nonspecific interstitial pneumonia and usual interstitial pneumonia with mutation in surfactant protein C in familial pulmonary fibrosis. Mod. Pathol. 2004;**17**:973–80.

85. Young LR, Nogee LM, Barnett B, Panos RJ, Colby TV, Deutsch GH. Usual interstitial pneumonia in an adolescent with ABCA3 mutations. Chest 2008;**134**:192–5.

86. Galambos C, Levy H, Cannon CL, *et al*. Pulmonary pathology in thyroid transcription factor-1 deficiency syndrome. Am. J. Respir. Crit. Care Med. 2013;**182**:549–54.

87. Tryka AF, Wert SE, Mazursky JE, Arrington RW, Nogee LM. Absence of lamellar bodies with accumulation of dense bodies characterizes a novel form of congenital surfactant defect. Pediatr. Dev. Pathol. 2000;**3**:335–45.

88. Doan ML, Guillerman RP, Dishop MK *et al*. Clinical, radiological and pathological features of ABCA3 mutations in children. Thorax 2008;**63**:366–73.

89. Hamvas A, Deterding RR, Wert SE, *et al*. Heterogeneous pulmonary phenotypes associated with mutations in the thyroid transcription factor gene NKX2–1. Chest 2013;**144**:794–804.

90. Wert SE, Whitsett JA, Nogee LM. Genetic disorders of surfactant dysfunction. Pediatr. Dev. Pathol. 2009;**12**:253–74.

91. Cutz E, Wert SE, Nogee LM, Moore AM. Deficiency of lamellar bodies in alveolar type II cells associated with fatal respiratory disease in a full-term infant. Am. J. Respir. Crit. Care Med. 2000;**161**:608–14.

92. Guillot L, Carre A, Szinnai G, *et al*. NKX2–1 mutations leading to surfactant protein promoter dysregulation cause interstitial lung disease in "Brain-Lung-Thyroid Syndrome". Hum. Mutat. 2010;**31**:E1146–62.

93. Gillett ES, Deutsch GH, Bamshad MJ, McAdams RM, Mann PC. Novel *NKX2.1* mutation associated with hypothyroidism and lethal respiratory failure in a full-term neonate. J. Perinatol. 2013;**33**:157–60.

94. Trapnell BC, Carey BC, Uchida K, Suzuki T. Pulmonary alveolar proteinosis, a primary immunodeficiency of impaired GM-CSF stimulation of macrophages. Curr. Opin. Immunol. 2009;**21**:514–21.

95. Parto K, Kallajoki M, Aho H, Simell O. Pulmonary alveolar proteinosis and glomerulonephritis in lysinuric protein intolerance: case reports and autopsy findings of four pediatric patients. Hum. Pathol. 1994;**25**:400–7.

96. Olivier KN, Weber DJ, Wallace RJ, Jr., *et al*. Nontuberculous mycobacteria. I: multicenter prevalence study in cystic fibrosis. Am. J. Respir. Crit. Care Med. 2003;**167**:828–34.

97. Rommens JM, Iannuzzi MC, Kerem B, *et al*. Identification of the cystic fibrosis gene: chromosome walking and jumping. Science 1989;**245**:1059–65.

98. Sheppard DN, Welsh MJ. Structure and function of the CFTR chloride channel. Physiol. Rev. 1999;**79**: S23–45.

99. Knowles MR, Daniels LA, Davis SD, Zariwala MA, Leigh MW. Primary ciliary dyskinesia. Recent advances in diagnostics, genetics, and characterization of clinical disease. Am. J. Respir. Crit. Care Med. 2013;**188**:913–22.

100. Jones VF, Eid NS, Franco SM, Badgett JT, Buchino JJ. Familial congenital bronchiectasis: Williams-Campbell syndrome. Pediatr. Pulmonol. 1993;**16**:263–7.

101. Morin FC, 3rd, Stenmark KR. Persistent pulmonary hypertension of the newborn. Am. J. Respir. Crit. Care Med. 1995;**151**:2010–32.

102. Haworth SG. Primary and secondary pulmonary hypertension in childhood: A clinicopathological reappraisal. Curr. Top. Pathol. 1983;**73**:91–152.

103. Murphy JD, Rabinovitch M, Goldstein JD, Reid LM. The structural basis of persistent pulmonary hypertension of the newborn infant. J. Pediatr. 1981;**98**:962–7.

104. Haworth SG, Hislop AA. Pulmonary vascular development: normal values of peripheral vascular structure. Am. J. Cardiol. 1983;**52**:578–83.

105. Hislop A, Reid L. Pulmonary arterial development during childhood: branching pattern and structure. Thorax 1973;**28**:129–35.

106. Stenmark KR, Fagan KA, Frid MG. Hypoxia-induced pulmonary vascular remodeling: cellular and molecular mechanisms. Circ. Res. 2006;**99**:675–91.

107. Faul JL, Berry GJ, Colby TV et al. Thoracic lymphangiomas, lymphangiectasis, lymphangiomatosis, and lymphatic dysplasia syndrome. Am. J. Respir. Crit. Care Med. 2000;**161**:1037–46.

108. Barker PM, Esther CR, Jr., Fordham LA, Maygarden SJ, Funkhouser WK. Primary pulmonary lymphangiectasia in infancy and childhood. Eur. Respir. J. 2004;**24**:413–9.

109. Esther CR, Jr., Barker PM. Pulmonary lymphangiectasia: diagnosis and clinical course. Pediatr. Pulmonol. 2004;**38**:308–13.

110. Moerman P, Van Geet C, Devlieger H. Lymphangiomatosis of the body wall: A report of two cases associated with chylothorax and fatal outcome. Pediatr. Pathol. Lab. Med. 1997;**17**:617–24.

111. Tazelaar HD, Kerr D, Yousem SA, Saldana MJ, Langston C, Colby TV. Diffuse pulmonary lymphangiomatosis. Hum. Pathol. 1993;**24**:1313–22.

112. Njolstad PR, Reigstad H, Westby J, Espeland A. Familial non-immune hydrops fetalis and congenital pulmonary lymphangiectasia. Eur. J. Pediatr. 1998;**157**:498–501.

113. Stevenson DA, Pysher TJ, Ward RM, Carey JC. Familial congenital non-immune hydrops, chylothorax, and pulmonary lymphangiectasia. Am. J. Med. Genet. A. 2006;**140**:368–72.

114. Soldatski IL, Onufrieva EK, Steklov AM, Schepin NV. Tracheal, bronchial, and pulmonary papillomatosis in children. Laryngoscope 2005;**115**:1848–54.

115. Freed GL, Derkay CS. Prevention of recurrent respiratory papillomatosis: role of HPV vaccination. Int. J. Pediatr. Otorhinolaryngol. 2006;**70**:1799–803.

116. Fletcher CDM, Bridge JA, Hogendoorn PCW, Mertens F, eds. *WHO Classification of Tumors of the Soft Tissue and Bone*, fourth edn. Lyon: WHO Press; 2013.

117. Siminovich M, Galluzzo L, Lopez J, Lubieniecki F, de Davila MT. Inflammatory myofibroblastic tumor of the lung in children: Anaplastic lymphoma kinase (ALK) expression and clinico-pathological correlation. Pediatr. Dev. Pathol. 2012;**15**:179–86.

118. Alaggio R, Cecchetto G, Bisogno G et al. Inflammatory myofibroblastic tumors in childhood: A report from the Italian Cooperative Group studies. Cancer 2010;**116**:216–26.

119. Dishop MK, McKay EM, Kreiger PA et al. Fetal lung interstitial tumor (FLIT): A proposed newly recognized lung tumor of infancy to be differentiated from cystic pleuropulmonary blastoma and other developmental pulmonary lesions. Am. J. Surg. Pathol. 2010;**34**:1762–72.

120. de Chadarevian JP, Liu J, Pezanowski D et al. Diagnosis of "Fetal lung interstitial tumor" requires a FISH negative for trisomies 8 and 2. Am. J. Surg. Pathol. 2011;**35**:1085; author reply 1086–7.

121. Hill DA, Jarzembowski JA, Priest JR, et al. Type I pleuropulmonary blastoma: pathology and biology study of 51 cases from the international pleuropulmonary blastoma registry. Am. J. Surg. Pathol. 2008;**32**:282–95.

122. Hill DA, Ivanovich J, Priest JR et al. DICER1 mutations in familial pleuropulmonary blastoma. Science 2009;**325**:965.

123. Priest JR, Williams GM, Hill DA, Dehner LP, Jaffe A. Pulmonary cysts in early childhood and the risk of malignancy. Pediatr. Pulmonol. 2009;**44**:14–30.

124. Cummings NM, Desai S, Thway K, et al. Cystic primary pulmonary synovial sarcoma presenting as recurrent pneumothorax: report of 4 cases. Am. J. Surg. Pathol. 2010;**34**:1176–9.

125. Askin FB, Rosai J, Sibley RK, Dehner LP, McAlister WH. Malignant small cell tumor of the thoracopulmonary region in childhood: A distinctive clinicopathologic entity of uncertain histogenesis. Cancer 1979;**43**:2438–51.

126. Whang-Peng J, Triche TJ, Knutsen T, et al. Cytogenetic characterization of selected small round-cell tumors of childhood. Cancer Genet. Cytogenet. 1986;**21**:185–208.

127. Yoshida A,Sekine S, Tsuta K, Fukayama M, Furuta K, Tsuda H. NKX2.2 is a useful immunohistochemical marker for Ewing sarcoma. Am. J. Surg. Pathol. 2012;**36**:993–9.

128. Folpe AL, Schmidt RA, Chapman D, Gown AM. Poorly differentiated synovial sarcoma: immunohistochemical distinction from primitive neuroectodermal tumors and high-grade malignant peripheral nerve sheath tumors. Am. J. Surg. Pathol. 1998;**22**:673–82.

Endocrine

María T. G. de Dávila, Laura Galluzzo, Derek de Sa, and Irene Scheimberg

The pituitary gland

The hypothalamo-hypophyseal axis plays a central role in endocrine control at all ages, and there are numerous instances where the function of this integrated system may be deranged. The diagnosis of the majority of these disease processes falls outside the realm of surgical pathology and this chapter will not attempt to discuss them.

There remain several conditions where the examination of surgical biopsy material from the pituitary and its immediate surrounds provides the cornerstone of diagnosis. The vast majority of pituitary lesions seen by surgical pathologists are tumors of the pituitary gland or of the adjacent suprasellar and parasellar regions that affect or even destroy the pituitary.

The pituitary lies in the sella turcica, a depression in the sphenoid bone below the hypothalamus and the base of the brain. Traditional light microscopy using hematoxylin and eosin (H&E) staining of the anterior pituitary gland delineated three main types of epithelial cells: acidophilic cells, basophilic cells, and chromophobes (cells with no proclivity for either type of stain).

In practical terms, good clinico-pathological correlation can be achieved in the vast majority of cases using: (a) light microscopy including the periodic acid–Schiff (PAS) stain; (b) immunohistochemistry with antibodies raised against the adenohypophyseal hormones (prolactin, adrenocorticotrophin, growth hormone, thryrotrophin, follicle-stimulating hormone, luteinizing hormone, and the glycoprotein-α subunit); and (c) electron microscopy.

Five main secretory cell types are recognized in the anterior pituitary: somatotrophs, lactotrophs, corticotrophs, gonadotrophs (cells which produce both follicle-stimulating and luteinizing hormone), and thyrotrophs. With traditional H&E staining, the somatotrophs and lactotrophs are acidophilic (eosinophilic), while the others are basophilic. Variable degrees of degranulation are responsible for the appearance of the chromophobes on routine microscopy.

Other cells within the adenohypophysis include specialized folliculo-stellate cells that express glial fibrillary acidic protein (GFAP), S100 protein, vimentin, and keratin. Other non-granulated cells produce nestin (1).

The neurohypophysis is made up of the infundibular eminence, the infundibular stem (pituitary stalk), and the pars nervosa (posterior pituitary). The infundibular stem (pituitary stalk) carries the long axons and the long vessels of the hypothalamo-hypophyseal portal system. The pars nervosa contains the terminal areas of the axons, the short hypothalamo-hypophyseal vessels, and specialized glial cells called pituicytes.

The axons of the magnocellular neurons carry oxytocin and vasopressin by axonal transport to the pars nervosa. The parvicellular neurons are linked to the release of the trophic hormones that are passed into the long hypothalamo-hypophyseal portal vessels and exert their effects on the cells of the adenohypophysis. The anatomical location of the pituitary gland is responsible for many of the clinical manifestations associated with a pituitary lesion.

Congenital anomalies of the pituitary

The majority of the congenital pituitary anomalies are of no concern for the surgical pathologist, except for *remnants of Rathke's pouch* within the cranium and along its migration. Small nodules of adenohypophyseal tissue have been described as incidental findings in the pharynx in many normal patients at all ages. They are derived from remnants of Rathke's pouch, and are rarely symptomatic. The exact incidence of the finding is not clear, because the lesion is located high in the nasopharynx, between the vomer and the sphenoid bone. All cell types common to the adenohypophysis have been identified, and the remnant may even be the site for an adenoma. Usually these adenohypophyseal foci are non-functioning, but the removal of a pharyngeal mass, in an otherwise normal child, which proved to be an ectopic pharyngeal pituitary was followed by the development of hypopituitarism (2,3).

Duplication of the pituitary gland is exceptionally rare, but may accompany nasopharyngeal teratoma or oral dermoids with callosal agenesis, and may be associated with precocious puberty (1).

Cysts of the sellar and parasellar area

Rathke's pouch cysts are small cystic structures between the adenohypophysis and neurohypophysis and are very frequent at all ages (1). These are usually incidental findings, but in a few patients the remnant of Rathke's pouch enlarges to form a cyst of sufficient size to become symptomatic and cause hypopituitarism (4). These cysts are filled with mucinous colloid, and the lining epithelium may have the same characteristics as the interglandular cleft lining (mucinous, cuboidal, or columnar cells with variable numbers of ciliated cells).

The sellar and parasellar region may be the site for *dermoid cysts* and *epidermal cysts*. Clinically they are very similar, and are discrete, slow-growing lesions. The lesions are identical to those in the skin. Most of these cysts are asymptomatic, but if large enough they may cause symptoms in the same manner as the craniopharyngioma (see Chapter 13).

Tumors of the adenohypophysis

Adenomas of the adenohypophysis are rare in prepubertal children, but become more frequent in adolescents and young adults. In children, the majority of the adenomas are functional (5–9; see also Chapter 13).

The first task for the surgical pathologist is to decide whether an adenoma is present or not. This can be very difficult if only small fragments are available, the only true indicator of an adenoma is the monomorphic cell population and the lack of any acinar pattern, in contrast to the mixed cell population and well-defined acinar nature of the normal gland. Reticulin preparations are sometimes very helpful in making the distinction between the normal gland and the adenomas.

The types of adenomas seen in the pediatric age group do not differ from those seen in adults. In some

studies adrenocorticotrophin (ACTH)-producing adenomas presented at an earlier age than other adenomas. Several of them may produce more than one hormone, particularly with prolactin being co-produced with ACTH. This was more likely to be seen in macroadenomas (Figure 6.1).

Microadenomas are intraglandular, < 10 mm in maximum dimension, and by definition do not have any suprasellar extension. Macroadenomas are > 10 mm and are more varied in their disposition. They may elevate the sella diaphragm or may have suprasellar extension and may invade adjacent structures. Invasiveness may be "localized" erosive invasion of the sella, or "diffuse" with invasion of bony structures outside the sella turcica (5). In children, plurihormonal tumors are usually macroadenomas (5). Microadenomas are associated with Cushing's disease (7; Figure 6.2).

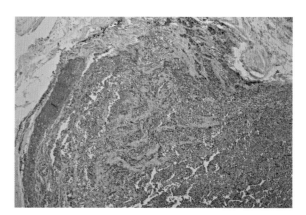

Figure 6.1 Pituitary basophilic adenoma extending outside the confines of the gland capsule. Compressed non-tumoral gland is seen on the right (H&E × 20).

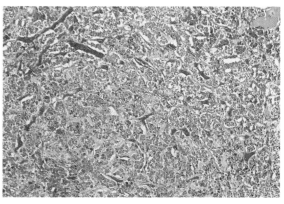

Figure 6.2 Pituitary microadenoma in a 15-year-old with Cushing's disease (H&E × 20).

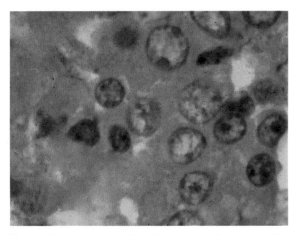

Figure 6.3 Prolactinoma with nucleoli in nuclei of varying size. This is not a definitive indicator of aggressiveness (H&E × 60).

The usual histological criteria that predict aggressiveness (mitotic activity, nuclear pleomorphism, cellularity, hemorrhage, necrosis) are of limited use in pituitary neoplasms, since they may all be present in tumors that behave in a slow-growing, non-aggressive fashion (Figure 6.3). The best method of judging aggressiveness in pituitary lesions is the use of immunohistochemical markers against antigens expressed in proliferating cells (Ki-67), replicating cells (proliferating cell nuclear antigen (PCNA)), or mutant tumor-suppressor genes (p53) (10,11). p53 is expressed in the more invasive adenomas and all of the extremely rare carcinomas of the pituitary. Fortunately, carcinoma arising in the pituitary of children is unknown. Proliferating cell nuclear antigen (PCNA) staining is technically more difficult, but PCNA positivity was seen in adenomas with extension outside the sella (12).

Adenomas made up of acidophilic cells may produce growth hormone, prolactin, or both, or be clinically silent. An adenoma made up of basophilic cells and secreting ACTH is the classic lesion associated with Cushing's disease, and with the less well-recognized Nelson syndrome (basophil adenomas developing or progressing after bilateral adrenalectomy for Cushing's disease). Many adenomas associated with Cushing's disease in children are microadenomas (7), while those of Nelson's syndrome are usually macroadenomas, and more aggressive (6).

It has been assessed that as many as 5% of all adenomas may be familial (8) and that this may be associated with an earlier age of presentation and more aggressive tumors. Pituitary tumors may be triggered by increased signaling of the *Wingless (Wnt)* gene (13).

Plurihormonal adenomas occurred in 9 of 36 pediatric patients reported from the Mayo Clinic (5). Plurihormonal tumors were usually macroadenomas. The combination includes somatotrophs with varying numbers of lactotrophs and gonadotrophs. Apart from the somatotrophic effect, the other hormones are not usually expressed.

Adenomas of the adenohypophysis are part of the multiple endocrine neoplasia I syndrome (MEN I syndrome), which has been mapped to 11q.13 (14). The adenomas may be of all types, especially prolactinomas and somatotrophic tumors, but plurihormonal adenomas may occur as well. The lesions are large (macroadenomas) and aggressive, and the pituitary adenoma can precede the other manifestations of the syndrome (15). Pituitary adenomas may also form part of the Carney complex, or be associated with familial acromegaly, and McCune–Albright syndrome (16,17). A growing body of information is becoming available regarding germline mutations in aryl-hydrocarbon receptor-interacting protein (AIP), as well as in a variety of other genetic syndromes (18,19).

So-called "collision" tumors of the pituitary region refer to two separate simultaneously occurring lesions interacting in the pituitary area; they are not common. The commonest combinations would appear to be the co-existence of a Rathke's cleft cyst with an adenoma. Less frequent is the association of an adenoma with a craniopharyngioma (20,21).

Secondary involvement of the pituitary by parasellar lesions

The pituitary is prone to be damaged by a large variety of other intracranial lesions, including intracranial germ-cell tumors (22), gliomas of the optic chiasm and hypothalamus, chordomas (arising from the adjacent clivus), as well as infiltrative lesions like Langerhans-cell histiocytosis, lymphocytic hypophysitis (23), and leukemia. This incomplete list is provided solely as a reminder that not all symptomatology that points to the pituitary is necessarily due to a primary lesion of the gland (see Chapter 13).

Tumors of the neurohypophysis

In children, as in adults, primary tumors (gliomas) of the neurohypophysis are uncommon and neurohypophyseal damage is seen in relation to infiltrative gliomas arising in the hypothalamus or optic chiasma, and infiltrative processes such as Langerhans-cell histiocytosis, lymphocytic hypophysitis, and sarcoidosis. Destruction is also seen with craniopharyngiomas. There is usually destruction of the adenohypophysis as well, and the patients present with diabetes insipidus.

A rare lesion that may be found near the neurohypophysis is the hypothalamic neuronal hamartoma (24). The lesion, which is attached to the ventral hypothalamus, is made up of mature neurons with axons and relatively few scattered glial cells. Some tumors have been associated with precocious puberty in boys. This lesion should be distinguished from the hypothalamic hamartoblastoma of the Pallister–Hall syndrome (25), a lesion of the neonatal period, which, although it destroys the gland, is not a problem in surgical pathology.

The thyroid gland

The thyroid gland, the first major endocrine gland to develop in the fetus, is functional *in utero*, and plays an important role in thermogenesis in the newborn. Normally the thyroglossal duct is resorbed by 7-weeks' gestation, but its persistence, in whole or part in many fetuses, infants, children, and even adults, is the source of several significant lesions that confront the surgeon. The caudal remnant of the duct may be seen in the pyramidal lobe, which is attached to the isthmus of the fully formed gland. What was initially a midline structure assumes the configuration of a paired, bilobar gland connected by an isthmus.

Developmental disorders

Dysgenesis of the thyroid is a generic designation for anomalies in the development of the gland, from complete failure in formation (*agenesis*) to absence of a lobe (*hemiagenesis*). In 50% of patients with left hemiagenesis, an absent thyroid isthmus is also found (26). Absence of the thyroid isthmus and sometimes part of a lobe may form part of the DiGeorge (III–IVth pharyngeal pouch) sequence (27). While parafollicular cells may be reduced in these cases, the presence of some "C" cells is suggestive that they can be derived from thyroid endodermal precursors (28).

Heterotopic thyroid glands are rare; in 90% of the cases the thyroid is found at the base of the tongue (*lingual thyroid*). However, it may be placed in any location from the foramen cecum to the mediastinum (29).

A *thyroglossal duct cyst (TDC)* results from the failure of the thyroglossal duct to undergo obliteration

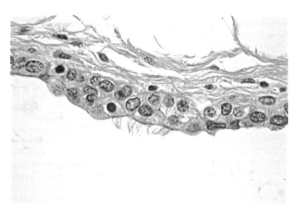

Figure 6.4 Thyroglossal duct cyst lining (H&E × 40).

during fetal life. These cysts usually present as a midline mass, but a minority of TDCs can be located along the course of the duct, including the base of the tongue, the floor of the mouth, or within the thyroid itself (29). Most TDCs are diagnosed at or before five years of age. The hyoid bone should accompany the surgical specimen. Microscopically, non-inflamed cysts are lined by columnar-to-cuboidal epithelium with cilia (Figure 6.4); pseudostratified and non-keratinizing squamous epithelium may be present. Fibrosis and chronic inflammation are usually present, and thyroid remnants are seen in 20% or less of TDC. In rare cases, the thyroid tissue may undergo malignant transformation, papillary carcinoma being the most common histological type (30; see also Chapter 4).

Heterotopias of normal tissues in the thyroid include parathyroid, salivary glands, and thymus.

Branchial pouch anomalies (BPAs) may present as a patent fistula, a simple sinus, a blind cyst, or an island of cartilage (see also Chapter 4). Those related to the first pouch appear in the preauricular area or beneath the posterior half of the mandible; one-third of them are located in the area of the parotid gland (31). The lining of these lesions is usually squamous epithelium, but columnar ciliated epithelium is also common. These BPAs may also have adnexal skin structures, and abundant lymphoid tissue is observed beneath.

The anomalies related to the second pouch are the most common; they are sited in the mid-neck, anterior to the sternocleidomastoid muscle. Those related to the third and fourth pouch are rare, they are found in the lower neck, supra- or infraclavicular. They usually present as an inflammatory neck mass, almost always involving the thyroid gland (32). These cysts may also contain mucinous, seromucinous, and sebaceous glands. Secondary infection may obscure the histological picture.

When the thyroid exhibits an epithelial-lined cyst with an associated lymphoid component, the lesion is called *lymphoepithelial cyst*.

Autoimmune-associated inflammatory conditions

Chronic lymphocytic thyroiditis (CLT), commonly diagnosed in children and *Hashimoto thyroiditis (HT)*, a disease of women over 40 years of age, represent different phases of the same disorder. Diagnosis is based on clinical and biochemical manifestations (33). Fine needle aspiration (FNA) is recommended to rule out a possible neoplasm and surgical resection is only reserved for selected circumstances. Grossly, the thyroid is generally symmetrically enlarged, may be vaguely nodular in CLT and could have a multinodular quality in HT.

Histologically, the common feature in these entities is the extensive lymphocytic infiltration of the gland associated with germinal center formation. Follicles are generally small and uniform in CLT, while in HT they are small, atrophic, and lined by Hürthle or oncocytic cells. Sometimes, optically clear nuclei similar to those seen in papillary carcinoma are present. Complications of HT include papillary carcinoma and much less commonly follicular carcinoma, lymphoma, Hürthle cell neoplasms, and others (33,34).

Graves' disease (diffuse toxic hyperplasia/goiter) may be associated with McCune–Albright syndrome. Diagnosis is based on clinical and biochemical manifestations of hyperthyroidism. Grossly, the gland shows diffuse enlargement.

Histologically, the follicles are hyperplastic, with prominent papillary infoldings, which unlike papillary carcinoma, lack fibrovascular cores. The epithelium is columnar, nuclei are basally located, and have a clear or microvacuolated cytoplasm. Some oncocytic cells may be present. The colloid is pale and has prominent scalloped margins. The stroma contains aggregates of lymphoid tissue with germinal center formation. There is a lower incidence of thyroid carcinoma than in HT (35–37).

Thyroid hyperplasia (goiter)

Enlargement of the thyroid – goiter – is the most common manifestation of thyroid disease. Goiters

can be: (1) endemic, which is secondary to low iodine content in the water and soil, or (2) sporadic, secondary to a number of conditions, including enzymatic defects and intake of substances which interfere with thyroid hormone synthesis. In children, a sporadic goiter caused by a congenital biosynthetic defect may cause cretinism.

Simple goiter is defined as gland enlargement (nodular or diffuse), ≥ 40 g, without evidence of hyperthyroidism. Simple goiter eventually evolves with time into multinodular goiter (≥ 100 g), which means an irregular enlargement of the thyroid due to repeated episodes of hyperplasia and involution. Some cases initially diagnosed as simple goiter in children may develop positive thyroid antibodies after some years, with the diagnosis changing to CLT (38).

Histologically, the simple goiter shows a diffuse enlargement with follicles of varying size, flattened epithelium, and formation of colloid cysts. Smaller follicles have a more columnar epithelium, lined by crowded columnar cells, which may form papillary projections similar to those seen in Graves' disease. Multinodular goiter may resemble a neoplasm with multiple variable-sized follicular nodules. Some follicles are lined by flattened epithelium, some are hyperplastic, and others may be mostly composed of Hürthle cells. Dilated follicles may have a conglomerate of small active follicles at one pole, so-called Sanderson's polsters (Figure 6.5).

Degenerative changes such as scarring, hemorrhage, calcifications, and cystic changes may be present. Rupture of dilated follicles with a colloid leak may lead

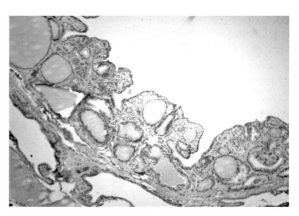

Figure 6.5 Sanderson polsters made up of clusters of follicles projecting into a cystic area of a nodular goiter. Note the rounded nature of the follicles in the polster and the elongated elliptical shape of the follicles at the base of the polster (H&E × 20).

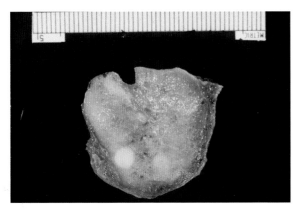

Figure 6.6 Dyshormonogenic goiter in a 15-year-old patient.

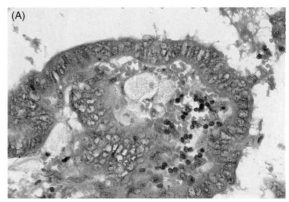

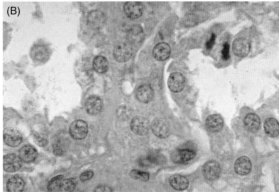

Figure 6.7 (a) Histology shows blunt papillary projections lined by cuboidal cells (H&E × 20); (b) at higher power, cuboidal cells with a rare mitotic figure (H&E × 40).

to a granulomatous reaction. The distinction between an adenoma and a hyperplastic nodule is a problem in any endocrine organ and nowhere more so than in the thyroid. Useful points of distinction are: (1) the fact that inflammatory changes within the nodule favor the likelihood of the nodule being hyperplastic; (2) the presence of Sanderson's polsters and blunt papillary projections within dilated follicles are indicative of a hyperplastic nodule; and (3) smaller nodules of similar histologic appearance are present in the remainder of the gland away from the main nodule. Adenomas are encapsulated with a relatively homogeneous appearance on the cut surface, lack the usual lobulated appearance of nodular hyperplasia, and collapsed and compressed acini of a different histologic appearance are seen around the nodule (39). Needless to say, many of these features may not be seen in FNA biopsies, and in some cases it may be impossible to make the distinction.

Dyshormonogenic goiters are due to abnormalities in the synthesis and metabolism of thyroid hormones (Figure 6.6). Most of these are inherited as autosomal recessive conditions, but they are a very heterogeneous group of defects related to synthesis of thyroglobulin, and some are inherited in an autosomal dominant fashion (40). The pathology of the gland in these disorders can be very striking, especially in older patients who have a deiodination defect (41). There are multiple hyperplastic nodules within the gland with variable reduction of colloid, closely packed aggregates of follicles, variable cystic change, and even papillary formations. Cellular pleomorphism and nuclear hyperchromatism tend to be worrying histologic features (Figure 6.7).

Neoplasms of the thyroid

Thyroid cancer is the most common endocrine malignancy in pediatric patients. Age at diagnosis is usually between 10 and 18 years. Females have a higher incidence than males. Radiation therapy and multiple endocrine neoplasia (MEN), are associated with an increased incidence of thyroid malignancy. Twenty-five years after the nuclear fallout of Chernobyl, data indicate that thyroid cancer in children has dramatically increased in the area. The histology distribution in those (pediatric) residents is the same as in the general population, although some isolated cases were anaplastic carcinoma, or mixed types of tumor (medullary/follicular and papillary/anaplastic). Even though the clinical presentation in many cases was severe, after 20 years, all children were alive except one (42).

Neoplasms are also more likely to happen in patients with a family history of thyroid cancer or HT (43). Compared to adults, thyroid nodules in children

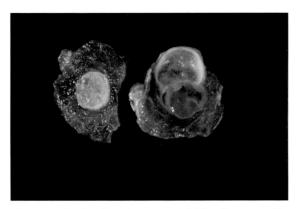

Figure 6.8 Papillary thyroid carcinoma. Left lobe of a 14-year-old girl's thyroid showing a partially cystic, clearly demarcated nodular lesion. MEN-1 associated tumors in family members.

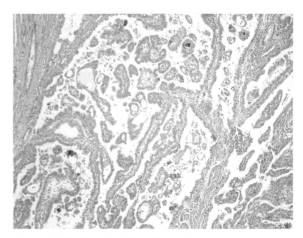

Figure 6.9 Papillary thyroid carcinoma showing a classic pattern with slender papillary projections and a few psammoma bodies (H&E × 10).

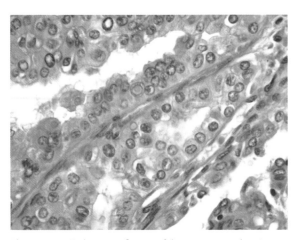

Figure 6.10 Higher magnification of the same tumor showing nuclear pseudoinclusions (H&E × 40).

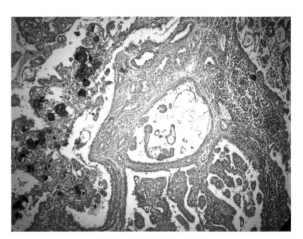

Figure 6.11 Papillary thyroid carcinoma showing numerous psammoma bodies and a germinal center (H&E × 20).

have an increased risk of being malignant (44). Fine needle aspiration is useful for preoperative planning, if the lesion is identified as papillary, but the lesion may be identified as benign, indeterminate, or follicular. Follicular lesions cannot be differentiated as benign or malignant by this method, as it cannot assess capsular invasion. Accuracy of FNA is very sensitive for the diagnosis of thyroid carcinomas in children (45).

Papillary thyroid carcinoma (PTC) is the most common neoplasia in children and has an excellent prognosis (46). The lesion may be solitary or multifocal and some tumors can be well circumscribed and even encapsulated (Figure 6.8).

Histologically, the tumor is diagnosed based on architectural and especially cytological features. In the most common architectural pattern numerous true and complex papillae with dense fibrovascular

cores are easily recognized (Figure 6.9). The epithelium is cuboidal, either simple or stratified. Associated tubular or branching follicles are almost always present. Cytological features include overcrowded ground-glass nuclei, optically clear nuclei (only evident in formalin-fixed tissue), irregular nuclear contours, nuclear grooves, and intranuclear cytoplasmic inclusions (present in fixed tissue, cytology, and frozen sections) (Figure 6.10). Squamous metaplasia is a common feature in children. The presence of psammoma bodies is a very helpful clue to diagnosis (Figure 6.11). The *follicular* variant of PTC is composed entirely or almost entirely of follicles, and the diagnosis is based on nuclear features, the invasive pattern of growth and psammoma bodies. The *solid variant of PTC* is a tumor with nuclear features of papillary carcinoma, but with

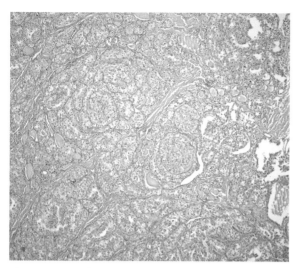

Figure 6.12 Papillary thyroid carcinoma showing a solid pattern (H&E × 10).

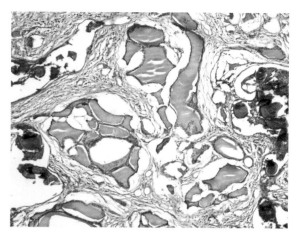

Figure 6.13 Papillary thyroid carcinoma diffuse sclerosing variant showing typical dense fibrosis and psammoma bodies (H&E × 20).

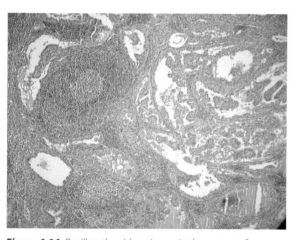

Figure 6.14 Papillary thyroid carcinoma in the context of Hashimoto thyroiditis (H&E × 20).

a solid pattern of growth. These tumors are particularly more common in children, especially those exposed to radiation (Figure 6.12) and account for approximately 25% of PTC.

The *oncocytic (oxyphilic) variant* of *PTC* has lining cells with abundant eosinophilic and granular cytoplasm. The pattern may be papillary or follicular, and the tumor may be encapsulated. An oncocytic tumor with a heavy infiltrate of lymphocytes in the stroma of the papillae is called Warthin-like tumor of the thyroid and is associated with an excellent prognosis. The typical nuclear features of PTC must be present.

When conventional PTC or its follicular variant have clear cells with typical nuclear features it is called

the *clear-cell variant.* Alcian-blue-positive mucin is occasionally seen.

The *diffuse sclerosing variant* tends to occur in young patients, without forming a dominant mass. Dense fibrosis replaces the gland and may extend to the surrounding soft tissues. The presence of numerous psammoma bodies, squamous metaplasia, dense lymphocytic infiltration, and stromal fibrosis is characteristic (Figure 6.13). The remnant thyroidal parenchyma may show features of chronic lymphocytic thyroiditis and patients have serologic evidence of autoimmune thyroid disease (Figure 6.14). Papillary thyroid carcinoma may occur as part of MEN-1 (47) and other familial cancer syndromes (48).

Follicular neoplasms of the thyroid

Follicular adenomas (FAs) may present sporadically in children as part of nodular goiters or in dyshormonogenesis. FA is usually a solitary nodule, which measures 1–3 cm, but may be larger. The tumor has a delicate continuous or interrupted fibrous capsule of variable thickness. The capsule separates relatively monotonous follicular architecture from the more variably sized follicles of the surrounding thyroid tissue. The cells are cuboidal or columnar, with uniform, dark round nuclei. Mitotic figures are rare. Secondary changes (stromal edema, calcification, cyst formation, etc.) may be found. By definition, no capsular or vascular invasion is present. This main feature emphasizes the importance of an adequate sampling of any suspicious tumor.

Follicular carcinomas (FCs) rarely occur in children (49). The frequency has decreased since the recognition

205

of the follicular variant of PTC. Follicular carcinomas have a thick circumscribed fibrous capsule with transcapsular invasion. Minimally invasive FCs have limited capsular and/or vascular invasion (grossly indistinguishable from FA). Widely invasive FCs have widespread infiltration of adjacent thyroid tissue and/or blood vessels. Capsular invasion is defined by mushroom-like tumor penetration through the capsule – not associated with the site of a previous FNA biopsy. Vascular invasion is defined by the presence of intravascular tumoral cells covered by endothelium or associated with a thrombus. The involved vessel must be within or beyond the tumor capsule. The probability of aggressive behavior increases with the extent of vascular invasion (50).

Histologically, the tumor cells lack the typical nuclear features of PTC, showing a wide range of patterns, from well-formed colloid-containing follicles to solid or trabecular growth. Nuclei are usually round to oval with granular chromatin.

Follicular tumors may be seen in Cowden syndrome (51), after pleuropulmonary blastoma treatment, or as part of familial cancer syndromes.

There are some histological variants, such as oncocytic/oxyphilic/Hürthle-cell carcinoma. Although this variant is very rare in childhood, the authors have seen one after radiation therapy of a medullobastoma. The nuclei in the oncocytic form tend to be hyperchromatic with prominent single nucleoli (Figure 6.15).

Unlike PTC, follicular carcinomas only uncommonly involve regional lymph nodes. The most common sites of distant metastases are lung and bone. Minimally invasive FCs have an excellent prognosis (3–5% mortality). Widely invasive FCs, however, have a long-term mortality approaching 50%.

Medullary thyroid carcinoma (MTC) This is a carcinoma with C-cell differentiation and represents a neuroendocrine neoplasm of the thyroid. MTC accounts for 5–10% of all thyroid tumors. Approximately 75% of MTC are sporadic. The remaining ones are heritable, caused by germline mutations in the *RET* proto-oncogen, in the setting of MEN type 2 (A and B) and familial MTC, with an autosomal dominant mode of inheritance (52).

The clinical presentation of MTC strongly depends on the familial/sporadic nature of the tumor. Mean age at presentation is 50 years in sporadic forms, but when associated with MEN-2A the usual age is the third decade of life, and MTC occurring in MEN-2B usually presents in infancy or childhood. Virtually all thyroids in the setting of MEN-2A, MEN-2B, and familiar MTC have at least microscopic multifocal C-cell hyperplasia (53).

Patients have elevated serum calcitonin levels, which have become an important marker to determine the presence of residual tumor or metastases. Grossly, MTC is a well-circumscribed, but not encapsulated tumor. Familial tumors are characteristically multifocal and bilateral.

Histology (Figure 6.16) shows several patterns, from compact solid-rounded nests to lobular, insular, or trabecular profiles. Tumor cells may be spindle or rounded and the polygonal nuclei usually have fine chromatin and prominent nucleoli. Many variants have been described: papillary, plasmacytoid, glandular, spindle cell, small cell, pigmented, etc. Mitotic activity is not brisk. Small psammoma-like concretions may be seen. The tumor usually infiltrates the

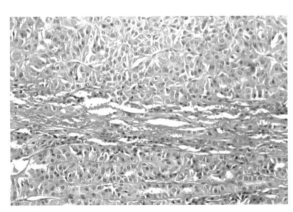

Figure 6.15 Hürtle-cell carcinoma showing a trabecular pattern and absent colloid (H&E × 40).

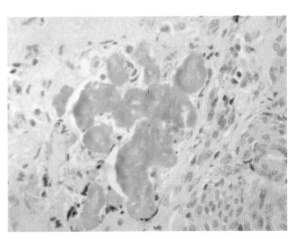

Figure 6.16 Medullary thyroid carcinoma showing a small amyloid deposit staining positive with Congo red (× 40).

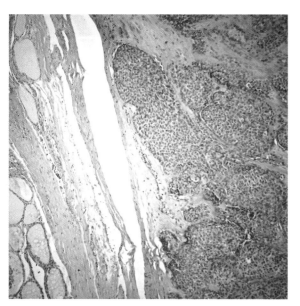

Figure 6.17 Medullary thyroid carcinoma showing an insular pattern and irregular interface between the tumor and the adjacent thyroid (H&E × 20).

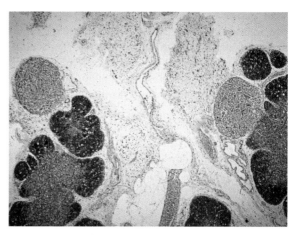

Figure 6.18 Paired ectopic parathyroid glands near the tongues of the thymic primordium within the anterior mediastinum. An incidental finding at autopsy in an infant of 27-weeks' gestation (H&E × 10).

surrounding thyroid tissue and lacks a true capsule (54). Larger tumors may exhibit fibrous bands and amyloid stroma (Figure 6.17). Immunohistochemistry shows positivity for calcitonin, synaptophysin, chromogranin-A, and CEA, but is negative for thyroglobulin (55). S100-positive sustentacular cells may occur at the periphery of the nests.

The tumor is very aggressive and prophylactic thyroidectomy is recommended in MEN-2 patients. The surgery depends basically on the *RET* codon mutation involved. Carriers of mutations in extracellular *RET* codons 634, 620, 618, and 609 should be operated on before five years of age. Preventive thyroidectomy at three years of age is recommended for germline mutations in codon 634. Individuals carrying mutations in intracellular *RET* codons, such as 804, should undergo total thyroidectomy before the age of 10 years. Carriers with the *RET 918* mutation (MEN-2B), should be operated on by six months of age (56).

Undifferentiated (anaplastic) carcinoma is an extremely aggressive malignant tumor of the elderly and will not be discussed.

The parathyroid glands

Calcium is very closely regulated in all species studied, and the parathyroid glands are essential for proper calcium regulation and metabolism. However,

parathyroid disorders are uncommon and the lesions that are of greatest interest to surgeons and surgical pathologists are those relating to primary hyperparathyroidism, namely adenomas and hyperplasia of the glands (57). Numerically, there are more patients with secondary hyperparathyroidism related to renal disease and hypocalcemia from a multitude of causes. Hyperplasia of the parathyroid glands is common in such a setting, and since the histological features of hyperplastic glands are the same, irrespective of cause, clinico-pathological correlation is critical.

There are many sites where parathyroid tissue may be found (58). This anomalous distribution of ectopic glands is easily understood, when the migratory routes of the glands are recalled. The parathyroid glands may be found within the substance of the thyroid and/or thymus, or within the submucosa of the esophagus or hypopharynx (59). The carotid artery's sheath may also be the site of a heterotopic parathyroid (60). There are other less frequently reported sites of heterotopic parathyroid glands, including the axilla and a single report in the vagina (61).

The number of glands may vary. The glands are paired and usually symmetrically situated in most patients, even in some ectopic glands (1); (Figure 6.18). Heterotopia is, by definition, not a symmetrical process. The exact size of the gland at different ages is uncertain, but glands larger than 1 cm in any dimension are unlikely to be normal at any age (57).

Supernumerary glands probably arise from splitting of developing primordia by vascular bundles, and the term parathyromatosis has been coined to describe supernumerary glands along the course of migration of the glands (62). The supernumerary glands have sometimes been strung out like a string of pearls.

Several genes interact in the development of parathyroid glands and the thymus. Mutations, either singly or in combination, may lead to ectopia, hypoplasia, or even absence of one or both glands. The genes identified include *Hox3a*, *Pax1*, *Eya 1*(on 8q13.3), and *Six-1*(chromosome 14q23) (63, 64). *Eya 1* mutations are implicated in branchio-oto-renal dysplasia, but somewhat surprisingly parathyroidism appears to be absent (65).

Each parathyroid gland has a delicate capsule, and a very vascular stroma, giving it a brown–red color in pediatric patients. The gland is made up of closely packed lobules of epithelial cells, with a vascular stroma surrounded by loose fibrous tissue. The parathyroid gland in neonates does not have significant numbers of intraglandular fat cells, oxyphilic (oncocytic) cells or follicles. These features appear with increasing age, starting with the appearance of fat cells in the late stages of the first decade, oxyphilic oncocytic cells in adolescence, and colloid follicles in adults (66, 67).

The fetal parathyroid gland is known to be active, as shown by the development of hyperparathyroidism in infants of mothers with hypoparathyroidism (68), backed by a multiplicity of reports outlining a close inter-relationship between maternal calcium homeostasis and fetal parathyroid hormone levels (69–72).

Cystic lesions associated with the parathyroid

Cysts of normally located parathyroid glands may be encountered and they may be confused with thyroid cysts, particularly since they are non-functional in the majority of cases (73, 74). Some may contain parathyroid hormone in the cyst fluid; compressed chief cells are present in at least part of the wall of the cyst. These probably represent remnants of the branchial clefts. Parathyroid cysts have been described in the mediastinum (75).

The parathyroid glands or supernumerary glands may be part of the wall of a thymic duct cyst. This lesion of the lower part of the neck may be clinically mistaken for a branchial cleft cyst (76). Thymic remnants may be seen in some cysts and it may be debated as to whether the primary lesion is of thymic or parathyroid origin. Given the complex nature of the ontogenetic development of the parathyroid gland, the distinction may be impossible to make.

Hemorrhage into an adenoma may, rarely, produce a cystic lesion, or be associated with a parathyroid crisis (77).

Primary hyperparathyroidism

Adenomas and hyperplasia of the parathyroid glands are the main lesions associated with primary hyperparathyroidism in children, as they are in adults. In the pediatric population, carcinomas of the parathyroid are, fortunately, excessively rare, but do exist, sometimes in ectopically located glands (78–81)

Parathyroid adenomas

In children with primary hyperparathyroidism, adenomas are far commoner than hyperplasia (82). The distinction between an adenoma and hyperplasia is at least as difficult in children as it is in adults. Fat is not a feature of the gland in preadolescents and this feature cannot be used as a distinction between the two. The size of the individual glands and their total combined weight may be of use: under the age of 20 years the combined weight of the glands should not exceed 100 mg (83).

For the surgical pathologist there are no true differences seen between the patterns of adenomas in children when compared to adults. Chief-cell adenomas are the main variety encountered and, within some tumors, occasional water clear cells may be encountered. Oxyphil nodules or collections are not features of lesions in prepubertal children, but are occasionally present in the post pubertal age groups. Adenomas are usually solitary. The adenomas may involve any parathyroid tissue, irrespective of location, and ectopic adenomas are seen especially within the anterior mediastinum.

In any adenoma, occasional nucleomegaly may be encountered in some cells, and occasional mitoses may also be seen (Figure 6.19). These should not be interpreted as evidence of malignancy in the absence of invasion outside the capsule (84).

A parathyroid adenoma leading to hyperparathyroidism with the probable production of an aberrant

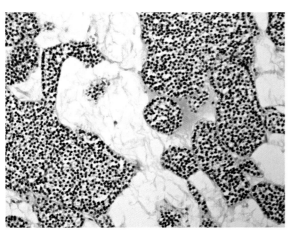

Figure 6.19 Chief-cell adenoma of parathyroid gland with a trabecular and solid pattern. This child had MEN I, confirmed by molecular studies (H&E × 40).

parathyroid hormone molecule that could not be detected with the usual assays has been reported in a child (85).

Parathyroid hyperplasia

There are many causes of secondary hyperparathyroidism in children, especially renal disease, malabsorption, vitamin-D-deficient rickets, and osteomalacia. Renal disease is by far the commonest cause of diffuse parathyroid gland hyperplasia; in children it leads to osetodystrophy (86, 87). The hyperplasia, by definition, affects all parathyroid tissue, and theoretically it should be easy to distinguish between a discrete adenoma and diffuse hyperplasia of all four glands. This is not always the case, and while a clearly enlarged gland may be easy to diagnose as an adenoma, the distinction can often be very difficult. Many cases of parathyroid hyperplasia seem to have a familial pattern, and there are examples of familial syndromes that may have hyperplasia or adenoma formation.

All cell types may be encountered, including chief-cell hyperplasia, water clear cells, and even oxyphilic nodules within chief-cell adenomas.

Neonatal primary hyperparathyroidism, a potentially fatal disease, is associated with an inactivating homozygous mutation in the calcium-sensing receptor (CaSR) and chief cell-hyperplasia of the parathyroid glands. Surgical removal of nearly all parathyroid tissue is the treatment of choice; a recent report

outlines some success with calcimimetic therapy after surgery for removal of hyperplastic glands (88). Interestingly, cases of familial neonatal hyperparathyroidism are homozygous for the CaSR mutation, while cases of familial benign hypercalcemia (familial hypocalciuric hypercalcemia) are heterozygous with no major morbidity (89).

Parathyroid disease is very often part of a number of complex MEN syndromes (90–92). The lesions seen within the gland may be either hyperplasia or adenoma. While there is often good correlation of phenotype with genotype, there are some cases with unusual combinations of lesions. *Classic MEN-1* is associated with inactivating mutations of the MEN-1 gene that maps to chromosome 11q.13 (93–95). The gene codes for a 610-amino-acid protein (menin) that is probably involved in DNA replication and repair, and transcriptional machinery. The disease is characterized by the presence of tumors of the parathyroid, anterior pituitary, and endocrine pancreas (the three "p"s). "Sporadic" cases have two or more tumors, while "familial" cases are defined as having at least one first-degree relative of a patient with MEN-1 who has one of the characteristic endocrine tumors. Other tumors that may be seen in these patients include carcinoid tumors, angiofibromas, collagenomas, lipomas, and meningiomas, with a combination of up to 20 endocrine and non-endocrine tumors.

MEN-2 is associated with a germline mutation in the *RET* proto-oncogene located on chromosome 10q.11.2, with overlap with genes of neurofibromatosis-1 and von Hippel–Lindau disease. The three main tumor components are MTC, pheochromocytoma, and parathyroid disease. There are three subtypes, MEN-2A (Sipple's syndrome), MEN-2B, and familial MTC. Medullary thyroid carcinoma presents with all three subtypes and the likelihood of medullary thyroid carcinoma in MEN-2 syndromes is almost 100% (96,97). Differences are seen between the two subtypes. Patients with MEN-2A have cutaneous lichen amyloidosis, and clinically significant hyperparathyroidism that may be due to either hyperplasia or adenoma (98). Patients with MEN-2B have marfanoid habitus, mucosal neuromas of the tongue, lips, and conjunctiva, and diffuse gastrointestinal tract ganglioneuromas (99). MEN-2B is less frequent than MEN-2A but tends to manifest at an earlier age and to be more aggressive (100).

Different mutations in various parts of the *RET* domain have been linked to the variations in clinical presentation (101).

The adrenal glands

The paired adrenal glands are each made up of two distinct components: the cortex, which produces steroids, and the medulla, which produces catecholamines. Each component has a different embryologic origin and a different structure.

The cortex is traditionally divided into three zones, which extend from the central region to the capsule and are called, from the medulla to the capsule, the zonae reticularis, fasciculata, and glomerulosa.

Medullary cells are situated in the central region of the gland, especially in the head and body of the gland. There is usually no intervening connective tissue between the zona reticularis and the medulla, but because of the different cellular characteristics, the boundary between them is easily identified. The majority of medullary cells, the pheochromocytes, are chromaffin cells. Admixed with these cells are occasional ganglion cells that are like their counterparts elsewhere in the autonomic nervous system. Their numbers vary greatly in individual cases. Variations of the medullary anatomy are important when assessing medullary hyperplasia.

The zona glomerulosa produces aldosterone in response to plasma volume depletion, decreased renal perfusion or potassium depletion through the production of renin, which in turn triggers the angiotensin pathway. The production of cortisol and 18-hydroxycorticosterone is effected in the zonae fasciculata and reticularis under the influence of corticotropin release from the hypothalamus, leading to ACTH secretion from the pituitary. Negative feedback to this system is provided by a rise in cortisol.

Congenital disorders of the adrenal gland

Most of the anomalies of the adrenal gland (1) are of little significance in the field of surgical pathology. It is necessary to recognize the existence of rare examples of fused adrenal glands anterior or posterior to the aorta, but these cases occur in association with other malformation syndromes. *Fusion* of the adrenal gland with adjacent organs, particularly the liver, kidney, or even lung may offer some challenge if a complete removal of the gland is required.

Ectopic adrenal cortical nodules may be found in many sites from the para-aortic region to the gonad in both sexes. They may be affected in processes that are associated with hyperplastic cortical reactions. They are seen most often in association with hernial sacs or the epididymal region of undescended testes, or in the para-ovarian tissue of adult females. Adrenal cortical rests have been seen in the vicinity of the diaphragmatic opening for the aorta or within the liver or as part of the wall of a mediastinal cyst (1,102–104). In treated and surviving cases of congenital adrenal hyperplasia, caused by interruption of adrenal corticosteroid synthesis pathways, due to specific enzymatic deficiencies, adrenal rests in the testis are often very prominent. These *testicular adrenal rest tumors (TART)* have assumed increasing importance in recent years due to prolonged survival of patients. They appear to be commoner in patients with the *CYP21A2* mutation (and steroid 21-hydroxylase deficiency) and may cause severe testicular damage (105–107).

The *enlarged adrenals* in Beckwith–Wiedemann syndrome (BWS, characterized by exomphalos, macroglossia, and organomegaly are very abnormal (Figure 6.20). Diffusely scattered cells within the fetal cortex have large, hyperchromatic nuclei with folded cytoplasm producing pseudonuclear inclusions and vacuoles. This striking feature of "adrenal cytomegaly" is the most readily identified histologic feature of the syndrome (108–109). The survivors, especially those with a hypermethylation alteration (IC1), have a higher risk of developing tumors of various types (110). Wilms tumors and adrenocortical carcinomas are the most frequent tumors, but pituitary amphophilic hyperplasia and testicular interstitial cell hyperplasia may occur. Adrenal cortical cytomegaly as seen in BWS may be found, but in

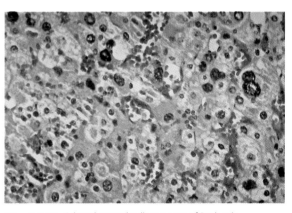

Figure 6.20 Adrenal cortical cells in a case of Beckwith–Wiedemann syndrome. Note marked variation in nuclear size, some showing pseudoinclusions (H&E × 40).

lesser numbers, in many other clinical settings (111–115), and ectopic foci of adrenal cortical tissue may show similar nuclear changes. The most important non-oncologic associations of adrenal cortical cytomegaly not associated with BWS is with diaphragmatic hernia (116).

Symptomatic hyperplasia that may affect the pediatric age group includes adrenocortical hyperplasia and adenomas in MEN-1 syndrome (118), where it may be associated with Cushing's syndrome in up to 40% of cases. Nodular hyperplasia and Cushing's syndrome may form part of the presentation of McCune–Albright syndrome (118). Primary pigmented micronodular adrenocortical disease may be part of the of the Carney complex; in this situation the adrenal cortex is disrupted by nodules of cortical cells with abundant lipofuscin. The intervening areas of the cortex are largely atrophic (119).

Cystic structures affecting the adrenal gland may be encountered throughout childhood, and the main diagnostic problem is in separating them from a cystic neuroblastoma (120). Calcification of old hemorrhages may also be encountered in the investigation of an abdominal lesion; most of these are the end result of old hemorrhages.

Adrenal agenesis is a rare developmental anomaly that presents in isolation or in combination with gonadal and pituitary disease (121). If undetected, it carries a high rate of fatality due to severe fluid and electrolyte imbalance. Bilateral adrenal agenesis is usually discovered at post-mortem examination. It has been associated with Ivemark Syndrome and anomalies of kidneys, lungs, spleen, and blood vessels (121).

Adrenal cortical tumors

Both *adenomas* and *carcinomas* of the adrenal gland may be seen in children. As in the thyroid gland, the distinction between a hyperplastic nodule and adenoma is not easy. An adenoma may be encapsulated, and with a different cellular appearance when compared to the adjacent gland. Nodules are not encapsulated and merge with the cells of the adjacent cortex. In children, most adrenocortical adenomas present with hormonal activity, virilization being the commonest manifestation followed by Cushing's disease (122–124). Functioning tumors are associated with an atrophic cortex, while in non-functioning tumors the cortex has normal thickness. Aldosterone-producing adenomas are an execption (Figure 6.21).

Virilizing tumors are often large at the time of presentation (> 175 g and up to 2000 g, ≥ 12 cm greatest diameter), relatively pale in color, except where secondary hemorrhagic necrosis has occurred (125; Figure 6.22a). The cells are usually compact and small with eosinophilic cytoplasm (Figure 6.22b). If

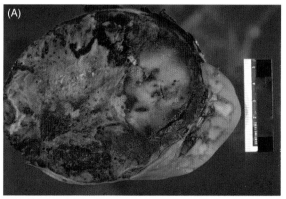

(A)

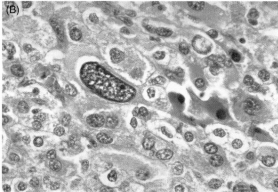

(B)

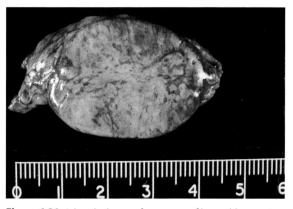

Figure 6.21 Adrenal adenoma from a case of hyperaldosteronism in a 19-year-old girl. Note the bright yellow color of the adenoma, its relatively small size and the non-atrophic cortex away from the adenoma.

Figure 6.22 (a) Adrenal lesion from a 14-month-old male with signs of virilization. The tumor was necrotic, weighed 220 g and had destroyed the left adrenal gland. (b) Occasional giant nuclei were seen in a tumor showing multiple areas of necrosis and hemorrhage (H&E × 40).

there is co-existent glucocorticoid excess, the adjacent cortex may be atrophic. In pediatric patients cases of virilization outnumber cases of feminization by a wide margin.

In children, 50–70% of cases of Cushing's syndrome are caused by an adrenal cortical neoplasm (126,127), while in adults the proportion is less than 20%. The adenomas are yellowish-brown and often variably mottled in appearance. The cells are a mixture of compact and clear cells, sometimes arranged in short cords or trabeculae. The adjacent cortex is atrophic. There may be nuclear hyperchromatism and pleomorphism, but in children, these are not indicators of malignancy of themselves. Mitoses are usually sparse (Figure 6.23).

Unlike the situation in most adult neoplasms, differentiating between a benign or malignant adrenal cortical tumor is compounded by the fact that the greatly respected and valuable Weiss score, as well as several related modifications, have not been found to be reliable predictors in children

(128–133). Other than metastases at the time of presentation, no single clear pathologic feature has emerged as being a reliable indicator of malignancy. Clinically, tumors with virilizing or feminizing effects are particularly indicative of a malignant potential. Conran *et al.* presented a working guide for the assessment of pediatric adrenal neoplasms (39). The risk factors for malignancy include: the presence of virilization or feminization, macroscopic invasion of adjacent structures, weight > 300 g, and the presence of necrosis. Histologic features suggestive of malignancy included broad fibrous bands, diffuse (i.e., non-trabecular) growth pattern histologically; vascular invasion; mitotic rate > 10 per high power field at ×40 magnification; atypical mitoses and predominance of compact cells. These criteria are not absolute, especially with smaller tumors (< 300 g). Larger tumors often do not pose a problem, as they manifest their malignant behavior clinically (134,135).

In addition to the association with BWS, MEN-1 syndrome and Carney's complex, adrenal cortical tumors, especially carcinomas, are associated with the familial cancer syndrome originally described by Li and Fraumeni in 1969 (136) and other cancer susceptibility syndromes (137). In southern Brazil, there is an inordinately high incidence of adrenocortical cancers in children (137) due to a unique germline mutation (TP53-R337H). The recognition of this mutation allows for the possibility of early diagnosis at a time when the tumors are small and completely resectable, when outcomes can be as high as 80% survival (138).

Attempts to differentiate and offer useful prognostic information in cases of adrenocortical tumors in children include attempts to study DNA methylation using microarrays (139) and screening for genetic variants in phosphodiesterase 8B (PDE8B) (140), as well as dysregulation of microRNAs (141).

Tumors of the adrenal medulla

Pheochromocytoma

These tumors are derived from the pheochromocytes (the catecholamine-producing cells of the adrenal medulla). Since catecholamine-producing cells are seen in the para-adrenal region, as well as in the para-aortic ganglia, pheochromocytomas may also develop in those sites, and on occasion it can be difficult to distinguish between an adrenal lesion and a para-adrenal lesion.

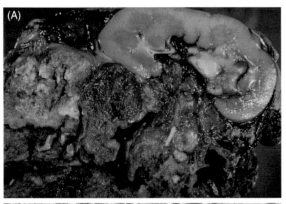

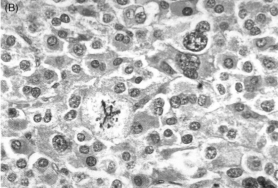

Figure 6.23 (a) Massive carcinoma replacing and destroying the adrenal gland in a three-year-old boy with rapidly developing virilization. (b) Atypical mitoses were seen among the sheets of compactly arranged polyhedral tumor cells (H&E × 40).

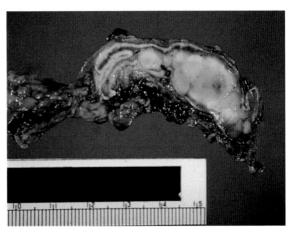

Figure 6.25 Small pheochromocytoma from the right adrenal gland of a 17-year-old with a family history of MEN-2B. Note the distortion of the gland by a yellow fleshy medullary tumor.

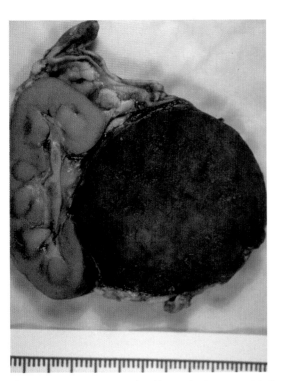

Figure 6.24 Large congested and hemorrhagic tumor originally thought to be of adrenal cortical origin. The lesion, however, was a pheochromocytoma. The child had hypertension and a family history of Li–Fraumeni syndrome.

Clinical presentation: Pheochromocytoma has been called the "10% tumor": 10% bilateral, 10% extra-adrenal, 10% malignant, and 10% in children (142). There is an elevation of the relative levels of epinephrine (adrenaline) to norepinephrine (noradrenaline) in the urine. In children there is a greater chance of association with a syndromic condition. The relationship with MEN must be considered in each patient and a careful evaluation of the presence or absence of medullary hyperplasia must be made. In patients with MEN-2A and MEN-2B, tumors may occur against a background of diffuse medullary hyperplasia, and sometimes the tumor may be relatively small, multifocal, and bilateral. Generally the presence of medullary hyperplasia is not difficult to find if thoroughly sought for in a fully sampled gland, since the expansion of the medulla is usually marked. Some patients with symptoms suggestive of pheochromocytomas, but no other manifestations of MEN have been shown to have medullary hyperplasia (143). Familial pheochromocytoma may be associated with neurofibromatosis, Beckwith–Wiedemann syndrome, von Hippel–Lindau syndrome, Carney complex, and familial pheochromocytoma and

neurofibromatosis (144). Cushing's syndrome associated with a pheochromocytoma has been reported, even in children (145).

Genetics: Familial cases may have *RET*, *VHL (von Hippel–Lindau)*, *SDHD (succinate dehydrogenase subunit D)*, and *SDHB (succinate dehydrogenase subunit B)* mutations. Somatic mutations in genes responsible for syndromic pheochromocytoma may be found in sporadic cases (146).

Macroscopy: Most tumors measure 3–5 cm and are generally solitary and well circumscribed. On cut section, the tumor is firm and dark, and may be completely hemorrhagic with cystic changes (Figure 6.24). In some cases it is difficult to distinguish between diffuse medullary hyperplasia and small tumors, and an arbitrary cut-off of > 1 cm diameter has been used to describe a nodule as a tumor, while lesions < 1 cm are classified as hyperplastic areas (147). Medullary hyperplasia can be asymmetrical, unilateral, or bilateral. The nodules can be variegated in color and texture, and can show similar patterns to those seen in larger tumors (Figure 6.25).

Histology: The tumor cells are arranged in nests surrounded by a fibrovascular stroma ("zelballen"); solid, trabecular, and areas with spindled cells are common variants. Very frequently hyperchromatic large nuclei with pseudoinclusions are found, and there are sometimes even admixed ganglion cells. Hyaline inclusions, as seen in some medullary cells in adults, may be present in many of the larger tumors. There can even be some diagnostic confusion with adrenal cortical lesions. The use of immunohistochemistry is useful, since the medullary cells are positive for neuron-specific enolase

213

(NSE), synaptophysin, chromogranin, neurosecretory protein-55 (NESP-55), and other markers (148). Ultrastructurally the presence of the characteristic neurosecretory granules is diagnostic. "Black" pheochromocytomas, where the tumors contain abundant granular pigment are reported in adults, but not in children.

Prognosis: Predicting the pattern of behavior of pheochromocytomas is very difficult. Larger tumors seem to have more malignant potential, but the incidence varies widely between series, and the presence of metastases to sites where chromaffin tissue is not normally found may be the only true test (149). Recurrences may be delayed by many years so that cases need a long follow-up (150).

Neuroblastoma–ganglioneuroma spectrum

Neuroblastoma (NB) is the commonest non-hemopoietic malignant tumor of childhood, and the majority (around 70%) present by the age of two years. There is no sex predilection. The cells of neuroblastoma share the same embryonic origin as the cells that will produce the sympathetic nervous system and the related paraganglionic structures elsewhere in the body. As a consequence, neuroblastoma may arise in many different parts of the body, but the majority arise within the adrenal gland. The relationship with the sympathetic nervous system is expressed in the production of catecholamines and related metabolites, forming the basis of the many screening programs and early biochemical detection. For NB staging see Table 6.1.

Macroscopy: The tumor may vary in size from minute lesions to very large masses. Some NBs have a fibrous pseudocapsule, while others are more infiltrative. The tumor has a tan color and generally shows cystic areas, as well as areas of hemorrhage and necrosis (Figure 6.26). Sometimes dystrophic calcification is obvious macroscopically.

Histology: Neuroblastomas' classic feature is the presence of sheets and clusters of "small, round cells" with a high nuclear-cytoplasmic ratio, feathery nuclear chromatin, little or no cytoplasm, poorly defined cell margins, and classically resembling the migratory neuroblast of embryologic importance (Figure 6.27). In most tumors there are areas where the cells may be arranged in small radial or elliptical clusters around a central area of neuropil (Figure 6.28). These are the classic "pseudorosettes." Many neuroblastomas do not have rosettes at all, and this can be particularly evident

Table 6.1 International neuroblastoma staging

Stage	Description
I	Localized tumor with complete gross excision, with or without microscopic residual disease; representative ipsilateral lymph nodes negative for tumor microscopically (nodes attached to and removed with the primary tumor may be positive).
IIA	Localized tumor with incomplete gross excision; representative ipsilateral non-adherent lymph nodes negative for tumor microscopically.
IIB	Localized tumor with or without complete gross excision, with ipsilateral nonadherent lymph nodes positive for tumor. Enlarged contralateral lymph nodes must be negative microscopically.
III	Unresectable unilateral tumor infiltrating across the midline, with or without regional lymph node involvement; or localized unilateral tumor with contralateral regional lymph node involvement; or midline tumor with bilateral extension by infiltration (unresectable) or by lymph node involvement. The midline is defined as the vertebral column. Tumors originating on one side and crossing the midline must infiltrate to or beyond the opposite side of the vertebral column.
IV	Any primary tumor with dissemination to distant lymph nodes, bone, bone marrow, liver, skin, and/or other organs (except as defined for stage 4S).
IV S	Localized primary tumor (as defined for stage 1, 2A, or 2B), with dissemination limited to skin, liver, and/or bone marrow (limited to infants younger than one year). Marrow involvement should be minimal (< 10% of total nucleated cells identified as malignant by bone biopsy or by bone marrow aspirate). More extensive bone marrow involvement would be considered to be stage 4 disease. The results of the MIBG (meta-Ido-benzyl-guanidine) scan (if performed) should be negative for disease in the bone marrow.

when dealing with small biopsies. Many tumors may have a very vascular pattern that may take on the appearance of sinusoids, reminiscent of the very vascular developing medulla. Neuroblastoma stains with a wide range of antibodies against neuronal markers (NB84, synaptophysin, chromogranin, NSE, PGP9.5, antibodies against neurofilament proteins) (Figure 6.29).

Differentiation in neuroblastoma is the synchronous development of nucleus and cytoplasm with progressive vesicular enlargement of the nucleus, appearance of nucleoli, and increasing cytoplasm so that the cell progressively resembles a ganglion cell (Figure 6.30). The fully differentiated form is the ganglioneuroma. In between these two extremes there is

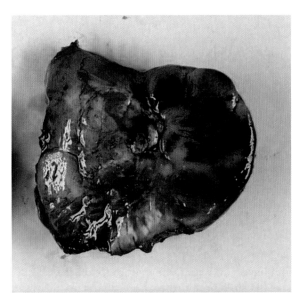

Figure 6.26 Cut surface of a neuroblastoma showing focal hemorrhage and calcification.

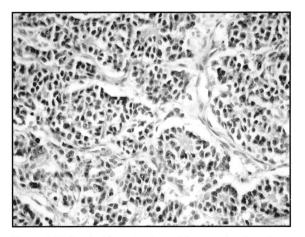

Figure 6.28 Poorly differentiated neuroblastoma, showing a few pseudorosettes (H&E × 40).

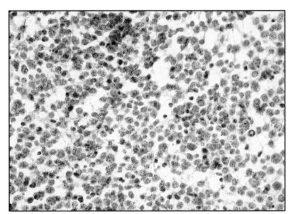

Figure 6.27 Undifferentiated neuroblastoma. Note the monomorphous blue round cells (H&E × 40).

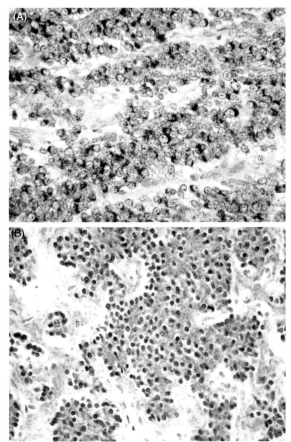

Figure 6.29 Neuroblastoma immunocytochemistry: (a) NB84 (× 40) and (b) synaptophysin (× 40).

considerable variation. The tumors are classified according to the International Neuroblastoma Pathology Classification (151; see Table 6.2).

Stromal development is important. Immature tumors are arranged in nests and clusters separated by variable amounts of fibrovascular tissue, and the groups are separated by variable amounts of neuropil, which is not accompanied by Schwann cells ("naked neuropil"). The emergence of Schwann cells marks a major change. The neuropil becomes organized into parallel fascicular bundles, with increasing proportions of Schwann cells. At the most extreme end of the spectrum, the tumor is composed of ganglion cells, mature bundles of Schwann cells intimately admixed with neuropil, akin to the ganglia of the sympathetic nervous system.

215

Table 6.2 International neuroblastoma pathology classification and prognostic evaluation (modified from 132)

International NB pathology classification		Prognosis
Neuroblastoma (Schwannian stroma-poor)		
< 1.5 years	Poorly differentiated & low or intermediate MKI	Favorable
1.5–5 years	Differentiating & low MKI	Favorable
< 1.5 years	(a) Undifferentiated (b) High MKI	Unfavorable
1.5–5 years	(a) Undifferentiated or poorly differentiated (b) Intermediate or high MKI	Unfavorable
≥ 5 years	All tumors	Unfavorable
Ganglioneuroblastoma, intermixed	*(Schwannian stroma-rich)*	Favorable
Ganglioneuroma	*(Schwannian stroma-dominant)*	
Maturing	Well differentiated	Favorable
Mature		Favorable
Ganglioneuroblastoma, nodular	*(composite Schwannian stroma)*	Unfavorable

MKI: mitosis-karyorrhexis index

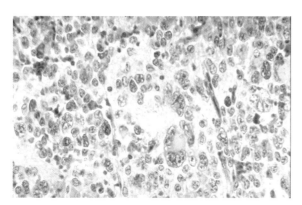

Figure 6.30 Neuroblastoma: differentiation is seen here with progressive enlargement of tumor cells and acquisition of increasing amounts of cytoplasm, as well as nuclear changes suggesting ganglion cells (H&E × 40).

The tumor must be inspected carefully and sampled thoroughly. Tumors are "stroma-rich" if they have large numbers of Schwann cells. These tumors are usually large, with a rubbery consistency,

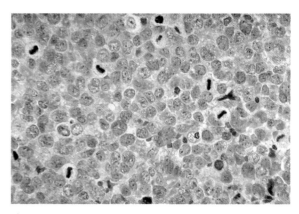

Figure 6.31 High mitotic karyorrhectic index (MKI) in a neuroblastoma (H&E × 40).

and have a very uniform appearance on the cut surface. Histologically, they have abundant Schwann cells with neuritic processes organized into fascicles. Cases lacking Schwann cells are "stroma-poor." This is not applicable if the tumor has been treated.

Neuroblastoma

The tumors that do not have Schwannian stroma (the "stroma-poor" tumors) are recognizable as neuroblastic tumors by standard histologic methods. In this group the age at diagnosis has prognostic significance. There are three important subsets: (a) over 5 years, (b) age between 18 months and 5 years, (c) age under 18 months.

In patients under five years of age the number of mitotic and karyorrhectic cells must be counted. This provides the "mitotic-karyorrhectic index" or "MKI" (Figure 6.31). The index is based on counting 5000 cells, which, depending on the cellularity of the tumor, can be done by reviewing 10–20 high-power fields (×40).

A practical and useful approach to identifying the MKI has been described (152), but usually high-MKI tumors (> 200/5000 cells) are easy to differentiate from low (< 100/5000 cells). The intermediate category (MKI > 100 < 200/5000 cells) is a problem and requires considerable effort. This is the step that causes most disagreement between observers. Care must be taken to exclude leukocytes from being counted in the MKI group. Joshi's approach is practical and useful (152).

Ganglioneuroblastoma (GNB)
Nodular GNB

The stroma-rich group may have grossly visible nodules that are clearly separate from the remainder of the

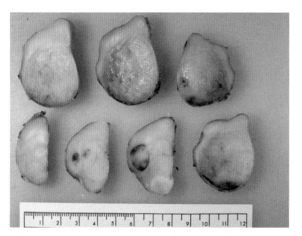

Figure 6.32 Stroma-rich ganglioneuroblastoma nodules.

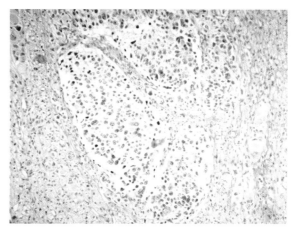

Figure 6.33 Nodular ganglioneuroblastoma. Note the immature nodule within the mature tumor (H&E × 20).

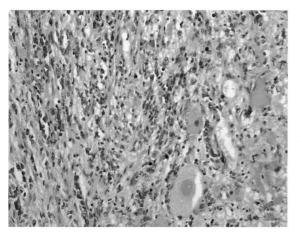

Figure 6.34 Intermixed ganglioneuroblastoma. Note the close association between the immature (left) and mature (right) components (H&E × 20).

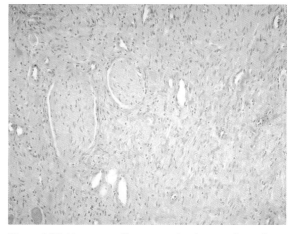

Figure 6.35 Mature ganglioneuroma showing ganglion cells (H&E × 20).

tumor (Figure 6.32). These nodules are often hemorrhagic and not difficult to identify, even when small. Histologically, the nodules are demarcated from the rest of the tumor by clearly defined fibrous bands of varying thickness (Figure 6.33). The nodules are islands of poorly differentiated or undifferentiated neuroblastic cells with neuropil set apart from a predominantly Schwannian stroma-rich tumor with gangliomatous cells.

Diffuse GNB

The diffuse form of GNB has islands of neuroblasts that merge imperceptibly with the Schwannian-rich zone, without nodule formation. This forms the "intermixed ganglioneuroblastoma" (Figure 6.34).

Ganglioneuroma (GN)

If there are no neuroblast islands, then the lesion is classified as a "stroma- rich" or Schwannian-dominant ganglioneuroma of the INPC (Figure 6.35).

Congenital neuroblastomas

Congenital tumors are rare, but, together with teratomas, NB is one of the most common congenital tumors (153). They may be very vascular and appear almost hemorrhagic. While most adrenal glands of fetuses and neonates studied at autopsy have scattered neuroblastic elements that appear to be situated in atypical sites within the cortex of the gland (154), these islands, rarely > 100 μm in diameter, should not be confused with the congenital

217

neuroblastoma *in situ* (155), which is defined as being > 2 mm in diameter. Many infants have evidence of focal calcification in their adrenals, which may represent regressed neuroblastoma (156).

IV S neuroblastoma

These present at birth with multiple lesions in skin, liver, and bone marrow, but not in bone or any viscera other than liver. The amount of bone marrow involvement is restricted: 10% or less of the marrow is infiltrated by neuroblasts and there must be no bone destruction. Any excess over this amount or any visceral involvement disqualifies the case as being in stage IV S, but places the case in the disseminated category of stage IV of the International Criteria for Staging of Neuroblastomas (157–159). However, a poor prognosis has been reported in patients with IV S NB, with unfavorable prognostic factors such as *MYCN* amplification (160).

Genetics: The recognition of cytogenetic abnormalities, such as abnormalities of the *MYCN* gene copy number, *TrkA* expression, multidrug resistance gene *MDR1*, and multidrug resistance-associated protein (MRP) have added to our knowledge of the molecular biology of this tumor (161–166). Genetic changes have prognostic importance. Hyperdiploid (near-triploid) NBs show better prognosis than diploid or tetraploid tumors (167). *MYCN* amplification is one of the strongest indicators of aggressive behavior, and patients with amplified *MYCN* have generally undifferentiated or poorly differentiated features with high MKI (168). Elevated expression of survivin, repp86, and PRAME correlates with bad prognosis(169–171), while TrkA, CD44, and CAMTA1 (calmodulin-binding transcription activator 1) correlate with favorable prognosis (172–174).

A consensus approach for pretreatment risk stratification has been developed, incorporating staging, histological classification, and genetic alterations (175).

Progression in neuroblastoma can be by direct invasion, lymph node metastases, or hematogenous spread. Hepatic and skull metastases have been known. A wide range of associations with neuroblastic tumors that include opsoclonus-myoclonus-ataxia syndrome, Hirschsprung's disease, congenital hypoventilation syndrome, intractable diarrhea syndrome, and an increased risk of thyroid cancer in irradiated patients are reported (39, 176).

Adrenal myelolipomas

These have been described in children (177–179), and may coexist with the BWS or adrenal cortical hyperplasia. While they are not functional they can cause diagnostic confusion, and when hemorrhage occurs they may cause flank pain. Rarely myelolipomas may be generalized (180) with pelvic, abdominal thoracic, or retro-orbital involvement.

The endocrine pancreas

Islet hypertrophy and hyperplasia

The relative underdevelopment of the acinar tissue in early infancy makes the islets appear more prominent. The term *islet hypertrophy* should be used in infants under two months of age when more than 10% of islets are over 200 mm in diameter, sparing the nesting architecture (181).

Islet hypertrophy (increased size) and *islet hyperplasia* (increased number of β-cells or of all cells) occur together in some newborn conditions, the best known being maternal diabetes.

The typical histological picture of the *infant of a diabetic mother (IDM)* is hypertrophy and hyperplasia of islets with concentric fibrosis and eosinophilic-rich inflammatory infiltrate around the islets (eosinophilic insulitis). Nowadays, the florid picture of IDM is seen less frequently, due to controls in maternal blood sugar during pregnancy (182). Other conditions in which islet-cell hypertrophy may be found are Beckwith–Wiedemann syndrome (with or without hyperinsulinemic hypoglycemia) (183), Perlman syndrome (patients also have renal dysplasia, Wilms tumor, and other congenital abnormalities) (184), Zellweger syndrome (185), tyrosinemia (186), leprechaunism (Donohue syndrome), Costello syndrome (187), and congenital hemochromatosis (188), among others.

Congenital hyperinsulinism (CH)

This comprises a group of different genetic disorders with the common finding of inappropriate secretion of insulin by pancreatic β-cells.

In 1938, Laidlaw described a diffuse neoformation of islet tissue (189) later called nesidioblastosis (190). The condition is also known as persistent neonatal hyperinsulinemic hypoglycemia and idiopathic hypoglycemia of infancy.

The estimated incidence is 1/50 000 live births (higher in societies with a high rate of consanguinity). Clinical manifestations include macrosomia, sweating, seizures, motor abnormalities, and somnolence.

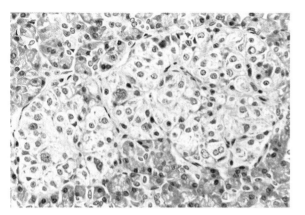

Figure 6.36 Diffuse congenital hyperinsulinemia showing pancreatic endocrine cells with large nuclei (H&E × 40).

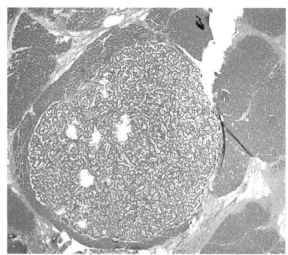

Figure 6.37 Pancreas showing an adenomatous nodule (H&E × 10).

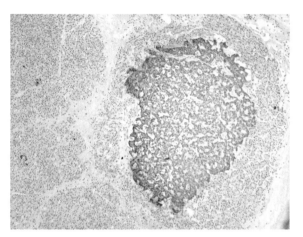

Figure 6.38 Insulin immunostaining in a case of focal congenital hyperinsulinism (×10).

Seventy percent of cases start during the neonatal period (191–192).

The histological abnormalities may be diffuse or focal (islet cell adenomatosis) and determining the histopathological form is important for surgical treatment (193).

The *diffuse* form shows an increase in the number of small-cell islet clusters, ductulo-insular complexes, and large islets of Langerhans, characterized by the presence of abnormally large islet-cell nuclei. The frequency of these enlarged nuclei varies from case to case. These nuclei should be four times the size of the nearby acinar-cell nuclei or nuclei occupying an area more than three times larger than the surrounding endocrine nuclei (194); (Figure 6.36).

Focal forms (or *adenomatous hyperplasia*) are usually small areas of the pancreas, with large endocrine cells, irregular- and angular-shaped nuclei, which are three to five times the size of the nearby acinar cells. Forty percent of the affected area may comprise endocrine cells, and insulin cells predominate. The focus retains a nested pattern, but it is poorly delimited. There may be satellites in the nearby pancreas, or more than one focus. True adenomas are composed entirely of β-cells, with no exocrine pancreas (Figure 6.37).

The abnormalities vary in intensity from one islet to another, but can be detected by immunohistochemical stains for insulin and glucagon (Figure 6.38).

A mosaic pattern showing the co-existence of two different types of islets different from the focal form has recently been described (195).

Differentiation between the two forms is important because focal lesions are cured by limited pancreatic resection, whereas diffuse lesions require a subtotal pancreatectomy with a high risk of diabetes mellitus.

A DOPA PET-scan is highly accurate in localizing *focal* lesions as part of the preoperative diagnosis. The combination of genetic analysis, 18F-fluoro-L-DOPA PET-scan, and intraoperative ultrasonography shows great potential for the identification and location of the lesion, and as a guideline for surgery in CH (196). Preoperative pancreatic ultrasonography is also useful to determine size, shape, and topography of *focal CH* (197). In *focal* forms it is possible to find a small

219

endocrine neoplasm-like nodule, but otherwise the organ looks normal in both types of lesions.

The PAS stain is very useful in intraoperative biopsies. The cytoplasm of pancreatic acinar cells is PAS-positive and islet cells are negative. This highlights the poorly delimited focal hyperplasia and helps to identify the nuclear abnormalities that will be present in the *diffuse* form.

Congenital hyperinsulinism can be classified according to the etiopathogenic process into channelopathies, enzyme anomalies, and transcription factor deficits (198,199).

Channelopathies are associated with recessive mutations of the β-cell ATP-sensitive potassium channel (K-ATP). The channel is composed of two subunits, *SUR1* and *Kir6.2*, encoded by adjacent genes (*ABCC8* and *KNCJ11*) on chromosome 11p15.1. In cases of *diffuse CH*, infants have mutations of both K-ATP parental alleles. Recessive K-ATP mutations may also cause *focal CH*, in which there is an area that expresses a paternally derived ATP-sensitive potassium-channel mutation due to embryonic loss of heterozygosity for the maternal 11p region. Because both diffuse and focal forms are mostly resistant to diazoxide treatment, surgical intervention is often indicated.

Enzyme anomalies incude mutations in glucokinase (GCK), glutamate dehydrogenase, and short-chain L-3-hydroxyacyl-CoA dehydrogenase or other metabolic defects involving the β-cells. These cases present as diffuse diazoxide-responsive CH, with the exception of GCK mutations, which can be unresponsive in some patients.

Transcription factor defects involve the hepatocyte nuclear factor α gene. This dominantly inherited CH is diazoxide responsive and is a diffuse form of the disease.

Pancreatic tumors are described in Chapter 3.

References

1. Lacsan A, de Sa DJ. Endocrine system. In Gilbert-Barness E, editor, *Potter's Pathology of the Fetus, Infant and Child*, second edn. New York: Mosby Elsevier; 2007;1595–605.

2. McPhie JL, Beck JS. The histological features and human growth hormone content of the pharyngeal pituitary gland in normal and endocrinologically-disturbed patients. *Clin.* Endocrinol 1973;**2**:157–73.

3. Weber FT, Donnelly WH, Bejar RL. Hypopituitarism following extirpation of a pharyngeal pituitary. *Am. J. Dis. Child.* 1977;**131**:525–8.

4. Bizzarri C, Marini R, Ubertini G, Cappa M. Partially reversible hypopituitarism in an adolescent with a Rathke cleft cyst. *Clin. Pediatr. Endocrinol.* 2012;**21**:75–80.

5. Partington MD, Davis DH, Laws ER Jr, Scheithauer BW. Pituitary adenomas in childhood and adolescence. Results of transsphenoidal surgery. *J. Neurosurg.* 1994;**80**:209–16.

6. Dyer EH, Civit T, Visot A, Delalande O, Derome P. Transsphenoidal surgery for pituitary adenomas in children. *Neurosurgery* 1994;**34**;207–12.

7. Pandey P, Ojha BK, Mahapatra AK. Pediatric pituitary adenoma: A series of 42 patients. *J. Clin. Neurosci.* 2005;**12**:124–7.

8. Harrington MH, Casella SJ. Pituitary tumors in childhood. *Curr. Opin. Endocrinol. Diabetes Obes.* 2012;**19**:63–7.

9. Jackman S, Diamond F. Pituitary adenomas in childhood and adolescence. *Pediatr. Endocrinol. Rev.* 2013;**10**:450–9.

10. Chiloiro S, Bianchi A, Doglietto F, *et al.* Radically resected pituitary adenomas: prognostic role of Ki 67 labeling index in a monocentric retrospective series and literature review. *Pituitary* 2013;**17**:267.

11. Pawlikowski M, Gruszka A, *et al.* Proliferating cell nuclear antigen (PCNA) expression in pituitary adenomas: relationship to the endocrine phenotype of adenoma. *Folia Histochem. Cytobiol.* 2006;**44**:37–41.

12. Hsu DW, Hakim F, Biller BM, *et al.* Significance of proliferating cell nuclear antigen index in predicting pituitary adenoma recurrence. *J. Neurosurg.* 1993;**78**:753–61.

13. Gaston-Massuet C, Andoniadu CL, Signore M, *et al.* Increased Wingless (Wnt) signaling in pituitary progenitor cells gives rise to pituitary tumors in mice and humans. *Proc. Natl. Acad. Sci. USA* 2011;**108**:11482–7.

14. Gaztambide S, Vazquez F, Castaño L. Diagnosis and treatment of multiple endocrine neoplasia type 1 (MEN1). *Minerva Endocrinol.* 2013;**38**:17–28.

15. Delemer B. MEN 1 and pituitary adenomas. *Ann. Endocrinol. (Paris)* 2012;**73**:59–61.

16 Raff SB, Carney JA, Krugman D, Doppman JL, Stratakis CA. Prolactin secretion abnormalities in patients with the "syndrome of spotty skin pigmentation, myxomas, endocrine overactivity and schwannomas" (Carney complex). *J. Clin. Endocrinol. Metabol.* 2000;**13**:373–9.

17. Cohen MM Jr, Howell RE. Etiology of fibrous dysplasia and McCune- Albright syndrome. *Int. J. Oral Maxillofac. Surg.* 1999;**28**:366–71.

18. Stratakis CA, Tichomirowa M, Boikos S, *et al.* The role of germline *AIP, MEN1, PRKAR1 A, CDKN 1B, CDKN*

2C mutations causing pituitary adenomas in a large cohort of children, adolescents, and patients with genetic syndromes. *Clin. Genet.* 2010;**78**:457–63.

19. Leontiou CA. The role of the aryl hydrocarbon receptor-interacting protein gene in familial and sporadic pituitary adenomas. *J. Clin. Endocrinol. Metabol.* 2008;**93**:2390–401.

20. Noh SJ, Ahn JY, Lee KS, Kim SH. Pituitary adenoma and concomitant Rathke's cleft cyst. *Acta Neurochir. (Wien)* 2007;**149**:1223–8.

21. Karavitaki N, Scheithauer BW, Watt J, *et al.* Collision lesions of the sella: coexistence of craniopharyngioma with gonadotroph adenoma and of Rathke's cleft cyst with corticotroph adenoma. *Pituitary* 2008;**11**:317–23.

22. Furtado SV, Thakar S, Ghosal N, Hegde AS. Atypical presentation of pediatric mixed germ cell tumors in the sellar and suprasellar region. *Neurol. India* 2012;**60**:90–3.

23. Cemeroglu AP, Blaivas M, Muraszko KM, Robertson, PL, Vazquez DM. Lymphocytic hypophysitis presenting with diabetes insipidus in a 14 year-old girl: case report and review of the literature. *Eur. J. Pediatr.* 1997;**156**:684–8.

24. Rousseau-Nepton I, Kaduri S, Garfield N, Krishnamoorthy P. Hypothalamic hamartoma associated with central precocious puberty and growth hormone deficiency. *J. Pediatr. Endocrinol. Metab.* 2013;**10**:1–5.

25. Stoll C, De Saint Martin A, Donato L, *et al.* Pallister-Hall syndrome with stenosis of the cricoid cartilage and microphallus without hypopituitarism. *Genet. Couns.* 2001;**12**:231–5.

26. Peña S, Robertson H, Walvekar RR. Thyroid Hemiagenesis: Report of a Case and Review of Literature. *Indian. J. Otolaryngol. Head Neck Surg.* 2011;**63**:198–200.

27. Robinson HB Jr. Di George's or the III-IV pharyngeal pouch syndrome: pathology and a theory of pathogenesis. *Perspect. Pediatr. Pathol.* 1975;**3**:173–206.

28. Pueblitz S, Weinberg G, Albores Saavedra J. Thyroid C cells in the Di George syndrome. *Pediatr. Pathol.* 1993;**13**:463–73.

29. Altay C, Erdogan N, Karasu S, *et al.* CT and MRI findings of developmental abnormalities and ectopia varieties of the thyroid gland. *Diagn. Interv. Radiol.* 2012;**18**:335–43.

30. Dzodic R, Markovic I, Stanojevic B, *et al.* Surgical management of primary thyroid carcinoma arising in thyroglossal duct cyst: An experience of a single institution in Serbia. *Endocr. J.* 2012;**59**:517–22.

31. Triglia JM, Nicollas R, Ducroz V. *et al.* First branchial cleft anomalies: A study of 39 cases and a review of the literature. *Arch. Otolaryngol. Head Neck Surg.* 1998;**124**:291–5.

32. Thomas B, Shroff M, Forte V, Blaser S, James A. Revisiting imaging features and the embryologic basis of third and fourth branchial anomalies. *Am. J. Neuroradiol.* 2010;**31**:755–60.

33. Michels AW, Eisenbarth GS. Immunologic endocrine disorders. *J. Allergy Clin. Immunol.* 2010;**125**(Suppl 2): S226–37.

34. Ahn D, Heo SJ, Park JH, *et al.* Clinical relationship between Hashimoto thyroiditis and papillary thyroid cancer. *Acta Oncol.* 2011;**50**:1228–34.

35. Mukasa K, Noh JY, Kunii Y, *et al.* Prevalence of malignant tumors and adenomatous lesions detected by ultrasonographic screening in patients with autoimmune thyroid diseases. *Thyroid* 2011;**21**:37–41.

36. Mssrouri R, Benamr S, Essadel A *et al.* Thyroid cancer in patients with Grave's Disease. *J. Chir. (Paris)* 2008; **145**:244–6.

37. Rago T, Fiore E, Scutari M, Santini F, *et al.* Male sex, single nodularity, and young age are associated with the risk of finding a papillary thyroid cancer on fine-needle aspiration cytology in a large series of patients with nodular thyroid disease. *Eur. J. Endocrinol.* 2010;**162**:763–70.

38. Bradly DP, Reddy V, Prinz RA, Gattuso P. Incidental papillary carcinoma in patients treated surgically for benign thyroid diseases. *Surgery* 2009;**146**:1099–104.

39. Conran RM, Askin FB, Dehner LP. The pineal, pituitary, parathyroid, thyroid and adrenal glands. In: Stocker JT, Dehner LP, editors, *Pediatric Pathology*, second edn. Philadelphia: Lippincott Williams & Wilkins; 2001;1028–40.

40. Park SM, Chatterjee VK. Genetics of congenital hypothyroidism. *J. Med. Genet.* 2005;**42**:379–89.

41. Kennedy JS. The pathology of dyshormonogenetic goiter. *J. Pathol.* 1969;**99**:251–64.

42. Piciu D, Piciu A, Irimie A. Thyroid cancer in children: A 20-year study at a Romanian oncology institute. *Endocr. J.* 2012;**59**:489–96.

43. Jaruratanasirikul S, Leethanaporn K, Khuntigij P, Sriplung H. The clinical course of Hashimoto's thyroiditis in children and adolescents: 6 years longitudinal follow-up. *J. Pediatr. Endocrinol. Metab.* 2001;**14**:177–84.

44. Roy R, Kouniavsky G, Schneider E, *et al.* Predictive factors of malignancy in pediatric thyroid nodules. *Surgery* 2011;**150**:1228–33.

45. Redlich A, Boxberger N, Kurt Werner S, *et al.* Sensitivity of fine-needle biopsy in detecting pediatric differentiated thyroid carcinoma. *Pediatr. Blood Cancer* 2012;**59**:233–7.

46. Collini P, Mattavelli F, Pellegrinelli A, *et al*. Papillary carcinoma of the thyroid gland of childhood and adolescence: Morphologic subtypes, biologic behavior and prognosis: A clinicopathologic study of 42 sporadic cases treated at a single institution during a 30-year period. *Am. J. Surg. Pathol.* 2006;**30**:1420–61.

47. Desai D, McPherson LA, Higgins JP, Weigel RJ. Genetic analysis of a papillary thyroid carcinoma in a patient with MEN1. *Ann. Surg. Oncol.* 2001;**8**:342–6.

48. Nosé V. Familial non-medullary thyroid carcinoma: An update. *Endocr. Pathol.* 2008;**19**:226–40.

49. Enomoto K, Enomoto Y, Uchino S, Yamashita H, Noguchi S. Follicular thyroid cancer in children and adolescents: clinicopathologic features, long-term survival, and risk factors for recurrence. *Endocr. J.* 2013;**60**:629–35.

50. Lloyd RV, Philipp U. Heitz, Charis E. *WHO Tumors of Endocrine Organs. World Health Organization Classification of Tumors* DeLellis RA, editor. Lyon: IARC Press, 2004.

51. Hall JE, Abdollahian DJ, Sinard RJ. Thyroid disease associated with Cowden syndrome: A meta-analysis. *Head Neck* 2013;**35**:1189–94.

52. Wells SA Jr, Pacini F, Robinson BG, Santoro M. Multiple endocrine neoplasia type 2 and familial medullary thyroid carcinoma: An update. *J. Clin. Endocrinol. Metab.* 2013;**98**:3149–64.

53. Mete O, Asa SL. Precursor lesions of endocrine system neoplasms. *Pathology* 2013;**45**:316–30.

54. Williams ED, Brown CL, Doniach I. Pathological and clinical findings in a series of 67 cases of medullary carcinoma of the thyroid. *J. Clin. Pathol.* 1966;**19**:103–13.

55. Pacini F, Basolo F, Elisei R, *et al*. Medullary thyroid cancer. An immunohistochemical and humoral study using six separate antigens. *Am. J. Clin. Pathol.* 1991;**95**:300–8.

56. Tavares MR, Toledo SP, *et al*. Surgical approach to medullary thyroid carcinoma associated with multiple endocrine neoplasia type 2. *Clinics (Sao Paulo)* 2012; **67** Suppl 1:149–54.

57. Roth S, Abu–Jawdeh GM. Parathyroid glands. In S.S. Sternberg, editor, *Histology for Pathologists*, second edn. Philadelphia: Lippincott-Raven 1997:1093–105.

58. Wang C-A. The anatomic basis of parathyroid surgery. *Ann. Surg.* 1976;**183**:271–75.

59. Lack EE, Delay S, Linnoila RI. Ectopic parathyroid tissue within the vagus nerve. *Arch. Pathol. Lab. Med.* 1988;**112**:304–6.

60. Neumann DR, Esselstyn CB Jr, Madera A, Wong CO, Lieber M. Parathyroid detection in secondary hyperparathyroidism with 123I/99m Tc-sestamibi subtraction single photon emission computed tomography. *J. Clin. Endocrinol. Metabol.* 1998;**83**:3867–71.

61. Kurman RJ, Prabha AC. Thyroid and parathyroid glands in the vaginal wall: report of a case. *Am. J. Clin. Pathol.* 1973;**59**:503–7.

62. Reddick, RL, Costa JC, Marx SJ. Parathyroid hyperplasia and parathyromatosis. *Lancet* 1977;**1**:549 (letter).

63. Su D, Ellis S, Napier A, Manley NR. *Hoxa3* and *pax1* regulate epithelial cell death and proliferation during thymus and parathyroid organogenesis. *Dev. Biol.* 2001;**236**:316–29.

64. Zou D, Silvius D, Davenport J, *et al*. Patterning of the third pharyngeal pouch into the thymus/parathyroid by Six and Eya 1. *Dev. Biol.* 2006;**293**:499–512.

65. Rodriguez Soriano J. Branchio-oto-renal syndrome. *J. Nephrol.* 2003;**16**:603–5.

66. Shannon WA, Roth SI. Ultrastructural study of acid phosphatase activity in normal, adenomatous and hyperplastic (chief cell type) human parathyroid glands. *Am. J. Pathol.* 1974;**77**:493–506.

67. DeLellis RA. *Atlas of Tumor Pathology: Tumors of the Parathyroid Gland 3rd Series*. Washington DC: Armed Forces Institute of Pathology,1991.

68. Bronsky D, Kiamko RT, Moncada R, Rosenthal IM. Intrauterine hyperparathyroidism secondary to maternal hypoparathyroidism. *Pediatrics* 1968;**42**:606–8.

69 Okonofua F, Menon RK, Houlder S, *et al*. Parathyroid hormone and neonatal calcium homeostasis: evidence for secondary hyperparathyroidism in the Asian neonate. *Metabolism* 1986;**35**:803–6.

70. Fukuoka H, Mukai S, Kobayashi Y, Jimbo T. Dynamic changes in serum osteocalcin levels in the perinatal period. *Nihon Naibuni Gakkai Zasshi* 1989;**65**:1116–22.

71. Sulaiman RA, Sharratt CL, Lee PW, *et al*. Ethnic differences in umbilical cord blood vitamin D and parathyroid hormone – South Asians compared to Whites born in the UK. *J. Matern. Fetal Neonatal Med.* 2010;**23**:1315–17.

72. Lothe A, Sinn J, Stone M. Metabolic bone disease of prematurity and secondary hyperparathyroidism. *J. Paediatr. Child. Health* 2011;**47**:550–3.

73. Keynes WM, Truscott BM. Large solitary cysts of the parathyroid gland. *Br. J. Surg.* 1956;**44**:23–4.

74. Lydiatt DD, Byers RM, Khouri KG, Whitworth PW, Sellin RV. Functional parathyroid cyst and hypocalciuric hypercalcemia. *Ear Nose Throat J.* 1993:**72**:142–4.

75. Dell'amore A, Asadi N, Bartalena T, Bini A, Stella F. Thoracoscopic resection of a giant mediastinal

parathyroid cyst. *Gen. Thorac. Cardiovasc. Surg.* 2013 (Epub ahead of print).

76. Gayatri P, Sanjay D, Ajay N, Amrut A. Mixed multilocular ectopic thymic cyst with parathyroid element presenting as neck mass. *Ann. Acad. Med. Singapore* 2012;**41**:271–2.

77. Daum F, Rosen JF, Boley SJ. Parathyroid adenoma, parathyroid crisis, and acute pancreatitis in an adolescent. *J. Pediat.* 1973;**83**:273–5.

78. Young TO, Saltzstein EC, Boman DA. Parathyroid carcinoma in a child: unusual presentation with seizures. *J. Pediatr. Surg.* 1984;**19**:194–200.

79. Meier DE, Snyder WH 3rd, Dickson BA, Margraf LR, Guzzetta PC Jr. Parathyroid carcinoma in a child. *J. Pediatr. Surg.* 1999;**34**:606–8.

80. Fiedler AG, Rossi C, Gingalewski CA. Parathyroid carcinoma in a child: An unusual case of an ectopically located malignant parathyroid gland with tumor invading the thymus. *J. Pediatr. Surg.* 2009;**44**:1649–52.

81. Herrera-Hernandez AA, Aranda-Valderrama P, Diaz-Perez JA, Herrera LP. Intrathyroidal parathyroid carcinoma in a pediatric patient. *Pediatr. Surg. Int.* 2011;**27**:1361–5.

82. Li CC, Yang C, Wang S, *et al.* A 10 year retrospective study of primary hyperparathyroidism in children. *Exp. Clin. Endocrinol. Diabetes* 2012;**120**:229–33.

83. Grimelius L, Akerstrom G, Johansson H, Juhlin C, Rastad J. The parathyroid glands. In Kovacs K, Asa S, editors, *Functional Endocrine Pathology.* Boston: Blackwell Scientific, 1990:375–95.

84. Ippolito G, Palazzo FF, Sebag F, De Micco C, Henry JF. Intraoperative diagnosis and treatment of parathyroid cancer and atypical parathyroid adenoma. *Br. J. Surg.* 2007;**94**(5):566–70.

85. Benaderet AD, Burton AM, Clifton-Bligh R, Ashraf AP. Primary hyperparathyroidism with low intact PTH levels in a 14- year-old girl. *J. Clin. Endocrinol. Metabol.* 2011;**96**:2325–9.

86. Wesseling K, Bakkaloglu S, Salusky I. Chronic kidney disease mineral and bone disorder in children. *Pediatr. Nephrol.* 2008;**23**:195–207.

87. Wesseling-Perry K. Bone disease in pediatric chronic kidney disease. *Pediatr. Nephrol.* 2013;**28**:569–76.

88. Wilhelm-Bals A, Parvex P, Magdelaine C, Girardin E. Successful use of biphosphonate and calcimimetic in neonatal severe primary hyperparathyroidism. Pediatrics 2012;**129**:812–16.

89. Hannan FM, Thakker RV Calcium-sensing receptor (CaSR) mutations and disorders of calcium, electrolyte and water metabolism. *Best. Pract. Res. Clin. Endocrinol. Metab.* 2013;**27**:359–71.

90. Giusti F, Marini F, Brandi ML. Multiple endocrine neoplasia type 1. In Pagon RA, Adam MP, Bird TD, Dolan CR, Fong CT, Stephens K, editors, *GeneReviews™* (Internet). Seattle, WA: University of Washington, Seattle, 1993–2013.

91. Lipps CJ, Dreijerink KM, Hoppener JW. Variable clinical expression in patients with a germline MEN1 disease gene mutation: clues to a genotype – phenotype correlation. *Clinics (Sao Paulo)* 2012;**67**:(S1) 49–56.

92. Marini F, Falchetti A, Del Monte F, *et al.* Multiple endocrine neoplasia type 2. *Orphanet. J. Rare Dis.* 2006;**2**:1–38.

93. Chandrasekharappa SC, Guru SC, Manickam P, *et al.* Positional cloning of the gene for multiple endocrine neoplasia-type 1. *Science* 1997;**276**:404–407.

94. Dreijerink KM, Lips CJ, Timmers HT. Multiple endocrine neoplasia type 1: A chromatin writer's block. *J. Intern. Med.* 2009;**266**(1):53–9.

95. Thakker RV, Newey PJ, Walls GV, *et al.* Clinical practice guidelines for multiple endocrine neoplasia type 1 (MEN1). *J. Clin. Endocrinol. Metab.* 2012;**97**:2990–3011.

96. Wagner SM, Zhu S, Nicolescu AC, Mulligan LM. Molecular mechanisms of RET receptor-mediated oncogenesis in multiple endocrine neoplasia 2. *Clinics (Sao Paulo)* 2012;**67** Suppl 1:77–84.

97. Zenaty D, Aigrain Y, Peuchmar M, *et al.* Medullary thyroid carcinoma identified within the first year of life in children with hereditary multiple endocrine neoplasia type 2A (codon 634) and 2B. *Eur. J. Endocrinol.* 2009;**160**:807–13.

98. Jabbour SA, Davidovici BB, Wolf R. Rare syndromes. *Clin. Dermatol.* 2006;**24**:299–316.

99. Lora MS, Waguespack SG, Moley JF, Walvoord EC. Adrenal ganglioneuromas in children with multiple endocrine neoplasia type 2: A report of two cases. *J. Clin. Endocrinol. Metab.* 2005;**90**:4383–7.

100. Lee NC, Norton JA. Multiple endocrine neoplasia type 2B–genetic basis and clinical expression. *Surg. Oncol.* 2000;**9**:111–8.

101. Raue F, Frank-Raue K. Genotype-phenotype correlation in multiple endocrine neoplasia type 2. *Clinics (Sao Paulo)* 2012;**67** Suppl 1:69–75.

102. Willis RA. *The Borderland of Embryology and Pathology.* London: Butterworths, 1958:326–9.

103. Vestfrid MA. Ectopic adrenal cortex in neonatal liver. *Histopathology* 1980;**4**:669–72.

104. Wright JR Jr, Gillis DA. Mediastinal foregut cyst containing an intramural adrenal cortical rest: A case report and review of supradiaphragmatic adrenal rests. *Pediatr. Pathol.* 1993;**13**:401–7.

223

105. Knape P, Reisch N, Dorr HG, *et al.* Testicular rest tumors (TART) in adult men with classic congenital adrenal hyperplasia (CAH). *Urologe A* 2008:**1596**–7,1599–602.

106. Claahsen-van der Grinten HL, Otten BJ, Stikkelbroek MM, Sweep FC, Hermus AR. Testicular adrenal rest tumors in congenital adrenal hyperplasia. Best *Pract. Res. Clin. Endocrinol. Metab.* 2009;**23**:209–20.

107. Mouritsen A, Jorgensen N, Main KM, Schwartz M, Juul A. Testicular adrenal rest tumors in boys, adolescents and adult men with congenital adrenal hyperplasia may be associated with the CYP21A2 mutation. *Int. J. Androl.* 2010;**33**:521–7.

108. Wiedemann HR. Complex familiale avec hernie ombilicale et macroglossie –un sybndrome nouveau. *J. Genet. Hum.* 1964;**13**:223–32.

109. Beckwith JB. Macroglossia, omphalocele, adrenal cytomegaly, gigantism and hyperplastic visceromegaly. *Birth Defects Orig. Artic. Series* 1969;**5**:188–96.

110. Cooper WN, Luharia A, Evans GA, *et al.* Molecular subtypes and phenotypic expression of Beckwith-Wiedemann syndrome. *Eur. J. Hum. Genet.* 2005;**13**:1025–32.

111. Aterman K, Kerenyi N, Lee M. Adrenal cytomegaly. *Virchows Arch. A* 1972;**355**:105–22.

112. Esterly JR, Oppenheimer EH. Intrauterine rubella infection. *Perspect. Pediatr. Pathol.* 1973;**1**:313–38.

113. Nakamura Y, Komatsu Y, Yano H, *et al.* Non immunologic hydrops fetalis; a clinicopathologic study of 50 autopsy cases. *Pediatr. Pathol.* 1987;**7**:19–30.

114. Camuto PM, Wolman SR, Perle MA, Greco MA. Flow cytometry of fetal adrenal glands with adrenocortical cytomegaly. *Pediatr. Pathol.* 1989;**9**:551–8.

115. Favara BE, Steele A, Grant JH, Steele P. Adrenal cytomegaly: quantitative assessment by image analysis. *Pediatr. Pathol.* 1991;**11**:521–36.

116. Ong BB, Wong KT. Adrenal cytomegaly associated with diaphragmatic hernia: report of a case. *Malays. J. Pathol.* 1996;**18**:121–123.

117. Skogseid B, Larsson C, *et al.* Clinical and genetic features of adrenocortical lesions in multiple endocrine neoplasia type 1. *J. Clin. Endocrinol. Metab.* 1992;**75**:76–81.

118. Kirk KM, Brain CE, Carson DJ, Hyde JC, Grant DB. Cushing's syndrome caused by nodular adrenal hyperplasia in children with McCune-Albright syndrome. *J. Pediatr.* 1999;**134**:789–92.

119. Stratakis CA, Jenkins RB, Pras E, *et al.* Cytogenetic and microsatellite alterations in tumors from patients with the syndrome of myxomas, spotty skin pigmentation, and endocrine overactivity (Carney complex). *J. Clin. Endocrinol. Metab.* 1996;**81**:3607–14.

120. Croitoru DP, Sinsky AB, Laberge JM. Cystic neuroblastoma. *J. Pediatr. Surg.* 1992;**27**:1320–1.

121. Sethuraman C, Rutter S, Drut R, *et al.* Bilateral absence of adrenal glands: A case series that expands the spectrum of associations and highlights the difficulties in prenatal diagnosis. *Fetal Pediatr. Pathol.* 2011;**30**:137–43.

122. Agrons GA, Lonergan GJ, Dickey GE, Perez-Monte JE. Adrenocortical neoplasm's in children: radiologic-pathologic correlation. *Radiographics* 1999;**19**:989–1008.

123. Michalkiewicz E, Sandrini R, *et al.* Clinical and outcome characteristics of children with adrenocortical tumors: A report from the International Pediatric Adrenocortical Tumor Registry. *J. Clin. Oncol.* 2004;**22**:838–45.

124. Che QL, Su Z, Li YH, *et al.* Clinical characteristics of adrenocortical tumors in children. *J. Pediatr. Endocrinol. Metab.* 2011;**24**:535–41.

125. Micic D, Zoric S, Popovic V, *et al.* Androgen-producing bilateral large cortical adrenal adenomas associated with polycystic ovaries in a young female. *Postgrad. Med. J.* 1992;**68**:219–22.

126. Driver CP, Birch J, Gough DC, Bruce J. Adrenal cortical tumors in childhood. *Pediatr. Hematol. Oncol.* 1998;**15**:527–32.

127. Bornstein SR, Stratakis CA, Chrousos GP. Adrenocortical tumors: recent advances in basic concepts and clinical management. *Ann. Intern. Med.* 1999;**130**:759–71.

128. Sasano H, Suzuki T, Moriya T. Recent advances in histopathology and immunohistochemistry of adrenocortical carcinoma. *Endocr. Pathol.* 2006;**17**:345–54.

129. van't Sant HP, Bouvy ND, Kazemier G, *et al.* The prognostic value of two different histopathological scoring systems for adrenocortical carcinomas. *Histopathology* 2007;**51**:239–45.

130. Lau SK, Weiss LS. The Weiss system for evaluating the adrenocortical neoplasms: 25years later. *Hum. Pathol.* 2009;**40**:757–68.

131. Papotti M, Libe R, Duregon E, *et al.* The Weiss score and beyond – histopathology for adrenocortical carcinoma. *Hum. Cancer* 2011;**2**:333–49.

132. Faria AM, Almeida MQ. Differences in the molecular mechanisms of adrenocortical tumorigenesis between children and adults. *Mol. Cell. Endocrinol.* 2012;**351**:52–7.

133. de Krijger RR, Papathomas TG. Adrenocortical neoplasia; evolving concepts in tumorigenesis with an

emphasis on adrenal cortical carcinoma variants. *Virchows Arch.* 2012;**460**:9–18.

134. Cagle PT, Hough AJ, Pysher TJ, *et al*. Comparison of adrenal cortical tumors in children and adults. *Cancer* 1986;**57**:2235–7.

135. Lack EE, Mulvihill JJ, Travis WD, Kozakewich HP. Adrenal cortical neoplasms in the pediatric and adolescent age group. Clinicopathologic study of 30 cases with emphasis on epidemiological and prognostic factors. *Pathol. Annu.* 1992;**27**:1–53.

136. Li FP, Fraumeni JF Jr. Rhabdomyosarcoma in children: epidemiologic study and identification of a familial cancer syndrome. *J. Natl. Cancer Inst.* 1969;**43**:1365–73.

137. Else T. Association of adrenocortical carcinoma with familial cancer susceptibility syndromes. *Mol. Cell. Endocrinol.* 2012;**351**:66–70.

138. Rodriguez-Galindo C, Figueiredo BC, Zambetti GP, Ribeiro RC. Biology, clinical characteristics and management of adrenocortical tumors in children. *Pediatr. Blood Cancer* 2005;**45**:265–73.

139. Fonseca AL, Kugelberg J, Starker LF, Scholl U, Choi M, *et al*. Comprehensive DNA methylation analysis of benign and malignant adrenocortical tumors. *Genes Chromosomes Cancer* 2012;**51**:949–60.

140. Rothenbuler A, Horvath A, Libe R, *et al*. Identification of novel genetic variants in phosphodiesterase (PDE8B), a camp-specific phosphodiesterase highly expressed in the adrenal cortex, in a cohort of patients with tumors. *Clin. Endocrinol. (Oxf)* 2012;**77**:195–9.

141. Singh P, Soon PS, Feige JJ, *et al*. Dysregulation of microRNAs in adrenocortical tumors. *Mol. Cell. Endocrinol.* 2012;**351**:118–28.

142. Lack EE. The adrenal gland. In Silverberg SS, De Lellis RA, Frable WJ, editors, *Principles and Practice of Surgical Pathology and Cytopathology*, third edn. New York: Churchill-Livingstone, 1997:2751–99.

143. DeLellis RA, Wolfe H, Gagel RT, *et al*. Adrenal medullary hyperplasia. A morphometric analysis in patients with familial medullary thyroid carcinoma. *Am. J. Pathol.* 1976;**83**:177–96.

144. Erlic Z, Neumann HP. Familial pheochromocytoma. *Hormones (Athens)* 2009;**8**:29–38.

145. Kumar M, Kumar V, Talukdar B, Mohta A, Khurana N. Cushing syndrome in an infant due to cortisol secreting adrenal pheochromocytoma: A rare association. *J. Pediatr. Endocrinol. Metab.* 2010;**23**:621–5.

146. Amar L, Bertherat J, Baudin E, *et al*. Genetic testing in pheochromocytoma or functional paraganglioma. *J. Clin. Oncol.* 2005;**23**:8812–18.

147. Carney JA, Sizemore GW, Sheps SG. Adrenal medullary disease in multiple endocrine neoplasia 2. *Am. J. Clin. Pathol.* 1976;**66**:279–90.

148. Rosai J. Adrenal and other paraganglia. In *Rosai and Ackerman's Surgical Pathology*, tenth edn. Oxford: Elsevier Mosby; 2011;1076–8.

149. Neville AM. The adrenal medulla. In Symington T, editor, *Functional Pathology of the Adrenal Gland*. Baltimore: Williams and Wilkins; 1969;219–34.

150. Scott HW Jr, Halter SA. Oncologic aspects of pheochromocytoma: the importance of follow-up. *Surgery* 1984;**96**:1061–6.

151. Shimada H, Ambros IM, Dehner LP, *et al*. Terminology and morphologic criteria of neuroblastic tumors: Recommendation by the International Neuroblastoma Pathology Committee. *Cancer* 1999;**86**:349–93.

152. Joshi VV. Peripheral neuroblastic tumors: pathologic classification based on recommendations of International Neuro blastoma Pathology Committee (modification of Shimada classification). *Pediatr. Dev. Pathol.* 2000;**3**:184–99.

153. Orbach D, Sarnacki S, Brisse HJ, *et al*. Neonatal cancer. *Lancet Oncol.* 2013;**14**(13):e609–20.

154. Turkel SB, Itabashi HH. The natural history of neuroblastic cells in the fetal adrenal glands. *Am. J. Pathol.* 1974;**76**:225–44.

155. Beckwith JB, Perrin EV. In situ neuroblastomas: A contribution to the natural history of neural crest Tumors. *Am. J. Pathol.* 1963;**43**:1089–104.

156. Kincaid OW, Hodgson JR, Dockerty MB. Neuroblastoma: A roentgenologic and pathologic study. *Am. J. Rontgenol. Radium Ther. Nucl. Med.* 1957;**78**:420–36.

157. Evans AE, D'Angio GJ, Randolph J. A proposed staging for children with neuroblastoma. *Cancer* 1971;**27**:374–8.

158. Brodeur GM, Pritchard J, Berthold F, *et al*. Revisions of the international criteria for neuroblastoma diagnosis, staging and response to treatment. *J. Clin. Oncol.* 1993;**11**:1466–77.

159. Hachitanda Y, Hata J. Stage IV S neuroblastoma: A clinical, histological and biological analysis of 45 cases. *Hum. Pathol.* 1996;**27**:1135–8.

160. Schneiderman J, London WB, Brodeur GM, *et al*. Clinical significance of MYCN amplification and ploidy in favorable-stage neuroblastoma: A report from the Children's Oncology Group. *J. Clin. Oncol.* 2008;**26**:913–18.

161. Brodeur GM, Green AA, *et al*. Cytogenetic features of human neuroblastomas and cell lines. *Cancer Res.* 1981;**41**:4678–86.

162. Gilbert F, Balaban G, Moorhead P, Bianchi D, Schlesinger H. Abnormalities of chromosome 1p in human neuroblastoma Tumors and cell lines. *Cancer Genet. Cytogenet.* 1982;7:33–42.

163. Brodeur GM, Seeger RC, Schwab M, Varmus HE, Bishop JM. Amplification of N-myc in untreated human neuroblastomas correlates with advanced disease stage. *Science* 1984;**224**(4653):1121–4.

164. Seeger RC, Brodeur GM, Sather H, *et al.* Association of multiple copies of the N-myc oncogene with rapid progression of neuroblastomas. *N. Engl. J. Med.* 1985;**313**:1111–16.

165. Nakagawara A, Arima-Nakagawara M, Scavarda NJ, *et al.* Association between high levels of expression of the TRK gene and favorable outcome in human neuroblastoma. *N. Engl. J. Med.* 1993;**328**:847–54.

166. Chan H, Haddad G, Thorner PS, *et al.* P-glycoprotein expression as a predictor of the outcome of therapy for neuroblastoma. *N. Engl. J. Med.* 1991;**325**:1608–14.

167. George RE, London WB, Cohn SL, *et al.* Hyperdiploid plus non amplified MYCN confers a favorable prognosis in children 12 to 18 months old with disseminated neuroblastoma: A Pediatric Oncology Group study. *J. Clin. Oncol.* 2005;**23**(27):6466–73.

168. Goto S, Umehara S, Gerbing RB, *et al.* Histopathology and MYCN status in peripheral neuroblastic tumors: A report from the Children's Cancer Group. *Cancer* 2001;**92**:2699–708.

169. Miller MA, Ohashi K, Zhu X, *et al.* Survivin mRNA levels are associated with biology of disease and patient survival in neuroblastoma: A report from the Children's Cancer Group. *J. Pediatr. Hematol. Oncol.* 2006;**28**:412–17.

170. Krams M, Heidebrecht HJ, Hero B, *et al.* Repp86 expression and outcome in patients with neuroblastoma. *J. Clin. Oncol.* 2003;**21**:1810–18.

171. Oberthuer A, Hero B, Spitz R, *et al.* The tumor-associated antigen PRAME is universally expressed in high stage neuroblastoma and associated with poor outcome. *Clin. Cancer Res.* 2004;**10**:4307–13.

172. Shimada H, Nakagawa A, Peters J, *et al.* TrkA expression in peripheral neuroblastic tumors: prognosis, significance and biological relevance. *Cancer* 2004;**101**;1873–81.

173. Kai-Oliver H, Bauer T, Schulte J, *et al.* CAMTA1, a 1p36 tumor suppressor candidate, inhibits growth and activates differentiations programs in neuroblastoma cells. *Cancer Res.* 2011;**15**:3142–51.

174. Wei JS, Greer BT, Westermann F, *et al.* Prediction of clinical outcome using gene expression profiling and artificial neural networks for patients with neuroblastoma. *Cancer Res.* 2004;**64**:6883–91.

175. Cohn SL, Pearson ADJ, London WB, *et al.* The International Neruoblastoma Risk Group (INRG) Classification System: An INRG task force report. *J. Clin. Oncol.* 2009; **27**:289–97.

176. De Vathaire F, Francois P, Schlumberger M, *et al.* Epidemiological evidence for a common mechanism for neuroblastoma and differentiated thyroid tumor. *Br. J. Cancer* 1992;**65**:425–8.

177. Hadjigeorgi C, Lafoyianni S, Pontikis Y, Van Vliet-Constantinidiou C. Asymptomatic myelolipoma of the adrenal. *Pediatr. Radiol.* 1992;**22**:465–6.

178. Cobanoglu U, Yaris N, Cay A. Adrenal myelolipoma in a child. *Pediatr. Surg. Int.* 2005;**21**:500–2.

179. Cardinalli IA, de Oliveira-Filho AG, Mastellaro MJ, Ribeiro RC, Aguilar SS. A unique case of synchronous functional adrenocortical adenoma and myelolipoma within the ectopic adrenal cortex in a child with Beckwith-Wiedemann Syndrome. *Pathol. Res. Pract.* 2012;**208**:189–94.

180. Arzanian MT, Khaleghnejad-Tabari A, *et al.* Generalized myelolipoma. *Arch. Iran. Med.* 2006;**9**:274–6.

181. Munns CFJ, Batch JA. The endocrine pancreas of the neonate and infant. *Perspect. Pediatr. Pathol.* 1982:7:137–65.

182. Milner RD, Wirdnam PK, Tsanakas J. Quantitave morphology of B, A, D, and PP cells in infants of diabetic mothers. *Diabetes* 1981;**30**:271–4.

183. Fukuzawa R, Umezawa A, *et al.* Nesidioblastosis and mixed hamartoma of the liver in Beckwith-Wiedemann syndrome: case study including analysis of H19 methylation and insulin-like growth factor 2 genotyping and imprinting. *Pediatr. Dev. Pathol.* 2001;**4**:381–90.

184. Neri G, Martini-Neri ME, Katz BE, Opitz JM. The Perlman syndrome: Familial renal dysplasia with Wilms tumor, fetal gigantism and multiple congenital anomalies. *Am. J. Genet. A* 2013;**161**:2691–6.

185. Patton RG, Christie DL, Smith DW, Beckwith JB. Cerebro-hepato-renal syndrome of Zellweger. Two patients with islet cell hyperplasia, hypoglycemia, and thymic anomalies, and comments on iron metabolism. Am. J. Dis. Child. 1972;**124**:840–4.

186. Halvorsen S, Pande H, Loken AC, Gjessing LR. Tyrosinosis. A study of 6 cases. *Arch. Dis. Child.* 1966;**41**:238–49.

187. Dickson PI, Briones NY, *et al.* Costello syndrome with pancreatic cell hyperplasia. *Am. J. Genet. A* 2004;**130A**:402–5.

188. Suh YL, Khang SK, Kim KN. Neonatal hemochromatosis- a report of an autopsy case. *J. Korean Med. Sci.* 1999;**6**:267–72.

189. Laidlaw, GF. Nesidioblastoma, islet tumor of pancreas. *Am. J. Pathol.* 1938;**14**:125–34.

190. Yakovac WC, Baker L, Hummeler K. Beta cell nesidioblastosis in idiopathic hypoglycemia of infancy. *J. Pediatr.* 1971;**79**:226–31.

191. Aynsley-Green, Hussain K, *et al.* Practical management of hyperinsulinism in infancy. *Arch. Dis. Child. Fetal Neonatal Ed.* 2000;**82**:F98–107.

192. Dunne MJ, Cosgrove KE, Shepherd RM, Aynsley-Green A, Lindley KJ. Hyperinsulinism in Infancy: From basic science to clinical disease. *Physiol. Rev.* 2004;**84**:239–75.

193. Rahier J, Sempoux C, Fournet JC, *et al.* Partial or near total pancreatectomy for persistent neonatal hyperinsulinaemic hypoglycaemia: the pathologist's role. *Histopathology* 1998; **32**:15–19.

194. Jack MM, Walker RM, Thomsett MJ, Cotterill AM, Bell JR. Histologic findings in persistent hyperinsulinemic hypoglycemia of infancy: Australian experience. *Pediatr. Devel. Pathol.* 2000;**3**:532–47.

195. Sempoux C, Capito C, Bellané-Chantelot *et al.* Morphological mosaicism of the pancreatic islets: A novel anatomopathological form of persistent hyperinsulinemic hypoglycemia of infancy. *J. Endocrinol. Metab.* 2011;**96**:3785–93.

196. Arbizu Lostao J, Fernandez-Marmiesse A, *et al.* 18F-fluoro-L-DOPA PET-CT imaging combined with genetic analysis for optimal classification and treatment in a child with severe congenital hyperinsulinism. *Ann. Pediatr.* 2008;**68**(5):481–5.

197. Von Rohden L, Mohnike K, Mau H, *et al.* Intraoperative sonography: A technique for localizing focal forms of congenital hyperinsulinism in the pancreas. *Ultraschall. Med.* 2011;**32**:74–80.

198. Arnoux JB, Verkarre V *et al.* Congenital hyperinsulinism: current trends in diagnosis and therapy. *Orphanet. J. Rare Dis.* 2011;**6**:63.

199. Giurgea I, Bellane-Chantelot C, Ribeiro M, *et al.* Molecular mechanisms of neonatal hyperinsulinism. *Horm. Res.* 2006;**66**:289–96.

Lymph nodes, bone marrow, and immunodeficiencies

Bo-Yee Ngan, Jo-Anne Vergilio, and Megan S. Lim

Lymph node pathology

Introduction

Overview of pediatric lymphoma

Lymphoma is a malignant clonal lymphoid neoplasm. It manifests initially within lymph node(s); the abnormal unregulated lymphoid proliferations markedly enlarge and destroy the normal architecture. As the disease progresses the proliferative process may also disseminate into other nodal sites or other hematopoietic organs such as the spleen and bone marrow, and systemically into many other extranodal sites. Sometimes it may transiently disseminate into the blood stream, and this is referred to as a leukemic phase of the lymphoma. Accurate diagnosis and the most reproducible result requires a surgical biopsy (or other multiple core biopsies) that should be obtained from the largest lymph node detected clinically and not simply from any lymph node that is the most surgically accessible. This is fundamental for accurate diagnose of subtypes. A minority of lymphomas may present primarily outside of the lymph nodes and they are termed extranodal lymphomas. When there is no lymph node involvement after six months this is called a primary extranodal lymphoma.

Epidemiological and clinical features

Lymphoma is the third most common cancer in children and adolescents. It comprises two major disease categories: Hodgkin's lymphoma (HL) and non-Hodgkin's lymphoma (NHL) (1–3). Both lymphomas have unique differences in their histopathological features, pathological subtypes, incidences, treatment requirements, and survival outcomes. Many of the epidemiological and clinical features in the pediatric population (age 0–19 years) are distinct from the adults. In NHL (4), for example, between the ages of 0–19, 79.5% are precursor B-cell type and only 13.8% are mature B-cell NHL, as compared with adults where the percentages are 2.3 and 85.5, respectively. The differences in the cases recorded remain the same when the percentages of precursor lymphoma (both B- and T-cell types) and leukemia are combined and compared between pediatric and adults, i.e., 80% vs. 4.4%. Diffuse large B-cell lymphoma (DLBCL) and Burkitt's lymphoma (BL) are almost equally prevalent (40% and 41.1%, respectively) in children; whereas within the adult group, the percentages for DLBCL vs. BL are 28% and 2.2%, respectively. However, when the age group 0–19 years is further divided, BL occurs more frequently in children between 5 and 14 years old and DLBCL in 15–19-year-olds. Follicular lymphoma is more prevalent in adults than in children (18.2% vs. 4.5%). Similarly, anaplastic large T-cell lymphoma represents 47% of mature T-cell lymphomas in children, whereas it only accounts for 15.2% in the adult population. As for HL, it has a bimodal distribution and the incidence peaks in the 20–24 years age group and again in the 75–79 years age group. Hodgkin's lymphoma accounts for 21% of all lymphoid neoplasm in the 0–19 age group and 13.4% in the 20–40 years age group.

Current concepts on the pathogenesis of B-cell lymphomas/HL

Lymphoma originates from malignant transformation of a single B-cell, T-cell, or natural killer (NK)-T-cell that undergoes clonal proliferation. The initiating transformation and the subsequent proliferation processes exhibit one or several hallmarks of cancer development (5). The hallmarks of cancer development in different types of lymphoma are listed in Table 7.1 (6–20).

Essentials of Surgical Pediatric Pathology, ed. Marta C. Cohen and Irene Scheimberg. Published by Cambridge University Press.
© Cambridge University Press 2014.

Table 7.1 Pathogenesis of lymphoma: insights from recent molecular pathology studies (see text for details) (6–20)

Cancer hallmarks	Abnormal alterations	Potential effects	Lymphoma types
Proliferative or receptor signaling	- CD79Aor B ITAM (del);CD79B ITAM mutation - oncogenic mutation of signaling complex CARD11-MALT1 or BCL10 - *A20* del	Chronic active B-cell receptor signaling, increased/constituitive activation of NF-κB followed by increase IRF4 inducing further differentiation; NK-κB mediates clonal proliferation	Germinal-center type B-NHL; activated B-cell-like NHL; MALT lymphoma
Proliferative or receptor signaling	*MYD88 (L265)* mutation and the associated *IRAK1* phosphorylation /4 kinase activity	Mediates toll and (IL)-1 receptor-mediated signaling, NF-κB signaling and JAK kinase activation of STAT3, secretion of IL-6, IL-10 and (IF)β-associated lymphoma cell survival	Germinal-center type B-NHL; <10% MALT lymphoma
Proliferative or receptor signaling	*JAK-STAT, AP-1, Notch-1, MAPK/ERK, PIK3/AKT, NF-κB* and receptor kinases; amplification of c-rel locus on 2p	Constituitive activation leading to enhanced cell survival	
Proliferative or receptor signaling	-EBV associated LMP-1 expression	LMP-1 activation of NF-κB	EBV+ve HD
Proliferative or receptor signaling	Nuclear *p50/p65* heterodimerization or *NFKB1A* inactivating mutation or deletion association with inactivation of *I-κB* or *A20* mutation	Associated with NF-κB activation	EBV–ve HD
Proliferative or receptor signaling	Unknown	Constitutive activation of NK-κB	LPHD
Proliferative or receptor signaling	*NOTCH1* mutation/ translocation	Activation (via γ-secretase) and subsequent transcriptional activation of downstream targets such as Myc oncogene or others	T-ALL; or t(7;9) ALL
Proliferative or receptor signaling	-*miR-17–92* amplification	mTOR signaling	Germinal-center type B-NHL
Proliferative or receptor signaling	Amplification of 9p24 with the tyrosine kinase *JAK2* within	Subsequent activation of transcription factor STAT6	Primary mediastinal lymphoma and Hodgkin's
Proliferative or receptor signaling	Translocation activation or amplification of 8q24	Activation of c-Myc	Burkitt's lymphoma
Evasion of growth suppressor	EVB-associated proteins	Evade immune surveillance	Post-transplant lympho-proliferative disease/lymphoma
Evasion of growth suppressor/ regulation	Increased STAT3; increased IL6 &10 or IRF4, both from NF-κB induction	Alteration of immune regulatory network	Activated B-cell-like NHL
Evasion of growth suppressor/ regulation	19q gain or amplification	Increased SPIB associated alteration of immune regulatory network	Activated B-cell-like NHL
Evasion of growth suppressor	*Blimp-1* del or mutation *BCL6* translocation *BCL6* mutation *SPIB* amplification	Differentiation arrest due to decreased Blimp-1	Activated B-cell-like NHL
Evasion of growth suppressor/ regulation	Trisomy 3	Increased FOXP1 associated alteration of immune regulatory network	Activated B-cell-like NHL
Evasion of growth suppressor/ regulation	9p24 amplicon	Increased PDL2 that inhibits immune surveillance	Primary mediastinal lymphoma
Resisting cell death/ apoptosis	*BCL2* translocation	Abort apoptosis	Germinal-center type B-NHL

Table 7.1 (cont.)

Cancer hallmarks	Abnormal alterations	Potential effects	Lymphoma types
Resisting cell death/apoptosis	BCL2 amplification	Abort apoptosis	Activated B-cell-like NHL
Resisting cell death/apoptosis	Increased NF-κB	Inhibit apoptosis	Activated B-cell-like NHL, primary mediastinal lymphoma and Hodgkin's
Resisting cell death/apoptosis	Amplification of 9p24 with the tyrosine kinase JAK2 within or mutation or del of SOCS1 mutation	Inhibition of apoptosis secondary to JAK 2 activation	Primary mediastinal lymphoma and Hodgkin's
Replicative immortality	EBV associated LMPs	Enhanced immortalization	Post-transplant lympho-proliferative disease/lymphoma
Enhanced genomic instability	PTEN, or ING1,or p53, or MDM2 del or amplification	Enabling acquisition of genomic instability	Germinal-center type B-NHL
Enhanced genomic instability	INK4-ARF del	Enabling acquisition of genomic instability	Activated B-cell-like NHL
Enhanced genomic instability	Increased activation-induced cytidine deaminase	Aberrant switch translocations	Activated B-cell-like NHL

Molecular studies on pediatric B-cell NHL are few. Some distinctive features are emerging in the characterization of pediatric and adult BL and DLBCL (21,22).

As for HL, since its identification by Thomas Hodgkin in 1832 (23), and the subsequent recognition of the Reed–Sternberg cell as the diagnostic hallmark cell of HL(24,25), its pathogenesis has remained unclear. The neoplastic Hodgkin cell has features of a germinal center or postgerminal center B-cell (24). Furthermore, the diagnostic cells of a subtype of HL, lymphocyte-predominant HL, were found to have features of a germinal center B-cell capable of undergoing somatic hypermutation of the immunoglobulin-gene VH segment, as well as other genes (26–29). These results provide support for the current concept that biologically, HL is really two disease entities: nodular lymphocyte-predominant HL and classical HL (30).

These studies, together with others, have shown that each subtype of HL and NHL is distinct and each of them exhibits unique molecular, immunological, and some cytogenetic abnormalities that are currently included as diagnostic criteria in the WHO classification of lymphoma (30).

General approaches to the histopathological analyses of lymph-node biopsies: tissue handling, triage, and histostains

All lymph-node biopsies should be submitted fresh in a sterile container, and examined and triaged in a sterile environment, observing biohazard protocols. For core biopsies, a minimum of six to eight cores should be submitted in chilled tissue culture media (such as RPMI) or buffered physiological saline. Lymph nodes are measured and bisected on a non-absorbent surface or on saline-soaked telfa gauze, and the gross features described. At least two touch imprints (one fixed for H&E; one air-dried for Wright–Giemsa stain) should be prepared. Thin slices sampled from the center and some from the periphery of the lymph node are fixed in formalin. The remaining should be divided up for cytogenetic analysis and snap freezing for molecular analyses. If there is sufficient tissue left, it can be used for flow cytometry. For core biopsies, at least 50% of the cores are used for formalin fixation, one core each for snap freezing, cytogenetics, and/or flow-cytometry analysis. If molecular analyses require complex analytical procedures to be performed by a laboratory at an academic health science center, the snap-frozen tissue should be shipped in a dry-ice pack. Cytogenetic specimens should stay chilled in sterile tissue culture media and be shipped in a crushed ice (or +4 ºC coolant gel) package.

Lymphoma diagnosis today and in the near future in the molecular pathology and molecularly targeted therapy era

The diagnostic practice incorporates additional immunohistological, cytogenetic, and molecular features to identify and subclassify lymphoma. Many of them had been incorporated into the WHO lymphoma classifications (30,31). The new discoveries in molecular pathogenetic mechanisms in lymphoma will no doubt be useful to provide therapeutic guidance for personalized and targeted drug therapy (32).

Benign lymph-node conditions

Reactive lymphoid hyperplasia

Clinical presentation: Non-specific; may include history of fever, swelling, fatigue, malaise; may have other underlying medical conditions. There are associations with rare conditions such as autoimmune lymphoproliferative syndrome (ALPS).

Subtypes: (1) Non-specific (unknown etiology); (2) infections; (3) dermatological; (4) post-therapy, such as postvaccination, allergies, and drug reaction; (5) rheumatological, autoimmune diseases, inflammatory bowel disease.

Macroscopic features: Cut surface is smooth to granular; multiple small nodules may be visible.

Histology: The best approach is to evaluate the patterns of changes according to the architectural components and domains, i.e., follicular; follicular and paracotical; paracortical; sinusoidal. The microscopic features according to the subtype of conditions are as follows.

Non-specific lymphoid hyperplasia

The changes are that of a near-balanced enlargement of germinal centers coupled with an expansion of the paracortex. The follicles are clearly defined by mantle zones, and within the germinal center there is polarization of the centrocytes (small and large cleaved cells) and centroblasts (non-cleaved cells) with a pale zone. Often this zone can be obscured by a prominent proliferation of tingible body macrophages. The

marginal zone may be slightly expanded. At low magnification, the paracortex may appear mottled, due to an increase in reactive histiocytes and macrophages. The lymphoid cellular population in the paracortex comprises increased numbers of immunoblasts and para-immunoblasts. The sinusoids are patent and they may contain increased numbers of sinusoidal histiocytes and lymphocytes. In the medulla, plasma cells are present.

Infection-associated lymphoid hyperplasia

Virus infections

The most frequent type of infection-related lymph-node changes seen in immunocompetent adolescents is that of Epstein–Barr virus (EBV). During the early phase, there is florid follicular hyperplasia, together with an exuberant colonization of the paracortex by viral transformed lymphocytes with cytological features of reactive centroblasts (non-cleaved cells), para-immunoblasts, and immunoblasts. Some may have a prominent nucleolus. The histopatholgical features may mimic lymphoma (33). Despite their large cell size and crowding within the paracortex, there is no destruction of the stroma and the lymphoid cells are not monomorphic, rather a spectrum of lymphoid cellular transformations from small, to intermediate, to large lymphoid cells should be present. Expansion of the marginal zone may be seen in some areas and occasional reactive epithelioid histiocytes may be present. Immunohistological stain should reveal a mixed population of T-cells and B-cells in the paracortex. *In situ* hybridization for EBV-encoded RNA (EBER) will be strongly positive. In the resolving phase of EBV infection, the reactive features are much subdued and only some foci of EBV-positive cells in both germinal centers and paracortex remain. Other viral infections, such as cytomegalovirus (CMV) or adenovirus will result in a similar non-specific lymphoid hyperplasia. Immunostains for these viruses will enable a specific diagnosis. In herpes lymphadenitis, syncytial giant cells may be present. Immunostain for herpes antigen can confirm the viral infection.

Protozoan infections

Toxoplasma will result in lymphoid follicular and paracortical hyperplasia. In addition, microaggregates of reactive epithelioid histiocytes may decorate the parafollicular location of some of the reactive germinal centers.

Mycobacterial infections

These will elicit a granulomatous inflammatory reaction within the paracortex. Mycobacterial infections are associated with necrotic granulomata (caseating necrosis), where small geographic foci of necrotic stroma that may or may not be demarcated by histiocytes or multinucleated giant cells, are present. A positive Ziel–Neelson stain can establish the presence of acid-fast mycobacteria, but is insufficient to rule out mycobacterial infection if the stain result is negative.

Fungal infections more commonly seen in lymph nodes include *Histoplasma*, *Cryptococcus*, *Blastomyces*, and *Coccidio*, and for the immunosuppressed, *Candida*, *Aspergillius*, and *Sporotrichum*. Formations of granuloma are common. A positive Gomori's silver methanamine or a periodic acid–Schiff-diastase (PAS-D) stain can give a diagnosis of fungal infection by revealing the presence of fungal spores, mycelium, or hyphae.

Bacterial, spirochetes, and others

Cat-scratch disease, tularemia, yersinia, and brucellosis: Gram-negative bacteria *Bartonella henselae*, *Francisella tularensis*, *Yersinia enterolitica*, *Yersinia pseudotuberculosis* and *Brucella suis*, *B. melitensis*, *B. abortus*, and *B. canis* are the causative agents for these, respectively.

Histopathological changes in the lymph node in all of these infections share similarities with cat-scratch disease (34): well-defined paracortical microabscesses surrounded by a cuff of palisading histiocytes (stellate abscesses) with granulomas. For the first three infections cited above, Gram, Warthin–Starry, or Steiner stains may be positive. For brucellosis, Gram stains can be difficult. For bartonellae, three diagnostic modalities (Steiner silver stain, immunohistochemistry with antibodies to *B. henselae*, or polymerase chain reaction (PCR) that target *B. henselae* and *B. Quintana*) are available (35).

Borrelia burgdorferi is the causative agent for Lyme's disease. The involved lymph node has follicular hyperplasia parafollicular necrotizing microabscesses infiltrated and surrounded by eosinophils. Stains such as Warthin–Starry, Dieterle, or immunostain for the spirochete may be negative. Reactive serology titer by immune-sorbent test is best to confirm exposure to the infectious agent. *Treponema pallidum*, the agent for syphilis, is associated with plasmacytic sinusoidal infiltrates and can have granulomatous lymphadenitis; it can be detected by Warthin–Starry or Steiner stains.

Dermatopathic change

In addition to the reactive changes described above, the distinguishable feature is the presence of small numbers of pigmented macrophages amongst the reactive lymphoid proliferations within the paracortex.

Post-therapy such as postvaccination, allergies, and drug reaction

Other than reactive lymphoid hyperplasia, there are no specific or additional histopathological features associated with postimmunization. Allergic reactions may be associated with a mild increase in eosinophils, but concern should be raised that the lymph node material is not obtained at draining sites of other diseases such as Hodgkin's lymphoma, eosinophilic granuloma, Kimura's disease, lymphomatoid papulosis, or Lyme's disease and is thus non-diagnostic. Drug reaction can be associated with florid paracortical lymphoid hyperplasia (e.g., hydantoin-associated lymphadenopathy). The presence of epithelioid histiocytes amongst reactive lymphoid infiltrates can be secondary to some immunosuppressive drugs.

Rheumatological, autoimmune diseases, inflammatory bowel disease

Non-specific reactive lymphoid follicular and paracortical hyperplasia are the predominant histological features. Microganulomas may be present in the paracortex from patients with inflammatory bowel disease, such as Crohn's disease. The presence of necrosis with prominent apoptosis and plasma cells, with or without neutrophils, can be a manifestation of systemic lupus erythematosis.

Autoimmune lymphoproliferative syndrome (ALPS)

This is an apoptosis defect in maintaining lymphocyte homeostasis due to germline mutations of the *FAS* (CD95/APO-1) genes (in a majority of cases), or somatic *FAS* mutation, or germline mutation of *FASL* or *CASP10*.

Clinical presentation: A rare condition associated with chronic (> six months) non-malignant lympadenopathy, hepatosplenomegaly, and multilineage cytopenia (often associated with autoimmune manifestations) in the vast majority of cases and frequently associated with the presence of a rare T-cell population known as CD4 and CD8 double-negative cells (36). The risk of ALPS patients developing Hodgkin's

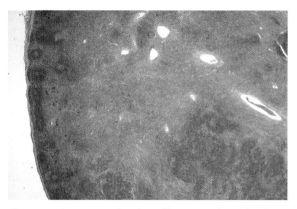

Figure 7.1 Autoimmune lymphoproliferative syndrome (ALPS) from a patient with a nonsense mutation in *TNFSF6* resulting in an immediate stop codon at position 467 in exon 3, encoding the extracellular portion of *FAS*. Note the presence of expansion of paracortex (3.9% double negative CD4/8 T-cells by flow cytometry), reactive germinal centers, and a concomitant LPHD nodule in the lower right corner.

lymphoma or non-Hodgkin's lymphoma is increased 50-fold and 14-fold, respectively, compared to the general population (36).

Genetics: A majority of cases are due to autosomal dominant transmission of heterozygous germline *FAS* gene mutations. Somatic *FAS* variants of ALPS are due to haplosufficiency, as mechanisms of decreased FAS expression also exist. Patients with Evans syndrome and common variable immune deficiencies have been found to have ALPS (37). Two main and six additional criteria are required for the diagnosis of ALPS (38).

Histology: Vast expansion of the paracortex due to marked paracortical hyperplasia, resulting in wide separation of reactive cortical lymphoid follicles (39; Figure 7.1). High magnification shows predominance of paraimmunoblasts and immunoblasts within a background of small and mid-sized lymphocytes. Some may contain reactive epithelioid histiocytes near to the reactive lymphoid follicles. Sinuses may be patent with reactive sinus histiocytosis. As ALPS patients have an increased risk of lymphoma, the presence of nodular lymphocyte-predominant Hodgkin's lymphoma or non-Hodgkin's lymphoma must be ruled out from the biopsy. Key findings are the presence of double-negative CD4 and CD8 T-cells, and a reduction or absence of CD45RO T-cells (40). However, not all cases are CD4- and CD8-negative. DNA analysis for T- or B-cell clonality is negative. Deleterious mutations that correspond to the region that code for the intracellular domain of *FAS* are diagnostic; polymorphisms

in *FAS* are not uncommon. A reference database for pathogenic ALPS-FAS is available via the NIH/USA website (http://www3.niaid.nih.gov/topics/ALPS/, accessed May 2014).

Differential diagnosis: Patients with ALPS-like syndromes can harbor germline mutations in *CASP8* and somatic mutations in *NRAS* and *KRAS* (36).

Progressive transformation of germinal centers (PTGC)

This is an uncommon benign condition associated with distinct clinicopathological features.

Clinical presentation: Chronic lymphandenopathy over one month. Occurs commonly (over 50%) in the cervical lymph node. Is seen in approximately 3–15% of non-specific lymphadenitis (41,42) One study showed a median age of 11.5 years, with clinical lymphadenopathy recurring within four years (42%), and 17% had histological confirmation of recurrent PTGC. Fourteen percent were associated with Hodgkin's lymphoma (especially nodular lymphocyte-predominant Hodgkin's lymphoma). Twenty four percent had associated immune disorders, including SLE (lupus), Castleman's disease, and probable ALPS (43).

Histology: There are one or more atypical large reactive lymphoid follicles (typically three to five times larger) amongst a background of secondary follicles within a lymph node, with features of marked reactive lymphoid follicular hyperplasia. A prominent thick, expanded mantle delineates this follicle and often there is some evidence of B-lymphocyte infiltration into the germinal center. Atypical lymphohistiocytic cells are absent, and expansion, but not disruption of the dendritic follicular cell network of the lymphoid follicle is seen (Figure 7.2).

There is an immunostaining pattern of the follicle by B-cell markers CD20, BCL-6, and CD21, with scattered CD57 T-cells, very few CD3 T-cells, complete lack of BCL2 expression in the germinal center B-cells, and absence of CD30 cells, with atypical cytological features in the parafollicular areas. T-cell rosettes formed around large lymphoid cells may be present, but the large cells do not have popcorn cell-like transformation. No epithelial membrane antigen (EMA)-positive large cells are seen (44) and *in-situ* hybridization (ISH) for EBV is negative.

Differential diagnosis: Nodular lymphocyte-predominant Hodgkin's lymphoma or, less frequently, other HL.

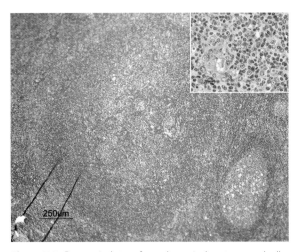

Figure 7.2 Progressively transformed germinal center: a markedly enlarged germinal center with expanded mantle-cell zone that invaginates into the germinal center or fuses with its neighboring follicles. Inset: occasional reactive histiocytes (or immunoblasts or RS-like cells not shown) may be present.

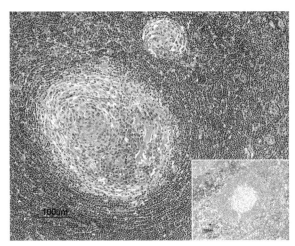

Figure 7.3 Castleman's disease: concentric arrays of small lymphocytes surround the involuted germinal center (GC) that contains condensation of follicular dendritic cells. Prominent small blood vessels with hyalinized wall and deposits emanate from the GC into the parafollicular areas. Inset: CD123+ plasmacytoid dendritic cells cluster around high endothelial venules in the paracortex.

Castleman's disease

This is a rare lymphoproliferative disorder; immune dysregulation either primary or secondary to HSV may have a pivotal role in producing IL6 or other B-cell growth factors and releasing angiogenic factors. IL6 may play a role in aiding lymphoid proliferation and plasma cell differentiation (45). The exact etiology and pathogenesis is unknown.

Clinical presentation: There are two clinical entities that correlate with histological variants. Localized or unicentric types usually have hyaline vascular histological features and the systemic/multicentric variant has plasma cells or mixed variants. The former presents with minimal symptoms and can be cured by surgical excision, whereas the latter requires systemic treatment with a guarded prognosis. In the systemic form, the patient may present with fever, fatigue, rash, and increased acute-phase reactants. In children the prognosis is better than in adults (45–47).

Histology: In the *hyaline vascular type*, there is formation of hypervascular germinal centers that are replaced by a compact concentric array of atypical dendritic reticulum cells. The germinal centers are poorly formed, atrophic-like, with mostly mantle B-cells. A few small blood vessels often emanate from the center of the germinal center and anastomose with the peri-follicular small blood vessels. The paracortex is hypervascular, with increased numbers of high endothelial venules, with clusters of plasmacytoid dendritic cells gathering around them (48,49). Hyaline

material is deposited in the perivascular area within the germinal center (Figure 7.3). In the *plasma cell variant*, hyperplastic germinal centers with plasma cell aggregates between high endothelial venules, partially sparing the sinuses, are the features of the plasma cell variant (50). In adults, hemophagocytic syndrome, autoimmune hemolytic anemia, and lymphoma are the commonest complications and Kaposi sarcoma is also reported (51).

Immunohistochemistry is not essential for diagnosis. For the hyaline vascular type, the hypervascular poorly formed germinal centers with predominant mantle cells are positive for B-cells marker such as CD20. CD123+ plasmacytoid dendritic cells are noted to be present in tight clusters (Figure 7.3 inset) more frequently than other reactive/autoimmune lymphadenopathies (49). The excessive concentric arrays of follicular dendritic reticulum cells can be demonstrated by antibodies to follicular dendritic cells (FDC), such as D2-40. In the plasmacytic variant, antibodies to immunoglobulin light chains κ and λ can demonstrate polyclonal plasma cells. In multicentric CD tested in adults, immunostain with anti-human herpes virus type 8 (HHV8) LANA-1 stains plasmablasts and PCR of blood is positive (51). Unfortunately, IL6 cannot be detected by immunohistochemisrty.

Differential diagnosis: Late phase of lymphadenopathy with regressing germinal centers, non-specific plasmacytosis, and plasmacytic neoplasms.

Kikuchi–Fujimoto disease

This is a self-limiting benign histiocytic necrotizing lymphadenopathy of unknown etiology.

Clinical presentation: There is a higher prevalence in Asia than elsewhere, mostly affecting patients under 40, with no male or female predominance. It presents as a benign unilateral tender cervical lymphadenopathy over a course of 2–3 weeks, painful in 59% patients. Generalized lymphadenopathy is much less frequent (1–20%). Half may have low-grade fever, with upper respiratory symptoms. Rare patients may have weight loss, nausea, vomiting, sore throat, or night sweats (52,53).

Histology: The disease has three histopathological phases: proliferative, necrotizing, and xanthomatous (53). Foci of coagulative necrosis, which can be extensive, typically develop within the paracortex. Abundant apoptotic histiocytes, plasmacytoid monocytes, and immunoblasts are seen within the lesional areas (Figure 7.4). Prominent numbers of plasmacytoid dendritic cells can be seen around the high endothelial venules. Different types of reactive histiocytes may be present, including phagocytotic (tingible body), non-phagocytotic (crescentic), and foamy (xanthomatous) types. Neutrophils are absent. The adjacent paracortex shows reactive changes; large numbers of immunoblasts may be present and may be mistaken for lymphoma cells (53). Other parts of the lymph node may have follicular hyperplasia.

The necrotic foci are infiltrated predominantly by CD8+, TiA1+, granzyme B+, and perforin+ cytotoxic T-cells (CD56+ NK cells are rare), amongst many CD68+ histiocytes (Figure 7.4 inset). Aggregates or single CD123+ plasmacytoid dendritic cells are also present (48,49,52).

Differential diagnosis: Systemic lupus erythematosus or other autoimmune diseases such as phospholipid syndrome, polymyositis, systemic juvenile idiopathic arthritis, bilateral uveitis, arthritis, cutaneous necrotizing vasculitis, and pulmonary hemorrhage have been linked to Kikuchi's. Non-Hodgkin's lymphoma may present as a histopathological challenge due to the presence of atypical lymphoid cells and immunoblasts when these cells are numerous (53). Kawasaki disease has perifollicular geographic necrosis, but the lesion contains neutrophils and fibrinoid thrombi.

Kimura disease

This is a rare, unique idiopathic chronic inflammatory disorder that clinically simulates a neoplasm.

Clinical presentation: Kimura disease is frequent in, but not exclusive to, Asians in middle age; it can occur in children and adolescents. It affects mostly head and neck skin and regional lymph nodes, and occurs less frequently in salivary glands. Elevated serum IgE levels and peripheral eosinophilia are common (54–56), and the condition can be recurrent.

Histology: Lymphoid follicular hyperplasia is seen, with prominent perifollicular and paracortical eosinophil infiltrates and proliferation of postcapillary venules, (Figure 7.5; 54).

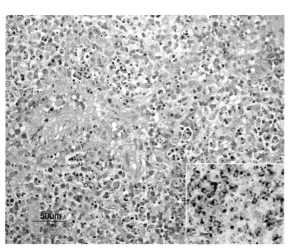

Figure 7.4 Kikuchi's disease: within the necrotic foci in the paracortex, marked increases in lymphocyte apoptosis result in the prominence of apoptotic nuclear debris within the affected areas. Neutrophils and plasma cells are completely absent and cytotoxic T-cells are increased (inset, showing granzyme B+ cytotoxic cells) and activated macrophages (not shown).

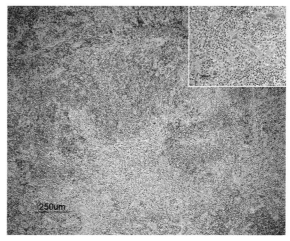

Figure 7.5 Kimura disease: marked infiltrates of eosinophils in the paracortex that shows reactive features. Inset shows that the high endothelial venules have reactive endothelium.

235

Differential diagnosis: Angiolymphoid hyperplasia with eosinophilia.

Kawasaki disease

This was first described as an acute febrile mucocutaneous syndrome with lymphoid involvement. Initially it was thought to be self-limiting and benign, but it was subsequently recognized that, if untreated, patients may develop coronary aneurysms and thrombo-embolic occlusions, leading to sudden death.

Clinical presentation: There is high prevalence in the Japanese population (57). Presentation is related to hyperactivation of the immune system, i.e., an acute systemic vasculitis of infancy and early childhood. Patients have prolonged fever, conjunctivitis, oropharyngeal inflammation, rash, erythematous induration of the distal extremities, and cervical lymphadenopathy (58,59).

Genetics: Non-conclusive; recent reports of several susceptibility genes (57).

Histology: Severe acute phase lymph nodes show variable geographic subcapsular, cortical, or paracortical necrosis, within which are fibrin thrombi in small blood vessels and nuclear debris. No immunoblasts are present. Active vasculits, arteritis, and phlebitis, and infiltrates of chronic inflammatory cells can be seen in the extranodal tissues (58). Immunohistochemistry and molecular analyses are not contributory; the bacterial genome is detected in a small percentage (59).

Differential diagnosis: Acute infectious or autoimmune non-granulomatous lymphadenopathies. Clinical correlations are necessary.

Benign histiocytic disease

Rosai–Dorfman disease

This is a worldwide, unique disease of unknown etiology, with childhood predilection. Its hallmark histological feature is sinus histiocytosis with massive lymphadenopathy, as this condition has also been appropriately termed.

Clinical presentation: Affects all ages. Peripheral lymphadenopathy is most common, but 40% of reported cases present with extranodal manifestations such as skin, upper respiratory/sinonasal tract, skeletal, central nervous system (CNS), extraorbital, oral cavity, genitourinary system, lower respiratory tract, and soft tissues. Involvement of the kidney, liver or lower respiratory tract was found to be a poor prognostic sign (60,61). Occurrence together with

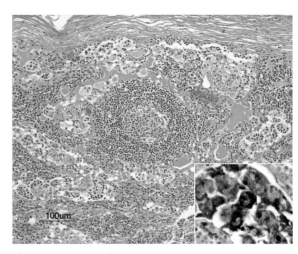

Figure 7.6 Rosai–Dorfman disease: lymph node displays a sinusoidal pattern of change with expansion into the sinus by markedly increased numbers of activated histiocytes that exhibit emperipolesis. Insert shows the activated histiocytes are from a subset that is S100+ (inset) and CD163+ (not shown).

lymphoma pre- or post-treatment, or ALPS has been reported (62–68).

Histology: There is expansion of lymph node sinusoids by large numbers of histiocytes. Many histiocytes exhibit emperipolesis (Figure 7.6). The remainder of the lymph-node compartments are normal and may show mild reactive lymphoid hyperplasia (60). The immunohistological hallmark of the sinus histiocytes is that they belong to a subset of histiocytes that express S100 protein (Figure 7.6 inset) and are CD1a-negative. The phagocytosed lymphocytes are usually T-cells. Activated histiocytes that exhibit emperipolesis are CD163+.

Differential diagnosis: Non-specific sinusoidal histiocyte hyperplasia, other histiocytic diseases such as Langerhans-cell histiocytosis, leukemic infiltrates, or metastatic tumors, and occasionally glycogen storage disease.

Histiocytic neoplasms

Langerhans cell histiocytosis (LCH)

This consists of clonal malignant proliferation of Langerhans cells that express CD1a, S100, and Langerin proteins, and show Birbeck granules by electron microscopy.

Clinical presentation: Most cases occur in childhood, with a male to female ratio of 3.7:1. It may be solitary or in multiple sites; the dominant site is in bone and adjacent soft tissues, lymph nodes, skin, and

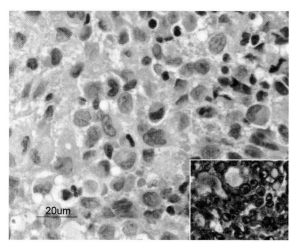

Figure 7.7 Langerhans-cell histiocytosis: characteristic histiocytes with nuclear grooves and linear nuclear folds are shown. Inset shows they are Langerin+.

lungs (manifesting as pulmonary cystic formations) being less frequent. The disseminated form or visceral involvement is termed Letterer–Siwe disease, and involvement of multiple sites is Hand–Schuller–Christian disease.

Genetics: Rare in black people; higher concordance rate has been observed in identical twins, but not in dizygous pairs and there is no vertical inheritance.

Histology: There are sinusoidal infiltrates of medium-sized oval histiocytes with folded, indented, or coffee bean-like nuclei with a nuclear groove (Figure 7.7). These cells also spill into the paracortex. There are prominent eosinophils and small numbers of plasma cells in the background. Other histiocytes and some osteoclast-like cells can be present (69). Large sheet-like or bulky aggregates of histiocytes with nuclear grooves that co-express S100, CD1a, and langerin (Figure 7.7 inset) may be seen. Expression of CD68 alone is insufficient to make this diagnosis.

Differential diagnosis: Dermatopathic lymphadenopathy, other benign histiocytic infiltrates, Rosai–Dorfman disease, and metastatic neoplasms.

Follicular dendritic cell sarcoma

This is a neoplastic proliferation of spindled to ovoid cells showing morphologic and immunophenotype features of follicular dendritic cells.

Clinical presentation: A rare neoplasm affecting lymph nodes and tonsils with a median age of 40 years (70), where extranodal manifestations can occur. A small number of cases in children have been

reported (71) and it has been reported as a rare complication of Castleman's disease in adults (70,72,73). Large tumor size of over 6 cm with intra-abdominal involvement bears a poor prognosis.

Histology: Tumor cells are spindle to ovoid or polygonal, and have oval nuclei, vesicular fine granular chromatin, and small distinct nucleoli. The cells have eosinophilic cytoplasm and indistinct cell borders. They form whorled-sheet, follicular-like structures, diffuse trabeculae, or pseudovascular spaces and may appear infiltrative. High mitotic activity (<10 per high-power field) with cytological atypia and necrosis can be associated with aggression and poor prognosis (70). Regarding immunocytochemistry, CD21+, CD23+, CD35+, EMA, S100, and/or CD68 positivity may be variable; CD1a is negative (70,72,75).

Differential diagnosis: Angiomatoid fibrohistiocytoma, secondary lymph node involvement by fibrosarcoma or atypical spitzoid tumors; ectopic thymoma.

Precursor T-cell or B-cell lymphomas

T-lymphoblastic lymphoma (T-LBL)

The T-lymphoblastic lymphoma is a precursor T-lineage neoplasm.

Clinical presentation: This is the commonest T-cell lymphoma in children and in the Western hemisphere; its prevalence is second to Burkitt's lymphoma for pediatric NHL and decreases with age (1,2). Common presentation includes supradiaphragmatic/mediastinal mass (70%), bulky cervical and supraclavicular lymph node leading to airway obstruction and superior vena cava syndrome (2,76). Involvement of liver and spleen may also develop and most present at stage 3–4. The testicular site is rare as the primary presentation, but is a common site of relapse.

Genetics: T-cell receptor (TCR) gene translocations are common. Identified transcription factors TAL1, HOX11, LYL1, NOTCH 1, SIL1, TAL1, 2, RHOMB1, B2, and TAN have been reported (1,2,76,77). In contrast to T-acute lymphoblastic leukemia (ALL), markedly few notable genetic anomalies are found and none are of prognostic importance.

Histology: There are small to medium-sized cells with hyperchromatic and hematoxyphilic nuclei and small amounts of cytoplasm. The nuclei are small, round, and lobated to slightly irregular. Thin sections reveal fine stippled-to-powdery chromatin without nucleoli. Some may have larger blasts with nucleoli

237

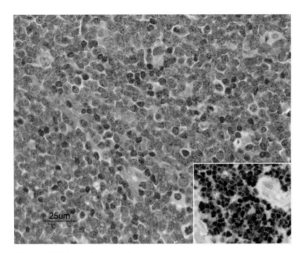

Figure 7.8 Lymphoblastic lymphoma: monomorphous small lymphoblasts with small nucleolus with fine stippled chromatin and scant amounts of cytoplasm. Inset shows they are nuclear terminal di-deoxytidyl transferase enzyme positive, indicating that they are precursor lymphoid cells.

and mitotic figures are frequent (Figure 7.8). Minute cytoplasmic lipid may be present and some may present with a starry sky pattern associated with abundant reactive histiocytes. The morphological and immunological features between T-LBL and T-ALL are indistinguishable from each other, only the presence of more than 25% malignant cells in the bone marrow distinguishes them (2). Stage 4 T-LBL has less than 25% malignant cells.

There is retention of nuclear expression of terminal deoxytidyl transferase (TdT) (Figure 7.8 inset). Cells express pan T-cell antigens (CD43, cytoplasmic CD3, CD45RO), as well as CD99, and will exhibit aberrant lineage antigen deficits; they can be CD4+8−; CD8+/4−; CD4−/8− or CD4+/8+, and some can be CD10+. Mib-1 is nearly 95%+ (77).

Differential diagnosis: T-ALL with nodal infiltration.

B-Lymphoblastic lymphoma (B-LBL)

This is a precursor B-lineage neoplasm.

Clinical presentation: Only 10% to 15% of lymphoblastic lymphomas are B-cell type. Its presentation is more limited than T-LBL. Localized disease involves usually a single peripheral nodal site, skin, soft tissues, tonsil, or bone (2).

Genetics: Rearrangement of immunoglobulin (Ig) gene with or without translocation can occur, but in contrast to B-ALL, markedly few notable genetic anomalies are found and none are of prognostic importance (2,77).

Histology: Similar to T-LBL, with monomorphic small cells with hyperchromatic chromatin, grayish deep-blue color, finely stippled, with small but distinct nucleoli. Cells are small to medium with scant amounts of cytoplasm. The nuclear contours vary from round to lobated to convoluted and there are frequent mitoses. Some may have a starry sky appearance due to the presence of reactive histiocytes. Immunohistochemistry is similar to T-LB: these cells express TdT and may express CD99. All express pan B markers, such as PAX-5, CD79a, CD19, CD22, but CD20 may be variable. They may express CD99 and CD10; Mib-1 is nearly 95%+ (77).

Differential diagnosis: Similar to T-LBL vs. T-ALL: morphological and immunological features of B-LBL are also similar to B-ALL. It is important to differentiate from B-ALL with nodal infiltration.

Post-thymic/peripheral T-cell lymphoma

Anaplastic large-cell lymphoma (ALCL)

This is a distinct type of T-cell lymphoma with large anaplastic cells expressing CD30 (Ki-1 antigen) (78).

Clinical presentation: Anaplastic large-cell lymphoma is the most prevalent post-thymic pediatric T-cell lymphoma, comprising approximately 10–15% of pediatric NHL. Patient ages range from 0.8 to 18 years (median 10 years). There is frequent extranodal involvement as compared with other pediatric NHL (skin bone and soft tissue) and frequent B symptoms and 56–70% are boys. Peripheral nodes are most frequent, followed by retroperitoneal lymph nodes, and a mediastinal mass (1,76). Bone marrow and CNS involvement is less frequent. The presence of B symptoms, mediastinal mass, skin lesions, CNS involvement, and histological subtypes, such as large cell histiocytic or small-cell variants, are associated with a high risk of failure. Newly emerging, poor prognostic factors, such as the combined presence of positive circulating t(2;5)+ cells or occult bone marrow involvement detected by molecular analysis, and a low ALK oncoantigen autoantibody titer have been described (79,80). Unlike other NHL, relapses can be treated effectively with salvage chemotherapy or bone-marrow transplant (1). A primary cutaneous clinical subtype has the same histopathology features as the systemic form, but has a favorable prognosis. Some patients have a history of lymphomatoid papulosis.

Another subtype is the clinically more aggressive small-cell variant of ALCL (81).

Genetics: There is a clonal TCR gene rearrangement, but the hallmark molecular abnormality is the presence of various chromosomal translocations involving the *ALK (anaplastic lymphoma kinase)* gene located on 2p23. The most frequent is t(2;5)(p23;q35), which fuses the *ALK* gene to the *nucleophosmin (NPM)* gene (76,77). Very diverse types of translocation partners with the *ALK* gene have been noted in the literature (76). There is no difference in clinical outcomes of patients with these alternative translocations (1).

Histology: The common form has large cells with ample amounts of pale eosinophilic to amphophilic cytoplasm. Each cell may have one, two, or multiple (in a wreath-like arrangement) nuclei, each containing a prominent nucleolus resembling the Reed–Sternberg cell of classical Hodgkin's lymphoma (CHL). Distinct from CHL, the background lymphocytes are atypical and, despite the presence of eosinophils, the background cells do not appear inflammatory (Figure 7.9). There are several other less frequent cytological variants: small cells (10%) (81) and others (5%): giant cells, mixed, neutrophil-rich, signet ring, and sarcomatoid (76).

The translocation abnormality results in the expression of the tyrosine kinase ALK protein in these neoplastic cells (Figure 7.9 inset). For the most frequent type of translocation that involves fusion to the *NPM*

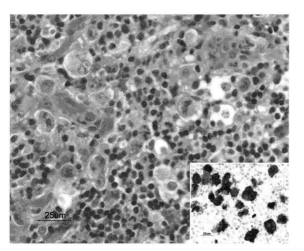

Figure 7.9 Anaplastic large-cell lymphoma: large cells with cellular and nuclear anaplasia. Cells have a close resemblance to Reed–Sternberg cells with the exception that their nucleoli are smaller than those in RS cells. The lymphoid cells in the background are also atypical. Inset shows ALK-1+ staining as a consequence of translocation/activation of the *ALK* gene in chromosome 2.

gene, ALK is expressed in the nucleus of the ALCL cells; for other types of translocations, ALK is expressed in the cytoplasm. In addition, ALCL is CD30+, CD15+/−, EMA+ (40–50%), CD25+, and HLA/DR+, with expression of most T-lineage antigens, and can exhibit aberrant T-lineage antigen loss similar to peripheral T-cell lymphoma (PTCL) (76,77); 10% may be null. By definition, ALCL is CD20−. Some express TiA-1 antigens (82), 10% ALCL may be ALK−. Proteomic signatures of NPM/ALK-positive ALCLs that differ from NPM/ALK-negative ALCLs and Hodgkin's lymphoma have been observed (83).

Differential diagnosis: Lymphocyte-depleted CHL, gray-zone lymphoma, indeterminate HL.

Small-cell variant of ALCL

The small-cell variant is a rare histopathological and clinical distinct subtype of ALCL (81).

Clinical features: Young patients (median of 14 years), presenting with B symptoms, skin, and lymph-node disease. It is more aggressive than ALCL and may transform the large-cell ALCL over a period of 60 months. Transformation signals a rapid clinical course, with death within a year (84).

Genetics: There are clonal *TCR* gene rearrangements and they also have the t(2;5)(p23;q35) abnormality.

Histology: There are small cells with marked nuclear irregularities, their infiltrates have inflammatory features, and they have a component of intra/perivascular infiltrate of CD30+ large cells. These small cells are CD30−, exhibit an aberrant T-cell phenotype, and have TiA-1+ cytotoxic granules (82).

Peripheral T-cell lymphoma

This is a malignant post-thymic (mature) T-cell lymphoma of clonal origin. This category likely encompasses clonal proliferations of diverse morphological small, medium-to-large T-cell types, and T-cell immunological subsets, as there are insufficient defining immunologic, cytogenetic, or molecular features to further subclassify them.

Clinical presentation: Overall it is an uncommon lymphoma in the Western hemisphere as compared to the Far and Middle East. It represents only 1% of pediatric NHL and is the second most common pediatric T-cell lymphoma after ALCL (76,85–87).

Patients present with generalized lymphadenopathy or extranodal disease of liver, spleen, skin, or bone marrow. Advanced-stage disease is associated with B symptoms (fever, night sweats, and/or weight loss) and high lactate dehydrogenase (LDH). Some may have hemophagocytic syndrome(76,86,88). Clinical aggressiveness can be defined by the stage of presentation.

Genetics: Diverse and sporadic cytogenetic abnormalities occur in a small proportion of cases. Molecular analysis for T-cell clonality may show rearrangement at the TCR γ, δ, or β loci.

Subtypes: This is a heterogeneous group of mature T-cell neoplasms. Three morphological variants have been noted: *lympho-epithelioid* (*Lennert lymphoma*), *follicular*, and *T-zone*. The latter two are exceedingly rare in children in the Western hemisphere.

Histology: Effacement of the lymph node begins within the paracortical T-cell domain. Some of the affected areas may have diminished cellularity within a background of stromal vascular prominence. The small blood vessels, high endothelial venules, may exhibit a unique arborizing pattern (Figure 7.10). In some cases perivascular/angiocentric lymphoma cells may infiltrate small arterial walls partially or fully. Cytologically, the lymphoma cells can be small or medium to large, with several types of atypical cytological features, such as clear cells, polymorphic cells with abnormal indentations on the nuclear membrane, paraimmunoblasts, plasmacytoid cells, or immunoblasts (Figure 7.10 inset). Immunohistochemistry shows expression of pan T-cell markers, such as CD43 and CD45RO, and there may be aberrant loss of one or

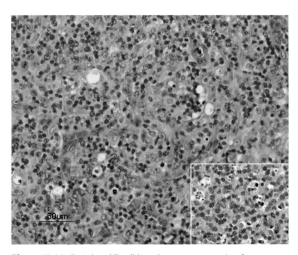

Figure 7.10 Peripheral T-cell lymphoma: an example of a morphologically heterogeneous group showing atypical lymphoid cells infiltrating the lymph node paracortex causing a characteristic arborizing pattern of small blood vessel proliferations. Inset shows small cells with atypical nuclear contours, less condensed chromatin, and some cells have water-clear cytoplasm. The presence of histiocytes can give a misleading impression of Burkitt's lymphoma.

several T-lineage markers. Typically, less than 40% of the lymphoma cells express CD7, CD2, CD3, and/or CD5. Some may retain CD4 or CD8, but some may be CD4+/CD8+ or CD4–/8–, and some may not express βF1. They should not express precursor marker TdT, ALCL marker CD30, or NK T-cell marker CD56 (31).

Differential diagnosis: Rare aggressive EBV-associated T-cell lympho-proliferative disease of childhood, immunodeficiency-associated lymphomas, nodal adult T-cell leukemia/lymphoma (HTLV1-associated), nodal involvement by the small-cell variant of ALCL. Pediatric angioimmunoblastic T-cell lymphoma is rare (87), with immunophenotypic findings of CXCL13+, CD3+, CD10+ lymphoma cells, and CD21 dendritic cells entrapping the HEV within the paracortex (30).

Hepato-splenic (γ/δ) T-cell lymphoma

This is an aggressive small-to-medium size cytotoxic T-cell lymphoma with predilection for splenic sinusoids and liver, and frequently also the bone marrow (76,86), with limited and very infrequent involvement of regional lymph nodes.

Clinical presentation: It is a rare disease of young adults, with a male predominance presenting with hepatosplenomegaly without lymphadenopathy. Up to 20% occur after long-term immunosuppression, post solid-organ transplants or post infliximab treatment for inflammatory bowel disease (76,86).

Genetics: There are cytogenetic anomalies, such as isochromosome 7q and trisomy 8 (76). Clonal rearrangement of the δ/γ TCR is present.

Histology: Infiltration and marked expansion of splenic sinusoids by monomorphous mixed small-to-medium-sized lymphoid cells can be seen. Individual cells have mild nuclear atypia. In the liver, the lymphoma cells can involve both hepatic sinusoids and portal tracts (Figure 7.11). Hemophagocytosis is not a dominant feature. Regional lymph nodes can be involved, though not clinically apparent. Pan T-cell markers are positive (CD43, CD45RO, CD3); it may exhibit aberrant deficits in other T-lineage antigens. Most express the TCR δ-1 epitope, some can be the α-β phenotype; the NK cell marker may be CD56+/–, cytoplasmic cytotoxic granules TiA-1+ (see Figure 10.11 insert) and granzyme B, perforin may be negative. Some cases are EBV+ (by ISH-EBER) (31).

Differential diagnosis: Epstein–Barr virus-associated lympho-proliferative syndrome, hepatic hemophagocytic lymphohistiocytosis, secondary PTCL in liver or spleen.

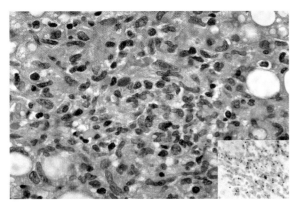

Figure 7.11 Hepatosplenic γ/δ T-cell lymphoma within the hepatic parenchyma: infiltrates of small- to medium-sized monomorphic lymphoid cells with atypical nuclei and nuclear profiles within the hepatic sinusoids, replacing some hepatocytes. Inset: lymphoma cells have TiA-1+ stained cytoplasmic granules.

Others: rare extranodal T- or T/NK-cell malignancies

Rare extranodal T-cell lymphomas in children, such as natural killer (NK) cell (CD56+) lymphomas (nasal and non-nasal types) and subcutaneous panniculitic T-cell lymphomas (CD56−), along with cutaneous lymphoma in children, such as hydroa vaccinforme-like lymphoma, an EBV-positive malignancy, and systemic EBV-positive T-cell lympho-proliferative disease of childhood (76) are beyond the scope of this chapter.

NK/T-cell lymphomas affect patients from the Far East, they are mostly episomal EVB-positive and have been found to express T/NK-associated transcription factor T-bet variably (89,90). Most have cytotoxic granules TiA-1, granzyme B; some have del 6q21, and T-cell clonality cannot be demonstrated in 70% of cases (29,31,91).

Mature B-cell lymphomas

Burkitt's lymphoma

Burkitt's lymphoma is an aggressive mature B-cell lymphoma with three variants: (1) endemic aggressive lymphoma associated with EBV in children of equatorial Africa, (2) non-endemic sporadic type, (3) human immunodeficiency virus (HIV)-associated or immunodeficiency-associated (primary or secondary, such as posttransplant lymphoproliferative disease (PTLD)) (1). It has medium-sized lymphoma cells with a high nuclear proliferative index and a high prevalence of *c-myc* translocation to the Ig gene loci (heavy- or light-chain genes).

Recent tumor biology studies have suggested that Burkitt's lymphoma might have its cellular origin from the developing B-cells from the dark zone of the germinal center. *c-myc* plus other genes that subsequently acquire mutations in the *TCF(E2A)* gene, resulting in augmentation of BCR signaling and phosphatidyl inositol 3-OH kinase, and in the *cyclin D3* gene, which confers a proliferative advantage, are crucial to the pathogenesis of Burkitt's lymphoma (9,92,93).

Clinical presentation: Burkitt's lymphoma has three peaks of occurrence at 5–9, 40–44, and 80–84 years, with a male predominance. There was a concurrent rise in BL cases with the HIV epidemic in North America. It can spread throughout the body (including the abdomen), CNS, lymph nodes, or bone marrow (BM) (1). Clinical BM involvement is present in approx 20% of pediatric patients (1).

Genetics: There is a high association with specific translocation of the *c-myc* gene to immunoglobulin genes amenable to detection by cytogenetic analyses. Approximately 80% of cases have t(8;14)(24;q32); 15% cases have t(2;8)(p12;q14), and the remaining 5% have t(8,22)(q24;q21) abnormalities. A small number (less than 5%) have no such abnormalities. Genomic profiling studies of 24 BL cases showed 96% had *c-myc* rearrangements (22). The presence of these translocation abnormalities has also been reported in 31% of pediatric DLBCLs (21). Del 13q and +7q are poor prognostic factors, with a significant inferior event-free survival outcome (94).

Subtypes: Typical forms have the microscopic features described below. There is an atypical variant termed non-Burkitt, Burkitt-like lymphoma, or atypical Burkitt (30).

Histology: Typical forms show diffuse monotonous proliferation of tightly packed medium-sized cells, some of them exhibiting squared-off borders of retracted cytoplasm. The cells have basophilic cytoplasm, and air-dry touch preparations reveal cytoplasmic lipid vacuoles. The nuclei are round and have fine or clumped chromatin. Nucleoli are small and basophilic and some are paracentrally located. They are associated with a histiocyte-rich background, which forms a starry sky appearance (Figure 7.12). There is frequent mitosis and apoptosis (Figure 7.12 inset). The atypical forms have larger cells with larger nuclei, which have more nuclear atypia and pleomorphism.

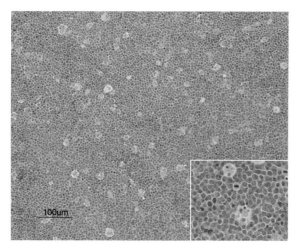

Figure 7.12 Burkitt's lymphoma: monomorphous small non-cleaved lymphoma cells that exhibit a mosaic pattern due to their squared-off cytoplasmic borders (see insert). Together with the mosaic pattern, the presence of prominent mitotic figures (inset), and infiltrates of reactive histiocytes, the triad of the diagnostic features of BL is met.

Small numbers of larger nucleoli are seen (76). Cells express pan B-cell antigens (CD19, 20, and 22) and are uniformly TdT-negative. They are also BCL6-positive, CD10-positive, surface IgM+, and weak to negative for BCL2. Aberrant co-expression of CD43 is present. Nuclear proliferative index is high (near 100%+) (31).

Differential diagnosis: There may be a significant overlap in the defining features of BL and DLBCL in some cases. The presence of shared histopathogical, immunohistochemistry, and cytogenetic features between BL and DLBC result in an indeterminate or unclassifiable lymphoma diagnosis. A subtype of lymphoma known as molecular Burkitt's lymphoma (mBL) is more prevalent in children (21,22. In a study, 31% of DLBCL were reclassified as mBL (21). Under the current treatment protocol for pediatric BL and DLBCL, this molecular subclassification has no impact on treatment and prognosis (21).

Diffuse large B-cell lymphoma (DLBCL)

This is a heterogeneous group of B-cell neoplasms that share in common large cell morphology and a diffuse growth pattern. Recent immunological and molecular studies suggest that both germinal-center B-cell lymphoma (GCB)/DLBCL and ABC/DLBCL may have their cellular origin in developing B-cells from the light zone of the germinal center (9).

Clinical presentation: Uncommon in children (only 3% under 5 years and 6% of all malignancies in children up to 14 years); incidence increases with age, rising to 25% in adolescents, and eventually becoming the most common type in young adults and adults. Extranodal involvement (head and neck regions, mediastinum, and abdomen) at presentation is common. Dissemination to BM and CNS is rare. More boys than girls (1.7:1) have DLBCL. Children have a significantly better prognosis than adults. Girls over 15 have worse outcomes than younger boys and girls. An underlying immunodeficiency is a significant risk factor for pediatric DLBCL (1–4).

Genetics: Clonal rearrangement in the immunoglobulin gene locus is the molecular hallmark. In addition, based on gene expression studies, DLBCL can be divided into germinal center (GC) B-cell-like and activation B-cell-like (95,96). In adults and young adults these subdivisions can predict outcome. A GC-like signature portends a favorable outcome (97). There is a striking prevalence of the GC type in children (6:1 of germinal-center B-cell subtype to activated B-cell subtype) (22). A high incidence of abnormalities in the 8q24/*Myc* locus is observed in pediatric DLBCL as part of a complex karyotype; event-free survival (EFS) is 34% in those with rearranged 8q24. Rearranged 8q24, +7q, and *del(13)(q34)* have independent prognostic significance (worse EFS). Alterations of *BCL6(3q27)* and *BCL2 (18q21)* are less than 7% and no concurrent t(14;18) and rearranged *8q24* have been detected (22,94). *IRF4-IgH* translocation was found in GC-type DLBCL, one follicular grade 3B and one follicular grade 3B/DLBCL pediatric lymphoma (age 4–15) (98).

Subtypes: Subclassification based on immunostaining for GC-like phenotype (such as BCL6 expression) has not been generally accepted. Expression of CD30 is not regarded as a diagnosis of anaplasia. Since the use of anti-CD20 antibody (rituximab) as an adjunct therapeutic agent, incorporation of this immunostaining feature has practical implications.

Histology: Cells are usually 3–4 times the diameter of a normal resting small lymphocyte and they proliferate in a diffuse manner. Frequently the large round-to-oval nuclei exhibit vesicular chromatin features of centroblasts or immunoblasts (characterized by a single prominent nucleolus). Not uncommonly in pediatric cases, the lymphoma nuclei are highly lobated or convoluted (Figure 7.13). Anaplastic cell types or RS-cell-like with multinucleation can occur, though frequently as a minor cell population. A majority expresses pan B-cell antigen CD20. CD20-negative cases can be identified by CD79a, CD19, and CD22 immunostains. A majority expresses BCL-6 and some express CD10; 30–40% show aberrant co-expression of CD43 and some may be BCL2-positive. Occasional cases express CD99(31,77).

Differential diagnosis: T-cell-rich B-cell lymphoma, progression lymphoma from NLPHL, anaplastic large-cell lymphoma, Hodgkin-like DLBCL, metastatic poorly differentiated alveolar rhabdomyosarcoma.

Primary mediastinal (thymic) large B-cell lymphoma (PMBCL)

This is a distinct clinicopathological subtype of DLBCL that occurs predominantly in the mediastinum. Recent molecular profiling analysis shows that PMBCL has a gene expression signature that shares more similarities to CHL than to DLBCL. The expressed gene contributes to the activation of NF-κB (99,100).

Clinical presentation: Rare in children, it presents in the mediastinum and may spread to adjacent pleura, pericardium, and/or pulmonary tissue; 48% have B symptoms. There is an absence of lymph node or BM involvement. Distinct from adults, where there is a high prevalence in women, there is a female to male ratio of 21:23 (N = 44; 3.3–18.7 years) (17). Half of the patients from this group had manifestations on both sides of the diaphragm.Treatment of pediatric patients with BL-like chemotherapeutic regimens showed an EFS of 70%. The results were worse than other pediatric DLBCL, as well as adults with similar lymphomas (17,100). Adding rituximab to dose-adjusted EPOCH (etoposide, vincristine, doxorubicin, cyclophosphamide, and prednisone) is now widely adapted; a favorable EFS and overall survival (OS) was noted (101).

Genetics: There may be 9p24 gain (75%), 2p16 gain (50%), MYC gain (20%), amplification (7%), and break (7%) (17). The frequency of gains and amplifications of *Rel* and *Jak2* observed in children is similar to the findings in adults.

Histology: Monomorphous large cells with pale eosinophilic cytoplasm forming cell nests, often sequestered by sclerotic hooks formed within the interstitium of the sclerotic stroma are seen (Figure 7.13 inset). Nuclear pleomorphism and multinucleation can occur, and such cells resemble the Reed–Sterngerg cell

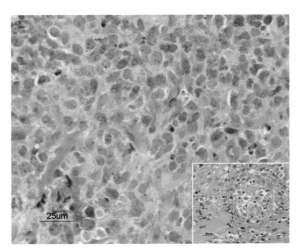

Figure 7.13 Diffuse large B-cell lymphoma: monomorphous population of large- to medium-sized non-cleaved (centroblastic) cells. Note the upper field also shows the frequent presence of lymphoma cells with poly-lobated nuclei (this appearance is similar to a subpopulation of cells found in the follicular/germinal center). The inset is a case of primary mediastinal large B-cell lymphoma with formations of sclerotic tissues that sequester the lymphoma cells into small compartments.

variant (102). The cells are all Pax 5+ and CD79a +, nearly all CD19+, CD20+, CD22+, CD23+ (85–67%), and CD30+ (80%). Frequent are MUM-1+ (70%), BCL-6+ (97%), and BCL2 expression is variable, CD10– mostly, CD15– and lacking surface immunoglobulin expression (17,31,103); EBER is negative. The tumor cells co-express Traf-1 and nuclear Rel and immunohistological features are similar to those in adults.

Differential diagnosis. Mediastinal classical Hodgkin's lymphoma, composite Hodgkin with DLBCL, anaplastic large-cell lymphoma, thymoma, or mediastinal gray-zone lymphoma.

Rare pediatric mature B-cell lymphomas

Follicular lymphoma (FL), pediatric type

A novel variant of the recognized form of follicular lymphoma (30,104), it is an indolent low-grade B-cell neoplasm of germinal-center origin (105).

Clinical presentation: Follicular lymphoma is rare in children (1–2% of lymphoma diagnosis) with increased prevalence in young adolescents (101). There is a male predominance, with the male:female ratio equalized in adolescents, and it usually presents at stage 1–2 cervical. Waldeyer ring and peripheral lymph node involvement have a better prognosis.

Occurrences in the GI tract, parotid gland, kidney, epididymis, and skin have been noted (101). Testicular FL in children has good outcomes after orchiectomy without radiation or chemotherapy treatment (104–106). Clinical utilization of the grading results remains discrepant (104,106).

Genetics: Children do not have the genetic hallmark t(14;18) translocation abnormality (which occurs in over 80% of adult grade 1–2 follicular lymphomas). However, molecular analysis of the Ig gene locus shows that cells are clonal B-cells. *C-Myc* is normal; one case of *BCL6-IgH* gene translocation was reported (104). In a rare number of cases of pediatric grade 3B with DLBCL, *IRF4* translocation was noted (107–108).

Subtypes: Grading is based on the assessment of the frequency of centroblasts per high-power field (based on 10 hpf of 10 follicles) into grades 1–3. Distinct from adults, children tend to be of high grade. There are distinct clinical pathological features in the younger age group to warrant the use of the term pediatric-type follicular lymphoma: it is defined by cases of stage 1 nodal FL with indolent clinical behavior, lacking the t(14;18) *BCL2-IgH* abnormalities by fresh tissue fluorescence *in-situ* hybridization (FISH), and having a high proliferation index by Ki-67 immunohistochemistry (105). Recently, microRNA profiles of adult t(14;18)-negative follicular lymphomas showed they have distinct microRNA profiles that are associated with an increased proliferative capacity and a "late" germinal-center B-cell phenotype (109).

Histology: There is lymph node effacement by crowded lymphoid follicles that lack polarization into light- and dark-zone centrocytes/centroblasts and reduced thinning of mantle or discordant presence of tingible body macrophages. Monomorphic populations of cytologically atypical centrocytes (with angulated nuclear or twisted profiles) and centroblasts of variable proportions that replace tangible body macrophages are present (Figure 7.14). Sheets of centroblasts may occur in some and are designated as grade 3B. Of note is that grade 3B is extremely rare in children and may have concurrent DLBCL (108).

Cells are CD19+, CD20+, CD22+, BCL6+, 80% CD10+, only 25–30% BCl2+ (Figure 7.14 inset); a minority of cases are CD43+ (24%) (106), CD5– (rare positive has been described), Ig-negative (10–15%), and 40% to 95% MiB-1 index. *IRF1* translocation-positive cases may be strongly MUM-1+ (107).

Differential diagnosis: Based on the presence of a follicular or pseudofolliclaur pattern: reactive follicular

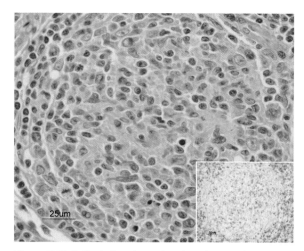

Figure 7.14 Follicular lymphoma: lymph-node parenchyma is replaced by closely packed (back-to-back) lymphoid follicles that have thin vague mantles with central regions that do not show features of polarization. The center comprises a dual population of centroblasts and centrocytes. Inset shows lack of BCL2 staining and CD10+ (not shown).

hyperplasia vs. grade 3a with high tingible body macrophage numbers, NLPDHL with or with progressively transformed germinal centers, NS-CHL, small lymphocytic lymphoma with pseudoproliferative centers, mantle-cell lymphoma, marginal-zone lymphoma, florid reactive follicular hyperplasia, or Castleman's disease.

Marginal-zone lymphoma, extranodal of mucosa-associated lymphoid tissues (MALT)

Marginal-zone lymphoma is an extranodal lymphoma of heterogeneous small B-cells, including marginal zone (centrocyte-like) cells, cells resembling monocytoid cells, small lymphocytes, scattered plasma cells and immunoblasts, and centroblast-like cells. The infiltrate is in the marginal zone of the reactive B follicle extending into the interfollicular region. In epithelial tissues, the neoplastic cells typically infiltrate the epithelium to form lympho-epithelial lesions (30).

Clinical presentation: The male:female ratio is 1.4:1, the median age is 24 (age range 1.5–29 years), and skin and soft tissue are the most common sites of presentation (110). The tumors occur in the stomach, breast, orbit, ocular adnexa, lip, sinonasal, parotid, and submandibular glands, and are highly localized (111). There are rare recurrences and many are treated with surgical excision only or with radiation; additional treatment is with rituximab for more advanced types (101). A mediastinal (thymic) type is reported most frequently in Asians with autoimmune antibodies, hyperimmunoglobulinemia, monogammopathy, and the lymphoma mass is usually cystic (112).

Genetics: Chromosomal aberrations are rare, but when present are similar to adult patients. They are, however, different from those occurring in the primary nodal type. The frequency of aberrations varies depending on the site of involvement. In adults, t(11;18)(q21;q21) is the most prevalent in luminal (e.g., gastrointestinal) *MALT* (53%), with an overall prevalence of 14%. T(14;18), involving *IGH* and *MALT1* genes is most common in ocular adnexa. One study found 18% of pediatric cases had genetic aberrations (110).

Subtypes: Pediatric nodal marginal-zone lymphoma (MZL) (see the following section) or splenic MZL (rare with no recent reports in the pediatric age range) (101).

Histology: There is effacement and expansion of the paracortex, and where residual follicles are present (not completely over-run), colonization and expansion of the marginal zone by monomorphous small lymphoid cells with small cleaved centrocytoid nuclei surrounded by narrow rim of pale eosinophilic cytoplasm. Nuclei are more spherical and have dispersed chromatin with small inconspicuous nucleoli. Monocytoid B-cells can be present. In extranodal tissues, colonization in mucosa with intraepithelial infiltrates (lympho-epithelial lesion) by a similar small lymphoma cell infiltrate is seen (Figure 7.15). Small lymphocytes, cells with plasmacytic differentiation, and centroblast-like cells can be present (Figure 7.15 inset) (30).

Immunohistochemistry: Nodal-type: Ig light-chain restriction, some are IgD+; extranodal type: light-chain restriction, some are IgA+; CD20+, CD10−, CD5−, CD23−, cyclinD−, and BCL6−.

Differential diagnosis: Associations with hepatitis C virus, *Helicobater pylori*, or HIV infections have been noted (101,113).

Marginal-zone lymphoma (MZL), pediatric nodal type

This is a nodal-type primary non-germinal center small B-cell neoplasm. It resembles lymph nodes that are secondarily involved by extranodal MZL or splenic MZL.

Clinical presentation: Predominantly in males (ratio 20:1), asymptomatic, stage 1 disease located mainly in

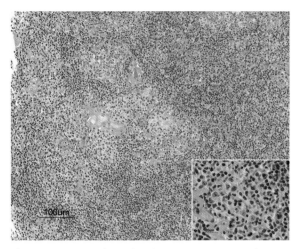

Figure 7.15 Marginal-zone lymphoma–mucosa associated lymphoid tissues (MALT) lymphoma: mucosal lymphoma involving the thymus. Abnormal cells cluster around the subtotally destroyed thymic epithelium. Inset shows the lymphoma comprises a monomorphous population of small centrocyte-like cells with pale to clear eosinophilic cytoplasm and nuclear atypia.

the head and neck lymph nodes. It has an excellent prognosis with low relapse and long survival.

Genetics: Genetic aberrations comprising t(14;18)/ *IGH-MALT1*, t(*BCL10*), t(*ODZ2*), t(*JMJD2C*) and t(*CNN3*) have been reported, as well as trisomies 8, 3, and 13 (114).

Histology: This is similar to those described in adults, and may be associated with a progressively transformed germinal center. Immunohistochemistry is similar to the adult type: CD20+, CD10−, CD5−, CD23−, cyclinD− (115). One pediatric study showed expression of CD43, BCL-2, and IgD in 25% of cases; BCL6 and CD10 were negative (110).

Mediastinal gray-zone lymphoma

This is an extremely rare lymphoma in children that shows transitional morphology and immunophenotypic features between CHL and PMBCL (e.g., RS cells within PMBCL, or detection of CD15+, EBER+ cells). Histologically it may also present with CHL in one area and mediastinal thymic large B-cell lymphoma in another. There is a close relationship between gray-zone lymphoma, CHL, and PMBCL (116–118).

Clinical presentation: The mediastinal type manifests in young adolescents and young adults (median age 29). The male:female ratio is 2:1.3 (119).

Genetics: 9p24.1 (*JAK2*, *PDL2*) is found in 61%; 2p16.1 (*BCL11*, *REL*) gain, 8q24 (*MYC*) gain, and

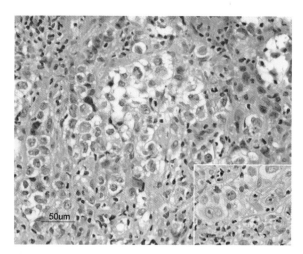

Figure 7.16 Gray-zone lymphoma: histopathological features are indeterminate between mediastinal B-cell lymphoma with sclerosis and Hodgkin's lymphoma (inset).

16p13.13(*CIITA*) gain in approximately 30% cases of mediastinal type; less frequently found in the non-mediastinal type (17,117).

Subtypes: Mediastinal and non-mediastinal.

Histology: Indeterminate between DLBCL and CHL (Figure 7.16; 17, 116–119. Immunohistochemistry is also indeterminate between DLBCL and CHL. In cases that are more DLBCL-like: CD30+ (100%) and cyclinE + (93%), HLA-DR with viable% cells+, most cases (80–70%) are CD20+, CD15+,CD79a+, Bob-1+, and Oct-2+; 60% are p63+. In cases that are more CHL-like, the numbers of CD15+ cells are less (58 vs. 80%). The positivity of these markers is lower in the non-mediastinal type. PAX5+, MUM-1+, OCT-2+, and CD23+ were reported to be 100% in four pediatric mediastinal cases (median age 13.7 years), EBER+ in 67%, BCL6+ in 33%, and CD15+ in 25% pediatric cases (17).

Differential diagnosis: Extremely rare entities, such as mediastinal composite lymphoma and mediastinal synchronous/metachronous lymphoma (117,120).

Hodgkin's lymphoma

Hodgkin's lymphoma was originally described in 1832 (23), although similar cases were described in 1856 (121,122); the histology was described later (24,25). Hodgkin's disease in the current nomenclature is defined as Hodgkin's lymphoma (HL) and comprises four histological subtypes. In pediatric HL, it encompasses two major diseases: classical Hodgkin's lymphoma (CHL), which is malignant (and shares similar tumor biology with the other histological subtypes) and nodular lymphocyte-predominant Hodgkin's lymphoma (NLPHD), which is indolent and has its own distinct tumor biological features. Hodgkin's lymphoma is a clonal proliferative malignancy (27). In CHL, the Reed–Sternberg cells originate from germinal-center B-cells that have lost their immunoglobulin gene (Ig) translational ability, due to functional defects in the regulatory elements (28) or due to an inactivation of the transcriptional machinery (123). Reed–Sternberg cells lack Ig transcription factors (124). Rare cases of CHL have been reported to be derived from post-thymic T-cells (125).

The lymphohistiocytic (L&H) cells of NLPHL are B-cells that show ongoing somatic mutations with interclonal diversity, suggesting that they are derived from selected germinal-center B-cells (126–127).

Clinical presentation: Ninety percent of children present with painless adenopathy in the neck and 60% have involvement of the anterior mediastinum, paratracheal, or hilar lymph nodes. B symptoms are present in 30% of newly diagnosed pediatric cases. They include unexplained fever, drenching night sweats, and weight loss in excess of 10% bodyweight. Hodgkin's lymphoma limited to the spleen is rare, and involvement of the liver is also rare and almost never seen without splenic involvement. Bone marrow infil tration is focal and is associated with extensive disease (1). Staging is based on the Cotswood modification of the Ann Arbor Staging System. Stage 1: involvement of a single lymph-node region or lymph-node structure such as spleen, thymus, and Waldeyer's ring. Stage 2: involvement of two or more lymph-node regions or lymph-node structures on the same side of the diaphragm. Hilar nodes should be considered to be "lateralized," and when involved on both sides this constitutes stage 2. Stage 3: involvement of the lymph-node regions or lymphoid structures on both sides of the diaphragm. Stage 4: bone-marrow involvement. A = No symptoms; B = fever (> 38 °C), drenching night sweats, loss of > 10% bodyweight over the preceding six months; X = bulky disease widening of the mediastinum by more than one-third or greatest dimension > 10 cm; E = involvement of a single extra-nodal site (1). An international prognostic score has been developed to better identify patients who are likely to benefit from reduced treatment, or those who are unlikely to have a sustained response to standard therapy. Long-term childhood HL survivors face increased risk of secondary diseases such as cardiovascular disease and malignancies (128). Long-term remission has been observed in children with limited-stage lymphocyte-predominant Hodgkin's lymphoma who were treated by surgical resection alone (129).

In some cases, EBV is associated with HL. Reed–Sternberg cells show expression of latent membrane protein 1 and 2a and EBNA1. Previously EBV-exposed individuals have a three times increased risk of developing HL (130). One pediatric HL study showed no influence of EBV infection on EFS, but it was present in NSCHL; LMP positivity was an independent factor for adverse outcome (131). There is an association between EBV-positive CHL and a genetic variant within the HLA-Class I region, and between EBV-negative CHL and a locus within the HLA-Class II region. The latter is confined to the nodular sclerosis histological subtypes (132).

Genetics: Reed–Sternberg cells are reported to have multiple aberrations (amplifications, deletions of subregions of the chromosomes or numeric abnormalities). No simple translocations have been specifically associated with HL. Fresh tissue fluorescence *in situ* hybridization analyses detected alterations in chromosome 2p, 3q, 6q, 7q, 9p, 13p, 14p, and 17q, and non-random breakpoints in 3q27, 6q15, 7q22, 11q23, and 14q32 (1). Gains in chromosome 2q, 4q, 5q, 6q, and 11q appear to be unique to lymphocyte-predominant HL (1).

Classification: Hodgkin's lymphoma comprises *nodular lymphocyte-predominant HL* and *classical HL*. The latter also has four histological subtypes: nodular-sclerosis CHL (NSCHL), mixed-cellularity CHL (MCCHL), lymphocyte-rich CHL (LRCHL), and lymphocyte-depleted CHL (LDCHL) (30). Nodular-sclerosis CHL represents 60–75% of pediatric HL, mixed-cellularity HL, 20–25%, and the remaining two subtypes are uncommon and extremely rare, respectively. Approximately 5% of the pediatric HL cases are NLPHL (1).

Histology: In *nodular lymphocyte-predominant HL*, the lymph-node parenchyma contains nodular aggregates of small lymphocytes with uniform size and shape, mixed with small numbers of larger lymphoid cells, histiocytes, and, specifically, cells with the appearance of lympho-histiocytic cells (also known as L&H cells). There may be the concomitant presence of reactive germinal centers, progressively transformed germinal centers within the lymph-node parenchyma. The nuclei of the L&H cells characteristically have a broadly lobated nuclear contour, with

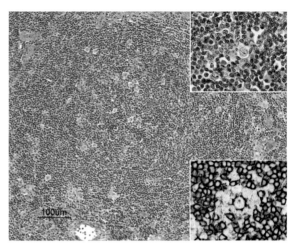

Figure 7.17 Nodular lymphocyte-predominant Hodgkin's lymphoma: lymph-node parenchyma is replaced by large nodular lymphoid aggregates within which abnormal lympho-histiocytic cells can be found. Upper inset shows L&H cells or popcorn cells amongst small lymphoid cells with no cytological atypia. They express pan B-cell antigen CD20 (lower inset).

some nucleoli adherent to the nuclear membrane, giving them a them a popcorn appearance (popcorn cells) (Figure 7.17). They are CD20+ and are frequently surrounded by a ring of CD3+/CD57+ PD−1 + T-cells (Figure 7.17 inset). Classic Reed-Sternberg (RS) cells are very rare, large transformed RS-like cells or reactive histiocytes may be present. Peudogranulomatous aggregates of epithelioid histiocoytes and, very infrequently, polykaryocytes may be present.

In *classical HL*, Reed–Sternberg cells (mononuclear or multinucleated) must be seen in an appropriate background of non-neoplastic inflammatory cells. These cells have deep eosinophilic cytoplasm as they become mummified. Based on the characteristics of the infiltrate, the stroma that accompany the diagnostic RS cells and the morphology of the RS cells, four subtypes are distinguished. The key features of each are as follows:

(1) *NSCHL*: a broad collagen band surrounds at least one nodule; there is a high frequency of RS cells, with lacuna cells that show cytoplasmic retraction of some of the cytoplasmic membrane of RS cells; RS cells may have more lobations, smaller nucleoli, more generous cytoplasm and eosinophils, and neutrophils may be prominent. RS cells and lacuna cells may form syncytial clusters (Figure 7.18).

(2) *MCCHL*: non-thickened lymph-node capsule and absent fibrotic bands; scattered RS cells in a mixed inflammatory lymphocytic infiltrate (diffuse or

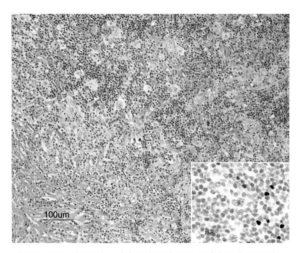

Figure 7.18 Classical Hodgkin's lymphoma, nodular sclerosis: the lymph-node paracortex is replaced by infiltrates of Reed–Sternberg cells within a background of small lymphocytes, plasma cells, and eosinophils. In association with these infiltrates, sclerotic tissue bands are formed within the stroma. Inset shows that Reed–Sternberg cells express B-cell transcription factor PAX-5.

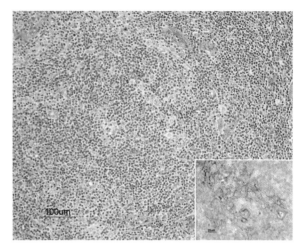

Figure 7.19 Classical Hodgkin's lymphoma, lymphocyte rich: Hodgkins infiltrates imparts a vague nodular appearance to the paracortex due to the presence of aggregates of expanded dendritic reticulum cells. Reed–Sternberg cells may be less prevalent than the other forms of Hodgkins and they are located in the vicinity of the dendritic reticulum network. Inset shows double immunostaining with CD30+ RS cells in red and CD21+ dendritic reticulum cell network in brown.

pseudonodular) containing eosinophils+/–, plasma cells+/–, macrophages; granulomatous epithelioid histiocytes may be present.

(3) *LRCHL* (uncommon in children): scattered RS cells in a nodular background of inflammatory small lymphocytes without eosinophils or neutrophils.

(4) *LDCHL* (extremely rare in children): abundant RS cells some appearing bizarre or sarcomatoid within an inflammatory-cell-depleted background of non-neoplastic lymphocytes and fibrillary matrix. Often resembles anaplastic large-cell lymphoma (1,30,122).

The Reed–Sternberg cells of CHL subtypes share the same immunophenotype. They are CD30+ (Figure 7.19 inset), CD15+ (membrane and/or Golgi+ in a majority of cases), MUM-1+, PAX-5+ (usually staining is weaker than normal or neoplastic B-cells) (Figure 7.18 inset), CD45–, EMA–, ALK–, OCT-2–, and BOB1–. Approximately 20% of cases are CD20+ and 25% of cases overall are EBV+ (LMP-1-positive or by ISH-EBER), and EBV+ cases are highest in MCCHL (75%) (30).

Nodular lymphocyte-predominant HL has a distinct immunophenotype. The diagnostic L&H cells are CD45+, CD20+ (Figure 7.17 inset), CD79a+, OCT-2+, BOB1+, BCL6+, and PAX-5+; 50% are MUM-1+. CD15 and ALK are negative; CD30 is generally negative, but rare positive cases can occur and some transformed B-cells (non-L&H cells) may express CD30 (30).

Differential diagnosis: Includes ALCL, PTCL, T-cell-rich B-cell lymphoma, CD30+ large B-cell lymphoma, EBV lymphadenopathy, drug reaction and metastatic neoplasms, such as melanoma or nasopharyngeal carcinoma. For mediastinal sites, metastatic CD30-positive germ-cell tumors and thymomas should be considered. When the immunotype findings are unusual, the very rare entities such as mediastinal (thymic) large B-cell lymphomas should then be considered.

Immunodeficiencies

Rare lymphoid malignancies associated with primary immunodeficiencies

In common variable immunodeficiency (CVID) and others: Zap-70 deficiency, Nijmegan breakage syndrome (NBS), and Ataxia Telangiectasia (ATM), patients have low levels of immunoglobulin, are unable to make specific antibodies in response to immunization or infection, and may exhibit variable T-cell abnormalities.

Clinical presentation: Most patients are diagnosed between the ages of 20–40; however, it can present in children. There can be three types of clinical manifestation: mulitsystemic ganulomatosis, autoimmune disorders secondary to immune dysregulations, and pre-disposition to malignancy such as NHL. There seems to be a 10-fold increased risk of NHL, as compared with the healthy population in patients with CVID (133).

Genetics: Genetic inheritance is complex and variable, and 10% of patients may exhibit a familial inheritance. Mutations have been observed within at least one of the four gene clusters: tumor necrosis factor (TNF), superfamily receptor transmembrane activator and calcium-modulating ligand interactor (*TACI*), B-cell activation factor of the TNF family (*BAFF-R*), the CD19 B-cell antigen, and the co-stimulator molecule, inducible co-stimulator (ICOS). Only *TACI* mutations have been found in a significant number of CVID cases. A deficiency of TACI is also associated with autoimmunity and lymphoprolifera-tive diseases. Mutations in the other three are rare, and *TACI*, *BAFFR*, and CD19 mediate B-cell development, and ICO deficiency causes deficiency in T-cells helping to render B-cells unable to undergo a class switch within the germinal center (133). Recently a patient thought to have CVID was found to have a -70 gene mutation (zeta chain-associated protein of the TCR complex) and developed DLBCL in early life (134).

Histology: Most lymphomas are B-NHL and sec-tions exhibit cytological monomorphism, most being EBV-negative. Hodgkin's lymphoma is extremely rare. However, in biopsies that show features of polymor-phous lympho-proliferations, with appearances simi-lar to polymorphous PTLD, an accurate diagnosis of malignancy remains a challenge without clinical correlations. Immune-deficient lymphoid cells can exhibit marked cytological atypia in response to anti-genic exposure. These can have the appearance of lymphoid follicular hyperplasia, atypical lymphoid hyperplasia, or chronic granulomatous inflammation. In some, EBV can be detected. Oligoclonal B-cell pro-liferations, and the presence of B- or T-cell antigen-deficit lymphoid cells, with or without positive T- or B-cell-antigen receptor monclonality by PCR analyses can be observed. If discordances between histopatho-logical features are found, correlations with other clinical features are crucial.

Combined immunodeficiency in chromosomal breakage syndrome: Nijmegen breakage syndrome (NBS)

This is an extraordinarily rare autosomal recessive syndrome of chromosomal instability due to a loss-of-function mutation of the nibrin gene. Nibrin functions as a part of the DNA repair complex.

Clinical presentation: Microcephaly and a small anterior fontenele at birth. A cleft palate, and minor skeletal anomalies in fingers and toes may be present. Also, there is facial dysmorphism, and prominent mid-face with sloping forehead as the child matures. Microcephaly persists and is progressive with age. They may exhibit mild growth retardation and intellectual impairments. Young and adolescent girls have hyper-gonadotrophic hypogonadism. The patient has com-bined cellular and humoral immunodeficiency, and an increased risk of development of a variety of malignan-cies, commonly lymphoma (40% by age 20) (135).

Genetics: Five base-pair deletion in exon 6 of the nibrin gene is most common. This mutation results in two truncated fragments of nibrin. Nibrin protein forms a trimeric complex with *MRE11* and *RAD50* (the MRN complex) (135,136). This complex is involved in the repair of DNA damage and the activa-tion of cell-cycle checkpoints via *ATM* (ataxia-telangiectasia, A–T gene) (136,137).

Histology: Mild to strong lymphopenia is present. Low CD4 with reduced to absent naïve CD4+ T-cells expressing CD45RA and low (75% reduction) B-cell numbers are seen. Peripheral T-cells are prone to rearrangements involving chromosomes 7 and 14. The histopathological features of all types of lympho-mas reported are similar to non-syndromic patients. B- and T-cell NHL are most frequent and among B-cell lymphomas, DLBCLs are most frequent. Burkitt or Burkitt-like lymphomas, HL, lymphoblastic leuke-mias, and acute myeloblastic leukemia are infrequent (135,136). Immunophenotypic features are similar to those of non-immunodeficient lymphomas.

Differential diagnosis: Based on the presence of immunodeficiency: A–T, DNA ligase IV-deficiency, LIG4 syndrome, Fanconi anemia, NHEJ1 syndrome, severe combined immunodeficiency (136).

Histiocytic disease associated with immunodeficiencies

Chronic granulomatous disease

Originally described as a fatal granulomatous disease of childhood, it is now established as a genetic neutrophil disease and it thus not part of the severe combined immunodeficiency group.

Genetics: It is a single disease with four genetic etiologies that affect the structure and function of the

NADPH oxidase enzyme complex essential for the production of microbial killing agents within the phagosome (138). Mutations in all of the four structural genes encoding NADPH oxidase have been found to cause CGD. Mutations of *gp91 (phox)* account for 65% of cases, mutations in *p47(phox)* about 25%, and the remainder is divided between *p67(phox)* and *p22(phox)*. There are no autosomal dominant cases and X-linked *gp91(phox)*-deficiency cases have earlier and more severe infections and earlier deaths than the *p47(phox)*-deficient patients (138).

Macroscopic features: Granulomatous lesions affect lung, skin, lymph nodes, and liver. When the GI tract is involved it mimics Crohn's disease and patients may present with gastric obstruction.

Histology: Infectious granulomas are the hallmarks. Some may appear dimorphic, where an abscess is present within a palisading granuloma. In North America, the most frequent infections are due to *Staphylococcus aureus*, *Burkholderia cepacia*, *Serratia marcescens*, *Nocardia*, and *Aspergillus*. In other parts of the world, *Salmonella*, Bacille Calmette–Guerin (BCG), and tuberculosis may be the infectious agents. The diagnosis is made by direct measurement of superoxide production, ferricytochrome c reduction, chemoluminescence, nitroblue tetrazolium reduction, or dihydrorhodamine oxidation.

Differential diagnosis: Myeloperoxidase deficiency can give abnormal DHR, but NBT and ferricytochrome c testing are normal. G6PD deficiency can lead to a decreased respiratory burst and increased susceptibility to infections (138).

Hemophagocytic lymphohistiocytosis (HLH)

This is a life-threatening clinical syndrome that manifests as severe hyperinflammation caused by immune-dysregulations leading to the uncontrolled proliferation of activated lymphocytes and histiocytes secreting high levels of inflammatory cytokines (139–141).

Clinical presentation: A majority of patients develop fever, cytopenia, hypertriglyceridemia, elevated ferritin, and elevated soluble α-chain of CD25 (139). They may have splenomegaly, skin rashes, and additional abnormalities in liver and bone marrow (140). Additionally, they may have sepsis-like or Kawasaki-like symptoms, acute respiratory failure, brain, ophthalmic, and neuromuscular symptoms (139).

Genetics: The various genetic mutations identified in familial HLH (FHL) are related to those that lead to loss of function of perforin, or the impairment of the mechanisms essential to the exocytosis of cytotoxic

granules in natural killer cells or cytotoxic T-cells. Examples of the gene mutations associated with FHL2, 3, 4, and 5 are *PRF1*, *UNC13*, *STX11*, or *STXBP2* genes, respectively; the gene alteration in FHL1 is unknown (139,141). Primary HLH is linked to familial/genetic aberrations, where HLH is the primary manifestation. Primary HLH is a genetic disorder of lymphocyte cytotoxicity that usually presents in children within the first two years of life. Sporadic HLH can occur in immunodeficiency disorders such as Chediak–Higashi syndrome 1 (*LYST* mutation), Griscelli syndrome 2 (*RAB27A* mutation), and X-linked lymphoproliferative syndromes I (*SH2D1A* mutation) and 2 (*XIAP* mutation). The latter two have similar severe inflammatory manifestations that are set off by a variety of triggers (infections, viral, or others) (139–141).

There are no primary immunodeficiencies or family history in secondary; patients are older children. Their disease is most likely triggered by infections and concurrent medical conditions (such as autoimmune disease and malignancies) (139).

Histology: Histopathology alone is not diagnostic. Assessment of family history, serum soluble α-chain of CD25, detection of low or absent NK-cell activity and molecular analysis of the candidate genes in familial types are essential to provide the diagnosis. Non-specific pathological changes, such as the presence of hemophagocytosis may be seen in the bone-marrow biopsy and the lymph-node sinusoids. Some patients with NHL may present with non-specific hemophagocytosis. Rare cases may have florid EBV-associated aggressive lympho-proliferations, notably those with X-linked lymphoproliferative disease. Most HLH affects the liver and causes liver enzyme abnormalities that lead to liver biopsies, which show severe chronic persistent hepatitis and severe steatosis. In early manifestations, the presence of sinusoidal hemophagocytosis is best detected by electron microscopy. Immunostain reveals increased CD163+ macrophages in the sinusoids (Figure 7.20). Decreased expression of impaired cytotoxicities markers such as perforin, *SAP*, *XIAP*, or mobilization of CD107a may be present (141).

Lymphomas associated with secondary immunodeficiencies

Post-transplant lymphoproliferative disease (PTLD)

Best defined as polyclonal or monoclonal B-cell or T-cell proliferations of donor or recipient origin,

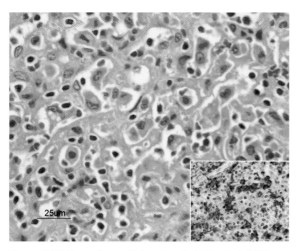

Figure 7.20 Hemophagocytic lymphocytic histiocytosis (HLH): increased activated macrophage/histiocytes displaying hemophagocytotic activities within the hepatic sinusoids. In advanced disease (not shown), massive bystander injuries by induction of apoptosis to hepatocytes can cause progressive disappearance of the hepatic parenchyma. Inset shows marked increase in activated CD163+macrophages in the hepatic sinusoids.

which occur either at an early or at a late stage after solid-organ transplantation. The majority of PTLD are of B-cell origin. As well as the immunosuppression burden of the patient, there is an overwhelming association with EBV in most cases.

Clinical features: The prevalence of PTLD in pediatric solid-organ transplant recipients is approximately 9%. This is higher than the 2% prevalence rate in adult recipients (142). Young Caucasian males are at the highest risk for PTLD development among solid-organ transplant recipients (143). Transplant recipients have a higher risk of developing lymphoma from PTLD. There is a 23–37-fold rise in lymphoma in recipients under 35 years of age (144), and recipients under 10 years of age have a 200- to 1200-fold increased incidence (145). Lymphomas arising from PTLD are 7- to 11-fold higher, as compared to the general population, and the degree of elevation in incidence varies with recipient age (145).

The overall median time to PTLD for pediatric transplant recipients is 5.5–25 months (25–72 months in adults) (146). This can vary according to the type of organ transplant, the availability of data from various registries, and the era of the study series. This disease can occur at any time post-transplant and the cumulative incidence increases over time (146). Early PTLD tends to be EBV-positive and late PTLD is EBV-negative (146). There are five risk factors associated with the development of PTLD (146): (1) EBV

infection; an EBV seronegative recipient has a 24-fold higher risk than an EBV-seropositive recipient. (2) Host-related factors such as young age (<18 years), male sex, Caucasian race, pretransplant malignancy, and fewer HLA matches. (3) Primary disease-related risk factors, such as pediatric liver recipients who have prior hepatic Langerhans-cell histiocytosis. (4) Graft organ-related factors. (5) Immunosuppression-related risk factors due to the increasing potency of immunosuppression protocols. While a number of retrospective studies showed increased risk of PTLD, prospective study results differ, and no increase in PTLD risk with any particular immunosuppressive agents could be found (3). Overall, the magnitude of risk with an immunosuppressive agent, in almost all cases, is much lower than the risk from an EBV seromismatch.

Pathological classification of PTLD (30,31):

1. Early lesions

    1.1 Plasmacytic hyperplasia

    1.2 Infectious mononucleosis-like PTLD

2. Polymorphic PTLD
3. Monomorphic PTLD (B- and T/NK-cell types); specify subtype
4. Classical Hodgkin's lymphoma-type PTLD

Histology: Early lesions of PTLD show mononucleosis-like reactive lymphoid follicular hyperplasia and paracortical hyperplasia or plasma-cell hyperplasia. These early lesions entail proliferations of lymphoid cells that do not show evidence of stromal effacement. The lymphoid cells show no atypia and comprise the full spectrum of various reactive lymphoid cell types. Small lymphocytes usually predominate and paraimmunoblasts and immunoblasts are the least frequent cell types. In the plasmacytic hyperplasia type, plasma cells predominate and in the infectious mononucleosis-like PTLD, the mixture of lymphoid cell types with appearances of transformed lymphoid cells is indistinguishable from that of mononucleosis (Figure 7.21). As most PTLD is EBV-associated (at least 75% of cases), ISH-EBER for location and density of EBV-containing lymphoid cells is an important diagnostic tool. Typically, aggregates of positive lymphoid cells with transformed nuclei or positive plasma cells are seen admixed with other reactive lymphoid cells in the parafollicular domains or the paracortices. Negative cases from EBV-positive allograft recipients will show sporadic single positive cells randomly distributed in various domains of the lymph node. Routine use of T- and B-cell markers or activation antigens such as

251

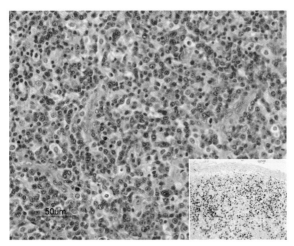

Figure 7.21 Post-transplant lymphoproliferative disease (PTLD), polymorphic: diffuse infiltrates of mixed infiltrates of small- and medium-sized cells with atypia. Occasional immunoblasts are present. This case is monoclonal for B cells by molecular analysis. Insert: another case with similar histological features, but is monoclonal for T-cells by molecular analyses. Both cases are EBV- by ISH-EBER.

CD30 is not warranted. CD30 stains a subset of plasma cells and reactive histiocytes, which may lead to a mistaken interpretation of HL Reed–Sternberg cells. Demonstration of κ or λ light-chain expression restriction is also error-prone, due to the insensitivity of the procedure or the presence of high background staining.

In *polymorphic PTLD*, effacement of tissue stroma is one of the most important features. The infiltrate always comprises a mixture of lymphoid cells with cytological atypia, which will not show the spectrum of lymphoid cell types that is seen in normal reactive lymphoid transformation (Figure 7.21). Plasma cells may also be present. Some of the atypical cells are large and may resemble either immunoblasts or Reed–Sternberg-like cells. For those that are EVB-associated, ISH-EBER will show a large number of positive atypical nuclei within the infiltrate, and this feature will aid the diagnosis.

In *monomorphic PTLD*, effacement of tissue stroma is also one of the important hallmarks. Cytologically, most of the B-cell lesions comprise monomorphous lymphoid-cell or plasma-cell-rich infiltrates, and a small number of this latter type resemble extramedullary plasmacytomas. For the lymphoid cell types, most monomophic PTLD essentially is indistinguishable from large B-cell lymphomas, Burkitt's lymphomas, or T-cell lymphomas of the non-immune-suppressed hosts. Currently, only cases that resemble small B-cell lymphomas are excluded. T-cell lymphomas are usually not monomorphic and

have atypical mixed cells, and various subtypes that aree similar to T-cell lymphomas of the non-immune suppressed hosts.

In *classical HL-type PTLD*, the diagnosis of Hodgkin's requires the fulfillment of the same diagnostic criteria as HL that occurs in a non-immunosuppressed host. Hodgkin's lymphoma post-transplantation is uncommon.

Immunohistochemistry: In the early lesions, as most of these proliferations are driven by EBV, *in situ* hybridization of EBV-encoded RNA (ISH-EBER) may show an increase in positive cells. In non-PTLD tissues of EBV-exposed patients, a smaller number of EBV carrier cells will be noted. Immunophenotyping shows an increase in B-cells amongst the infiltrates and PCR for B-clonality will always be negative.

In *polymorphic PTLD* and cases that are EVB-associated, ISH-EBER will show large number of positive atypical nuclei within the infiltrate and this feature will aid the diagnosis. The immunophenotype shows a mixture of B- and T-cells. A majority of these lesions are B-cell-rich; however, analysis for B-cell clonality may not be definitive, as a proportion of this type of PTLD can be clonal. Apart from BCL6 mutations, other oncogene abnormalities are usually absent.

In *monomorphic PTLD*, the histologic, immuno-histologic, and molecular characteristics of the various types of monomorphic PTLD fulfill the diagnostic criteria of the WHO classification of non-Hodgkin's lymphoma (30) and the diagnostic work-up should follow the most recent CAP recommendations for the examination of specimens from patients with non-Hodgkin's lymphoma/lymphoid neoplasms (31).

Genetics: Recent molecular studies of post-transplant diffuse large B-cell lymphoma in adults using single nucleotide polymorphism arrays showed a genomic profile with specific features, such as small interstitial deletions targeting known fragile sites such as *FRA1b*, *FRA2E*, and *FRA3B*. Deletions at 2p16 (*FRA2E*) were the most common lesion. These lymphomas also lack del (13q14.30)(*MIR15/16*) and a copy of neutral LOH affecting the 6p MHC locus (147).

Others

Human immunodeficiency virus (HIV)-associated lymphomas

This refers to Hodgkin's (HL) or non-Hodgkin's lymphomas (NHL) arising in a patient with HIV (before, at, or after AIDS onset).

Clinical presentation: Most of these are aggressive lymphomas presenting at advanced clinical stage. Burkitt's lymphoma arises during early onset of HIV, whereas DLBCL occurs in long-standing AIDS patients, especially those with low CD4-T-cell counts. Improvement of CD4 counts could influence both the occurrence and the survival with HIV lymphomas.

Prevalence of malignancies such as Kaposi's sarcoma (KS) and HIV-lymphoma in industrialized countries differs from developing countries. Kaposi's sarcoma is most prevalent in developing countries. The AIDs-Cancer Match Registry Study group reported in 2000 that amongst 4954 children with AIDS, 100 had NHL, 8 had KS, 4 had leiomyosarcoma and 2 had HD (148). The overall lymphoma prevalence resembled that of adults; however, KS is rare in children in the industrialized world (149). Combined reports from Malawi, South Africa, and Uganda showed KS with the highest prevalence, followed by Burkitt's lymphoma (amongst NHL), and other types of NHL and HL (150–152).

Genetics: Recently genome-wide DNA profiling studies were performed on adult HIV B-NHL. Varied genomic complexities were found across HIV-NHL subtypes. HIV Burkitt's lymphoma showed a significantly lower number of lesions than HIV-DLBCL (153). Genomic aberrations affecting the poor outcome of immunodeficiency-related DLBCL, such as gains at 1q or at 18q, the presence of del(3p13.2), or of +2p23.1 have been observed in adult HIV-DLBCL (154).

Classification: A spectrum of HIV-NHL subtypes has been reported in children. Similar to adults, the majority of them are Burkitt's, followed by DLBCL, plasmablastic lymphoma (oral and non-oral), T-cell lymphomas and HL (149–160), primary effusion lymphoma (HHV8-EBV co-infection), CNS lymphomas, and others.

Histology: With the exception of HIV-plasmablastic lymphoma (which is a distinct subtype of NHL) (161), other HIV-associated NHL are similar to the various types occurring in immunocompetent patients. Plasmablastic lymphomas are very rare in HIV children. Similar to adults, it can present in the oral cavity (155). HIV-plasmablastic lymphomas express all plasma cell markers (CD138), but can show variable expression of B-cell markers. In adults, EBV is detectable in approx 74% of cases.

Differential diagnosis: In non-industrialized countries, metastatic KS in lymph nodes is more frequent than HIV-NSHL.

Bone-marrow pathology

Comprehensive bone-marrow examination is essential for the diagnosis and classification of various stem-cell disorders within the pediatric age group. Acute leukemia is the most common, representing approximately 30% of pediatric cancer and is of lymphoid, as opposed to myeloid, origin in 80% and 20% of cases, respectively (162–163). Other, much less common precursor neoplasms are restricted to specific patient populations, e.g., myeloid proliferations in Down syndrome, or are of unique and still poorly understood origin, e.g., blastic plasmacytoid dendritic cell neoplasms. Still other stem-cell disorders specific to the pediatric age group, such as juvenile myelomonocytic leukemia, exhibit myeloproliferative (full spectrum of maturation without immature arrest) and myelodysplastic (aberrant cytomorphology with ineffective hematopoiesis) features without an acute leukemic presentation. In contrast, the broad category of marrow failure syndromes manifesting with cytopenias of varying degrees, encompass both primary (e.g., constitutional) and secondary (e.g., refractory cytopenia of childhood, aplastic anemia) disorders and are important to recognize and discriminate, as these entities warrant distinct clinical and therapeutic approaches.

An important step in the evaluation of bone-marrow (BM) specimens is the initial triage of material for ancillary studies that are critical to both diagnosis and prognosis. Acquisition of both an aspirate and a biopsy is necessary for comprehensive assessment. The marrow aspirate should be allocated for cytomorphologic, flow cytometric, cytogenetic, and molecular diagnostic analyses. Air-dried touch imprints of a fresh core should be routinely prepared, as these slides can be stained for immediate cytologic assessment or can be held and submitted for cytogenetic/FISH or molecular analysis, as needs dictate. Biopsy cores can also be submitted fresh on saline-soaked gauze or in tissue media for flow cytometric or cytogenetic analysis. Up-front triage, in this way, allows for expeditious and comprehensive marrow assessment.

Precursor B-lymphoid neoplasms

B-lymphoblastic leukemia/lymphoma (B-ALL) is a neoplasm of B-cell progenitors (e.g., B-lymphoblasts). Bone marrow involvement is usually pronounced, hence the leukemic designation; however, extramedullary (lymphomatous) manifestations may also occur.

Clinical presentation: Bone-marrow replacement typically results in peripheral cytopenias, with consequent infection, fatigue, and/or mucosal bleeding, secondary to neutropenia, anemia, and thrombocytopenia, respectively. The white blood cell count may be markedly elevated or depressed, with varying numbers of circulating lymphoblasts. Aleukemic presentations are uncommon, but can occur, and circulating normoblasts may be a harbinger of underlying disease. Hepatosplenomegaly, lymphadenopathy, and testicular enlargement reflect tissue infiltration, while bone pain may be experienced secondary to periosteal involvement or tumor necrosis. Unexplained fever may also precipitate clinical investigation.

Classification: Precursor B-lymphoid neoplasms are segregated into two broad categories of disease: B-lymphoblastic leukemia/lymphoma, with recurrent genetic abnormalities, and B-lymphoblastic leukemia/lymphoma, not otherwise specified (NOS) (30). Distinguishing features of the genetically defined entities are detailed in Table 7.2; neoplasms within the NOS category lack unique characteristics (164–176).

Histology: In smear preparations, lymphoblasts are characteristically intermediate-sized cells (1.5–2 times the size of a small mature lymphocyte) with convoluted nuclei, finely dispersed chromatin, inconspicuous-to-small (generally single) nucleoli, and scant cytoplasm, with occasional cytoplasmic vacuoles. The blasts may be

Table 7.2 Characteristics of B-lymphoblastic leukemia/lymphoma with genetically defined abnormalities as defined within the WHO 2008 classification scheme (30,164–176)

Recurrent genetic abnormality	Frequency	Unique clinical manifestations	Most common phenotypic characteristics	Diagnostic or methodologic considerations	Prognosis
t(v;11q23); *MLL* rearranged	5–8% children 90% <6 mos 50% 6–12 mos 6% 12–24 mos	Disease of infancy Hyperleukocytosis (WBC >150 K/ul) Hepatosplenomegaly CNS involvement	CD10– CD20– CD15+ CD13CD33–	Most often t(4;11) May be cryptic	Poor EFS 10–30% (worse with younger age) Early relapse (within 2 yrs)
t(12;21)(p13;q22); *TEL-AML1* (*ETV6-RUNX1*)	25% children (most common translocation)	1–10 yrs Leukopenia	CD10 + CD20– CD15– CD13CD33 dim	Cryptic lesion	Favorable 5-yr EFS 80–95%
t(9;22)(p34;q11.2); *BCR-ABL1*	3–5% children	Older age Hyperleukocytosis	CD10 bright CD20 dim CD15– CD13CD33+	Exclude CML	Poor 3 yr EFS 35% 3 yr EFS 80% with TKI
t(1;19)(p23;q13.3); *E2A-PBX1* (*TCF3-PBX1*)	5% children	African American	CD10–/dim CD20 dim/+ CD15 neg CD13CD33– cyt IgM–	May be cryptic	Was poor, improved with intensive therapy EFS 80–85% Increased risk of CNS relapse observed in some trials
t(5;14)(p31;q32); *IL3-IGH*	Rare <1%	Eosinophilia		Detectable on routine karyotype	Unclear
Hyperdiploidy >50–65 chromosomes DNA index ≥1.16	25% children	1–10 yrs Leukopenia	CD10 bright CD20 dim/+ CD15– CD13CD33–	+4, +10, +17* portend best outcome	Favorable 5-yr EFS 80–90%
Hypodiploidy <44–45 chromosomes	5–6% children				Poor EFS 30% (< 44 chrom) EFS 50% (≤ 44 chrom)

*Controversial in some trials

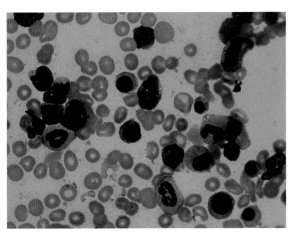

Figure 7.22 Lymphoblasts are intermediate in size and have convoluted nuclei, dispersed chromatin, inconspicuous to small nucleoli, and scant cytoplasm, with occasional cytoplasmic vacuoles.

heterogeneous in appearance, including small, intermediate, and large forms, the last of which may be mistaken for myeloblasts, given less irregular nuclear contours and more prominent nucleoli (Figure 7.22). Mitoses are easily identified and, given this high-proliferation fraction, tingible body macrophages may be seen in biopsy sections, conferring a "starry-sky" appearance at low power. Near-total marrow replacement is the norm, though megakaryopoiesis may be preserved. On rare occasions, marrow hypoplasia or aplasia may be seen (177,178). The involvement of the CNS is often asymptomatic, though detectable on microscopic review of cerebrospinal fluid.

Immunophenotypic characterization of lymphoblastic leukemia is important for diagnosis (e.g., lineage assignment), prediction of underlying genetic abnormalities, and prognosis (e.g., minimal residual disease detection). Flow cytometry offers more rapid and comprehensive assessment, as well as greater sensitivity for disease detection as compared to immunohistochemical methods. Although phenotypic profiles may resemble that of normal maturing B-cells (hematogones), inherent deviations distinguish these cells as neoplastic (179,180). CD34, TdT, and dim/absent expression of CD45 can all be used to identify blasts. CD19, CD20, CD22, CD10, cytoplasmic Igμ, and surface κ and λ immunoglobulin light chains assess B-cell differentiation and maturation. B-lymphoblasts characteristically uniformly express strong CD19, but lack expression of surface immunoglobulin. Myeloid antigens (CD13, CD15, and CD33) may be expressed to varying degrees and may offer clues to underlying genetic abnormalities.

Differential diagnosis: Neoplastic B-lymphoblasts must be distinguished from hematogones, their benign counterpart. Hematogones predominate in infancy and proportionately regress with development into adulthood. Hematogones progress through three predictable and reproduceable stages of maturation that are easily assessed using flow cytometric techniques (179,180). Expanded populations of hematogones may be observed during marrow regeneration, such as after infectious, toxin, or drug exposures. Differential diagnosis also includes the small round blue-cell tumors of childhood. These are most often cohesive and arrayed in clusters and clumps on smear preparations, while the textural chromatin of these non-hematopoietic tumors is more granular and not as finely dispersed as in lymphoblasts. Undifferentiated acute myeloid leukemias and plasmacytoid dendritic cell neoplasms must also be excluded.

Prognosis: Although childhood B-ALL has become highly treatable with overall 80% five-year event free survival (174), refractory disease and relapse are still problematic in a subset of patients. Multiple parameters are of prognostic significance and segregate patients into differential risk categories (Table 7.3; 174,176,181–183).

One of the most significant independent predictors of disease relapse is the assessment of minimal residual disease early in the course of therapy and/or at end remission-induction. Comprehensive analysis of patients with high-risk disease has identified additional abnormalities that portend a poor prognosis, suggest the presence of co-operative mutations in leukemogenesis, and warrant further multi-institutional investigation (Table 7.4; 174,176,184).

Acute myeloid leukemia (AML) and related precursor neoplasms

Acute myeloid leukemia is a neoplasm of a hematopoietic stem cell (blast) or a lineage-specific progenitor cell (blast equivalent) that together include myeloblasts, monoblasts, and megakaryoblasts, as well as malignant promyelocytes and promonocytes. In general, AML is defined by the presence of ≥ 20% blasts in blood and/or marrow; however, when specific genetically defined abnormalities are present, no minimum blast percentage is required.

Classification: Acute myeloid leukemia is segregated into several broad categories of disease: (1) AML with recurrent genetic abnormalities

Table 7.3 Prognostic factors in B-lymphoblastic leukemia/lymphoma (174,176,181–183)

	Favorable	Unfavorable
Age	1–10 yrs	<1 yr 10–21 yrs
Leukocyte count	< 50 ×10^9/L	≥50 ×10^9/L
Chromosomal abnormality	High hyperdiploidy (> 50, +4, +10, +17*) TEL-AML1 (ETV6-RUNX1)	Hypodiploidy MLL rearrangement BCR-ABL1
Cerebrospinal fluid status	CNS-1 (no blasts)	CNS-3 ≥5 WBC/ul with blasts)
Flow cytometric MRD in marrow (% blasts)		
Day 15 induction (rapidity of treatment response)	< 0.01%	≤ 10%
Day 29 induction (end of remission-induction)	< 0.01%	≥1%

*Favorable prognosticator only in some clinical trials

Table 7.4 Additional molecular genetic abnormalities that confer a poor prognosis in pediatric B-ALL (174,176,184)

	Frequency	Clinical associations	Other associations	Prognosis (5-yr EFS)
Intrachromosomal amplification of chromosome 21 (iAMP21)	2–3% children	Older children and adolescents		Poor 80–90%
IKZF1 deletions/ mutations	15%	80% BCR-ABL1 ALL	JAK1–3 activating mutations seen in 10% of cases (co-operative)	Poor 50–55%
CRLF2 rearrangement with overexpression	6–7% children	50–70% Down-associated ALL		Poor ?%

(Table 7.5; 30,164,174,185–193); (2) AML, not otherwise specified (NOS) (30; Table 7.6); (3) myeloid sarcoma; and (4) therapy-related myeloid neoplasms (Table 7.7; 30,194–198).

Clinical presentation: Patients generally present with hematopoietic failure manifest by peripheral cytopenia(s) with circulating myeloblasts and/or normoblasts. Extramedullary disease may also be present.

Histology: In general, myeloblasts are large cells that have dispersed chromatin, prominent single and occasionally multiple nucleoli, and typically scant cytoplasm. However, blasts may vary in appearance depending upon the AML subtype; likewise, varying degrees of associated granulocytic and monocytic differentiation may be present within some categories of disease (Figures 7.23–7.26). Blasts may contain a few fine or numerous coarse cytoplasmic granules. Auer rods may also be seen. Blast enumeration is based upon cytomorphologic assessment of a peripheral blood smear, aspirate smear, and/or core biopsy preparation. Flow cytometric quantitation is suboptimal, as the blast percentage may be falsely lowered or elevated as a consequence of hemodilution/cell loss during processing, or red-cell lysis.

The differential diagnosis includes other malignancies such as lymphoblastic leukemia, myelodysplastic/marrow failure syndromes with an expanded blast population, and solid tumors of childhood as well as non-neoplastic conditions such as megaloblastic anemia, growth-factor therapy effects, and recovery from toxic/infectious insults.

Prognosis varies based upon the specific AML subtype; however, the overall five-year event-free survival rate is approximately 60% in children less than 15 years of age (174). Flow cytometric or molecular diagnostic minimal residual disease assessment is important in the ongoing assessment of treatment response, and in predicting relapse as well as overall survival (199–201).

Table 7.5 Classification of acute myeloid leukemia, with recurrent genetic abnormalities, as designated within the 2008 WHO Classification (30,164,174,185–193)

Genetic abnormality	t(8;21)(q22;q22) RUNX1-RUNX1T1	inv(16)(p13.1q22) or t(16;16)(p13.1q22) CBFB-MYH11	t(5;17)(q22;q12) PML1-RARA	t(9;11)(p22;q23) MLLT3-MLL	t(6;9)(p23;q34) DEK-NUP214	t(1;22)(p13;q13) RBM15-MKL1
Incidence	10–15%	5–10%	10–15%	5–20%	1%	<1%
Caveats		Often cryptic (use FISH if suspected) Often associated with isolated trisomy 22	Variant translocations exist (unresponsive to ATRA)	Often cryptic (use FISH if suspected)	Often cryptic (use FISH if suspected)	
Clinical presentation	Young adults Myeloid sarcoma	Young adults Myeloid sarcoma	Two variants: — Classic: Leukopenia, Low platelets DIC — Microgranular: Hyperleukocytosis, Low platelets DIC	Children Myeloid sarcoma	Basophilia	Infants Young children (<3 yrs) Non-Down Organomegaly
Microscopic	Long thin tapered Auer rods present in blasts, neutrophils, and eosinophils Maturing granulocytes with salmon-colored granules and surrounding basophilia Dysgranulopoiesis	Typically myelomonocytic differentiation Abnormal eosinophilic-basophilic forms No peripheral eosinophilia	Promyelocytic maturation arrest Intense azurophilic Granules Occasional cells with multiple Auer rods Reniform, bilobed, folded nuclei (often confused with monocytes) Varied amounts of agranular cytoplasm	Monoblastic or promonocytic in appearance	Trilineage dysplasia Occasional ring sideroblasts	Megakaryoblasts (varied in size and nuclear pleomorphism, basophilic cytoplasm with cytoplasmic blebbing) Micromegas Marrow fibrosis
Flow cytometric features	TdT+, CD19+, CD56+	Immature population with granulocytic & monocytic differentiation & maturation asynchrony	CD34- HLA-DR- MPO bright Often CD34+ HLA-DR- CD2+ CD64+ MPO bright	CD34- CD117- HLA-DR bright MPO-/weak CD14 var/dim CD68+ Lysozyme+ NSE+	MPO&NSE+	CD34-/+ CD61+ CD41+ CD42 variable
Prognosis	Favorable	Favorable	Favorable	Intermediate	Poor	?
Differential			Transient agranulocytosis G-CSF effects			Down AMKL Metastatic tumor

Table 7.6 Classification of acute myeloid leukemia, not otherwise specified, as designated within the 2008 WHO Classification (30)

FAB	WHO Classification 2008	
	AML, NOS	Marrow findings
M0	AML, minimally differentiated	< 3% MPO positivity in blasts myeloid antigen expression
M1	AML, without maturation	≥ 3% MPO positivity in blasts blasts ≥ 90% non-erythroids
M2	AML, with maturation	≥ 3% MPO positivity in blasts ≥ 10% maturing myeloids < 20% monocytes
M3		
M4	Acute myelomonocytic leukemia	≥ 3% MPO positivity in blasts ≥ 20% maturing myeloids ≥ 20% maturing monocytes (NSE+)
M5	Acute monoblastic/monocytic leukemias	≥ 80% leukemic cells monocytic < 20% maturing neutrophils
M6	Acute erythroid leukemia	≥ 50% nucleated cells are erythroid ≥ 20% myeloblasts in non-erythroid
M7	Acute megakaryoblastic leukemia	≥ 50% blasts are megakaryocytic MPO/SBB negativity CD41, CD61, CD42 positivity

FAB – French-American-British; WHO – World Health Organization
Cytochemical studies: MPO = myeloperoxidase; SBB = Sudan black B; NSE = non-specific esterase

Table 7.7 Therapy-related myeloid neoplasms, two broad subsets of disease (194–198)

Therapeutic exposure		Alkylating agents and/or radiation	DNA topoisomerase II inhibitors
Clinical presentation	Latency period	5–10 years	< 1–3 years
	Onset	Prolonged myelodysplastic prodrome	Abrupt AML
	Peripheral blood features	Cytopenias	Leukocytosis
Common associated genetic abnormalities		Complex karyotypes with unbalanced chromosomal loss Chromosomes 5 and/or 7 commonly affected, as well as 13q, 20q, 11q, 3p, 17, 18, 21	Balanced chromosomal translocations Commonly: 11q23 Much less frequently: t(8;21) t(15;17) inv(16)
Cytomorphologic marrow findings		Uni-, bi-, trilineage dysplasia Marrow fibrosis	AML often monocytic Marrow fibrosis
Prognosis		Poor survival (< 1 year) Expression of multidrug resistance-associated proteins and drug efflux Co-operative class I and II mutations	Variable survival Achieve initial complete remission, but with high risk of relapse

Genetics: Two genetically defined entities are provisional categories within the current WHO 2008 classification system, but are of prognostic importance in adults and seemingly in children as well, though in the latter they have been studied less extensively, given their limited occurrence. These entities include mutations of nucleophosphmin (*NPM1*) and of the *CCAAT*/enhancer binding protein-α (*CEBPA*) gene. *NPM1* mutations occur in 10–20% of pediatric AML with a normal karyotype, but are rare in children

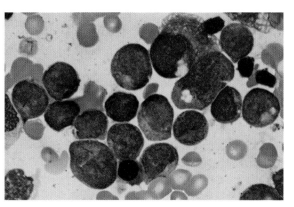

Figure 7.23 Myeloblasts are generally large and have round to irregular nuclei, fine chromatin, variably prominent nucleoli, and scant to moderate cytoplasm with occasional granules and/or vacuoles. The Auer rods in several of these cells confirm that these are of myeloid origin.

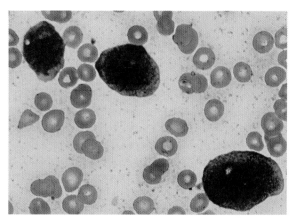

Figure 7.24 Acute promyelocytic leukemia (APML) with t (15;17)(q22;q12)(*PML-RARA*) exhibits maturation arrest at the promyelocyte stage of development. In the "classic" variant, the neoplastic cells exhibit round to ovoid eccentric nuclei and abundant cytoplasm, with numerous azurophilic granules.

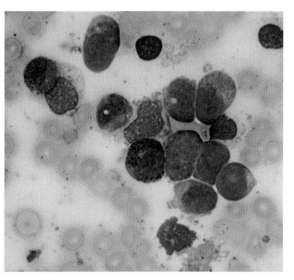

Figure 7.25 AML with inv(16)(p13.1;q22) demonstrates blasts, eosinophilic precursors, and aberrant "eos-baso" forms (center and upper right). The cytogenetic abnormality is defining of AML, regardless of blast count.

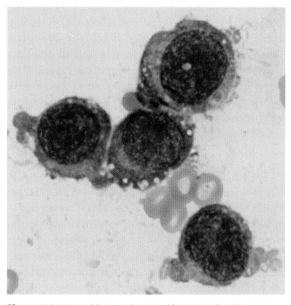

Figure 7.26 Monoblasts are large and have round nuclei, prominent and often central nucleoli, and abundant basophilic cytoplasm with occasional cytoplasmic granules and vacuoles. Monoblasts are often seen in the setting of *MLL* (11q23) rearrangement that can manifest with extramedullary infiltrates.

younger than two years of age (174). When present in isolation, they are associated with a favorable prognosis; otherwise, the prognosis is unclear. *CEBPA* mutations occur in 15% of pediatric AML with a normal karyotype (174); 70–80% of these patients exhibit double mutant alleles, which portends a favorable prognosis. Differing prognoses have been reported in the setting of single mutant alleles. Mutations of fms-like tyrosine kinase 3 (*FLT3*), typically involving internal tandem duplications (ITD), occur in 5–10% of pediatric AML and portend a poor

prognosis when present, though this is not currently a defined or provisional category within the WHO classification system (30,174).

Myeloid sarcoma

Myeloid sarcoma is a tumor mass, occurring at an anatomic site other than the bone marrow, that effaces tissue architecture, is composed of blasts or blast

259

equivalents, with or without maturation, and is equivalent to a diagnosis of AML.

Clinical presentation: Myeloid sarcoma can occur in any organ; however, skin, gingival mucosa, gastrointestinal tract, lymph node, and gonads are the most commonly involved sites of disease. Myeloid sarcoma can precede or can occur concurrently with a diagnosis of AML, or may be the initial, and perhaps isolated, manifestation of disease relapse. The presence of myeloid sarcoma generally portends a poor prognosis.

Histology: Monoblastic or myelomonocytic differentiation (with varying degrees of maturation) is most commonly observed. Diagnosis requires partial or total effacement of normal tissue architecture as leukemic infiltrates can be seen in association with AML, particularly in the setting of hyperleukocytosis.

The phenotypic profile is lineage dependent; however, CD43 and lysozyme are generally expressed. Myeloperoxidase, CD34, CD117, and CD33 are often expressed with granulocytic differentiation, while CD4 and CD68 are associated with monocytic differentiation. Cytochemical positivity for non-specific esterase is typically strongly positive in monoblastic lesions (202).

Differential diagnosis: Includes small round blue-cell tumors of childhood, blastic plasmacytoid dendritic cell neoplasms, and various lymphoid neoplasms (lymphoblastic, Burkitt's, diffuse large B-cell).

Therapy-related myeloid neoplasms

Therapy-related myeloid neoplasms encompass any AML, myelodysplastic syndrome (MDS), or myelodysplastic/myeloproliferative neoplasm (MDS/MPN) that develops as a consequence of prior cytotoxic chemotherapy or radiation. In this setting, these normally disparate entities are merged into one broad category, given that neither differing clinical manifestations nor varied blast counts are believed to be of prognostic or therapeutic significance.

Clinical presentation: Two subsets of disease are distinguished by their varied clinical presentations, associated genetic abnormalities, cytomorphologic features, prognosis, and underlying therapeutic exposures (Table 7.7). Overall, prognosis is poor, with less than 10% five-year survival in these patients. Those individuals with a myelodysplastic prodrome fair even worse with less than one year survival secondary to expression of multidrug resistance-associated proteins and drug efflux, while those with a leukemic presentation generally achieve an initial complete remission, but have a high likelihood of disease relapse.

Histology: When a myelodysplastic prodome exists, patients exhibit peripheral cytopenias secondary to ineffective hematopoiesis. Erythroid, myeloid, and megakaryocytic lineages may all be affected and may exhibit cytomorphologic dysplasia. Erythropoiesis may exhibit megaloblastoid maturation with nuclear contour irregularities, aberrant nuclear lobation, and/or detached nuclear fragments. Myelopoiesis may show nuclear hypolobation and cytoplasmic hypogranularity. Megakaryopoiesis may contain small hypolobated micromegakaryocytes or megakaryocytes with multiple separated nuclear lobes. In the absence of a myelodysplastic prodrome, leukocytosis with circulating blasts is typically seen.

No distinct immunophenotypic profile exists; however, various abnormalities have been described and include dys-synchronous expression of markers of maturation, lineage infidelity with aberrant expression of T-cell or B-cell markers on myeloid elements (e.g., CD7 and CD56), and aberrant over- or under-expression of surface proteins (203).

Myeloid proliferations related to Down syndrome

Transient abnormal myelopoiesis (TAM) and acute myeloid leukemia (AML)

Approximately 10% of newborns with constitutional trisomy 21 inherent to Down syndrome present with a transient myeloproliferative disorder indistinguishable from acute leukemia and termed transient abnormal myelopoiesis (TAM). While in most cases the proliferation resolves spontaneously, approximately 20% will develop acute megakaryoblastic leukemia (204,205). These are grouped as a separate clinicopathologic entity in the 2008 WHO classification (30).

Clinical presentation: Transient abnormal myelopoiesis presents in the newborn period with the median age at diagnosis of five days (205). There are asymptomatic abnormalities of peripheral blood, including neutrophilia, thrombocytopenia, and borderline polycythemia. Significant organomegaly, including hepatomegaly, with significant hyperbilirubinemia is characteristic. There is extramedullary involvement of soft tissues in rare cases. In Down syndrome, AML typically presents in the first three years of life. Most cases are preceded by prolonged periods of myelodysplasia.

Genetics: In addition to Down syndrome, those with mosaicism for trisomy 21 also have a high risk for TAM (206). Mutations in the megakaryocytic

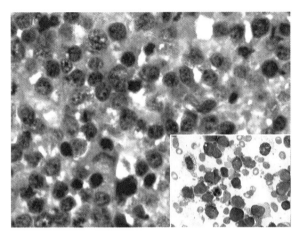

Figure 7.27 Transient abnormal myelopoiesis: bone-marrow core of transient abnormal myelopoiesis demonstrates sheets of large immature myeloid cells with variable amount of pink granular cytoplasm. Insert: Bone-marrow aspirate demonstrates numerous myeloid blasts with a subset showing cytoplasmic blebbing resembling megakaryocytes.

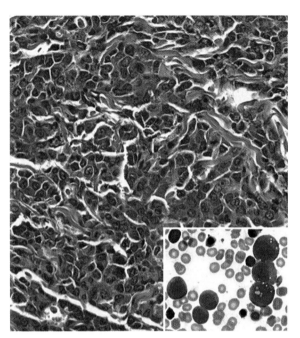

Figure 7.28 Skin biopsy of congenital leukemia: diffuse dermal infiltration by immature hematopoietic cells. The pleomorphic neoplastic cells exhibit large irregular blastic nuclei with prominent nucleoli and abundant basophilic cytoplasm. Insert: Wright–Giemsa stain of bone-marrow aspirate demonstrates large nuclei with prominent nucleoli, abundant cytoplasm, occasional cytoplasmic vacuoles, and fine esinophilic granules.

transcription factor *GATA1* (207) and *JAK3* are associated with TAM, as well as AML (208).

Histology: There is leukocytosis with increased numbers of blasts in the peripheral blood and bone marrow (Figure 7.27). The blasts are typically myeloid, with a subset that shows megakaryocytic differentiation. Some cases show basophilic cytoplasm with cytoplasmic projections (Figure 7.27 inset). Soft tissue and skin involvement (blueberry muffin syndrome) by acute myeloid leukemia can also be present. The blasts typically express moderate CD45, HLA-DR, and CD33, as well as CD34 and CD117. They show aberrant expression of CD7 and CD56, with variable expression of megakaryocytic antigens CD41, CD61, and CD71.

Differential diagnosis: Acute myeloid leukemia occurring in the setting of Down syndrome should be excluded. Typically they occur in the first three years of life and often follow a prolonged period of myelodysplasia.

Congenital acute leukemia with spontaneous remission

Congenital leukemia manifests within the first four weeks of life. It is rare and occurs at a rate of 1 per 5 million live births, and represents less than 1% of all childhood leukemia. Rarely, congenital leukemia exhibits a distinct natural history and is either transient or shows spontaneous remission. Congenital leukemia with t(8;16)(p11;p13) has a favorable prognosis,

with some demonstrating spontaneous remission (209,210).

Clinical presentation: Patients typically present with leukocytosis, hepatosplenomegaly, and CNS involvement. Over 60% of newborns with leukemia present with leukemia cutis (211).

Genetics: Children with Down syndrome have a 10- to 20-fold increased risk for congenital leukemia (212). Maternal exposure to radiation and high birth weight are other risk factors.

Histology: Peripheral blood and bone marrow show increased numbers of myeloid blasts (Figure 7.28 inset). Skin or soft tissues involved by leukemia show diffuse dermal infiltration by immature hematopoietic cells with open blastic chromatic appearance (Figure 7.28).

The neoplastic cells show expression of myeloid (CD33, HLA-DR) or monocytic (CD14, CD11c, CD56) cells, as well as antigens associated with immaturity (CD34). There may be a spectrum of myeloperoxidase or nonspecific esterase expression.

Differential diagnosis: Includes reactive monocytic proliferations, and reactive histiocytic proliferations such as juvenile xanthogranuloma. Other neoplasms

261

with aggressive histology such as diffuse large B-cell lymphoma, soft tissue neoplasms, and acute lymphoblastic leukemia/lymphoma should be considered. Cytogenetic evaluation and clinical correlation are critical to identify this entity.

Juvenile myelomonocytic leukemia

Juvenile myelomonocytic leukemia (JMML) is a clonal proliferation of granulocytic and monocytic lineage that occurs in early childhood. It has been previously referred to as juvenile chronic myeloid leukemia and represents an overlap between myelodysplastic/myeloproliferative neoplasms. The disease can occur in a sporadic form, but affects approximately 10% of children with neurofibromatosis-1, and more rarely Noonan syndrome.

Clinical presentation: It is an aggressive myeloid malignancy with a heterogeneous pattern of clinical manifestation. The disease presents in early childhood with 95% presenting before the age of six. There is an equal male: female ratio. Typical presentations include fever, hepatosplenomegaly, and high white blood cell count. The tumor also involves the gastrointestinal tract and lung.

Genetics: About 10% occur in children with neurofibromatosis-1 and more rarely Noonan syndrome. The main karyotypic abnormality is monosomy 7, detected in approximately 25% of patients (213). Deregulated activation of the RAS signaling pathway plays a central role in the pathogenesis of JMML. Genetic aberrations of *RAS*, *PTPN11*, or *NF1* genes are detected in 70–80% of JMML patients (214).

Histology: Peripheral blood demonstrates moderate leukocytosis, monocytosis, and immature neutrophils, including rare blasts. Bone-marrow aspirate demonstrates hypercellularity with a myeloid predominance. Blasts and promonocytes are increased, but typically are present at less than 20% (Figure 7.29). Hepatosplenomegaly is due to leukemic infiltration. Within the spleen, the blasts infiltrate predominantly within the red pulp and can compress the while pulp. There is periportal and sinusoidal infiltration by the neoplastic cells within the liver. The neoplastic cells express CD14, CD16, CD11b, CD68, and lysozyme, which can be detected in the tissue sections involved.

Differential diagnosis: The clinical and morphologic features may resemble a reactive process secondary to either infection or inflammation. Careful examination of peripheral blood and bone marrow, and evaluation for the presence of dysplasia is helpful.

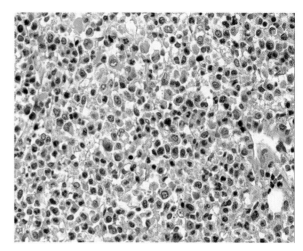

Figure 7.29 Juvenile myelomonocytic leukemia: bone-marrow clot section demonstrates hypercellularity with prominence of myeloid and monocytic cells with evidence of maturation.

The diagnosis of JMML requires integration of morphologic, flow cytometric, and molecular studies. Molecular studies should be performed to exclude a *BCR-ABL1*-positive chronic myeloid leukemia.

Blastic plasmacytoid dendritic cell neoplasm

Blastic plasmacytoid dendritic cell neoplasm (BPDCN) is a rare aggressive neoplasm with putative origin from immature plasmacytoid dendritic cells. They have been previously referred to as blastic NK-cell lymphomas (215), agranular CD4+ natural killer cell leukemias (216), and CD4+ CD56+ hematodermic neoplasm (217,218).

Clinical presentation: The disease occurs in the elderly, but can involve children (204–206), and typically presents with cutaneous, bone-marrow, and peripheral blood involvement at diagnosis. There is a male predilection, with a male:female ratio of 3.3:1 (218–220). The disease is clinically aggressive and many patients die within a year of diagnosis. Patients present with multiple skin lesions in the form of plaques or nodules. Peripheral cytopenias may be mild to severe depending on the extent of bone-marrow involvement. There may be lymph-node involvement in a subset of cases. Approximately 10% of patients develop acute myeloid leukemia (221).

Genetics: There are no characteristic hereditary or molecular features associated with BPDCN. IgH and TcR genes are typically in the germline configuration, though rare cases of clonal TCR gene rearrangements

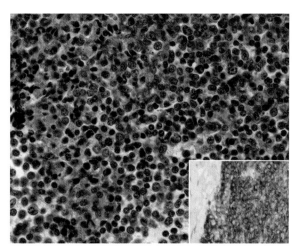

Figure 7.30 High-power magnification of blastic plasmacytoid dendritic-cell neoplasm involving the dermis of the skin: the neoplastic cells are intermediate in size and show a diffuse pattern of growth within the dermis. They are round to angulated with fine stippled to blastic chromatin. The tumor cells are CD123+ (inset) and TCL-1+ (not shown).

have been reported (218,222). The karyotypes of BPDCN are complex, with recurrent abnormalities targeting 5q21 or 5q34 (~75%), 12p13, and loss of chromosome 9 (221,223,224).

Histology: The skin infiltration demonstrates a "bottom-heavy" distribution of BPDCN blasts, which form aggregates in the dermis with extension into the subcutaneous adipose tissue. The epidermis is typically not involved. The neoplastic cells are monotonous, intermediate-sized cells with irregular indented nuclei and scant basophilic cytoplasm (Figure 7.30). In lymph nodes, the neoplastic cells exhibit an interfollicular, medullary, or "leukemic" distribution, or total effacement of the nodal architecture. Scattered mitoses and focal areas with tingible body macrophages containing karyorrhectic debris are seen.

The tumor cells are CD3–, CD4+, CD43, CD45RA, CD56+, TCL1+ (not shown), CD123+ (interleukin-3 α-chain receptor) (Figure 7.30 inset), CD303 (BDCA-2) + (218,225). A subset of tumors expresses CD68, TdT, CD2, CD7, CD33, and CD38.

Differential diagnosis: Blastic hematopoietic neoplasms such as precursor-B- and T-ALL, and AML should be considered. Extramedullary chronic myelomonocytic leukemia that evolves into extramedullary myeloid cell tumors needs to be distinguished from BPDCN.

Bone-marrow failure

The term "bone-marrow failure" represents a broad category of disease characterized by peripheral cytopenia(s) and generally, bone marrow that is hypocellular for age. This category encompasses the inherited bone marrow failure syndromes (e.g., Fanconi anemia, dyskeratosis congenita, Schwachman–Diamond syndrome, Diamond–Blackfan anemia, amegakaryocytic thrombocytopenia), the acquired myelodysplastic syndromes (e.g., refractory cytopenia of childhood), and idiopathic aplastic anemia. Although microscopic clues to underlying pathogenesis may exist on blood and marrow examination, definitive discrimination of these entities can be difficult. To this end, after exclusion of "reactive" (e.g., infectious, nutritional, metabolic, and autoimmune/rheumatologic) etiologies that can mimic marrow failure, classification of a bona fide marrow failure disorder then requires exclusion of the inherited syndromes, the diagnosis of which has clinical, therapeutic, and genetic ramifications for patients and their families. Comprehensive assessment of clinical and phenotypic features, cytogenetic and molecular abnormalities, as well as other specialized testing is mandatory. The presence of aberrant hematopoiesis characterized by myelodysplasia and/or markedly left-shifted erythropoiesis, as well as the presence of specific cytogenetic abnormalities may aid in the diagnosis of refractory cytopenia of childhood, while a diagnosis of idiopathic aplastic anemia remains a diagnosis of exclusion.

Inherited bone-marrow failure syndromes (IBFS)

Refer to Table 7.8 for a summary of the distinguishing clinical, hematologic, diagnostic, pathogenetic, and prognostic features of these inherited marrow failure syndromes (226–230).

Refractory cytopenia of childhood (RCC)

Although myelodysplasia is rare in the pediatric population, RCC is the most common subtype, arising in approximately 50% of cases (231).

Clinical presentation: Children may present with bleeding, infection, and fatigue, secondary to thrombocytopenia, neutropenia, and anemia, respectively. Macrocytosis is also common and hemoglobin F may be elevated. The presence of monosomy 7 portends a high likelihood of disease progression with a median

Table 7.8 Inherited marrow-failure syndromes (226–230).

	Fanconi anemia (FA)	Dyskeratosis congenita (DC)	Schwachman–Diamond syndrome (SDS)	Amegakaryocytic thrombocytopenia (AT)	Diamond–Blackfan anemia (DBA)
Hematologic abnormality Blood Marrow	Pancytopenia Macrocytosis Hypocellularity	Pancytopenia Macrocytosis Hypocellularity	Neutropenia Myeloid hypoplasia	Thrombocytopenia Megkaryocytic aplasia/hypoplasia	Anemia Macrocytosis Erythroid hypoplasia
Median age at diagnosis (range)	6.5 yrs (0–49 yrs)	14 yrs (0–75 yrs)	2 wks (0–11 yrs)	< 1 yr (NA)	3 mos (0–64 yrs)
Clinical features	Microsomia Short stature Hyperpigmentation Abnormal thumbs GU abnormalities	Triad: Dystrophic nails Reticular rash Oral leukoplakia	Exocrine pancreatic insufficiency	Petecchiae and/or hemorrhage	Craniofacial abnormalities Abnormal thumbs
Other malignancies Heme Non-heme	MDS/leukemia HNSCC, liver, brain, gynecol	MDS/leukemia HNSCC	MDS/leukemia	MDS/leukemia	MDS/leukemia Osteosarcoma
Underlying pathogenesis	Altered DNA repair signaling	Defective telomere maintenance	? Ribosomal maturation defect	Dysregulation of megakaryopoiesis	Altered ribosomal RNA processing
Screening tests	Chromosomal aberrations during culture with DNA crosslinkers	Shortened telomere length	Decreased serum trypsinogen and/or pancreatic isoamylase	Marrow for examination of megakaryocytes	Elevated red cell adenosine deaminase
Genes affected (inheritance pattern)	*FANCA, FANCC-M* Autosomal recessive *FANCB* X-linked	*DKC1* X-linked *TERT, TERC, TIN2* *Autosomal dominant* *NHP2, NOP10, TERT, TCAB1* *Autosomal recessive*	*SBDS* Autosomal recessive	*MPL* Autosomal Recessive	*RPS19* Autosomal Dominant

HNSCC = head and neck squamous cell carcinoma; MDS = myelodysplastic syndrome, gynecol; AR = autosomal recessive

time to progression of approximately two years (232,233).

Histology: The bone marrow is commonly, though not exclusively, hypocellular for age. Clusters of at least ten left-shifted erythroid precursors are present in the core biopsy and contain increased numbers of proerythroblasts. Dysplasia is evident within at least two myeloid lineages or comprises greater than 10% of one cell line. Dyserythropoiesis includes megaloblastoid maturation, multinucleation, aberrant nuclear lobulation, and late-appearing mitoses. Dysmyelopoiesis includes nuclear hypolobation, cytoplasmic hypogranlarity, and dys-synchronous nuclear and cytoplasmic maturation. Dysmegakaryopoiesis includes separated nuclear lobes and small microgakaryocytes that have unihypolobated nuclei.

"Dwarf" megakaryocytes can easily be missed on H&E marrow sections; therefore, CD61 is helpful to accentuate this abnormality. Blasts comprise less than 5% of marrow cellularity. Of note, hematopoiesis can be patchy in its distribution throughout the marrow. Therefore, two biopsies performed at least two weeks apart are recommended for representative sampling prior to establishment of a definitive diagnosis of myelodyspasia.

Differential diagnosis: Secondary myelodysplasia can mimic RCC and can be seen in the setting of viral infection (e.g., CMV, Epstein–Barr virus, HIV), nutritional deficiencies (e.g., folate, vitamin B12, vitamin B6), rheumatologic/autoimmune disorders, and inborn errors of metabolism. Likewise, cytomorphologic features indistinguishable from RCC can be seen in patients with idiopathic aplastic anemia who have been treated with immunosuppressive therapy.

Aplastic anemia (AA)

Clinical presentation: Infection, fatigue, bleeding, and petechiae occurs secondary to pancytopenia.

Histology: Peripheral blood typically contains a predominance of small mature lymphocytes with diminished numbers of cytologically unremarkable granulocytes and platelets. Red cells can be macrocytic or normocytic. Circulating myeloblasts or normoblasts are not present.

Bone-marrow biopsy reveals marrow hypocellularity for age with aplasia of all three cell lines, predominant adipose tissue, absence of reticulin fibrosis, and increased numbers of small mature lymphocytes, plasma cells, histiocytes, and mast cells.

The degree of peripheral cytopenias and marrow cellularity define the severity of disease (234):

Severe AA: Bone-marrow cellularity

- < 25% (of normal age-related values), or
- 25–50% with < 30% residual hematopoiesis

At least two of the following:

- Neutrophils $< 0.5 \times 10^9$/L
- Platelets $< 20 \times 10^9$/L
- Reticulocytes $< 20 \times 10^9$/L

Very severe AA: As above, with neutrophils $< 0.2 \times 10^9$/L

Flow cytometric analysis for detection of clones with the phenotype of paroxysmal nocturnal hemoglobinuria (e.g., absent or diminished expression of FLAER, CD55, CD59) is routinely performed; however, whether this is a cause or consequence of AA has not been clearly established.

Prognosis: The only curative treatment for AA is a hematopoietic stem-cell transplant (HSCT) and is usually the recommended first-line therapy for patients with severe or very severe AA, who have a matched sibling donor. Given more recent advances in transplant technology, overall survival approximates 80–90% in children, and improved outcomes are described in those with younger age at transplant and diminished interval from diagnosis to transplantation (221). For patients lacking a matched sibling donor, immunosuppressive therapy is the mainstay of treatment, with response rates of 50–80% (235–238).

Differential diagnosis: Idiopathic aplastic anemia cannot be definitively diagnosed with any single test; hence, it remains a diagnosis of exclusion. Comprehensive history and physical examination should be performed to elicit drug or toxin exposures that may cause marrow aplasia and to exclude phenotypic abnormalities that might suggest an underlying IBFS. Formal testing for IBFS, as previously discussed, must also be performed. Rare causes of marrow aplasia include pregnancy, systemic lupus erythematosus, and neoplasia (e.g., thymoma).

References

1. Jaglowski SM, Linden E, Termuhlen AM, *et al.* Lymphoma in adolescents and young adults. Semin. Oncol. 2009;**36**:381–418.

2. Shukla NN, Trippett TM. Non-Hodgkin's lymphoma in children and adolescents. Curr. Oncol. Rep. 2006;**8**:387–94.

3. Percy C, Smith MA, Linet M, *et al. Lymphomas and reticuloendothelial neoplasms*. ICCCII. National Cancer Institute SEER Pediatric Monograph. Bethesda, MD: NCI, 2009:35–50.

4. Surveillence Epidemiology and End Results. Seer Stat Fact Sheets: Non-Hodgkin Lymphoma or Hodgkin Lymphoma 2006–2009. http://seer.cancer.gov./statfacts/html/nhl.html (accessed May 28, 2012).

5. Hanahan D, Weinberg RA. Hallmarks of cancer: the next generation. Cell 2011;**144**:646–74.

6. Staudt LM. Oncogenic activity of NK- kB. Cold Spring Harbor Perspect. Bio. 2010;**2**:1–30.

7. Lenz G, Staudt LM. Aggressive lymphomas. N. Eng. J. Med. 2010;**362**:1417–29.

8. Ngo VN, Young RM, Schmitz R, *et al.* Nature 2011;**470**:115–19.

9. Shaffer AL, Staudt LM. The case of the missing c-Myc. Nat. Immunol. 2012;**13**:1029–31.

10. Basso K, Dalla-Favera R. Roles of BCL6 in normal and transformed germinal center B cells. Immunol.Rev. 2012:**247**:172–83.

11. Graber C, Von Boehmer H, Look T. Notch 1 activation in the molecular pathogenesis of T-cell acute lymphoblastic leukemia. Nat. Rev. Cancer 2006;**6**:347–59.

12. Jundt F, Schwarzer R, Dorken B. Notch signaling in leukemias and lymphomas. Curr. Mol. Med. 2008;**8**:51–9.

13. Armstrong F, Brunt de la Grange P, Gerby B, *et al.* Notch is a key regulator of human T-cell leukemia initiating cell activity. Blood 2009:**113**:1730–40.

14. Ventura A, Young AG, Winslow MM, *et al*. Targeted deletion reveals essential and overlapping functions of the miR-17 through 92 family of miRNA clusters. Cell 2008;**132**:875–86.

15. Lenz G, Wright GW, Emre NC, *et al*. Molecular subtypes of diffuse large B-cell lymphoma arise by distinct genetic pathways. Proc. Natl. Acad. Sci. USA 2008;**105**:13520–5.

16. Mottok A, Renne C, Seifert M, *et al*. Inactivating SOCS1 mutations are caused by aberrant somatic hypermutation and restricted to a subset of B-cell lymphoma entities. Blood 2009;**114**:4503–6.

17. Oschlies I, Burkhardt B, Salaverria I, *et al*. Clinical, pathological and genetic features of primary mediastinal large cell lymphoma and mediastinal gray zone lymphoma in children. Haematologica 2011;**96**:262–8.

18. Snow AL, Martinez OM. Epstein-Barr virus: evasive maneuvers in the development of PTLD. Am. J. Transplant. 2007;**7**:271–7.

19. Morscio J, Dierickx D, Tousseyn T. Molecular pathogenesis of B-cell posttransplant lymphoproliferative disorder: what do we know so far? Clin. Dev. Immunol. 2013:150835.

20. Rui L, Schmitz R, Ceribelli M, *et al*. Malignant pirates of the immune system. Nat. Immunol. 2011;**12**:933–40.

21. Klapper W, Szczepanowski M, Burkhardt B, *et al*. Molecular profiling of pediatric mature B-cell lymphoma treated in population-based prospective clinical trials. Blood 2008;**112**:1374–81.

22. Deffenbacher KE, Iqbal J, Sanger W, *et al*. Molecular distinctions between pediatric and adult mature B-cell non-Hodgkin lymphomas identified through genomic profiling. Blood 2012;**119**:3757–66.

23. Hodgkin T. On some morbid appearances of absorbent glands and spleen. Trans. Med. Chir. Soc. Lond. 1832;**17**:68.

24. Sternberg C. Ueber einer eigenartige, unter dem Bilde der Pseudoleukame verlaufende tuberkulose des lymphatischen Apparates. Zeitschrift für Heilkunde (Prague) 1898;**19**:21–90.

25. Reed DM. On the pathological changes in Hodgkin's disease with special reference to its relation to tuberculosis. Johns Hopkins Hosp. Rep. 1902;**10**:133–96.

26. Kuppers R, Rajewsky K, Zao M, *et al*. Hodgkin disease: Hodgkin and Reed-Sternberg cells picked from histological sections show clonal immunoglobulin gene rearrangements and appear to be derived from B cells at various stages of development. Proc. Natl. Acad. Sci. USA 1994;**91**:10962–6.

27. Kanzler H, Kuppers R, Hansmann ML, *et al*. Hodgkin and Reed-Sternberg cells in Hodgkin's disease represent the outgrowth of a dominant tumor clone derived from (crippled) germinal center B cells. J. Exp. Med. 1996;**184**:1495–1505.

28. Marafioti T, Hummel M, Foss HD, *et al*. Hodgkin and Reed-Sternberg cells represent an expansion of a single clone originating from a germinal center B-cell with functional immunoglobulin gene rearrangements but defective immunoglobulin transcription. Blood 2000;**95**:1443–50.

29. Liso A, Capello D, Marafioti T, *et al*. Aberrant somatic hypermutation in tumor cells of nodular-lymphocyte-predominant and classical Hodgkin lymphoma. Blood 2008;**108**:1013–20.

30. Swerdlow SH, Campo E, Harris NL, *et al*. *WHO Classification of Tumors of Haematopoietic and Lymphoid Tissues*, fourth edn. Lyon: IARC, 2008.

31. Hussong JW, Arber DA, Bradley KT, *et al*. Protocol for the examination of specimens from patients with Non-Hodgkin Lymphoma/Lymphoid neoplasms. Arch. Pathol. Lab. Med. 2010;**134**:e40–7.

32. Lim M, Cairo MS. New therapeutic frontiers for childhood non-hodgkin's lymphoma. In: Arceci, R Houghton, P editors, *Molecularly-Targeted Therapy for Childhood Cancer*. New York: Springer; 2010.

33. Louissant A Jr., Ferry JA, Soupir CP, *et al*. Infectious mononucleosis mimicking lymphoma: distinguishing morphological and immunophenotypic features. Mod Pathol 2012;**25**:1149–59.

34. Lamps LW, Scott MA. Cat scratch Disease: historic, clinical and pathologic perspectives. Am. J. Clin. Pathol. 2004;**121**(Supp 1):S71–80.

35. Caponetti GC, Pantanowitz L, Marconi S, *et al*. Evaluation of immunohistochemistry in identifying *Bartonella henselae* in cat-scratch disease. Am. J. Clin. Pathol. 2009;**131**:250–6.

36. Koneti V, Oliveira JB. How I treat autoimmune lymphoproliferative syndrome. Blood 2011;**118**:5741–51.

37. Teachey DT. New advances in the diagnosis and treatment of autoimmune lymphoproliferative syndrome. Curr. Opin. Pediatr. 2012;**24**:1–8.

38. Oliveira JB, Blessing JJ, Dianzani U, *et al*. Revised diagnostic criteria and classification for the autoimmune lymphoproliferative syndrome (ALPS): report from the 2009 NIH International Workshop. Blood 2010;**116**:e35–40.

39. Lim MS, Straus SE, Dale JK, *et al*. Pathological findings in human autoimmune lymphoproliferative syndrome. Am. J. Pathol. 1998;**153**:1541–50.

40. Kraus MD, Shenoy S, Chatila T, *et al*. Light microscopic, immunophenotypic and molecular genetic study of autoimmune lymphoproliferative syndrome caused by fas mutation. Pediatr. Dev. Pathol. 2000;**3**:101–9.

41. Hicks J, Flaitz C. Progressive transformation of germinal centers: review of histopathologic and clinic features. Int. J. Pediatr. Otorhinolaryngol. 2002;**65**:195–202.

42. Licup AT, Campisi P, Ngan B, *et al*. Progressive transformation of germinal centers, an uncommon cause of pediatric cervical lymphadenopathy. Arch. Otolaryngol. Head and Neck Surg. 2006;**132**:797–801.

43. Shaikh F, Ngan B, Alexander S, *et al*. Progressive transformation of germinal centers in children and adolescents: An intriguing cause of lymphadenopathy. Pediatr. Blood Cancer 2013;**60**:26–30.

44. Nguyen PL, Ferry JA, Harris NL. Progressive transformation of germinal centers and nodular lymphocyte predominance Hodgkin's disease: A comparative immunohistochemical study. Am. J. Surg. Pathol. 1999;**23**:27–33.

45. Palestro G, Turrini F F, Pagano M, *et al*. Castleman's disease. Adv. Clin. Pathol. 1999;**3**:11–22.

46. Salisbury JR. Castleman's disease in childhood and adolescence: report of a case and review of the literature. Pediatr. Pathol. 1990;**10**:609–15.

47. Parez N, Bader-Meunier B, Roy CC, *et al*. Paediatric Castleman disease: report of seven cases and review of the literature. Eur. J. Paediatr. 1999;**158**:631–7.

48. Jegalian AG, Facchetti F, Jaffe ES. Plasmacytoid dendritic cells: physiologic roles and pathologic states. Adv. Anat. Pathol. 2009;**16**:392–404.

49. Marian A, Rollins-Ravel MD, Marafioti T, *et al*. The number and growth pattern of plasmacytoid dendritic cells vary in different types of reactive lymph nodes: An immunohistochemical studies. Hum. Pathol. 2013;**44**:1003–10.

50. Hall PA, Donaghy M, Cotter FE, *et al*. An immunohistological and genotypic study of the plasma cell form of Castleman's disease. Histopathology 1989;**14**:333–46.

51. Dossier A, Meignin V, Fieschi C, *et al*. Human Herpes 8-related Castleman disease in the absence of HIV infection. Clin. Infect. Dis. 2013;**56**:833–42.

52. Bosch X, Guilabert A, Miguel R, *et al*. Enigmatic Kikuchi-Fujimoto Disease. A comprehensive review. Am. J. Clin. Pathol. 2004;**122**:141–52.

53. Hutchinson CB, Wang E. Kikuchi-Fujimoto disease. Arch. Pathol. Lab. Med. 2010;**134**:289–93.

54. Chen H, Thompson LD, Aguilera NS, *et al*. Kimura disease: A clinicopathological study of 21 cases. Am. J. Surg. Pathol. 2004;**28**:505–13.

55. Abuel-Haija M, Hurford MT. Kimura Disease. Arch. Pathol. Lab. Med. 2007;**131**:650–1.

56. Xu X, Fu J, Liang L. Kimura disease in children: A case report and a summary of the literature in Chinese. J. Pediatr. Hematol. Oncol. 2011;**33**:306–11.

57. Onouchi Y. Genetics of Kawasaki Disease–what we know and don't know. Circ. J. 2012;**76**:1561–86.

58. Yokouchi Y, Oharaseki T, Harad M, *et al*. Histopathological study of lymph node lesions in the acute phase of Kawasaki disease. Histopathology 2013;**62**:387–96.

59. Katano H, Sato S, Sekizuka T, *et al*. Pathogenic characterization of a cervical lymph node derived from a patient with Kawasaki disease. Int. J. Clin. Exp. Pathol. 2012;**5**:814–23.

60. Foucar E, Rosai J, Dorfman R. Sinus histiocytosis with massive lymphadenopathy (Rosai–Dorfman disease): review of the entity. Semin Diagn. Pathol. 1990;**7**:19–73.

61. McAlister WH, Herman T, Dehner LP. Sinus histiocytosis with massive lymphadenopathy (Rosai-Dorfman disease). Pediatr. Radiol. 1990;**20**:425–32.

62. Mala DM, Dorfman RF. Focal changes of sinus histiocytosis with massive lymphadnopathy (Rosai-Dorfman disease) associated with nodular lymphocyte predominant Hodgkin's disease. Hum. Pathol. 1995;**26**:1378–82.

63. Lu D, Estalilla OC, Manning JT, *et al*. Sinus histiocytosis with massive lymphadenopathy and malignant lymphoma involving the same lymph node:a report of four cases and review of the literature. Mod. Pathol. 2000;**13**:414–9.

64. Faulk S, Stutte HJ, Fizzera G. Hodgkin's disease and sinus histiocytosis with massive lymphadenopathy-like changes. Histopathology 1991;**19**:221–4.

65. Pang CS, Grier DD, Beaty MW. Concomitant occurrence of sinus histiocytosis with massive lymphadenopathy and nodal marginal zone lymphoma. Arch. Pathol. Lab. Med. 2011;**135**:390–3.

66. Lossos IS, Okon E, Bogomolski-Yahalom V, *et al*. Sinus histiocytosis with massive lymphadenopathy (Rosai-dorfman disease): report of a patient with isolated renotesticular involvement after cure of Hodgkin's lymphoma. Ann. Hematol. 1997;**74**:41–4.

67. Castro EC, Blazquez C, Boyd J, *et al*. Clinicopathologic features of histiocytic lesions following ALL, with a review of the literature. Pediatr. Dev. Pathol. 2010;**13**:225–37.

68. Maric I, Pittaluga S, Dale JK, *et al*. Histologic features of sinus histiocytosis with massive lymphadenopathy in patients with autoimmune lymphoproliferative syndrome. Am J. Surg. Pathol. 2005;**29**:903–11.

69. Favara BE, Jaffe R. The histopathology of Langerhans cell histiocytosis. Br. J. Cancer 1994;**70**:Suppl XXIII, S17–23.

70. Chan JK, Fletcher CD, Nayler SJ, *et al*. Follicular dendritic cell sarcoma. Clinicopathologic analysis of 17 cases suggesting a malignant potential higher than currently recognized. Cancer 1997;**79**:294–313.

71. Silver AL, Faquin WC, Caruso PA, *et al*. Follicular dendritic cell sarcoma presenting in the submandibular region of an 11 year old. Laryngoscope 2010;**120**:Suppl 4, S183.

72. Chan AC, Chan KW, Chan JK, *et al*. Development of follicular dendritic cell sarcoma in hyaline vascular Castleman's disease of the nasopharynx: tracing its evolution by sequential biopsies. Histopathology 2001;**38**:501–8.

73. Katano H, Kaneko K, Shimizu S, *et al*. Follicular dendritic cell sarcoma complicated by hyaline vascular type Castleman's disease in Schizophrenic patient. Pathol. Int. 1997;**47**:703–6.

74. Biddle DA, Ro JY, Yoon GS, *et al*. Extranodal follicular dendritic cell sarcoma of the head and neck region: three new cases, with a review of the literature. Mod. Pathol. 2002;**15**:50–8.

75. Wang H, Su Z, Hu Z, *et al*. Follicular dendritic cell sarcoma:are part of six cases and a review of the Chinese literature. Diagn. Pathol. 2010;**5**:67–72.

76. El-Mallawany NK, Fraser JK, Van Vlierberghe P, *et al*. Pediatric T- and NK-cell Lymphomas: new biologic insights and treatment strategies. Blood Cancer J. 2012;**2**:e65–82.

77. Perkins SL, Morris SW. Biology and pathology of pediatric Non-Hodgkin Lymphoma. In: Weinstein H, Hudson MM and Link MP, editors, *Pediatric Lymphoma*. Heidelberg: Springer-Verlag; 2007:91–140.

78. Stein H, Mason DY, Gerdes J, *et al*. The expression of the Hodgkin's disease associated antigen Ki-1 in reactive and neoplastic lymphoid tissue: evidence that Reed-Sternberg cells and histiocyte malignancies are derived from activated lymphoid cells. Blood 1985;**66**:848–58.

79. Moussolin L, Damm-Welk C, Pillon M, *et al*. Use of minimal disseminated disease and immunity to NPM-ALK antigen to stratify ALK-positive ALCL patients with different prognosis. Leukemia 2013;**27**:416–22.

80. Ait-Tahar K, Damm-Welk C, Burkhardt B, *et al*. Correlation of the autoantibody response to the ALK oncoantigen in pediatric anaplastic lymphoma kinase-positive anaplastic large cell lymphoma with tumor dissemination and relapse risk. Blood 2010;**115**:3314–9.

81. Kinney MC, Collins RD, Greer JP, *et al*. A small-cell-predominant variant of primary Ki-1 (CD30)+ T-cell lymphoma. Am. J. Surg. Pathol. 1993;**17**:859–68.

82. Felgar RE, Salhany KE, Macon WR, *et al*. The expression of TIA-1+ cytolytic granules and other cytolytic lymphocyte-associated markers in CD30+ anaplastic large cell lymphomas (ALCL): correlation with morphology, immunophenotype, ultrastructure, and clinical features. Hum. Pathol. 1999;**30**:228–36.

83. Lim MS, Carlson ML, Crockett DK, *et al*. The proteomic signature of NPM/ALK reveals deregulation of multiple cellular pathways. Blood 2009;**114**:1585–95.

84. Hodges KB, Collins RD, Greer JP, *et al*. Transformation of the small cell variant Ki-1+ lymphoma to anaplastic large cell lymphoma: pathologic and clinical features. Am. J. Surg. Pathol. 1999;**23**:49–58.

85. Windsor R, Stiller C, Webb D. Peripheral T cell lymphoma in childhood:population-based experience in the United Kingdom over 20 years. Pediatr. Blood Cancer 2008;**50**:784–7.

86. Mahmoud A, Weitzman S, Schechter T, *et al*. Peripheral T-cell lymphoma in children and adolescents:a single institution experience. J. Pediatr. Hematol. Oncol. 2012;**34**:611–16.

87. Kobayashi R, Yamato K, Tanaka F, *et al*. retrospective analysis of non-anaplastic peripheral T-cell lymphoma in pediatric patients in Japan. Pediatr. Blood Cancer 2010;**54**:212–5.

88. Rodriguez-Abreu D, Filho VB, Zucca E. Peripheral T-cell lymphomas, unspecified (or not other specified): A review. Hematol. Oncol. 2008;**26**:8–20.

89. Au WY, Weisenburger DD, Intragumtornchai T, *et al*. Clinical differences between nasal and extranasal natural killer/T cell lymphoma: A study of 136 cases from the international peripheral T-cell lymphoma project. Blood 2009;**113**:3931–37.

90. Ren Y, Nong L, Zhang S, *et al*. Analysis of 142 Northern Chinese patients with peripheral T/NK-cell lymphoma. Subtype distribution, clinicopathological features and prognosis. AmJ. Clin. Pathol 2012;**138**:435–47.

91. Pongpruttipan T, Sukpanichnant S, Assanasen T, *et al*. Extranodal NK/T-cell lymphoma, nasal type, includes cases of natural killer cells and αβ, γδ and αβ/γδ T-cell origin:a comprehensive clinicopathologic and phenotypic study. Am. J. Surg. Pathol. 2012;**36**:481–99.

92. Dominguez-Sola D, Victoria GD, Ying CY, *et al*. The proto-oncogene MYC is required for selection in the germinal center and cyclic reentry. Nat. Immunol. 2012;**13**:1083–91.

93. Calado DP, Sasaki Y, Godinho SA, *et al*. The cell-cycle regulator c-Myc is essential for the formation and

maintenance of germinal centers. Nat. Immunol. 2012;**13**:1092–100.

94. Poirel HA, Cairo MS, Heerema NA, *et al.* Specific cytogenetic abnormalities are associated with a significantly inferior outcome in children and adolescents with mature B-cell non-Hodgkin's lymphoma: results of the FAB/LMB 96 international study. Leukemia 2009;**23**:323–31.

95. Alizadeh AA, Eisen MB, Davis RE, *et al.* Distinct types of diffuse large B cell lymphoma identified by gene expression profiling. Nature 2000;**403**:503–11.

96. Rosenwald A, Wright G, Chan WC, *et al.* The use of molecular profiling to predict survival after chemotherapy for diffuse large B-cell lymphoma. N. Engl. J. Med. 2002;**346**:1937–47.

97. Oschlies I, Klapper W, Zimmermann M, *et al.* Diffuse large B-cell lymphoma in pediatric patients belongs predominantly to the germinal-center type B-cell lymphoma: A clinicopathologic analysis of cases included in the German BFM (Berlin Frankfurt-Munster) multicenter trial. Blood 2006;**107**:4047–52.

98. Salaverria I, Phillip C, Oschlies I, *et al.* Translocations activating IRF4 identify a subtype of germinal center-derived B-cell lymphoma affecting predominantly children and young adults. Blood 2011;**118**:139–47.

99. Calvo KR, Traverse-Glehen A, Paiitaluga J, *et al.* Molecular profiling of primary mediastinal large B-cell lymphoma as a distinct entity related to classical Hodgkin lymphoma: implications for mediastinal gray zone lymphomas as an intermediate form of B-cell lymphoma. Adv. Anat. Pathol. 2004;**11**:227–38.

100. Grant C, Dunleavy K, Eberle FC, *et al.* Primary mediastinal large B cell lymphoma, classical Hodgkin lymphoma presenting in the mediastinum, and gray zone lymphoma: what is the oncologist to do? Curr. Hematol. Malig. Rep. 2011;**6**:157–63.

101. Bhuvanna AS, Termuhlen AM. Rare Pediatric Non-Hodgkin Lymphoma. Curr. Hematol. Malig. Rep. 2010;**5**:163–168.

102. Pauli M, Strater J, Gianelli U, *et al.* Mediastinal B-cell lymphoma:a study of its histomorphological spectrum based on 109 cases. Hum. Pathol. 1999;**30**:178–87.

103. Salama ME, Mariappan M, Inamder K, *et al.* The value of CD23 expression as an additional marker in distinquishing mediastinal (thymic) large B cell lymphoma from Hodgkin Lymphoma. Int. J. Surg. Pathol. 2010;**18**:121–8.

104. Oschlies I, Salaverria I, Mahn F, *et al.* Pediatric follicular lymphoma-a clinico-pathologial study of a population based series of patients treated within the Non-Hodgkin's Lymphoma-Berlin –Frankfurt-Munster (NHL-BFM) multicenter trials. Haematologica 2010;**95**:253–9.

105. Louissaint A, Ackerman AM, Dias-Santagata D, *et al.* Pediatric type nodal follicular lymphoma:an indolent clonal proliferation in children and adults with high proliferation index and no BCL2 rearrangement. Blood 2012;**120**:2395–404.

106. Lorsbach RB, Shay-Seymore D, Moore J, *et al.* Clinicopathologic analysis of follicular lymphoma occurring in children. Blood 2002;**99**:1959–64.

107. Salaverria I. Phillipp C, Oschlies I, *et al.* Translocations activating IRF4 identify a subtype of germinal center-derived B-cell lymphoma affecting predominantly children and young adults. Blood 2011;**118**:139–47.

108. Salaverria I, Siebert R. Follicular lymphoma grade 3B. Best Pract. Res. Clin. Haematol. 2011;**24**:111–19.

109. Leich E, Zamo A, Horn H, *et al.* MicroRNA profiles of t(14;18)-negative follicular lymphoma support a late germinal center B-cell phenotype. Blood 2011;**118**:5550–8.

110. Rizzo KA, Streubel B, Pittaluga C, *et al.* Marginal zone lymphomas in children and the young adult population; characterization of genetic aberrations by FISH and RT-PCR. Mod. Pathol. 2010;**23**:866–73.

111. Claviez A, Meyer U, Dominick C, *et al.* Brief Report MALT lymphoma in children: A report from the NHL-BFM study group. Pediatr. Blood Cancer 2006;**47**:210–14.

112. Naithani R, Ngan BY, Roifman C, *et al.* Thymic mucosal associated lymphoid tissue lymphoma in an adolescent girl. J. Pediatr. Hematol. Oncol. 2012;**34**:552–7.

113. Mo JQ, Dimashkieh H, Mallery SR, *et al.* MALT lymphoma in children: case report and review of the literature. Pediatr. Dev. Pathol. 2004;**7**:407–13.

114. Elenitoba-Johnson KS, Kumar S, Lim MS, *et al.* Marginal zone B-cell lymphoma with monocytoid B-cell lymphocytes in pediatric patients without immunodeficiency. A report of two cases. Am J. Clin. Pathol. 1997;**107**:92–8.

115. Salama ME, Lossos IS, Warnke RA, *et al.* Immunoarchitectural patternas in nodal marginal zone B-cell lymphoma: A study of 51 cases. Am. J. Clin. Pathol. **132**:39–49.

116. Traverse-Glehen A, Pittaluga S, Gauland P, *et al.* Mediastinal Gray Zone Lymphoma, the missing link between Classical Hodgkin's Lymphoma and Mediastinal Large B-cell Lymphoma. Am J. Surg. Pathol. 2005;**29**:1411–21.

117. Eberle FC, Salaverria I, Steidl C, *et al.* Gray zone Lymphoma: chromosomal aberrations with immunophenotypic and clinical correlations. Mod. Pathol. 2011;**24**:1586–97.

269

118. Quintanilla-Martinez L, De Jong D, deMascarel A, *et al.* Gray zones around diffuse large B cell lymphoma. Conclusions based on the Workshop of the XIV meeting of the European Association for Hematology and the Society of Hematopathology in Bordeau, France. J. Hematopathol. 2009;**2**:211–36.

119. Dunleavy K, Grant C, Eberle FC, *et al.* Gray zone lymphoma: better treated like Hodgkin Lymphoma or Mediastinal Large cell Lymphoma? Curr. Haematol. Malig. Rep. 2012;**7**:241–7.

120. Gualco G, Natkunam Y, Bacchi CE. The spectrum of B-cell lymphoma, unclassifiable, with features intermediate between diffuse large B-cell lymphoma and classical Hodgkin lymphoma:a description of 10 cases. Mod. Pathol. 2012;**25**:661–74.

121. Wilks S. Cases of lardaceous disease and some allied affections: with remarks. Guy's Hosp. Rep. 1856;**2**:103–32.

122. Hutchison RE, Uner A. Biology and pathology of Hodgkin's disease. In Weinsten HJ, Hudson MM, Link M, editors, *Pediatric Lymphomas.* Heidelberg: Springer-Verlag, 2007:7–33.

123. Thomas RK, Wolf J, Diehl V. Part 1: Hodgkin's lymphoma molecular biology of Hodgkin and Reed Sternberg cells. Lancet Oncol. 2004;**5**:11–18.

124. Stein H, Marafioti T, Foss HD, *et al.* Down regulation of BOB.1/ and OCT 2 in classical Hodgkin disease but not in lymphocyte predominant Hodgkin disease correlates with immunoglobulin transcription. Blood 2001;**97**:496–501.

125. Seitz V, Hummel M, Marafioti T, *et al.* Detection of clonal T-cell receptor gamma chain gene rearrangements in Reed-Sternberg cells of classical Hodgkin Disease. Blood 2000;**95**:3020–24.

126. Marafioti T, Hummel M, Anagnostopoulos I, *et al.* Origin of nodular lymphocyte predominant Hodgkin's disease from a clonal expansion of highly mutated germinal center B cells. N. Eng. J. Med. 1997;**337**:453–58.

127. Braeuninger A, Kuppers R, Strickler JG. Hodgkin and Reed-Sternberg cells in lymphocyte predominant Hodgkin disease represent clonal populations of germinal center-derived tumor B-cells. Proc. Natl. Acad. Sci. USA 1997;**94**:9337–42.

128. Castellino SM, Gelger AM, Mertens AC, *et al.* Morbidity and mortality in long-term survivors of Hodgkin lymphoma:a report from the childhood Cancer Survivor Study. Blood 2011;**117**:1806–16.

129. Muaz-Korholz C, Gorde-Grosjean S, Hasenclever D, *et al.* Resection alone in 58 children with limited stage lymphocyte-predominant Hodgkin Lymphoma-Experience from the European Network Group on Pediatric Hodgkin Lymphoma. Cancer 2007:**110**:179–85.

130. Keegan TH, Glaser SL, Clarke CA, *et al.* Epstein-Barr virus as a marker of survival after Hodgkin's lymphoma: A population-based study. J. Clin. Oncol. 2005;**23**:7604–13.

131. Claviez A, Tiemann M, Lauders H, *et al.* Impact of latent Epstein-Barr virus infection on outcome in children and adolescents with Hodgkin's lymphoma. J. Clin. Oncol. 2005;**23**:4048–56.

132. Urayama KY, Jarrett RF, Hjalgrim H, *et al.* Genome-wide association study of classical Hodgkin lymphoma and Epstein-Barr virus status-defined subgroups. J. Natl. Cancer Inst. 2012;**104**:240–53.

133. Chua I, Isabella I, Grimbacher B. Lymphoma in common variable immunodeficiency:interplay between immune dysregulation, infection and genetics. Curr. Opin. Haematol. 2008;**15**:368–74.

134. Newell A, Dadi H, Goldberg R, *et al.* Diffuse large B-cell lymphoma as presenting feature of ZAP-70 deficiency. J. Allergy Clin. Immunol. 2011;**127**:517–20.

135. Chrzanowska KH. Gregorek H, dembowska-Baginska B, *et al.* Nijmegen breakage syndrome (NBS). Orphanet. J. Rare Dis. 2012;**7**:13–32.

136. de Miranda NF, Bjorkman A, Pan-Hammarstrom Q. DNA repair: the link between primary immunodeficiency and cancer. Ann. NY Acad. Sci. 2011;**1246**:50–63.

137. Stracker TH, Roig I, Knobel PA, *et al.* The ATM signaling network in development and disease. Front. Genet. 2013;**4**:37.

138. Holland SM. Chronic Granulomatous Disease. Clinic Rev. Allerg. Immunol. 2010,**38**.3–10.

139. Jordan MB, Allen CE, Weitzman S, *et al.* How I treat haemophagocytic lymphohistiocytosis. Blood 2011;**118**:4041–52.

140. Risma K, Jordan MB. Hemophagocytic lymphohistiocytosis:updates and evolving concepts. Curr. Opin. Pediatr. 2012;**24**:9–15.

141. Rosado FGN, Kim AS. Hemophagocytic lymphohistiocytosis An update on diagnosis and pathogenesis. Am. J. Clin. Pathol. 2013;**139**:713–727.

142. United Network of Organ Sharing Data (UNOS). http://www.unos.org (accessed January 2013).

143. Dharnidharka VR, Tejani AH, Ho P-L, *et al.* Post-Transplant lymphoproliferative disorder in the United States:young Caucasian males are at highest risk. Am. J. Transplant. 2002;**2**:993–8.

144. Webster AC, Craig JC, Simpson JM, *et al.* Identifying high risk groups and quantifying absolute risk of cancer risk after kidney transplantation: A cohort of 15,183 recipients. Am. J. Transplant. 2007;**7**:2140–51.

145. Opelz G, Dohler B. Lymphoma after solid organ transplantation: A collaborative transplant report. Am. J. Transplant. 2004;**4**:222–30.

146. Dharnidharka VR. Epidemiology of PTLD. In: Dharnidharka VR, Green M, Webber SA, editors, *Post-Transplant Lymphoproliferative Disorders*. Berlin, Heidelberg: Springer-Verlag; 2010:17–28.

147. Rinaldi A, Capello D, Scandurra M, *et al.* Single nucleotide polymorphism-arrays provide new insights in the pathogenesis of post-transplant diffuse large B-cell lymphoma. Br. J. Haematol. 2010:**149**:567–77.

148. Biggar RJ, Frisch M, Goedert JJ. Risk of cancer in children with AIDS. AIDS-cancer Match Registry Study Group. JAMA 2000;**284**:205–9.

149. Mueller BU. HIV-Associated malignancies in children. AIDS Patient Care STDS 1999;**13**:527–33.

150. Stefan DC, Wessels G, Poole J, *et al.* Infection with human immunodeficiency virus-1 (HIV) among children with cancer in South Africa. Pediatr. Blood Cancer 2011;**56**:77–9.

151. Tukei VJ, Kekitiinwa A, Beasley RP. Prevalence and outcome of HIV-associated malignancies among children. AIDS 2011;**25**:1789–93.

152. Sinfield RL, Molyneux EM, Banda K, *et al.* Spectrum and presentation of pediatric malignancies in the HIV era: experience from Blantyre, Malawi, 1998–2003. Pediatr. Blood Cancer 2007;**48**:515–20.

153. Capello D, Scandurra M, Poretti G, *et al.* Genome wide DNA profiling of HIV-related B-cell lymphomas. Br. J. Haematol. 2009;**148**:245–55.

154. Kwee I, Capello D, Rinaldi A, *et al.* Genomic aberrations affecting the outcomes of immunodeficiency-related diffuse large B-cell lymphoma. Leuk. Lymphoma 2012;**53**:71–6.

155. Radhakrishnan R, Suhas S, Kumar RV, *et al.* Plasmablastic lymphoma of the oral cavity in an HIV-positive child. Oral Surg. Oral Med. Oral Pathol. Oral Radiol. Endod. 2005;**100**:725–31.

156. Pather S, MacKinnon D, Padayachee RS. Plasmablastic lymphoma in pediatric patients:clinicopathological study of three cases. Ann. Diagn. Pathol. 2013;**17**:80–4.

157. Funkouser AW, Katzman PJ, Sickel JZ, *et al.* CD30-positive anaplastic large cell lymphoma (ALCL) of T-cell lineage in a 14 month-old infant with perinatally acquired HIV-1 infection. J. Pediatr. Hematol. Oncol. 1998;**20**:556–9.

158. Chiu SS, Chan GC, Loong F. Epstein-Barr virus (EBV) induced hemophagocytic syndrome followed by EBV associated T/NK lymphoma in a child with perinatal human immunodeficiency virus (HIV) infection. Med. Pediatr. Oncol. 2001:**36**:326–8.

159. Preciado MV, De Matteo E, Fallo A, *et al.* EBV-associated Hodgkin's disease in an HIV-infected child presenting with a hemophagocytic syndrome. Leuk. Lymphoma 2001;**42**:231–4.

160. Joshi VV, Gagnon GA, Chadwick EG, *et al.* The spectrum of mucosa-associated lymphoid tissue lesions in pediatric patients with HIV: A clinicopathologic study of six cases. Am. J. Clin. Pathol. 1997;**107**:592–600.

161. Castillo J, Pantanowitz L, Dezube BJ. HIV-associated plasmablastic lymphoma:lesons learned from 112 published cases. Am. J. Haematol. 2008;**83**:804–9.

162. Pui C-H, Evans WE. Treatment of acute lymphoblastic leukemia. N. Engl. J. Med. 2006;**354**:166–178.

163. Deschler B, Lubbert M. Acute myeloid leukemia: epidemiology and etiology. Cancer 2006;**107**:2099–107.

164. Hrušák O, Porwit-MacDonald A. Antigen expression patterns reflecting genotype of acute leukemias. Leukemia 2002;**16**:1233–58.

165. Sutcliffe MJ, Shuster JJ, Sather HN, *et al.* High concordance from independent studies by the Children's Oncology Cancer Group (CCG) and Pediatric Oncology Group (POG) associating favorable prognosis with combined trisomies 4, 10, and 17 in children with NCI Standard-Risk B-precursor acute lymphoblastic leukemia: A Children's Oncology Group (COG) initiative. Leukemia 2005;**19**:734 40.

166. Nachman JB, Heerema NA, Sather H, *et al.* Outcome of treatment in children with hypodiploid acute lymphoblastic leukemia. Blood 2007;**110**:1112–5.

167. Pieters R, Schrappe M, De Lorenzo P, *et al.* A treatment protocol for infants younger than 1 year with acute lymphoblastic leukemia (Interfant-99): An observational study and a multicenter randomized trial. Lancet 2007;**370**:240–50.

168. Rubnitz JE, Wichlan D, Devidas M, *et al.* Prospective analysis of TEL gene rearrangements in childhood acute lymphoblastic leukemia: A Children's Oncology Group study. J. Clin. Oncol. 2008;**26**:2186–91.

169. Jeha S, Pei D, Raimondi SC, *et al.* Increased risk for CNS relapse in pre-B cell leukemia with the t(1;19)/TCF3-PBX1. Leukemia 2009;**23**:1406–9.

170. Schultz KR, Bowman WP, Aledo A, *et al.* Improved early event-free survival with imatinib in Philadelphia chromosome-positive acute lymphoblastic leukemia: A children's oncology group study. J. Clin. Oncol. 2009;**27**:5175–81.

171. Vrooman LM, Silverman LB. Childhood acute lymphoblastic leukemia: update on prognostic factors. Curr. Opin. Pediatr. 2009;**21**:1–8.

172. Moorman AV, Ensor HM, Richards SM, *et al.* Prognostic effect of chromosomal abnormalities in childhood B-cell precursor acute lymphoblastic leukemia: results from the UK Medical Research Council ALL97/99 randomized trial. Lancet Oncol. 2010;**11**:429–38.

271

173. Silverman LB, Stevenson KE, O'Brien JE, *et al.* Long-term results of Dana-Farber Cancer Institute ALL Consortium protocols for children with newly diagnosed acute lymphoblastic leukemia (1985–2000). Leukemia 2010;**24**:320–34.

174. Pui C-H, Carroll WL, Meshinchi S, *et al.* Biology, risk stratification, and therapy of pediatric acute leukemias: An update. J. Clin. Oncol. 2011;**29**:551–65.

175. Schrappe M, Hunger SP, Pui C-H, *et al.* Outcomes after induction failure in childhood acute lymphoblastic leukemia. N. Engl. J. Med. 2012;**366**:1371–81.

176. Pui CH, Mullighan CG, Evans WE, *et al.* Pediatric acute lymphoblastic leukemia:where are we going and how do we get there? Blood 2012;**120**:1165–74.

177. Hasle H, Heim S, Schroeder H, *et al.* Transient pancytopenia preceding acute lymphoblastic leukemia (Pre-ALL). Leukemia 1995;**9**:605–8.

178. Horsley SW, Colman S, McKinley M, *et al.* Genetic lesions in a preleukemic aplasia phase in a child with acute lymphoblastic leukemia. Genes Chromosomes Cancer 2008;**47**:333–40.

179. McKenna RW, Asplund AL, Kroft SH. Immunophenotypic analysis of hematogones (B-lymphocyte precursors) and neoplastic lymphoblasts by 4-color flow cytometry. Leuk. Lymphoma 2004;**45**:277–85.

180. van Lochem EG, van der Velden VHJ, Wind HK, *et al.* Immunophenotypic differentiation patterns of normal hematopoiesis in human bone marrow: reference patterns for age-related changes and disease-induced shifts. Cytomet. B (Clin. Cytomet.) 2004;**60B**:1–13.

181. Borowitz MJ, Devidas M, Hunger SP, *et al.* Clinical significance of minimal residual disease in childhood acute lymphoblastic leukemia and its relationship to other prognostic factors: A Children's Oncology Group study. Blood 2008;**111**:5477–85.

182. Attarbaschi A, Mann G, Panzer-Grumayer R, *et al.* Minimal residua disease values discriminate between low and high relapse risk in children with B-cell precursor acute lymphoblastic leukemia and an intrachromosomal amplification of chromosome 21: the Austrian and German acute lymphoblastic leukemia Berlin-Frankfurt-Munster (ALL-BFM) trials. J. Clin. Oncol. 2008;**26**:3046–50.

183. Basso G, Veltroni M, Valsecchi MG, *et al.* Risk of relapse of childhood acute lymphoblastic leukemia is predicted by flow cytometric measurement of residual disease on day 15 bone marrow. J. Clin. Oncol. 2009;**27**:5168–74.

184. Winter SS. Pediatric acute leukemia therapies informed by molecular analysis of high-risk disease. Hematol. Am. Soc. Hematol. Educ. Program 2011;**2011**:366–73.

185. Ferrara F, Del Vecchio L. Acute myeloid leukemia with t(8;21)/AML/ETO:a distinct biological and clinical entity. Haematologica 2002;**87**:306–19.

186. Le Beau MM, Larson RA, Bitter MA, *et al.* Association of an inversion of chromosome 16 with abnormal marrow eosinophils in acute myelomonocytic leukemia. A unique cytogenetic-clinicopathological association. N. Engl. J. Med. 1983;**30**:630–6.

187. Wong KF, Kwong YL. Trisomy 22 in acute myeloid leukemia: A marker for myeloid leukemia with monocytic features and cytogenetically cryptic inversion 16. Cancer Genet. Cytogenet. 1999;**109**:131–3.

188. Davis KL, Marina N, Arber D, *et al.* Pediatric AML as classified using 2008 WHO criteria. Am. J. Clin. Pathol. 2013;**139**:818–25.

189. Wang ZY, Chen Z. Acute promyelocytic leukemia: from highly fatal to highly curable. Blood 2008;**111**:2505–15.

190. Rubnitz JE, Raimondi SC, Tong X, *et al.* Favorable impact of the t(9;11) in childhood acute myeloid leukemia. J. Clin. Oncol. 2002;**20**:2302–9.

191. Martinez-Climent JA, Espinosa R, Thirman MJ, *et al.* Abnormalities of chromosome band 11q23 and the MLL gene in pediatric myelomonocytic and monoblastic leukemias. Identification of the t(9;11) as an indicator of long survival. J. Pediatr. Hematol. Oncol. 1995;**17**:277–83.

192. Oyarzo MP, Lin P, Glassman A, *et al.* Acute myeloid leukemia with t(6;9)(p23;q34) is associated with dysplasia and a high frequency of flt3 gene mutations. Am. J. Clin. Pathol. 2004;**122**:348–58.

193. Bernstein J, Dastugue N, Haas OA, *et al.* Nineteen cases of the t(1;22)(p13;q13) acute megakaryoblastic leukaemia of infants/children and a review of 39 cases: report from a t(1;22) study group. Leukemia 2000;**14**:216–8.

194. Rowley JD, Olney HJ. International workshop on the relationship of prior therapy to balanced chromosome aberrations in therapy-related myelodysplastic syndromes and acute leukemia: overview report. Genes Chromosomes Cancer 2002;**33**:331–45.

195. Bloomfield CD, Archer KJ, Mrozek K, *et al.* 11q23 Balanced chromosome aberrations in treatment-related myelodysplastic syndromes and acute leukemia: report from an international workshop. Genes Chromosomes Cancer 2002;**33**:362–78.

196. Mauritzson N, Albin M, Rylander L, *et al.* Pooled analysis of clinical and cytogenetic features in treatment-related and de novo adult acute myeloid leukemia and myelodysplastic syndromes based on a consecutive series of 761 patients analyzed 1976–1993and on 5098 unselected cases reported in the literature 1974–2001. Leukemia 2002;**16**:2366–78.

197. Singh ZN, Huo D, Anastasi J, *et al.* Therapy-related myelodysplastic syndrome: morphologic subclassification may not be clinically relevant. Am. J. Clin. Pathol. 2007;**127**:197–205.

198. Pedersen-Bjergaard J, Andersen MK, Andersen MT, *et al.* Genetics of therapy-related myelodysplasia and acute myeloid leukemia. Leukemia 2008;**22**:240–8.

199. Inab HE, Coustan-Smith E, Cao X, *et al.* Comparative analysis of different approaches to measure treatment response in acute myeloid leukemia. J. Clin. Oncol. 2012;**30**:3625–32.

200. Loken MR, Alonxo TA, Pardo L, *et al.* Residual disease detected by multidimensional flow cytometry signifies high elapse risk in patients with de novo acute myeloid leukemia:a report from Children's Oncology Group. Blood 2012;**120**:1581–8.

201. Coustan-Smith E, Campana D. Should evaluation for minimal residual disease be routine in acute myeloid leukemia? Curr. Opin. Hematol. 2013;**20**:86–92.

202. Klco JM, Welch JS, Nguyen TT, *et al.* State of the art in myeloid sarcoma. Int. J. Lab. Hematol. 2011;**33**:555–65.

203. Wood BL. Flow cytometric diagnosis of myelodysplasia and myeloproliferative disorders. J. Biol. Regul. Homeost. Agents 2004;**18**:141–5.

204. Brink DS. Transient leukemia (transient myeloproliferative disorder, transient abnormal myelopoiesis) of Down syndrome. Adv. Anat. Pathol. 2006;**13**:256–62.

205. Bruwier A, Chantrain CF. Hematological disorders and leukemia in children with Down syndrome. Eur. J. Pediatr. 2012;**171**:1301–7.

206. Shen JJ, Williams BJ, Zipursky A, *et al.* Cytogenetic and molecular studies of Down syndrome individuals with leukemia. Am. J. Hum. Genet. 1995;**56**:915–25.

207. Alford KA, Reinhardt K, Garnett C, *et al.* Analysis of GATA1 mutations in Down syndrome transient myeloproliferative disorder and myeloid leukemia. Blood 2011;**118**:2222–38.

208. Sato T, Toki T, Kanezaki R, *et al.* Functional analysis of JAK3 mutations in transient myeloproliferative disorder and acute megakaryoblastic leukaemia accompanying Down syndrome. Br. J. Haematol. 2008;**141**:681–8.

209. Sainati L, Bolcato S, Cocito MG, *et al.* Transient acute monoblastic leukemia with reciprocal (8;16)(p11;p13) translocation. Pediatr. Hematol. Oncol. 1996;**13**:151–57.

210. Wu X, Sulavik D, Roulston D, *et al.* Spontaneous remission of congenital acute myeloid leukemia with t(8;16)(p11;13). Pediatr. Blood Cancer 2011;**56**:331–2.

211. Bresters D, Reus AC, Veerman AJ, *et al.* Congenital leukaemia: the Dutch experience and review of the literature. Br. J. Haematol. 2002;**117**:513–24.

212. Lange BJ, Kobrinsky N, Barnard OR, *et al.* Distinctive demography, biology, and outcome of acute myeloid leukemia and myelodysplastic syndrome in children with Down syndrome: Children's Cancer Group Studies 2861 and 2891. Blood 1998;**91**:608–15.

213. Bergstraesser E, Hasle H, Rogge T, *et al.* Non-hematopoietic stem cell transplantation treatment of juvenile myelomonocytic leukemia: A retrospective analysis and definition of response criteria. Pediatr. Blood Cancer 2007;**49**:629–33.

214. Loh ML. Recent advances in the pathogenesis and treatment of juvenile myelomonocytic leukaemia. Br. J. Haematol. 2011;**152**:677–87.

215. Jaffe E, Harris NL, Stein H, *et al. Pathology and Genetics of Tumors of the Haematopoietic and Lymphoid Tissues*, second edn. Lyon: IARC; 2001.

216. Brody JP, Allen S, Schulman P, *et al.* Acute agranular CD4-positive natural killer cell leukemia. Comprehensive clinicopathologic studies including virologic and in vitro culture with inducing agents. Cancer 1995;**75**:2474–83.

217. Petrella T, Comeau MR, Maynadie M', *et al.* Agranular CD4+ CD56+ hematodermic neoplasm' (blastic NK-cell lymphoma) originates from a population of CD56+ precursor cells related to plasmacytoid monocytes. Am. J. Surg. Pathol. 2002;**26**:852–62.

218. Herling M, Jones D. CD4+/CD56+ hematodermic tumor: the features of an evolving entity and its relationship to dendritic cells. Am. J. Clin. Pathol. 2007;**127**:687–700.

219. Feuillard J, Jacob MC, Valensi F, *et al.* Clinical and biologic features of CD4(+)CD56(+) malignancies. Blood 2002;**99**:1556–63.

220. Jacob MC, Chaperot L, Mossuz P, *et al.* CD4+ CD56+ lineage negative malignancies: A new entity developed from malignant early plasmacytoid dendritic cells. Haematologica 2003;**88**:941–55.

221. Reichard KK, Burks EJ, Foucar MJ, *et al.* CD4(+) CD56(+) lineage-negative malignancies are rare tumors of plasmacytoid dendritic cells. Am. J. Surg. Pathol. 2005;**29**:1274–83.

222. Petrella T, Bagot M, Willemz R, *et al.* Blastic NK-cell lymphomas (agranular CD4+CD56+ hematodermic neoplasms): A review. Am. J. Clin. Pathol. 2005;**123**:662–75.

223. Petrella T, Dalac S, Maynadie M', *et al.* CD4+ CD56+ cutaneous neoplasms: A distinct hematological entity? Groupe Francais d'Etude des Lymphomes Cutanes (GFELC). Am. J. Surg. Pathol. 1999;**23**:137–46.

224. Leroux DF, Mugneret F, Callanan M, *et al.* CD4(+), CD56(+) DC2 acute leukemia is characterized by recurrent clonal chromosomal changes affecting

273

6 major targets: A study of 21 cases by the Groupe Francais de Cytogenetique Hematologique. Blood 2002;**99**:4154–59.

225. Herling M, Teitell MA, Shen RR, *et al*. TCL1 expression in plasmacytoid dendritic cells (DC2s) and the related CD4+ CD56+ blastic tumors of skin. Blood 2003;**101**:5007–9.

226. Shimamura A, Alter BP. Pathophysiology and management of inherited bone marrow failure syndromes. Blood Rev. 2010;**24**:101–22.

227. Alter BP. Diagnosis, genetics, and management of inherited bone marrow failure syndromes. Hematol. Am. Soc. Hematol. Educ. Program 2007;**2007**:29–39.

228. Dokal I. Dyskeratosis congenita. Hematol. Am. Soc. Hematol. Educ. Program 2011;**2011**:480–6.

229. Ball S. Diamond Blackfan anemia. Hematol. Am. Soc. Hematol. Educ. Program 2011;**2011**:487–91.

230. Soulier J. Fanconi anemia. Hematol. Am. Soc. Hematol. Educ. Program 2011;**2011**: 492–7.

231. Niemeyer CM, Baumann I. Myelodysplastic syndrome in children and adolescents. Semin. Hematol. 2008;**45**:60–70.

232. Kardos G, Baumann I, Passmore SJ, *et al*. Refractory anemia in childhood: A retrospective analysis of 67 patients with particular reference to monosomy 7. Blood 2003;**102**:1997–2003.

233. Niemeyer CM, Baumann I. Classification of childhood aplastic anemia and myelodysplastic syndromes. Hematol. Am. Soc. Hematol. Educ. Program 2011;**2011**:487–91.

234. Davies JK, Guinan EV. An update on the management of severe idiopathic aplastic anemia in children. Br. J. Haematol. 2007;**136**:549–564.

235. Locasciulli A, Neto RO, Baciagalupo A, *et al*. Outcome of patients with acquired aplastic anemia given first line bone marrow transplantation or immunosuppressive treatment in the last decade: A report from the European Group for Blood and Marrow Transplantation. Haematologica 2007;**92**:11–18.

236. Scheinberg P, Wu CO, Nunez O, *et al*. Long-term outcome of pediatric patients with severe aplastic anemia trated with antithymocyte globulin and cyclosporine. J. Pediatr. 2008;**153**:814–19.

237. Yoshida N, Yagaski H, Hama A, *et al*. Predicting response to immunosuppressive therapy in childhood aplastic anemia. Haematologica 2011;**96**:771–4.

238. Fuhrer M, Ramf U, Baumann I, *et al*. Immunosuppressive therapy for aplastic anemia in children: A more severe disease predicts better survival. Blood 2005;**106**:2102–4.

Kidneys and lower urinary tract

Marie-Anne Brundler, Aurore Coulomb, and Gordan Vujanic

Non-neoplastic renal disease

Congenital developmental anomalies of the kidney

Introduction

Congenital developmental anomalies of the kidney and urinary tract (CAKUT) and renal cystic diseases (RCD) comprise a heterogeneous group of disorders. Of these CAKUT are relatively frequent, in particular when including minor anomalies of the urinary tract, and represent a major cause of end-stage renal disease in infants and children (1). Familial clustering is relatively common. Renal anomalies are often associated with anomalies of the urinary tract, and now are mostly identified on antenatal ultrasound. The term CAKUT was proposed in 2002 to underscore the importance of this association and to challenge existing ideas on their pathogenesis (2). Genetic factors, impaired urinary flow or urinary tract obstruction, and external factors, in isolation or combination, are thought to interfere with the normal nephrogenesis, possibly through overlapping molecular pathways (3,4). Significant advances were made in recent years with regards to the identification of underlying genetic defects and the understanding of pathogenetic mechanism (1,2,4–6).

Classification of CAKUT and RCD

There are numerous classification systems (reviewed in reference 6), with varying emphasis on morphological, clinical, pathogenetic, and or/genetic characteristics. Many of the more recent classification systems separate RCD and CAKUT. A recently proposed classification system (6), based on new genetic and path-

ogenetic insights, incorporates the following major categories; genetic and acquired renal cystic diseases, CAKUT, tubulointersitial syndromes and cysts, cystic neoplasm and neoplastic cysts, and miscellaneous cysts (Table 8.1).

In RCD the initial nephron formation is normal, but later the renal architecture is disrupted by the development of tubular and/or glomerular cysts. Renal dysplasia and other congenital renal developmental anomalies, on the other hand, are characterized by parenchymal maldevelopment. This may be caused either by a genetic defect, impaired urinary flow, or obstruction; external factors potentially may also play a role. Obstructive anomalies show a predilection for the regions of fusion or branching during embryogenesis (pyelo-ureteral, uretero-vesical, and vesical-urethral junctions). Renal developmental and urinary tract anomalies can occur in isolation or in combination. Ipsilateral, contralateral, or bilateral involvement is possible. Duplex anomalies are frequent. They may form part of a field defect, a genetic syndrome, or be associated with multiple other malformations (1–3). In the classification proposed by Bonsib (Table 8.1), medullary cystic diseases and nephronophthisis are categorized as tubulointerstitial syndromes and cysts, whilst in most other classification systems they are categorized as medullary cystic diseases.

Pathology and clinical presentation

Conditions relevant to pediatric surgical pathology practice are discussed in more detail. The most commonly encountered are multicystic dysplasia (and its variants) and obstructive dysplasia. Diffuse renal dysplasia is rarely seen in surgical practice, but its recognition and distinction from multicystic dysplasia or cystic renal disease is important because of the

Table 8.1 Classification of renal cystic disease and developmental anomalies of kidney and urinary tract (adapted from reference 6)

1 Polycystic renal diseases
  A: Autosomal recessive; neonatal, infantile, or childhood onset
  B: Autosomal dominant; adult or early childhood onset
  C: Acquired renal cystic disease
  D: Glomerulocystic Alomerulocystic disease; familial, hereditary with autosomal recessive or dominant polycystic disease, syndromic non-hereditary, sporadic, or acquired

2 Congenital developmental anomalies of kidney and urinary tract
  A: Renal agenesis and dysplasia; uni- or bilateral, sporadic, non-syndromic or syndromic, hereditary dysplasia
  B: Renal hypoplasia, uni-or bilateral, simple, or other
  C: Abnormalities in form, position, and number; in isolation or in combination with A, B, or D
  D: Ureteral, ureteropelvic, or urethral abnormalities; in isolation or in combination with A to C

3 Tubulointersitial syndromes and cysts
  A: Renal tubular dysgenesis, genetic or acquired
  B: Nephronophtisis
  C: Medullary cystic diseases
  D: Bardet–Biedl syndrome

4 Cystic neoplasm and neoplastic cysts (benign and malignant)

5 Miscellaneous

Table 8.2 Pathological classification of renal developmental anomalies

Dysplasia and variants
  Multicystic, diffuse or segmental
  Aplastic
  Hypoplastic

Obstructive

Hypoplasia

Abnormal position, duplication, or fusion

Supernumerary kidney

Tubular dysgenesis

divergent clinical and genetic implications (7–10). Renal developmental anomalies and associated urinary tract anomalies are frequently identified on prenatal ultrasound. Bilateral renal anomalies with oligo- or anhydramnios and Potter sequence have a very poor prognosis. Unilateral kidney anomalies or less severe urinary tract anomalies diagnosed on prenatal ultrasound are best managed by a multidisciplinary team. Presentation at birth with abdominal distension or renal failure is now extremely rare. In some cases, recurrent urinary tract infections lead to the discovery of urinary tract anomalies later in life, or the diagnosis is made coincidentally. It is important to obtain clinical, imaging, and surgical information, when assessing resections for CAKUT or RCD. Classification of renal developmental anomalies traditionally is based on morphological appearances. Clinical, radiologic, and genetic or molecular characteristics, however, are of increasing importance.

Surgical specimens, particularly renal resections for renal cystic disease are rarely encountered in the pediatric surgical pathology practice. The diagnosis is made clinically, by ultrasound examination or needle core biopsy. Even when the patients eventually undergo dialysis or renal transplantation for end-stage renal disease, the native kidneys are left *in situ*, unless they are massively enlarged, or the patient suffers from recurrent infections or refractory hypertension. A diagnosis of tubulo-interstitial and medullary cystic renal disease is generally made by needle core biopsy. Liver disease along the spectrum of congenital hepatic fibrosis is present in a wide range of renal cystic diseases and clinical syndromes found to have in common an underlying defect in primary cilia (ciliopathies) (8–9). There is no definite evidence that congenital developmental anomalies of the kidney are associated with an increased risk of renal malignancy (11). Rare cases of Wilms' tumor arising in multicystic kidneys or in association with contralateral developmental reports have been described (12–13, personal communication AC).

Renal dysplasia

Renal dysplasia is a congenital developmental anomaly resulting from abnormal development of the metanephric duct and the metanephric blastema. It is characterized by disorganization of the renal parenchyma and presence of primitive ducts (10,14–15). Cysts are common, but not an obligatory feature. Neither is divergent differentiation (e.g., the presence of cartilage) nor the presence of immature tubules or glomeruli. Associated abnormalities of the ureter or lower urinary tract are identified in > 50–75% of cases (16). Historically, the classification of renal dysplasia (Table 8.2) is based on morphological appearances (17).

Recent advances in unraveling the molecular mechanism and genetic factors leading to a perturbed renal development partly challenge the clinical validity of such a classification (3,4). In multicystic dysplasia, the renal pelvis and proximal ureter usually are atretic, and dysplasia involves the entire kidney (18). Ultrasound follow-up data suggest that hypoplastic or aplastic dysplasia represents regression of multicystic dysplasia (19–20). In obstructive dysplasia the abnormal renal development is due to congenital urinary tract obstruction or mega-ureter, resulting in impaired urinary flow and urinary retention (reflux). Segmental dysplasia occurs in duplex kidneys.

Clinical presentation: Renal dysplasia is one of the commonest urinary abnormalities detected on prenatal ultrasound (21–24). Associated urinary tract malformations or bilateral disease significantly determine the outcome (22,24,25). In addition, renal dysplasia may present later in life as a small, non-functioning kidney, with vesico-ureteric reflux, urinary tract obstruction, or recurrent infections (20,26). It can also be an incidental finding (24). Diffuse renal dysplasia is mostly bilateral and occurs in association with other malformations or forms part of genetic syndromes, notably Meckel–Gruber and Bardet–Biedl, which are caused by mutations in ciliary genes (8,9).

Macroscopy: In aplastic or hypoplastic dysplasia the kidney is very small, with little or no recognizable renal parenchyma. In multicystic dysplasia, the kidney is of variable size and shows an irregular shape (Figure 8.1). Multiple cysts of varying size are present. The renal pelvis is not identifiable or severely hypoplastic. The proximal ureter is small or atretic. In diffuse dysplasia the kidneys are typically enlarged and retain a reniform shape. The cysts are generally smaller and of more uniform size (Figure 8.2). The collecting system is better developed when compared to multicystic or aplastic dysplasia. Obstructive dysplasia (Figure 8.3) is often accompanied by hydronephrosis, hydroureter, or ureteric stenosis. Cysts are less conspicuous and of small size. In dysplasia associated with a duplex system there is segmental involvement, generally of the upper pole, thought to be related to obstruction.

(A)

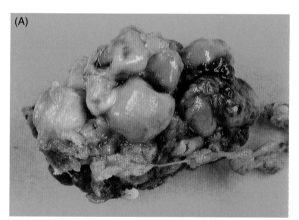

(B)

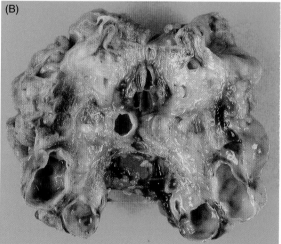

Figure 8.1 Multicystic renal dysplasia. Multiple cysts distort the kidney (A). The central portion of the kidney is fibrotic, renal pelvis, and proximal ureter are not identified (B).

(A)

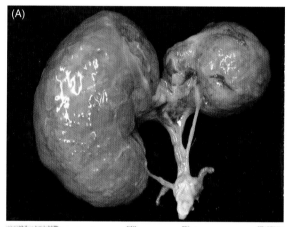

(B)

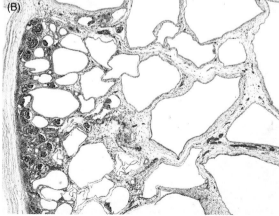

Figure 8.2 Bilateral diffuse renal dysplasia in Meckel–Gruber syndrome (A). The cysts are of smaller size and appear more rounded on microscopic examination (courtesy of Dr. C, Trevenen, Calgary, Canada) (B) (H&E × 40).

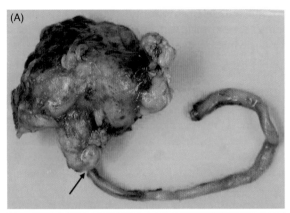

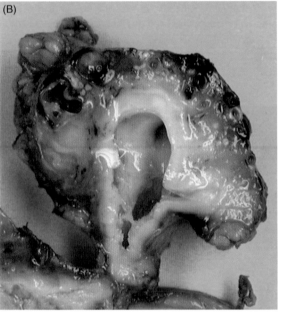

Figure 8.3 (A) Obstructive renal dysplasia due to pelviureteric obstruction. The kidney is small and shows multiple small peripheral cysts. The ureteropelvic junction is very narrow (arrow). (B) The cut surface shows a dilated renal pelvis.

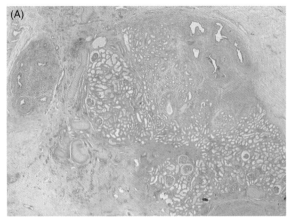

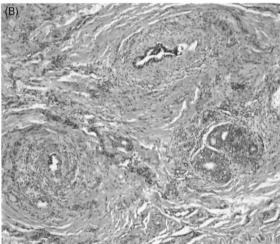

Figure 8.4 Renal dysplasia, microscopic features. The renal architecture is severely disorganized (A) (H7E × 10). Besides nodules of renal cortical tissue, cartilage and immature tubules (shown at higher magnification in B) are identified (H&E × 20).

Histology: Parenchymal maldevelopment with presence of primitive tubules and ducts is the hallmark of renal dysplasia (14,15,17; Figure 8.4). The primitive ducts are lined by cuboidal or columnar epithelium and are surrounded by a cuff of mesenchymal cells. Immature glomeruli and cartilage is variably present. The renal parenchyma is most severely disorganized in multicystic dysplasia. Dilated tubules and cysts of varying size are typically present. Only very scant amounts or no definite renal parenchyma may be identifiable (Figure 8.5a). In obstructive dysplasia, variable degrees of cortico-medullary differentiation are seen. The maldevelopment may be segmental (Figure 8.5b) or confined to outer cortex and/or renal medulla. In obstructive dysplasia, the architectural distortion may be less severe or patchy, and the cysts of smaller size and arranged more peripherally. Inflammation and scarring may be prominent and obscure underlying dysplastic changes. Cysts are more evenly distributed and usually show lesser variation in size in diffuse renal dysplasia (Figure 8.2b).

Renal hypoplasia

By definition, the kidneys are reduced in size. They weigh significantly less than the expected weight (mean) for age and show reduced numbers of lobules (≤ 5 compared to ≥ 10 in a normal kidney) (27–28). Compensatory hypertrophy or secondary

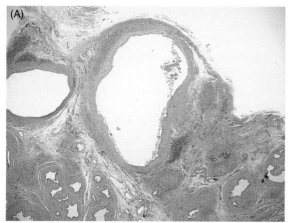

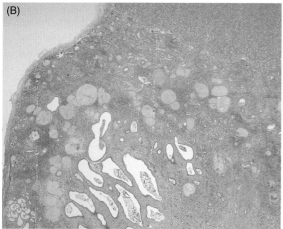

Figure 8.5 Variants of renal dysplasia. Only cysts and immature ducts are identified in hypoplastic dysplasia (A) (H&E × 10). Segmental dysplasia is seen in a duplex kidney (B) (H&E × 20).

focal segmental glomerulosclerosis (FSGS) may develop. True renal hypoplasia is rare, and must be distinguished from small kidneys due to atrophy or maldevelopment. In renal hypoplasia, the parenchyma is normally developed; no inflammation, maldevelopment, or scarring is seen. Oligometanephric hypoplasia, a distinct form of bilateral renal hypoplasia, is characterized by two small kidneys with a reduced number of nephrons, which are significantly enlarged with large glomeruli and dilated tubules (29). Most cases are sporadic. Association with other developmental anomalies and chromosome 4p deletion/4p ring chromosome has been reported in two cases (30). PAX-2 mutations were recently documented in three patients who in addition showed eye anomalies (31). The clinical presentation of renal hypoplasia is similar to juvenile nephronophthisis, but proteinuria is more prominent. End-stage renal disease may develop within months, or as late as early-mid adolescence (27–31).

Renal agenesis

Renal agenesis is defined as complete uni- or bilateral absence of the kidney. Bilateral renal agenesis is less common than unilateral agenesis and shows a clear male predilection. Absent or insufficient urinary production in bilateral renal agenesis (but also bilateral renal dysplasia, or autosomal recessive polycystic kidney disease) results in decreased production of amniotic fluid (oligohydramnios). The resulting Potter sequence, with characteristic facial and limb deformities and pulmonary hypoplasia, has a very poor prognosis. Unilateral renal agenesis mostly is an incidental finding. Renal function is maintained by a single kidney undergoing hypertrophy. Association with other urinary tract anomalies or malformation syndromes or sequences is common (3). The likeliest mechanism is failure of the ureteric bud to develop from the mesonephric duct, and consequently the metanephric blastema to differentiate into renal parenchyma (5). In some instances, unilateral renal agenesis may represent regression of renal dysplasia (19). Mutations in *RET* or *GDNF* are rarely associated with renal agenesis (32,33).

Abnormally positioned or shaped kidneys, renal duplication, and supernumerary kidneys

They often remain clinically asymptomatic. Associated urinary tract anomalies primarily account for the increased risk of recurrent urinary tract infections. Fused and duplex kidneys are thought to develop as a result of aberrant induction of metanephric blastema by a ureteric bud arising either proximal or distal to the normal mesonephric zone, or from ureteric buds developing in too close proximity (5,27). Ectopic non-fused kidneys mostly are located in the pelvis, and show an abnormal rotation. This is thought to result from abnormal caudal growth of the embryo (3). The kidney may be small in size, which possibly is due to a reduced vascular supply. The ureter may insert ectopically, on the same or cross over to the other side. Fused kidneys often are found closer to the midline. Concurrent urinary tract or urogenital anomalies and developmental abnormalities in other organs may be present.

A supernumerary kidney is distinct from a duplex system as it is completely separate, with its own pelvicaliceal system and separate vascular supply.

279

Reflux nephropathy

Reflux nephropathy results from non-obstructive urinary back flow at the level of the vesico-ureteric junction (34). Antenatal diagnosis of vesico-ureteric reflux is difficult. The diagnosis is made on retrograde cystography. The reflux may be congenital or acquired, uni- or bilateral, occur in isolation or in association with other urinary tract anomalies (posterior urethral valves, bladder diverticula, or duplex systems). In addition, it may be a manifestation of a bladder-emptying problem (such as neuropathic bladder).

Clinical presentation: Vesico-ureteric reflux with some degree of ureteric or pelvic dilatation is detected in about 1% of live births on prenatal ultrasound. In two-thirds of cases reflux is mild and will resolve by two years of age (35). The clinical presentation is very variable, ranging from asymptomatic reflux to recurrent urinary tract infections, and, in rare instances, renal failure (35,36). Reflux is confirmed by imaging studies and classified according to its severity into five grades. It is more frequent in male neonates and grade 5 is observed nearly exclusively in males (35). Familial occurrence of vesico-ureteric reflux is well documented, with a higher incidence of high-grade reflux in young children (< 2 yrs) leading to calls for screening of asymptomatic siblings (37). Surgical management with ureteric reimplantation and prophylactic antibiosis appear similarly effective (36).

Macroscopy: Nephrectomy is generally reserved for severe cases of reflux nephropathy with significant loss of renal function, or cases complicated by recurrent infections or hypertension. In most instances the kidney is small, but normally lobulated. The renal pelvis and calices are dilated with variable flattening or indentation of renal papillae. Scarring, segmental, or more diffuse is common. The ureter is dilated and may be tortuous (Figure 8.6).

Histology: Changes vary and in part overlap with those seen in urinary tract obstruction. The parenchyma is either more diffusely atrophic (Figure 8.7) or shows sharply demarcated areas of scarring with sclerosed glomeruli and atrophic tubules. Inflammation is variable. The microscopic appearances may overlap with those seen in urinary tract obstruction if there is an associated obstruction, such as posterior urethral valves or in the case of a duplex system.

Obstructive nephropathy

Hydronephrosis and obstructive nephropathy result from mechanical obstruction of the urinary flow at any level of the urinary tract. The accumulation of

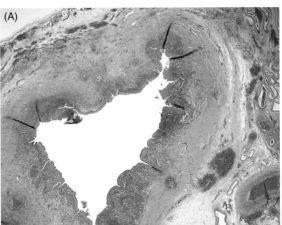

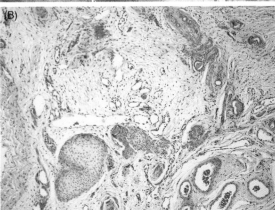

Figure 8.7 Severe reflux nephropathy. Renal pelvis and calices show marked chronic inflammation and fibrosis. The renal parenchyma is reduced to a narrow rim of loose fibro-vascular tissue (A) (H&E × 10). On higher magnification (B) only scant primitive tubules and cartilage are identified (H&E × 20).

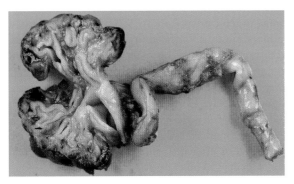

Figure 8.6 Severe reflux nephropathy. The kidney is small and shows a markedly thinned renal cortex. Renal pelvis and ureter are dilated.

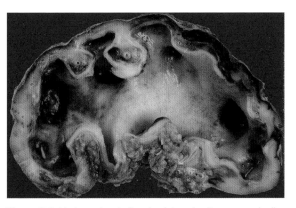

Figure 8.8 Hydronephrosis. Renal pelvis and calices are markedly dilated. The renal cortex is thin and renal papillae appear flattened.

urine leads to distension of the renal pelvis and/or renal calices. In children, obstruction of the pelviureteric junction (PUJ) is the commonest cause, occurring in as many as 1 per 1000–2000 newborns. Obstruction of the PUJ may occur in isolation or in association with vesico-ureteric reflux or duplex systems. Other more rare causes of hydronephrosis in children include ureteral valves, posterior urethral valves, or tumors (extrinsic or intrinsic).

Clinical presentation: The diagnosis of pelviureteric obstruction in most instances is made on prenatal ultrasound. Antero-posterior dilatation of the renal pelvis of >10 mm is considered significant (38). Postnatal presentations include urinary tract infection, abdominal pain, or hematuria. Pyeloplasty is the treatment of choice. Nephrectomy is performed only in severe cases, with significant impairment of the renal function, recurrent infections, nephrolithiasis, or hypertension.

Macroscopy: Typically, the resected kidney shows hydronephrosis (Figure 8.8). The renal pelvis and calices are dilated. Renal papillae are flattened and the renal parenchyma is markedly thinned. In some cases of pelviureteric obstruction, a small atrophic kidney is found (Figure 8.3). The pelviureteric junction is narrow and there may be thickening of the wall.

Histology: Examination of the resected pelviureteric junction shows disarray of the muscle layer and fibrosis of the wall. Smooth-muscle abnormalities appear to contribute to the pathogenesis of the pelviureteric obstruction (39). Inflammation, in our experience, is insignificant in most cases. Microscopic appearances of the resected kidney depend on the severity, duration, and age of onset of the obstruction. Findings include cortical atrophy with glomerulosclerosis, tubular atrophy, interstitial inflammation, and fibrosis. Dysplastic changes (parenchymal maldevelopment) may be present.

Urinary tract infections: pyelonephritis

Urinary tract and renal developmental anomalies predispose children and adults to recurrent urinary tract infections. Unless there is obstruction, massive pyonephrosis, or significant parenchymal destruction, pyelonephritis nowadays is rarely encountered by the surgical or pediatric pathologist. Most infections are caused by Gram-negative enteric bacteria (*E. coli*) and the commonest manifestation is pyelonephritis. The presentation may be acute or chronic. Fever, flank pain, and pyuria are common symptoms.

Macroscopy: The kidney appears swollen with abscesses or whitish areas on cut sections.

Histology: Typically, there is destructive acute inflammation of renal tubules, often with a stripy pattern. Interstitial and pelvicaliceal inflammation is variable. Papillary necrosis may be seen.

Xanthogranulomatous pyelonephritis

This is a distinct variant of chronic infectious pyelonephritis that most frequently affects middle-aged women, and rarely also manifests in childhood.

Clinical presentation: Patients present with a renal mass, accompanied by fever, pyuria or hematuria, and anemia (40–41). Given the often significant enlargement of the kidney, the main differential diagnosis is that of a renal neoplasm, notably Wilms tumor.

Macroscopy: Calices appear dilated, are filled with pus or calculi and are rimmed by yellowish tissue. Yellow areas also present in the remaining kidney.

Histology: Is characterized by sheets of foam cells with fine granular cytoplasm.

Malakoplakia

A rare inflammatory condition of possible infectious pathogenesis, which occurs in children and adults, it is characterized by an infiltrate of histiocytes with intracytoplasmic PAS-positive inclusions, so-called Michaelis–Gutman bodies. The clinical presentation, in cases of renal involvement, is that of a urinary tract infection.

Renal tubular dysgenesis (RTD)

Renal tubular dysgenesis is a fetal disorder characterized by either complete absence or poor development of proximal tubules (42). Hypoperfusion during renal development appears to play a crucial role in the pathogenesis. It may be inherited in an autosomal recessive mode or be acquired during fetal development. Inherited RTD is linked to mutations in genes of the renin-angiotensin system (42,43). Acquired forms are described in association with congenital cardiac malformations, neonatal hemochromatosis (44,45), placental pathologies, such as massive perivillous fibrin deposition (46,47), and treatment with ACE inhibitors during pregnancy (48). Renal hypoperfusion appears to be the common underlying pathogenetic mechanism.

Clinical presentation: Renal tubular dysgenesis usually manifests *in utero* with severe oligo- or anhydramnios and Potter sequence. In addition, ossification defects of the skull are commonly encountered. In most cases RTD is fatal, with death occurring *in utero* or shortly after birth.

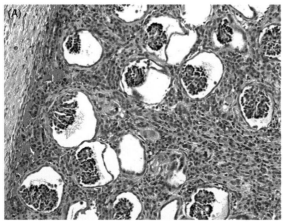

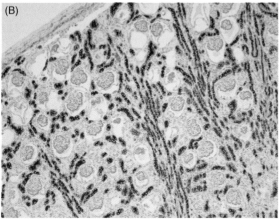

Figure 8.9 Renal tubular dysgenesis (RTD). Glomeruli appear crowded (A) (H&E × 20). Tubules are of uniform appearances and stain for epithelial membrane antigen (EMA) (B) (H&E × 10).

Macroscopy: Given the severity of the clinical manifestation, RTD is mostly encountered at autopsy. The kidneys are of normal size and shape.

Histology: Crowding of glomeruli is noted at microscopy. Tubules appear uniform, and epithelial membrane antigen (EMA) stains all tubules (Figure 8.9). This is in contrast to the normal kidney where tubules can easily be differentiated into proximal and distal tubules. In addition, normally only distal tubules stain for EMA, whilst proximal tubules remain unstained.

Renal cystic diseases (RCD)

Renal cystic diseases (RCD) represent a clinically, genetically, and morphologically heterogeneous group of disorders. They include autosomal recessive polycystic disease (ARPKD), autosomal dominant polycystic disease (ADPKD), glomerulocystic disease (GCKD), and nephronophtisis/medullary cystic disease (NPHP/MCDK). Pertinent clinical, genetic, and morphological features discussed below are summarized in Table 8.3.

Genetics: Autosomal recessive polycystic kidney disease and ADPKD, some forms of GCKD and nephronophtisis/medullary cystic disease (NPHP/MCK) are linked to mutations in genes coding for proteins located in the primary cilium (49–56). These genes regulate a wide range of cellular functions, including maintenance of cell polarity and proliferation. Primary cilia also act as chemo- and mechanoreceptors. Identification of mutations in ciliary genes as a common denominator in a wide spectrum of diseases and syndromes led to their designation as ciliopathies. Renal involvement, either in the form of renal maldevelopment or renal cystic disease, represents the most common manifestation of a ciliopathy. Other frequently affected organs include liver, eyes/retina, skeleton, and brain (8,9,57). The exact function of affected ciliary genes and the mechanism that leads to the formation of renal, and frequently also hepatic, cysts are still only partly understood. Also, the role of genetic modifiers contributing to phenotypic overlap and variability in ciliopathies remains largely speculative (56).

Clinical presentation: The clinical presentation, including age of onset, varies significantly, depending on the type of renal cystic disease. It also is influenced by the nature and severity of extrarenal manifestations. Typically, autosomal recessive polycystic disease is either diagnosed prenatally or manifests in the neonatal period. Later presentation, in adolescence or adulthood,

Table 8.3 Pertinent clinical, genetic, and morphological features of the commonest renal cystic diseases.

	Age	Inheritance	Gene	Macroscopy	Histology	Extrarenal manifestations
AR PKD	Congenital, neonatal > infancy, childhood	AR	PKHD1	Large kidneys, reniform shape retained, uniform fusiform cysts	Radiating tubular cysts, mainly collecting ducts	Liver, congenital hepatic fibrosis, Caroly syndrome
AD PKD	Adults > adolescence >> early childhood	AD	PKD1 PKD2	Large distorted kidneys, variable size cysts	Tubular cysts, glomerular (in early onset)	Biliary cysts and hamartoma (congenital hepatic fibrosis), brain aneurysm
GCKD with PKD GCKD	Variable	AD/AR AR	PKD1/PKHD1 NHF-β1	Enlarged small	Glomerular cysts (>5%)	Liver in PKD1/ PHKD1
Nephronophtysis	Variable	AR AD	NPHP1–11 (AR), MCKD1 & 2 (AD)	Small to normal in size	Tubular basement membrane disruption, interstitial fibrosis, tubular cysts, no dysplasia	Variable, liver, and other

is typical for autosomal dominant polycystic disease. Symptoms include hypertension, hematuria, abdominal distension, or pain. In some patients, the liver disease dominates the clinical picture (58). All patients with ARPKD show liver involvement, usually presenting as congenital hepatic fibrosis. Although less frequent, the latter also occurs in other forms of RCD. In ADPKD, biliary hamartomas or non-communicating biliary cysts are typically identified, but may remain clinically silent (8). In addition, patients with ADPKD develop cardiovascular complications later in life (58). Nephronophtisis is the commonest genetic cause of end-stage renal disease in children and adolescents. It typically manifests initially with polyuria and polydipsia (46,56).

Pathology: Polycystic kidneys are rarely resected, unless there are clinical complications, including pain, bleeding, or infection. In autosomal dominant polycystic disease, kidneys occasionally are removed prior to transplantation because of their large size. Renal biopsy may be performed to confirm a diagnosis of glomerulocystic kidney disease or nephronophthisis.

In ARPKD the kidneys are markedly enlarged, but retain their reniform shape. Cysts are radially arranged, and involve predominantly collecting ducts (Figure 8.10). In ADPKD, the kidney is markedly enlarged, the reniform shape is lost and the renal surface appears bosselated. The cysts may greatly vary in size. Cysts arise from all segments of the nephron and

may also involve glomeruli (Figure 8.11). Glomerular cysts are characterized by a dilatation of the Bowman space which exceeds 2–3 times its normal size (Figure 8.12). Glomerular cystic change (cysts in > 5% of glomeruli) may be seen in a range of developmental and cystic diseases of the kidney. The designation of GCKD, however, is usually restricted to familial glomerulocystic disorders (54). Nephronophtisis (Figure 8.13) is characterized by disruption of the tubular basement membrane, diffuse interstitial fibrosis, and cystic dilatation of tubules at the cortico-medullary junction or in the medulla, without associated dysplasia (59).

The pathological spectrum of liver disease in ciliopathies includes congenital hepatic fibrosis, Caroli syndrome, and polycystic liver disease. Variation in the severity of the ductal plate malformation and the involvement along the portobiliary system are thought to account for the morphological spectrum encountered across the various ciliopathies (60).

Primary glomerular and tubulo-interstitial disorders in children

These are primarily diagnosed by percutaneous renal biopsy. Due to their rarity, the technical complexity of the investigations required (microscopy, immunofluorescence or immunoperoxidase, and electron microscopy) and because close correlation with

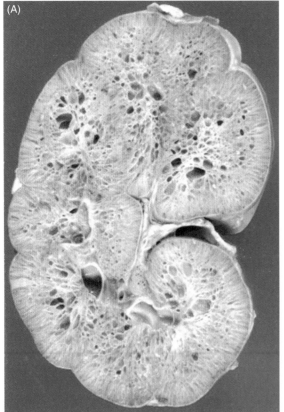

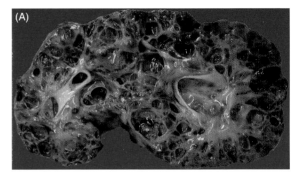

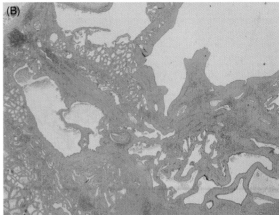

Figure 8.11 ADPKD. The kidney is severely distorted by variably sized cysts (courtesy of Dr. C. Treven, Calgary, Canada) (A). On microscopy they involve all segments and often show papillary infoldings. In between, areas of preserved renal parenchyma are identified (B) (H&E × 40).

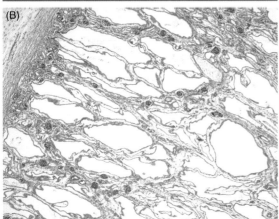

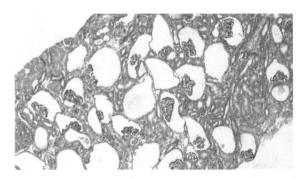

Figure 8.10 ARPKD. The kidney is markedly enlarged, but retains a reniform shape (A). The kidney is diffusely involved by relatively uniform radiating cysts. Collecting ducts are mainly affected and show fusiform dilatation on microscopy (B) (H&E × 40).

Figure 8.12 GCKD. Most of the glomeruli show marked dilatation of the Bowman space. Otherwise the kidney appears normally developed (H&E × 20).

clinical presentation, laboratory investigations including serological results is required, renal biopsies mostly are dealt with by highly specialized, renal or pediatric, pathologists. Whilst the microscopic features generally are identical to those seen in adults,

the spectrum of pathologies encountered in infants and children differs significantly from adults and includes a larger proportion of genetic disorders (Table 8.4). For further details the interested reader is referred to specialist textbooks on renal pathology.

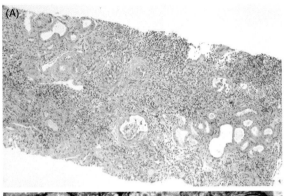

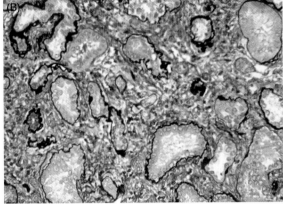

Figure 8.13 Nephronophthisis. The renal biopsy shows marked interstitial inflammation and fibrosis (A) (H&E × 10). Atrophy and focally cystic dilatation of tubules is demonstrated associated with disruption and in places lamellation of the tubular basement membranes (B) (Jones Silver stain × 20).

Table 8.4 Spectrum of glomerular and tubulo-interstitial disorders in children

Condition	Main presenting symptoms
Nephrotic syndrome*	Nephrotic range proteinuria
IgA nephropathy	Micro- or macroscopic hematuria
HSP nephritis	Micro- or macroscopic hematuria
Lupus nephritis	Hematuria, proteinuria
Basement membrane disorders (thin basement membrane disease, Alport's)	Micro- or macroscopic hematuria, deafness (Alport's)
Tubulo-interstitial nephritis	Variable, progressive renal failure, extrarenal manifestations
Nephronophthisis	Renal failure, polydipsia, polyuria

*Biopsied only if refractory or relapsing to exclude FSGS, or to assess for drug/cyclosporine toxicity

Table 8.5 Primary renal tumors of childhood

Tumors	Relative percentage
Wilms, non-anaplastic	80
Wilms, anaplastic	5
Mesoblastic nephroma	4
Clear-cell sarcoma	4
Rhabdoid tumor	2
Miscellaneous: – Renal-cell carcinoma – Primitive neuroectodermal tumor – Neuroblastoma – Synovial sarcoma – Others	5

Renal tumors of childhood

Renal tumors of childhood are rare, although they represent one of the most common solid tumors of childhood. The annual incidence is about seven per million (approximately 1 child per 10 000 births), with around 100 new cases diagnosed annually in the UK and around 500 cases in the USA (61,62). They comprise 6–7% of all tumors in children under 15 years of age, and many have a striking age distribution, which can be a helpful diagnostic clue in the differential diagnosis (see below). The most common renal tumor of childhood is Wilms' tumor (WT) (~85%), whereas all other tumors are much more rare (Table 8.5).

Nephroblastoma (Wilms' tumor)

Nephroblastoma is a malignant embryonal tumor, which develops from nephrogenic tissue and mimics events in normal and abnormal nephrogenesis.

Clinical presentation: Wilms' tumor (WT) has a peak incidence between three and four years of age, and the majority of patients (~90%) present before the age of six years (61). It is very uncommon in the neonatal period (0.16%) (63) and only 15% of cases present in the first year of life (61). It can rarely occur in adults, too (64). It is slightly more common in girls than in boys and their median age at presentation is 42.5 months, whereas it is 36.5 months for boys (61,65). In 5–10% of cases WT presents as bilateral disease and these patients are younger than those with unilateral tumors (the average

age at presentation is 30–33 months) (66). Very rarely it may present as an extrarenal tumor (67).

Wilms' tumor typically presents as an abdominal mass in an otherwise well-appearing child, but 25–30% of affected children may have other symptoms, including abdominal pain, fever, anemia, hematuria, and hypertension (68).

Genetic features: The genetics of WT is complex, with a significant degree of genetic heterogeneity involving various tumor-suppressor genes, different genetic mechanisms, with losses and gains of chromosomal material, some translocations, and notably methylation and imprinting changes, particularly involving 11p15 (the Beckwith–Wiedemann locus) (69,70). It appears that at least three types of genetic pathway are involved in the pathogenesis of WT (71). Similarly, there are at least three genes associated with familial WT (72).

It is believed that 10–15% of patients with WTs have a heritable cause. In 1–2% of cases WT is familial (72) and in around 5–10% is associated with syndromes and congenital anomalies (61). The commonest anomalies are hemihypertrophy and genitourinary anomalies, including hypospadias and cryptorchidism. There are more than 50 syndromes associated with WT, but the most common include Beckwith–Wiedemann syndrome (omphalocele, visceromegaly, hemihypertrophy), WAGR syndrome (Wilms, aniridia, mental retardation, and genitourinary anomalies) and Denys–Drash syndrome (mesangial sclerosis, pseudohermaphroditism), all of which carry a risk of developing WT of 10%, 30% and 90%, respectively (73). Other, rarely associated syndromes include Perlman syndrome, Simpson–Golabi–Behlem syndrome, Fraser syndrome, and Bloom syndrome (73). Through studies of these syndromes, genetic changes associated with the development of WT have been identified. The WT1 gene has been identified through its involvement in WAGR syndrome and is located on chromosome 11p13. The gene plays a key role in renal and gonadal development and its somatic and germ-cell mutations have been found in WT. In children with complete deletion of one WT1 allele, as in the WAGR syndrome, genitourinary abnormalities are less severe than in children with the typical intragenic WT1 mutations of Denys–Drash syndrome (73). About 2–3% of children carry a constitutional *WT1* mutation without any evidence of genitourinary malformation (71) and they are more likely to develop stromal-predominant WT, often with rhabdomyoblastic differentiation, and intralobar nephrogenic rests. However, mutations in the *WT1* gene do not explain

Table 8.6 COG and SIOP histological classifications of childhood renal tumors

COG	SIOP
Favorable histology	*Low risk*
Mesoblastic nephroma	Mesoblastic nephroma
CPDN	CPDN
	Completely necrotic type
Standard histology	*Intermediate risk*
Mixed	Mixed type
Epithelial predominant	Epithelial type
Stromal predominant	Stromal type
Blastemal predominant	Regressive type
	Focal anaplasia
Unfavorable histology	*High risk*
Focal and diffuse anaplasia	Diffuse anaplasia
CCSK	Blastemal type
RTK	CCSK
	RTK

COG: Children's Oncology Group; SIOP: International Society of Paediatric Oncology; CPDN – Cystic partially differentiated nephroblastoma; CCSK – Clear cell sarcoma of kidney; RTK – Rhabdoid tumor of kidney

the majority of cases of either the rare familial form or the more common sporadic form of the disease. It is believed that there is at least one more gene involved in Wilms tumorigenesis, and it is designated the *WT-2* gene. This gene has been mapped to chromosome 11p15, but still has not been isolated (70). Similarly, the familial Wilms' tumor genes, *FWT1* and *FWT2*, have been mapped to chromosomes 17q and 19q, respectively, but still remain to be identified.

Recent National Wilms' Tumor Study Group (NWTSG) studies showed that loss of heterozygosity at 1p and 16q is associated with adverse prognosis in children with non-anaplastic WT (74), and this has been taken as a prognostic parameter in the ongoing Children's Oncology Group (COG) trial.

Classification: At present, there are two major histological classifications of WT, including SIOP (International Society of Paediatric Oncology) and COG classifications (75,76). The COG classification is applicable to primarily operated tumors and distinguishes two major types: non-anaplastic and anaplastic WT. The SIOP classification is applicable to tumors that are treated with preoperative chemotherapy followed by surgery; in its criteria for subclassifying tumors, both chemotherapy-induced changes and the amount of viable tumor are taken into account. Tumors are stratified into three groups: low-risk tumors, intermediate-risk tumors, and high-risk tumors (Table 8.6; 75,76).

Table 8.7 SIOP WT 2001 histological criteria for subclassifying Wilms' tumors

Tumor type	Histological features (% of a tumor)			
	CIC	Blastema	Epithelium	Stroma
Completely necrotic	100	0	0	0
Regressive	> 66	0–33	0–33	0–33
Mixed	< 66	0–66	0–66	0–66
Stromal	< 66	0–10	0–33	67–100
Epithelial	< 66	0–10	67–100	0–33
Blastemal	< 66	67–100	0–33	0–33
Anaplasia (focal or diffuse)	Any of the above (excluding completely necrotic)			

SIOP: International Society of Paediatric Oncology; CIC – chemotherapy-induced changes

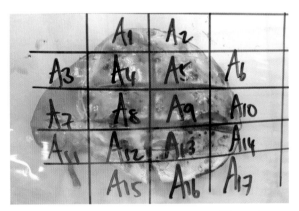

Figure 8.14 Sampling of a whole tumor slice with clear indication where blocks are taken from (courtesy of Dr M. McDermott, Our Lady Children's Hospital, Dublin, Ireland).

Since the accurate assessment of the components of different tumors is critical for SIOP subclassification, it is important to sample the tumor according to the established protocol (77), which requires that at least one whole slice of tumor surface is blocked (Figure 8.14). The first step in assessing a pretreated tumor is to determine the percentage of chemotherapy-induced changes. If there are no viable tumor elements in any section, the tumor is classified as completely necrotic (low-risk tumor). If there are viable tumor components, the tumor is further subclassified according to the SIOP criteria (Table 8.7; 77), which differ from the COG criteria. The criteria for subclassification used should be based on prenephrectomy treatment (primary surgery = COG criteria; preoperative chemotherapy = SIOP criteria).

Macroscopy: Wilms' tumor usually presents as a solitary, rounded mass arising from any part of the kidney. In some 10% of cases it may be multicentric and in ~7% of cases bilateral. The nephrectomy specimen may weigh from 60 g to 6350 g, with a median weight of 550 g (78). The cut surface is usually bulging, pale gray in color, soft, friable, and lobulated, with areas of necrosis and hemorrhage, especially in pretreated tumors. Some tumors may have cysts of different sizes and shapes. The tumor is usually sharply demarcated from the adjacent renal tissue by a pseudocapsule. In rare cases it may show an intrapelvic growth resulting in a botryoid appearance. It often invades the renal vein, and may extend up through the vena cava to the right atrium.

Histology: Classical WT consists of three different components: blastemal, epithelial, and stromal, which may be present in any proportion. In addition, epithelial and stromal components may show different lines and degrees of differentiation, whereas the blastemal component may show any of numerous patterns (see below). As a result, no two WT look the same, and the only other tumor with so many different histological patterns is a teratoma. In some WTs, a teratoid pattern may be very prominent (genuine primary renal teratomas are exceptionally rare), but it has no influence on prognosis and such tumors are subclassified on the basis of other components.

A blastemal component is an undifferentiated component composed of blastemal cells; these are small-to medium-sized and may form different patterns, namely diffuse, serpentine, and basaloid patterns (Figure 8.15A; (78). Although regarded as the most aggressive component, it is at the same time the most chemotherapy-sensitive, except for a small number of cases in which it persists after preoperative chemotherapy.

An epithelial component is present in most WT. As mentioned previously, it may show different lines and different degrees of differentiation, ranging from very early epithelial structures such as rosettes to well-differentiated tubules and glomeruli (Figure 8.15B). In addition, many other epithelial types may be found, including squamous epithelium, respiratory type, and gastrointestinal epithelium (78).

A stromal component may also show different patterns and degrees of differentiation, ranging from undifferentiated hypocellular stroma to well-differentiated stroma with rhabdomyoblastic differentiation (Figure 8.15C). In some tumors there might be numerous islands of cartilage, and even osteoid (78).

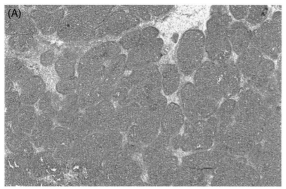

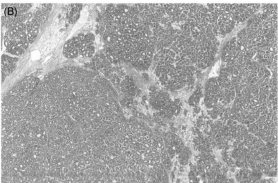

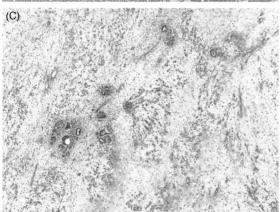

Figure 8.15 Histological components of Wilms' tumor. (A) Blastemal component showing the nodular pattern (H&E × 20). (B) Epithelial component consisting entirely of tubular structures (H&E × 20). (C) Stromal component with rhabdomyoblastic differentiation (H&E × 20).

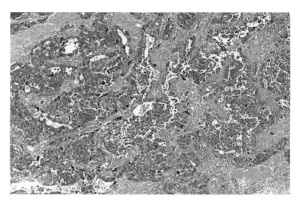

Figure 8.16 Anaplasia with atypical mitoses, nuclear enlargement, and hyperchromasia (H&E × 40).

Figure 8.17 Completely necrotic Wilms' tumor with no recognizable component (H&E × 20).

Anaplasia is a histological feature associated with adverse prognosis. It occurs in 5–8% of WT and can be focal or diffuse (79). Histological criteria for anaplasia include the presence of enlarged atypical mitotic figures, marked nuclear enlargement, and hyperchromasia (Figure 8.16). It may occur in any of the tumor components, but in order to fulfill the criteria for anaplasia, all three features have to be present. Anaplasia is associated with p53 mutation (80) and is often positive using p53 immunohistochemical staining. Focal (or localized) anaplasia is defined as the presence of anaplastic changes in one or a few sharply defined foci within the tumor, with no evidence of marked nuclear atypia elsewhere in the tumor. All other cases are regarded as diffuse anaplasia. Focal anaplasia is less common than diffuse anaplasia (21% vs. 79%, respectively) (81), and in the SIOP trials is treated the same as other intermediate-risk tumors, whereas in COG trials it is treated more aggressively. In rare cases prolonged chemotherapy for bilateral tumors may result in the development of anaplasia (82).

Chemotherapy-induced changes are seen in tumors treated with preoperative chemotherapy, as in the SIOP trials. They include necrosis, the presence of foamy histiocytes, hemosiderin deposits, and fibrosis (Figure 8.17). Other chemotherapy-induced changes include blastemal, epithelial, and stromal maturation, with striated muscle being the most frequent. Some tumors may show a remarkable responsiveness to

Table 8.8 SIOP WT 2001 staging criteria for renal tumors of childhood

Stage I
(a) The tumor is limited to kidney or surrounded with a fibrous (pseudo) capsule if outside of the normal contours of the kidney. The renal capsule or pseudocapsule may be infiltrated by the tumor, but it does not reach the outer surface.
(b) The tumor may be protruding ("bulging") into the pelvic system and "dipping" into the ureter, but it is not infiltrating their walls.
(c) The vessels or the soft tissues of the renal sinus are not involved.
(d) Intrarenal vessel involvement may be present.

Notes:
– Fine needle aspiration or percutaneous core needle ("tru-cut") biopsy does not upstage the tumor, but the size of the needle gauge should be mentioned to the pathologist.
– The presence of necrotic tumor or chemotherapy-induced change in the renal sinus and/or within the perirenal fat should not be regarded as a reason for upstaging a tumor providing it is completely excised and does not reach the resection margins.
– Infiltration of the adrenal gland does not upstage tumor if the external capsule of the adrenal gland is intact.
– Liver: tumor might be attached to the liver capsule and this should not be regarded as infiltration of the adjacent organ; only if clear infiltration of the liver parenchyma is present, tumor should be regarded as stage III.

Stage II
(a) Viable tumor penetrates through the renal capsule and/or fibrous pseudocapsule into perirenal fat but is completely resected (resection margins "clear").
(b) Viable tumor infiltrates the soft tissues of the renal sinus.
(c) Viable tumor infiltrates blood and lymphatic vessels of the renal sinus or in the perirenal tissue but it is completely resected.
(d) Viable tumor infiltrates the renal pelvic or ureter wall.
(e) Viable tumor infiltrates adjacent organs or vena cava, but is completely resected.

Stage III
(a) Viable or non-viable tumor extends beyond resection margins.
(b) Any abdominal lymph nodes are involved.
(c) Tumor rupture before or intraoperatively (irrespective of other criteria for staging).
(d) The tumor has penetrated through the peritoneal surface.
(e) Tumor implants are found on the peritoneal surface.
(f) The tumor thrombi present at resection margins of vessels or ureter, transected or removed piecemeal by surgeon.
(g) The tumor has been surgically biopsied (wedge biopsy) prior to preoperative chemotherapy or surgery.

Note: The presence of necrotic tumor or chemotherapy-induced changes in a lymph node or at the resection margins is regarded as proof of previous tumor with microscopic residue and therefore the tumor is assigned stage III (because of the possibility that some viable tumor is left behind in the adjacent lymph node or beyond resection margins).

Stage IV

Hematogenous metastases (lung, liver, bone, brain, etc.) or lymph node metastases outside the abdomino-pelvic region.

Stage V

Bilateral renal tumors at diagnosis. Each side should be substaged according to the above criteria.

chemotherapy, resulting in complete necrosis, and requiring minimal treatment after surgery (83). Preoperative chemotherapy makes an overall assessment of the tumor histology and its stage (Table 8.8) more difficult, since different components and criteria have to be taken into account, which may result in discrepancies in diagnosis and staging between the institutional pathologists and central pathology review (84).

Immunohistochemistry: Is not particularly helpful in the diagnosis of WTs, which in nephrectomy specimens should be reached on the basis of the histological features present. Blastemal cells may be positive for different markers, but apart from vimentin, which is virtually always positive, other markers may show variable and focal positivity. The WT1 marker shows characteristic nuclear positivity in ~80% of the cases. It is also positive in the epithelial cells. CD56 is positive in 100% of blastemal cells, whereas desmin, epithelial markers, and CD99 may be only focally positive (85).

Differential diagnosis: Triphasic or even biphasic WTs are usually easy to diagnose and typically represent no diagnostic difficulty, although their subclassification may be problematic (as discussed above). However, monophasic WT may be rather challenging to discriminate from other renal tumors that show the same or similar histological features. Pure blastemal WT may be difficult to distinguish on light microscopy from other undifferentiated tumors, such as primitive neuroectodermal tumors, desmoplastic small round-cell tumors of the kidney and even neuroblastomas. In such cases, immunohistochemistry and molecular biology may be of a great diagnostic help. Primitive neuroectodermal tumors show characteristic diffuse CD99 membranous positivity, and genetic studies reveal characteristic translocations, t(11;22)(q24;q12) being the most frequent. Desmoplastic small round-cell tumor has recently been described in the kidney and should be diagnosed only if the EWS-WT1 t(11;22)(q13;q12) translocation is demonstrated (86). Rarely, a rhabdoid tumor of the kidney may represent a differential diagnostic problem, but it shows characteristic negative INI1 immunostaining. In the differential diagnosis of pure epithelial WT, renal-cell carcinoma should be considered, although histological features of renal-cell carcinoma in children are rather distinctive (see below). Also, in rare cases metanephric adenoma may be difficult to distinguish from epithelial WT, but when the diagnostic criteria are strictly followed, the right diagnosis should be reached. In the differential diagnosis of pure stromal WT, a clear-cell sarcoma of the kidney and mesoblastic nephroma are included. In WTs treated with preoperative chemotherapy, the stroma may show a striking clear cell sarcoma-like appearance and extensive sampling may be required in order to find foci with other WT components.

Nephrogenic rests

Nephrogenic rests are foci of embryonal cells which are abnormally persistent after 36 weeks of gestation, and which are capable of developing into WT. They are found in ~40% of WTs and very rarely in routine infant post-mortem examinations. The term nephroblastomatosis is used to describe the presence of multiple nephrogenic rests. Two major types of nephrogenic rests are perilobar and intralobar nephrogenic rests, depending on their localization within the renal lobe. Both types may be further subclassified as dormant, sclerosing, adenomatous, or hyperplastic (87).

Perilobar and intralobar nephrogenic rests have different epidemiological and histological features. Perilobar nephrogenic rests are found at the periphery of the renal lobe, they are usually multifocal, sharply demarcated, and consist of blastema and tubules (Figure 8.18A). Perilobar nephrogenic rests are associated with an overgrowth syndrome, including hemihypertrophy and Beckwith–Wiedemann syndrome, and they have a lower malignant potential than intralobar nephrogenic rests.

Intralobar nephrogenic rests are randomly situated within the renal lobe, show poorly defined, irregular, and

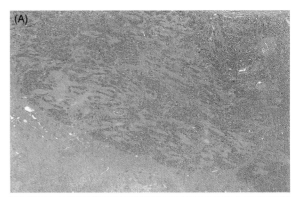

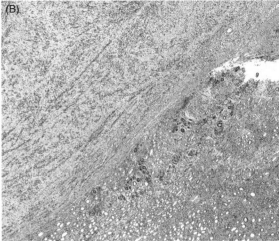

Figure 8.18 (A) Perilobar nephrogenic rest (H&E × 20). (B) Intralobar nephrogenic rest situated between tumor (up) and renal parenchyma (H&E × 20).

intermingling margins, and consist of stroma, blastema, and tubules (although stroma often predominates) (Figure 8.18B). They are associated with WAGR and Denys–Drash syndromes. Both perilobar and intralobar nephrogenic rests may become hyperplastic and it may be difficult to distinguish them from WT. However, most nephrogenic rests regress and do not develop into a tumor. If any type of nephrogenic rest is found in the kidney and/or WT, the child should be considered at increased risk for development of a tumor in the contralateral kidney. The risk is the greatest with intralobar nephrogenic rests and in children less than 12 months of age (88).

Cystic partially differentiated nephroblastoma and cystic nephroma

Cystic partially differentiated nephroblastoma and cystic nephroma are closely related completely cystic neoplasms (89). Molecular biological studies have

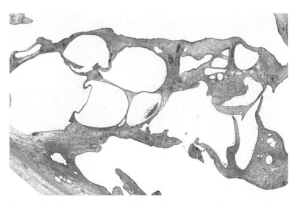

Figure 8.19 Cystic partially differentiated nephroblastoma with small groups of blastemal cells in the septa (H&E × 20).

confirmed that cystic nephroma is a neoplastic lesion rather than a congenital malformation (90). It is also associated with DICER1 mutations (91). Most cases of cystic nephroma occur under the age of four years, with a male-to-female ratio of 2:1 (92). The cystic nephroma that occurs in women over 30 years of age is now regarded as a different entity called a mixed epithelial and stromal tumor. There is also an association of cystic nephroma and pleuropulmonary blastoma, both showing DICER1 mutations (93). Cystic nephroma and cystic partially differentiated nephroblastoma occur as a solitary, unilateral, multilocular cystic lesion, usually measuring 5–10 cm in diameter, with cysts ranging in size from a few mm to 4 cm. They are sharply demarcated from the kidney, and the septa are the only solid portion of the tumor (Figure 8.19). Some WTs, and especially those treated with preoperative chemotherapy, may have a very prominent cystic appearance, which is of no prognostic significance since they require the same treatment as non-cystic WT. Other renal tumors such as mesoblastic nephroma, clear-cell sarcoma of the kidney, and rhabdoid tumor of the kidney may have a prominent cystic appearance, too. Still, the correct diagnosis can be reached if other histological features of these tumors are carefully searched for, which will be present in the septa and/or the tumor's solid areas. The prognosis for cystic nephroma/cystic partially differentiated nephroblastoma is excellent, and total nephrectomy is regarded as sufficient treatment (89).

Mesoblastic nephroma

Mesoblastic nephroma is a mesenchymal neoplasm with low malignant potential.

Clinical presentation: Mesoblastic nephroma comprises ~4% of renal tumors of childhood, but as many as 56% of renal tumors in the first three months of life, and 15% in the first six months of life (94). Nearly 90% of patients present in the first year, and the diagnosis should not be made in patients over three years of age. It usually presents as an abdominal mass and *in utero* it may present with polyhydramnios and fetal hydrops.

Genetic features: Mesoblastic nephroma is not associated with the congenital anomalies and genetic syndromes that are associated with WT. Cellular mesoblastic nephroma and infantile fibrosarcoma share the same characteristic chromosome translocation t(12;15)(p13,q25), which results in ETV6-NTRK3 gene fusion (95). Therefore, it seems logical to change terminology and rename cellular mesoblastic nephroma as infantile renal fibrosarcoma, and classical mesoblastic nephroma as infantile renal fibromatosis, but for now, the old terms are still used.

Classification: Histologically, mesoblastic nephromas can be divided into classical, cellular, and mixed types, and not infrequently more than one pattern is present.

Macroscopy: Mesoblastic nephroma appears as a unilateral, solitary mass macroscopically similar to WT. It is usually firm, but necrosis, hemorrhage, and cysts are not uncommon features. It usually grows near the renal sinus, which is often infiltrated.

Histology: There are two main histological types, including classical and cellular, but many tumors show features of both. The classical type (seen in about 22% of cases) resembles infantile fibromatosis and is composed of interlacing fascicles of bland, elongated spindle cells with rare mitoses (Figure 8.20A). It contains slit-like thin-walled blood vessels, which are scattered throughout the tumor. The tumor shows a very infiltrative growth resulting in entrapment of islands of normal renal parenchyma. The cellular type consists of densely packed, plump, slightly spindled cells with large vesicular nuclei and a moderate amount of cytoplasm (Figure 8.20B). Mitoses are usually frequent. Unlike the classical type, the cellular type has a pushing border with the renal parenchyma. The mixed type (~20% of cases) shows features of the classical and cellular types. Mesoblastic nephroma rarely presents in stage I, since in the absence of a capsule it easily infiltrates the renal sinus and perirenal fat (78).

Immunohistochemistry: It is consistently positive for markers of myofibroblasts (vimentin, desmin,

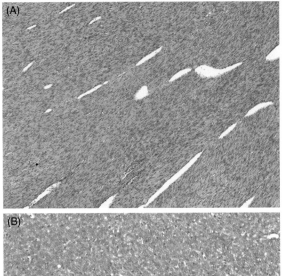

Figure 8.20 Classical (A) (H&E × 20) and cellular (B) mesoblastic nephroma (H&E × 40).

actin, and fibronectin), and negative for epithelial markers and WT (78).

Differential diagnosis: Other renal tumors of childhood have to be considered, since their treatment and prognosis vary considerably. They include pure stromal WT and clear-cell sarcoma of the kidney. It may also be difficult to distinguish metanephric stromal tumor from mesoblastic nephroma (96), but this is of no clinical significance, since their treatment and prognosis are the same. So-called "adult mesoblastic nephromas" are now recognized to represent other tumors, such as metanephric stromal tumors or mixed epithelial and stromal tumors (97).

Prognosis: Mesoblastic nephroma is generally regarded as a tumor with a very low malignant potential, and surgical removal is all that is required for its treatment. In rare cases, local recurrences and distant metastases have occurred with 12 months of the original diagnosis (98).

Clear-cell sarcoma of the kidney (CCSK)

Clear-cell sarcoma of the kidney is a malignant mesenchymal neoplasm that comprises about 3–5% of renal tumors of childhood.

Clinical presentation: It presents as an asymptomatic abdominal mass or abdominal pain. It is extremely rare in the first six months of life, and reaches its peak incidence between two and three years of age. Rare cases of CCSK in adults have also been described. It shows a male-to-female predominance of 2:1 (99).

Genetic features: Clear-cell sarcoma of the kidney is not associated with specific malformations, genetic abnormalities or syndromes associated with WT. No characteristic cytogenetic or molecular marker has been identified for clear-cell sarcoma of the kidney, but in some cases a t(10;17)(q22;p13/p12) translocation has been found, suggesting it may be involved in tumorigenesis (100). 17p13 is the site of the p53 gene, but this gene does not show abnormal expression in clear-cell sarcoma of the kidney and most likely is not involved.

Macroscopy: The tumor is always unicentric and unilateral. It varies in weight from 40 g to 3000 g. On cut surface, untreated tumors are homogeneous, firm and light brown. There is usually a distinct tumor–kidney border although there is no capsule. In some cases, when cysts are a predominant feature, it is important to distinguish CCSK from benign cystic renal lesions.

Histology: Clear-cell sarcoma of the kidney shows a spectrum of histological patterns, which are often found within the same tumor, explaining why it is one of the most commonly misdiagnosed renal tumors of childhood. The classical pattern consists of cell cords or nests separated by arborizing blood vessels within the fine septa ("chicken wire" pattern) (Figure 8.21). Tumor cells are uniform in size and distribution, with indistinct borders, and show no overlapping. The nuclei are uniform, pale with finely granular and evenly dispersed chromatin, and may appear "empty." Nucleoli are small and inconspicuous. "Clear cells" are a predominant feature in about 20% of cases, but they can be found in most tumors if adequately sampled. In many tumors there are entrapped nephrogenic elements, sometimes with cystically dilated tubules resulting in a cystic appearance. However, genuine neoplastic tubules are not a feature of CCSK. In addition to the classical pattern, CCSK may show numerous other patterns, including

Figure 8.21 Clear-cell sarcoma of the kidney (H&E × 20).

myxoid, sclerosing, cellular, epithelioid, palisading, spindled, storiform, and anaplastic (99).

Immunohistochemistry: There are no diagnostic immunohistochemical markers for CCSK. All are vimentin-positive and cytokeratin-negative, including the epithelioid pattern. WT1 and CD99 markers are also negative.

Differential diagnosis: As previously stated, CCSK is the most frequently misdiagnosed renal tumor of childhood. The main differential diagnoses include blastemal WT, rhabdoid tumor of the kidney, primitive neuroectodermal tumor, mesoblastic nephroma, and metanephric stromal tumor.

Prognosis: The majority of patients present with stage 2 (37%) or 3 (34%), while the tumor rarely presents with distant metastases (4% cases). However, subsequent metastases to various sites are seen in about 45% cases. The most common site of metastasis at the time of presentation are renal hilar lymph nodes, while bone metastases are the most common site of relapse, followed by lung metastases (99). Interestingly, in about 20% of cases metastases occur three years or more after diagnosis and some as long as 10 years later, which might be related to doxorubicin therapy, which seems to prolong the interval to relapse (99).

The only significant histological factor associated with poor prognosis in tumors that received no preoperative chemotherapy is the presence of necrosis. Favorable survival rate is associated with lower tumor stage, patient's age at diagnosis of 2–4 years of age, and treatment with doxorubicin, which improves significantly the overall survival, now around 70%, although it varies from 98% for stage I to 50% for stage 4 disease (99).

Renal rhabdoid tumor (RRT)

Renal rhabdoid tumor is a distinctive, highly malignant neoplasm that constitutes about 2% of pediatric renal tumors.

Clinical presentation: As with other renal tumors of childhood, RRT usually presents as an abdominal mass, with or without pain and hematuria. There are two striking clinical associations: hypercalcemia and the development of synchronous or metachronous primary brain tumors (101). It is never associated with nephrogenic rests or conditions and syndromes found in children with Wilms' tumor. Renal rhabdoid tumor has a distinctive predilection for infants with a median age of 11 months, with 60% of patients diagnosed under one year of age, and over 80% under two years of age. It virtually never occurs over five years of age, and in such cases other tumors showing rhabdoid-like features should be considered.

Genetic features: Molecular biology studies on RRT have shown chromosome 22q11.2 deletion, which led to the identification of the *hSNF5/INI1* tumor-suppressor gene, now regarded as the molecular hallmark of RRT. Extra-renal rhabdoid tumors that occur in soft tissue, brain, and other visceral sites share the same feature, confirming they represent the same tumor entity (102).

Macroscopy: Renal rhabdoid tumor is a unilateral and unicentric tumor, sharply demarcated from renal parenchyma; satellite nodules are frequently observed as an early manifestation of the aggressiveness of this neoplasm.

Histology: Classical RRT shows a diffuse pattern of non-cohesive sheets of cells with abundant eosinophilic cytoplasm and large eccentric nuclei with prominent eosinophilic central nucleoli (Figure 8.22). Tumor cells often have large oval intracytoplasmic hyaline inclusions composed of whorled masses of intermediate filaments. In addition, there are other patterns which may be present, with or without the classical pattern, including sclerosing, spindled, epithelioid, lymphomatoid, and vascular patterns, and which may cause diagnostic difficulties (103,104). The tumor shows a very invasive growth pattern with invasion of blood and lymphatic vessels, the renal parenchyma and the renal sinus.

Immunohistochemistry: Renal rhabdoid tumors express many markers, including vimentin, which is virtually always positive, whereas cytokeratin, epithelial membrane antigen, desmin, and neurofilaments are frequently (but not always) co-expressed, and

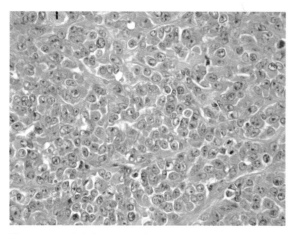

Figure 8.22 Rhabdoid tumor of the kidney with large cells and nuclei, and prominent nucleoli (H&E × 40).

they usually show patchy positivity (103,104). INI1 staining, which is positive in the nuclei of almost all other pediatric tumors, is characteristically absent in rhabdoid tumor cells.

Differential diagnosis: A number of other tumors have to be considered, including blastemal WT, cellular mesoblastic nephroma, CCSK, primitive neuroectodermal tumor, and renal carcinoma (105). However, absent INI1 immunostaining in rhabdoid tumor of the kidney is regarded as diagnostic.

Prognosis: Renal rhabdoid tumor is a very aggressive tumor with a poor prognosis, which has remained very poor, despite intensified therapeutic regimes. Over 75% of patients die within one year of diagnosis, with widespread hematogenous and lymphatic metastases (103,104). Age at diagnosis appears to be a significant factor – infants under the age of six months have a very poor prognosis (8.8% four-year survival), while survival for children two years of age or older is 41.1% (106).

Metanephric tumors

These tumors comprise a spectrum of recently recognized entities, which are classified according to the extent of their epithelial and stromal components. The entities include metanephric stromal tumor, metanephric adenofibroma, and metanephric adenoma.

Metanephric stromal tumor is composed entirely of the stromal component. The median age at diagnosis is 13 months (range 2 days to 13 years). It shows a nodular appearance resulting from hypo- and hypercellular areas. Histologically, the tumor is non-encapsulated, but with a very distinctive tumor–kidney border (unlike classical mesoblastic nephroma), and composed predominantly of spindle cells. Other characteristic features include an "onion-skin" appearance around entrapped renal tubules and blood vessels, angiodysplasia-type changes of intratumoral vessels, and juxtaglomerular cell hyperplasia. In about 20% of cases, foci of heterologous differentiation, in particular glial or cartilaginous nodules may be found. The diagnosis is based on morphological criteria and CD34 positivity of tumor cells (96).

Metanephric adenofibroma has stromal and epithelial components present in variable proportions (107). *Metanephric adenoma* is a purely epithelial lesion composed of small, well-differentiated, closely packed tubules with no nuclear atypia or mitoses. It is sharply demarcated from the adjacent renal parenchyma, but has no capsule. Age at presentation ranges from 5 to 80 years (108). Treatment of choice for all metanephric tumors is complete surgical removal and they have an excellent prognosis.

Renal-cell carcinoma (RCC) in children

Renal-cell carcinomas comprise around 1–2% of renal tumors of childhood, but present in older age than other typical pediatric renal tumors, usually around 10 years of age. They show many features not seen in adult RCCs, such as an association with congenital anomalies or syndromes (found in around one-third of cases) (109), different histological types and features (110), and specific translocations involving the *TFE3* gene located on Xp11.2 (111–114). These translocation-associated RCCs comprise over 33% of pediatric renal carcinomas, but may rarely also been seen in adults. Histologically, their typical appearance is a nested pattern, with large cells with granular eosinophilic or clear cytoplasm. Tumor cells show strong nuclear positivity for TFE3. Another translocation-associated RCC in children is t(6;11)-translocation renal cell carcinoma, which seems to be less aggressive than Xp11.2-translocation RCC (115).

Many of these tumors occur after chemotherapy treatment of neuroblastoma and WTs (116), but there is also a definite association of RCC developing after neuroblastoma, not necessarily after therapy (117), and RCC following WTs.

Adult-type renal cell carcinoma may also occur in childhood and show similar genetic changes to adult cases (118). Renal-cell carcinomas with lymph node metastases appear to have a better prognosis in children.

Renal medullary carcinoma is a highly aggressive tumor occurring in children and young adults with sickle-cell trait or disease (119,120). It belongs to the family of so-called INI1-deficient tumors, all of which show loss of INI1 protein expression, rhabdoid phenotype, and share the same poor prognosis (121). Immunohistochemistry for INI1 is negative and this is regarded as a diagnostic feature.

Other entities

Other renal tumors include very rare tumors that are either organ specific or have been known in other sites, but recently recognized in the kidney by the application of molecular biology techniques. The former group includes juxtaglomerular cell tumor (122), ossifying renal tumor of infancy (123), anaplastic sarcoma of the kidney (124), and mixed epithelial and stromal tumor of the kidney (97). The group of tumors identified by modern techniques includes primitive neuroectodermal tumor (125), synovial sarcoma (126) and desmoplastic small round-cell tumor (127).

Urinary bladder

Developmental anomalies

Bladder diverticulum

Primary bladder diverticula are thought to form because of an underlying defect in the muscular wall, usually close to the ureteral orifice. Secondary bladder diverticula result from an increased pressure within the bladder due to obstruction distal to the bladder. Causes in children include posterior urethral valves, urethral stenosis, and neurogenic bladder. Bladder diverticula also occur in association with a number of congenital syndromes (reviewed in reference 128). Excluding cases diagnosed incidentally, or in association with a congenital syndrome or a urinary tract anomaly, urinary tract infection and hydronephrosis are the commonest modes of presentation (129). The reported prevalence of bladder diverticula ranges from 1–10%; boys are three to four times more likely to be affected than girls (128,130).

Diverticula can vary significantly in size, ranging from 0.5 to 10 cm (129,130). The resected diverticulum shows an attenuated bladder wall with a thinned or absent muscle layer. Inflammation and fibrosis are also frequently encountered. Cystitis glandularis cystica and nephrogenic metaplasia (see below) are occasionally seen in children. Urothelial neoplasias, however, are highly unlikely to arise in bladder diverticula in the pediatric age group (130).

Cystitis

Infectious cystitis

Cystitis in most instances is a manifestation of a urinary tract infection caused by coliform bacteria. Underlying urinary tract abnormalities are a major predisposing factor in children. Adenovirus infection is an important cause of hemorrhagic cystitis in immunocompetent and immunocompromised children (131). Fungal infections, including candidiasis and aspergillosis, primarily occur in preterm infants or children with a primary or secondary immunodeficiency. Parasitic infections are rare in developed countries.

Cystoscopy or biopsy is not usually undertaken unless the clinical presentation is atypical or prolonged, or there is thickening of the bladder wall or a polyp or mass is apparent on imaging (bladder ultrasonography, CT or MRI), leading the clinician to suspect a malignancy.

Other inflammatory disorders of the bladder

Malakoplakia (see also above), a rare inflammatory disorder of possible infectious origin most commonly presents in the urinary bladder. Multiple soft yellow plaques or slightly raised nodules are typically seen on cystoscopy. Microscopic features are as described earlier. The differential diagnosis includes xanthogranulomatous cystitis and juvenile xanthogranuloma.

Eosinophilic cystitis is a rare cause of dysuria and hematuria in children and adults. Association with allergies and primary hypereosinophilic disorders is reported in children (132). In rare cases eosinophilic cystitis presents as an abdominal or bladder mass mimicking a malignancy (133,134). Bladder biopsy shows eosinophilic inflammation of bladder mucosa and underlying muscularis.

Interstitial cystitis is poorly recognized in children, the diagnosis is mainly based on clinical presentation with progressive, often debilitating bladder symptoms (135). Mast cells are thought to play a role in the pathogenesis of interstitial cystitis; increased numbers of mast cells and mast-cell activation are reported in bladder biopsy (136).

Tumors and tumor-like lesions

Contrary to adults, bladder tumors are rare in children. Also, the histological types encountered differ significantly from those in adults.

Epithelial (urothelial) neoplasms are rare in the pediatric population and mostly present with gross hematuria. They mostly manifest as polypoid lesions and are histologically benign or low-grade malignant lesions (137,138). Similar to adults they show a strong predilection for males, but are less likely to be multifocal, to recur, or to progress than tumors in adults. Also, the molecular pathogenesis of these tumors is thought to differ from their adult counterparts (138).

Embryonal rhabdomyosarcoma is by far the commonest bladder neoplasm children (136). Microscopic classification of rhabdomyosarcoma, molecular findings, and clinical outcome of rhabdomyosarcoma is discussed in more detail in Chapter 11.

Pseudosarcomatous myofibroblastic tumor or pseudosarcoma of the bladder is a rare but important differential diagnosis of rhabdomyosarcoma of the bladder. Unlike rhabdomyosarcoma it is usually cured by surgical excision alone (139,140). Inflammation or surgical trauma are documented as possible causative or triggering factors in some cases. Clinical presentation includes hematuria, dysuria, or bladder obstruction. Grossly, pseudosarcoma presents as a polypoid lesion or mass. Microscopic features in part overlap with those of inflammatory myofibroblastic tumor (IMFT) (140). Pseudosarcoma of the bladder typically shows a loose fascicular arrangement of large spindle cells with eosinophilic cytoplasm mimicking rhabdomyoblasts. Consistent with a myofibroblastic proliferation, there is usually staining for α-smooth-muscle and smooth muscle actin (SMA), and patchy staining for desmin. Staining for MyoD1 and myogenin, however, is always negative, allowing distinction from rhabdomyosarcoma. In inflammatory myofibroblastic tumor, immunohistochemical staining for Alk-1 and translocations involving the ALK-1 gene are demonstrated in > 50% of cases (140).

Reactive epithelial proliferations arising secondary to surgery or chronic inflammation caused by (recurrent) infection or in association with diverticula, bladder exstrophy, or stones, also can present as a polypoid lesion or mass mimicking a malignancy (141–145). Cystitis glandularis cystica is characterized by benign glandular proliferations of the bladder mucosa, rare cases presenting as a polypoid bladder mass are documented in children (141). Nephrogenic adenoma, also called nephrogenic or adenomatous metaplasia, may develop anywhere in the urinary tract. It mostly presents as a polypoid or raised lesion (142,143,145). Recurrence following surgical removal is possible

(143). Microscopic patterns described include a solid tubular, tubular cystic, papillary, or polypoid pattern (144). The lining cells are cuboidal and cytologically bland. Mitoses typically are absent or very sparse (144,145). In children, microscopic distinction from bladder carcinoma rarely is a concern, given the rarity of epithelial neoplasm in this age group.

References

1. Yosypiv IV Congenital anomalies of the kidney and urinary tract: A genetic disorder? Int. J. Nephrol, 2012:909083.

2. Ichikawa I, Kuwayama F, Pope IV JC, *et al.* Paradigm shift from classic anatomic to contemporary biological views of CAKUT. Kidney Int. 2002;**61**:889–98.

3. Liapis H, Wynyard P. Cystic diseases and developmental kidney defects. In Jennette JC, Olson JL, Schwartz MM, Silva FG, editors, *Heptinstall's Pathology of the Kidney*, sixth edn. Philadelphia, PA: Lippencott Williams & Wilkins; 2007;1257–306.

4. Pope JC VI, Brock JW III, Adams MC *et al.* How they begin and how they end: Classic and new theories for the development and deterioration of congenital anomalies of the kidney and urinary tract, CAKUT. J. Am. Soc. Nephrol. 1999;**10**:2018–28.

5. Glassberg KI. Normal and abnormal development of the kidney: A clinician's interpretation of current knowledge. J. Urol. 2002;**167**:2339–51.

6. Bonsib SM. The classification of renal cystic diseases and other congenital malformations of the kidney and urinary tract. Arch. Pathol. Lab. Med. 2010;**134**:554–68.

7. Renkema KY, Winyard PJ, Skovorodkin IN, *et al.* EUCAKUT consortium. Novel perspectives for investigating congenital anomalies of the kidney and urinary tract (CAKUT). Nephrol. Dial. Transplant. 2011;**26**:3843–51.

8. Gunay-Aygun M. Liver and kidney disease in ciliopathies. Am. J. Med. Genet. C Semin. Med. Genet. 2009;**151C**:296–306.

9. Hildebrandt F, Benzing T, Katsanis N. Ciliopathies. N. Engl. J. Med. 2011;**364**:1533–43.

10. Narchi H. Risk of Wilm's tumor with multicystic kidney disease: A systematic review. Arch. Dis. Child. 2005;**90**:147–9.

11. De Oliveira-Filho AG, Carvalho MH, Sbragia-Neto L, *et al.* Wilms tumor in a prenatally diagnosed multicystic kidney. J. Urol. 1997;**158**:1926–7.

12. Kirkpatrick B-E, El-Kechen D. A unique presentation of 22q13 deletion syndrome: multicystic kidney, orofacial clefting and Wilms tumor. Clin. Dysmorphol. 2011;**20**:53–4.

13. Glassberg KI, Stephens FD, Lebowitz RL, *et al.* Renal dysgenesis and cystic disease of the kidney: A report of the Committee on Terminology, Nomenclature and Classification, Section on Urology, American Academy of Pediatrics. J. Urol. 1987;**138**:1085–92.

14. Bernstein J. The morphogenesis of renal parenchymal maldevelopment (renal dysplasia). Pediatr. Clin. North Am., 1971;**18**:395–407.

15. Risdon RA. Renal dysplasia. I. A clinico-pathological study of 76 cases. J. Clin. Pathol. 1971;**24**:57–71.

16. Damen-Elias HA, Sotuentbeck PH, Visser GH, *et al.* Concomitant anomalies in 100 children with unilateral multicystic kidney. Ultrasound Obstet. Gynecol. 2005; **25**: 384–8.

17. Risdon RA, Young LW, Chrispin AR. Renal hypoplasia and dysplasia: A radiological and pathological correlation. Pediatr. Radiol. 1975;**15**:213–25.

18. de Klerk DP, Marshall FF, Jeffs RD. Multicystic dysplastic kidney. J. Urol. 1977;**118**:306–8.

19. Mesrobian H-G, Rushton HG, Bulas D. Unilateral regression of multicystic renal dysplasia. J. Urol. 1993;**150**:793–94.

20. Ranke A, Schmitt M, Didier F, *et al.* Antenatal diagnosis of multicystic renal dysplasia. Eur. J. Pediatr. Surg. 2001; **11**:246–54.

21. Sukthankar S, Watson AR. Unilateral multicystic kidney disease: defining the natural history. Acta Paediatr. 2000;**89**:811–13.

22. van Eijk L, Cohen Overbeek TE, den Hollander NS, *et al.* Unilateral multicystic dysplastic kidney: A combined pre- and postnatal assessment. Ultrasound Obstet. Gynecol. 2002;**19**:180–3.

23. Eckoldt F, Woderich R, Smith RD, *et al.* Antenatal diagnostic aspects of unilateral multicystic kidney dysplasia. Fetal Diagn. Therapy 2004;**19**:163–9.

24. Winyard P, Chitty LS. Dysplastic kidneys. Semin. Fetal Neonatal. Med. 2008;**13**:142–517.

25. Damen-Elias HA, De Jong TP, Stigter RH, *et al.* Congenital renal tract anomalies: outcome and follow up of 402 cases detected antenatally between 1986 and 2001. Ultrasound Obstet. Gynecol. 2005;**25**:134–43.

26. Kiyak A, Yilmaz A, Turhan P, *et al.* Unilateral multicystic kidney: single-center experience. Pediatr. Nephrol. 2009;**24**:99–104.

27. Baggenstoss AH. Congenital anomalies of the kidney. Med. Clin. North Am. 1951;**1**:987–1004.

28. Boissonat P. What to call hypoplastic kidney. Arch. Dis. Child. 1962;**37**:142–92.

29. Adelman RD, Shapiro S. Bilateral renal hypoplasia with oligomeganephromania. Urology 1977;**9**:571–5.

30. Park SH, Chi JG Oligomeganephromania associated with 4p deletion type chromosomal anomaly. Pediatr. Pathol. 1993;**13**:731–40.

31. Salomon R, Tellier AL, Attie-Bitach T, *et al.* PAX-2 mutations in oligomeganephromania. Kidney Int. 2001;**59**:457–62.

32. Skinner MA, Safford SD, Reeves JG, *et al.* Renal aplasia in humans is associated with RET mutations. Am. J. Hum. Genet. 2008;**82**:344–51.

33. Jeanpierre C, Macé G, Parisot M, *et al.* Société Française de Foetopathologie. RET and GDNF mutations are rare in fetuses with renal agenesis or other severe kidney development defects. J. Med. Genet. 2011;**48**:497–504.

34. Bailey RR. The relationship of vesico-ureteric reflux to urinary tract infection and chronic pyelonephritis-reflux nephropathy. Clin. Nephrol. 1973;**1**:132–41.

35. Yeung CK, Godley ML, Dhillon HK, *et al.* The characteristics of primary vesico-ureteric reflux in male and female infants with pre-natal hydronephrosis. Br. J. Urol. 1997;**80**:319–27.

36. Birmingham reflux study group. Prospective trial of operative vs. non-operative treatment of severe vesicourtecric rcflux in children: five year's observation. Br. Med. J. (Clin. Res. Ed.) 1987;**295**:237–41.

37. Chertin B, Puri P. Familial vesicoureteral reflux. J. Urol. 2003;**169**:1804–8.

38. Gramellini D, Fieni S, Caforio E, *et al.* Diagnostic accuracy of fetal renal pelvis anteroposterior diameter as a predictor of significant postnatal nephrouropathy: second vs. third trimester of pregnancy. Am. J. Obstet. Gynecol. 2006;**194**:167–73.

39. Pinter AB, Horvath A, Hrabovszky Z. The relationship of smooth muscle damage to age, severity of pre-operative hydronephrosis and post-operative outcome in obstructive uropathies. Br. J. Urol. 1997;**80**:227–33.

40. Quinn FMJ, Dick AC, Corbally MT, *et al.* Xanthogranulomatous pyelonephritis in childhood. Arch. Dis. Child. 1999;**81**:483–6.

41. Duffy SP, Capps S, Nouriquand D *et al.* Xanthogranulomatous pyelonephritis in childhood. J. Pediatr. Surg. 2001;**36**:598–601.

42. Gubler MC. Renal tubular dysgenesis. Pediatr. Nephrol. 2014;**29**:51–9.

43. Gribouval O, Moriniere V, Pawtoski A, *et al.* Spectrum of mutations in the renin-angiotensin system genes in autosomal recessive renal tubular dysgenesis. Hum. Mut. 2012;**33**:316–26.

44. Bonilla SF, Melin-Aldenha H, Whitington PF. Relationship of proximal tubular dysgenesis and fetal liver injury in neonatal hemochromatosis. Pediatr. Res. 2010;**67**:188–93.

45. Collardeau-Franchon S, Heissat S, Bouvier R, *et al.* French retrospective multicentric study of neonatal hemochromatosis: importance of autopsy and autoimmune maternal manifestations. Pediatr. Dev. Pathol. 2012;**15**:450–70.

46. Leong MY, Walford N, Varanasi VR, *et al.* Another case of concomitant fetal renal tubular dysgenesis and placental massive perivillous fibrin deposition. Pediatr. Dev. Pathol. 2013;**16**:447–9.

47. Linn RL, Kiley J, Minturn L. Recurrent massive perivillous fibrin deposition in the placenta associated with fetal renal tubular dysgenesis. A case report and literature review. Pediatr. Dev. Pathol 2013;**16**:378–86.

48. Buttar HS An overview of the influence of ACE inhibitors on fetal-placental circulation and perinatal development. Mol. Cell Biochem. 1997;**176**:61–71.

49. Watnick T, Germin G. From cilia to cyst. Nat. Genet. 2003;**34**:355–6.

50. Gresh L, Fischer E, Reimann A, *et al.* A transcriptional network in polycystic kidney disease. EMBO J. 2004;**23**:1657–68.

51. Hiesberger T, Bai Y, Shao X, *et al.* Mutation of hepatocyte nuclear factor-1beta inhibits Pkhd1 gene expression and produces renal cysts in mice. J. Clin. Invest. 2004;**113**:814–25.

52. Schieren G, Rumberger B, Klein M, *et al.* Gene profiling of polycystic kidneys. Nephrol. Dial. Transplant. 2006;**21**:1816–24.

53. Hildebrandt F, Zhou W. Nephronophthisis associated ciliopathies. J. Am. Soc. Nephrol. 2007;**18**:1855–71.

54. Lennerz JK, Spence DC, Iskandar SS, Dehner LP, Liapis H. Glomerulocystic kidney: one hundred-year perspective. Arch. Pathol. Lab. Med. 2010;**134**:583–605.

55. Deltas C, Papagregoriou G. Cystic diseases of the kidney: molecular biology and genetics. Arch. Pathol. Lab. Med. 2010;**134**:569–82.

56. Benzing T, Schermer B. Clinical spectrum and pathogenesis of nephronophthisis. Curr. Opin. Nephrol. Hypertens. 2012;**21**:272–8.

57. Ferkol TW, Leigh MW. Ciliopathies: the central role of cilia in a spectrum of pediatric disorders. J. Pediatr. 2012;**160**:366–71.

58. Salomon R, Saunier S, Niaudet P. Nephronophthisis. Pediatr. Nephrol. 2009;**24**:2333–44.

59. Dell KM. The spectrum of polycystic kidney disease in children. Adv. Chronic Kidney Dis. 2011;**18**:339–47.

60. Desmet VJ. Ludwig symposium on biliary disorders, part I. Pathogenesis of ductal plate abnormalities. Mayo Clin. Proc. 1998;**73**:80–9.

61. Birch JM, Breslow N. Epidemiological features of Wilms tumor. Hematol. Oncol. Clin. North Am. 1995;**9**:1157–78.

62. Stiller CA, Parkin DJ. International variations in the incidence of childhood renal tumors. Br. J. Cancer 1990;**62**:1026–30.

63. Ritchey ML, Azizkhan RG, Beckwith JB, Hrabovsky EE, Haase GM. Neonatal Wilms' tumor. J. Pediatr. Surg. 1995;**30**:856–59.

64. Reinhard H, Aliani S, Ruebe C, *et al.* Wilms' tumor in adults: results of the Society of Pediatric Oncology (SIOP) 93–10/Society for Pediatric Oncology and Hematology (GPOH) study. J. Clin. Oncol. 2004;**22**:4500–06.

65. Breslow N, Olshan A, Beckwith JB, Green DM. Epidemiology of Wilms tumor. Med. Pediatr. Oncol. 1993;**21**:172–81.

66. Coppes MJ, de Kraker J, Van Dijken PJ, *et al.* Bilateral Wilms' tumor: long-term survival and some epidemiological features. J. Clin. Oncol. 1989;**7**:310–15.

67. Coppes MJ, Wilson PC, Weitzman S. Extrarenal Wilms' tumor: staging, treatment, and prognosis. J. Clin. Pathol 1991;**9**:167–74.

68. Sinniah D, D'Angio GJ, Eds. *Atlas of Pediatric Oncology.* London: Arnold; 1996;129–43.

69. Pritchard-Jones K, Vujanic GM. Recent developments in the molecular pathology of paediatric renal tumors. Open Pathol. J. 2010;**4**:32–9.

70. Dome JS, Coppes MJ. Recent advances in Wilms tumor genetics. Curr. Opin. Pediatr. 2002;**14**:5–11.

71. Little SE, Hanks SP, King-Underwood L, *et al.* Frequency and heritability of WT1 mutations in nonsyndromic Wilms' tumor patients: A UK Children's Cancer Study Group. J. Clin. Oncol. 2004;**22**:4140–46.

72. Ruteshouser EC, Huff V. Familial Wilms tumor. Am. J. Med. Genet. C Semin. Med. Genet. 2004;**129**:29–34.

73. Scott RH, Stiller CA, Walker L, Rahman N. Syndromes and constitutional chromosomal abnormalities associated with Wilms' tumor. J. Med. Genet. 2006;**43**:705–15.

74. Grundy PE, Breslow NE, Li S, *et al.* Loss of heterozygosity for chromosome 1p and 16q is an adverse prognostic factor in favourable-histology Wilms tumor: A report from the National Wilms Tumor Study Group. J. Clin. Oncol. 2005;**23**:7312–21.

75. Vujanic GM, Sandstedt B, Harms D, *et al.* Revised International Society of Paediatric Oncology (SIOP) working classification of renal tumors of childhood. Med. Pediatr. Oncol. 2001;**38**:79–82.

76. Gratias EJ, Dome JS. Current and emerging chemotherapy treatment strategies for Wilms tumor in North America. Pediatr. Drugs 2008;**10**:115–24.

77. Vujanic GM, Sandstedt B. The pathology of nephroblastoma: the SIOP approach. J. Clin. Pathol. 2010;**63**:102–9.

78. Murphy WM, Grignon DJ, Perlman EJ. Kidney tumors in children. In *Tumors of the Kidney, Bladder, and Urinary Structures, Atlas of Tumor Pathology*, fourth series, fascicle 1, Washington DC: Armed Forces Institute of Pathology, 2004:1–47.

79. Faria P, Beckwith JB, Mishra K, *et al.* Focal vs. diffuse anaplasia in Wilms tumor – new definitions with prognostic significance. A report from the national Wilms study group. Am J. Surg. Pathol. 1996;**20**:909–20.

80. Bardeesy N, Falkoff D, Petruzzi MJ, *et al.* Anaplastic Wilms' tumor, a subtype displaying poor prognosis, harbours p53 gene mutation. Nat. Genet. 1994;**7**:91–7.

81. Dome JS, Cotton CA, Perlman EJ, *et al.* Treatment of anaplastic histology Wilms' tumor: results from the fifth national Wilms' tumor study. J. Clin. Oncol. 2006;**24**:2352–58.

82. Popov SD, Vujanic GM, Sebire NJ. Bilateral Wilms tumor with TP53 related anaplasia. Pediatr. Develop. Pathol. 2013;**16**:217–23.

83. Boccon-Gibod L, Rey A, Sandstedt B, *et al.* Complete necrosis induced by preoperative chemotherapy in Wilms' tumor as an indicator of low risk: Report of the International Society of Paediatric Oncology (SIOP) Wilms' tumor trial and study 9. Med. Pediatr. Oncol. 2000;**34**:183–90.

84. Vujanic GM, Sandstedt B, Kelsey A, *et al.* Central pathology review in multicentre trials and studies: lessons from nephroblastoma trials. Cancer 2009;**115**:1977–83.

85. Muir TE, Cheville JC, Lager DJ. Metanephric adenoma, nephrogenic rests, and Wilms' tumor: A histologic and immunophenotypic comparison. Am. J. Surg. Pathol. 2001;**25**:1290–96.

86. Wang LL, Perlman EJ, Vujanic GM, *et al.* Desmoplastic small round-cell tumor of the kidney in childhood. Am. J. Surg. Pathol. 2007;**31**:576–84.

87. Beckwith JB. Precursor lesions of Wilms tumor: clinical and biological implications. Med. Pediatr. Oncol. 1993;**21**:158–68.

88. Coppes MJ, Arnold M, Beckwith JB, *et al.* Factors affecting the risk of contralateral Wilms tumor development: A report from the National Wilms Tumor Study Group. Cancer 1999;**85**:1616–25.

89. Joshi VV, Beckwith JB. Multilocular cyst of the kidney (cystic nephroma) and cystic, partially differentiated nephroblastoma: terminology and criteria for diagnosis. Cancer 1989;**64**:466–79.

90. Kanomata N, Eble JN, Halling K. Nonrandom X chromosome inactivation in cystic nephroma demonstrates the neoplastic nature of these tumors. J. Urol. Pathol. 1997;**7**:81–9.

91. Schultze-Florey RE, Graf N, Vorwerk P, *et al.* DICER1 syndrome: A new cancer syndrome. Clin. Padiatr. 2013;**225**:177–8.

92. Eble JN, Bonsib SM. Extensively cystic renal neoplasms: cystic nephroma, cystic partially differentiated nephroblastoma, multilocular cystic renal cell carcinoma, and cystic hamartoma of renal pelvis. Sem. Diagn. Pathol. 1998;**15**:2–20.

93. Boman F, Hill DA, Williams GM, *et al.* Familial association of pleuropulmonary blastema with cystic nephroma and other renal tumors: A report from the International Pleuropulmonary Blastoma Registry. J. Pediatr. 2006;**149**:850–4.

94. Van den Heuvel-Eibrink MM, Grundy P, Graf N, *et al.* Characteristics and survival of 750 children diagnosed with a renal tumor in the first seven months of life: A collaborative study by the SIOP/GPOH/SFOP, NWTSG, and UKCCSG Wilms tumor study groups. Pediatr. Blood Cancer 2008;**50**:1130–4.

95. Knezevich SR, Garnett MJ, Pysher TJ, *et al.* ETV6-NTRK3 gene fusions and trisomy 11 establish a histogenetic link between mesoblastic nephroma and congenital fibrosarcoma. Cancer Res. 1998;**58**:5046–48.

96. Argani P, Beckwith JB. Metanephric stromal tumor: report of 31 cases of a distinctive pediatric renal neoplasm. Am. J. Surg. Pathol. 2000;**24**:917–26.

97. Michal M, Hes O, Bisceglia M, *et al.* Mixed epithelial and stromal tumors of the kidney: A report of 22 cases. Virchows Arch. 2004;**445**:359–67.

98. Beckwith JB. Letter to editor. Pediatr. Pathol. 1993;**13**:886–7.

99. Argani P, Perlman EJ, Breslow NE, *et al.* Clear cell sarcoma of the kidney: A review of 351 cases from the National Wilms Tumor Study Group Pathology Center. Am. J. Surg. Pathol. 2000;**24**:4–18.

100. Brownlee NA, Perkins LA, Stewart W, *et al.* Recurring translocation (10;17) and deletion (14q) in clear cell sarcoma of the kidney. Arch. Path. Lab. Med. 2007;**131**:446–51.

101. Bonnin JM, Rubinstein LJ, Palmer NF, *et al.* The association of embryonal tumors originating in the kidney and in the brain. Cancer 1984;**54**:2137–46.

102. Hoot AC, Rus P, Judkins AR, *et al.* Immunohistochemical analysis of hSNF5/INI1 distinguishes renal and extra-renal malignant rhabdoid tumors from other pediatric soft tissue tumors. Am. J. Surg. Pathol. 2004;**28**:1485–91.

103. Weeks DA, Beckwith JB, Mierau GW, *et al.* Rhabdoid tumor of kidney. A report of 111 cases from the

299

National Wilms' Tumor Study Pathology Center. Am. J. Surg. Pathol. 1989;**13**:439–58.

104. Vujanic GM, Sandstedt B, Harms D, *et al.* Rhabdoid tumour of the kidney: A clinicopathological study of 22 patients from the International Society of Paediatric Oncology (SIOP) nephroblastoma file. Histopathology 1996;**28**:333–40.

105. Weeks DA, Beckwith JB, Mierau GW, *et al.* Renal neoplasms mimicking rhabdoid tumor of kidney. A report from the National Wilms' Tumor Study Pathology Center. Am. J. Surg. Pathol. 1991;**15**:1042–54.

106. Tomplison GE, Breslow NE, Dome J, *et al.* Rhabdoid tumor of the kidney in the National Wilms' Tumor Group: Age at diagnosis as a prognostic factor. J. Clin. Oncol. 2005;**23**:7641–45.

107. Arroyo MR, Green DM, Perlman EJ, *et al.* The spectrum of metanephric adenofibroma and related lesions: clinicopathologic study of 25 cases from the National Wilms Tumor Study Group Pathology Center. Am. J. Surg. Pathol. 2001;**25**:433–44.

108. Davis CJ, Jr., Barton JH, Sesterhenn IA, *et al.* Metanephric adenoma. Clinicopathological study of fifty patients. Am. J. Surg. Pathol. 1995;**19**:1101–14.

109. Selle B, Furtwangler R, Graf N, *et al.* Population-based study of renal cell carcinoma in children in Germany, 1980–2005: more frequently localized tumors and underlying disorders compared with adult counterparts. Cancer 2006;**19**:1420–26.

110. Bruder E, Passera O, Harms D, *et al.* Morphologic and molecular characterization of renal cell carcinoma in children and young adults. Am. J. Surg. Pathol. 2004;**28**:1117–32.

111. Argani P, Antonescu CR, Couturier J, *et al.* PRCC-TFE3 renal carcinomas: morphologic, immunohistochemical, ultrastructural, and molecular analysis of an entity associated with the t(X;1)(p11.2; q21). Am. J. Surg. Pathol. 2002;**26**:1553–66.

112. Ramphal R, Pappo A, Zielenska M, *et al.* Pediatric renal cell carcinoma: clinical, pathologic, and molecular abnormalities associated with the members of the mit transcription factor family. Am. J. Clin. Pathol. 2006;**126**:349–64.

113. Argani P, Ladanyi M. Distinctive neoplasms characterised by specific chromosomal translocations comprise a significant proportion of paediatric renal cell carcinomas. Pathology 2003;**35**:492–98.

114. Renshaw AA, Granter SR, Fletcher JA, *et al.* Renal cell carcinomas in children and young adults: increased incidence of papillary architecture and unique subtypes. Am J. Surg. Pathol. 1999;**23**:795–802.

115. Argani P, Lae M, Hutchinson B, *et al.* Renal carcinomas with the t(6;11)(p21;q12):

clinicopathologic features and demonstration of the specific α-TFEB gene fusion by immunohistochemistry, RT-PCR, and DNA PCR. Am. J. Surg. Pathol. 2005;**29**:230–40.

116. Argani P, Lae M, Ballard ET, *et al.* Translocation carcinomas of the kidney after chemotherapy in childhood. J. Clin. Oncol. 2006;**24**:1529–34.

117. Medeiros LJ, Palmedo G, Krigman HR, *et al.* Oncocytoid renal cell carcinoma after neuroblastoma: A report of four cases of a distinct clinicopathologic entity. Am. J. Surg. Pathol. 1999;**23**:772–80.

118. Soller MJ, Kullendirf CM, Bekassy AN, *et al.* Cytogenetic findings in pediatric renal cell carcinoma. Cancer Genet. Cytogenet. 2007;**173**:75–80.

119. Davis CJ, Jr., Mostofi FK, Sesterhenn IA. Renal medullary carcinoma. The seventh sickle cell nephropathy. Am. J. Surg. Pathol. 1995;**19**:1–11.

120. Swartz MA, Karth J, Schneider DT, *et al.* Renal medullary carcinoma: clinical, pathologic, immunohistochemical, and genetic analysis with pathogenetic implications. Urology 2002;**60**:1083–89.

121. Hollmann TJ, Horncik JL. INI1-deficient tumors: diagnostic features and molecular genetics. Am. J. Surg. Pathol. 2013; **35**: e47–63.

122. Martin SA, Mynderse LA, Lager DJ, *et al.* Juxtaglomerular cell tumor: A clinicopathologic study of four cases and review of the literature. Am. J. Clin. Pathol. 2001;**116**:854 63.

123. Sotelo-Avila C. BJB, Johnson JE. Ossifying Renal Tumor of Infancy. Pediatr. Pathol. Lab. Med. 1995;**15**:745 62.

124. Vujanic GM, Kelsey A, Perlman EJ, *et al.* Anaplastic sarcoma of the kidney: A clinicopathologic study of 20 cases of a new entity with polyphenotypic features. Am J. Surg. Pathol. 2007;**31**:1459–68.

125. Jimenez RE, Folpe AL, Lapham RL, *et al.* Primary Ewing's sarcoma/primitive neuroectodermal tumor of the kidney: A clinicopathologic and immunohistochemical analysis of 11 cases. Am. J. Surg. Pathol. 2002;**26**:320–7.

126. Argani P, Faria PA, Epstein JI, *et al.* Primary renal synovial sarcoma: molecular and morphologic delineation of an entity previously included among embryonal sarcomas of the kidney. Am. J. Surg. Pathol. 2000;**24**:1087–96.

127. Wang LL, Perlman EJ, Vujanic GM, *et al.* Desmoplastic small round-cell tumor of the kidney in childhood. Am. J. Surg. Pathol. 2007;**31**:576–84.

128. Psutka SP, Cendron M. Bladder diverticula in children. J. Pediatr. Urol. 2013;**9**(2):129–38.

129. Alexander RE, Kum JB, Idrees M. Bladder diverticulum: clinicopathologic spectrum in pediatric patients. Pediatr. Dev. Pathol. 2012;**15**(4):281–5.

130. Idrees MT, Alexander RE, Kum JB, *et al.* The spectrum of histopathologic findings in vesical diverticulum: implications for pathogenesis and staging. Hum. Pathol. 2013;**44**(7):1223–32.

131. Allen CW, Alexander SI. Adenovirus associated haematuria. Arch. Dis. Child. 2005;**90**(3):305–6.

132. Thompson RH, Dicks D, Kramer SA. Clinical manifestations and functional outcomes in children with eosinophilic cystitis. J. Urol. 2005;**174**(6):2347–9.

133. Gerharz EW, Grueber M, Melekos MD, *et al.* Tumor-forming eosinophilic cystitis in children. Case report and review of literature. Eur. Urol. 1994;**25**(2):138–41.

134. Verhagen PC, Nikkels PG, de Jong TP. Eosinophilic cystitis. Arch. Dis. Child. 2001;**84**(4):344–6.

135. Yoost JL, Hertweck SP, Loveless M. Diagnosis and treatment of interstitial cystitis in adolescents. J. Pediatr. Adolesc Gynecol. 2012;**25**(3):162–71.

136. Sant GR, Kempuraj D, Marchand JE, *et al.* The mast cell in interstitial cystitis: role in pathophysiology and pathogenesis. Urology 2007;**69**(4 Suppl):34–40.

137. Huppmann AR, Pawel BR. Polyps and masses of the pediatric urinary bladder: A 21-year pathology review. Pediatr. Dev. Pathol. 2011;**14**(6):438–44.

138. Williamson SR, Lopez-Beltran A, MacLennan GT, *et al.* Unique clinicopathologic and molecular characteristics of urinary bladder tumors in children and young adults. Urol. Oncol. 2013;**31**(4):414–26.

139. Meyer S, Bruce J, Kelsey A, *et al.* Pseudosarcoma of the bladder associated with residual urachus in a 3-year-old girl. Pediatr. Surg. Int. 2000;**16**(8):604–6.

140. Alquati S, Gira FA, Bartoli V, *et al.* Low-grade myofibroblastic proliferations of the urinary bladder. Arch. Pathol. Lab. Med. 2013;**137**(8):1117–28.

141. Defoor W, Minevich E, Sheldon C. Unusual bladder masses in children. Urology 2002;**60**(5):911.

142. Jéquier S, Bugmann P, Bründler MA. Nephrogenic adenoma of the bladder: ultrasound demonstration. A case report. Pediatr. Radiol. 1999;**29**(3):185–7.

143. Crook TJ, Mead Z, Vadgama B, *et al.* A case series of nephrogenic adenoma of the urethra and bladder in children: review of this rare diagnosis, its natural history and management, with reference to the literature. J. Pediatr. Urol. 2006;**2**(4):323–8.

144. Kao CS, Kum JB, Fan R, *et al.* Nephrogenic adenomas in pediatric patients: A morphologic and immunohistochemical study of 21 cases. Pediatr. Dev. Pathol. 2013;**16**(2):80–5.

145. Oliva E, Young RH. Nephrogenic adenoma of the urinary tract: A review of the microscopic appearance of 80 cases with emphasis on unusual features. Mod. Pathol. 1995;**8**(7):722–30.

Reproductive system

Katja Gwin, Naveena Singh, Allison Cavallo, and Miguel Reyes-Múgica

Female reproductive system

Ovary

Non-neoplastic disorders of the ovary

Congenital anomalies of the ovary and the fallopian tube

Clinical presentation: The absence of ovaries and fallopian tubes may be caused by complete necrosis resulting from torsion or may be related to disturbed development of the Müllerian ducts (1). Additionally, tubal duplication or partial atresia can occur. Structural abnormalities of the fallopian tube have been described in association with *in utero* exposure to diethylstilbestrol (DES) (2).

Congenital and neonatal follicular ovarian cysts

Ovarian cysts are the most common cause of abdominal masses in newborns, and of adnexal lesions in adolescence (3). They develop in response to maternal hormonal stimulation and spontaneously resolve by six months due to decreasing hormone levels.

Hereditary/genetic features: Functional ovarian cysts with pseudoprecocious puberty may occur as part of McCune–Albright syndrome (polyostotic fibrous dysplasia, *café au lait* skin pigmentation, and endocrine hyperfunction) (4), caused by a mutation in the *GNAS1* gene (5).

Macroscopy: Follicular cysts are thin-walled, unilocular, and contain serosanguinous fluid.

Histology: Follicular cysts are composed of an inner layer of luteinized theca-granulosa cells and an outer theca interna layer.

Differential diagnosis: Cystic granulosa cell tumors are significantly larger than follicular cysts and present a disorderly pattern of granulosa and theca cells.

Polycystic ovarian syndrome (PCOS)

Criteria for the diagnosis of PCOS (6,7) are inappropriate gonadotropin secretion and hyperandrogenism, together with ovarian dysfunction.

Clinical presentation: In childhood, PCOS may present with pseudoprecocious puberty and obesity, while in adolescence, menstrual irregularities and androgenic symptoms dominate. The diagnosis is based on increased androgen levels, hyperinsulinemia, and elevated levels of luteinizing hormone (6). The presence of polycystic ovaries is not required.

Hereditary/genetic features: PCOS may show familiar clustering and is thought to be the result of an interplay of environmental factors with genetic predisposition (8).

Macroscopy: The ovaries are enlarged due to multiple symmetrically placed, even-sized follicles and exhibit thickened, capsule-like cortices.

Histology: The outer ovarian cortex reveals a fibrotic stroma that can extend to the medulla. The follicles exhibit prominent, luteinized outer theca interna layers and inner layers of granulosa cells.

Differential diagnosis: In contrast to PCOS, multiple sporadic follicular cysts are more variable in size and do not have the fibrotic superficial cortex.

Massive ovarian edema (including fibromatosis)

Ovarian tumor-like enlargement due to the accumulation of edematous fluid.

Clinical presentation: Massive ovarian edema typically occurs in adolescents and young women, but has been described in babies and infants (9,10). The clinical presentation is variable and includes pelvic pain, an abdominal mass, or hormonal manifestations. Massive ovarian edema and fibromatosis likely represent a spectrum of the same disease (11).

Essentials of Surgical Pediatric Pathology, ed. Marta C. Cohen and Irene Scheimberg. Published by Cambridge University Press.
© Cambridge University Press 2014.

Macroscopy: The ovary is enlarged with a smooth, gray, and edematous surface. In ovarian fibromatosis, the gray-white cut surface is smooth with a lobulated appearance.

Histology: Central edematous, hypocellular stroma that surrounds and separates the developing follicles, but spares the outer cortex. In ovarian fibromatosis, the follicular structures are preserved and surrounded by a diffuse, fibrotic spindle-cell proliferation.

Differential diagnosis: Massive ovarian edema can resemble sclerosing stromal tumors, Krukenberg tumors, and other ovarian neoplasms with edematous features. In massive edema and ovarian fibromatosis, the preserved follicular structures are diffusely surrounded by the stroma, which is not seen in the other entities.

Autoimmune oophoritis

Autoimmune-related inflammation resulting in ovarian failure.

Clinical presentation: Approximately 10% of cases of premature ovarian failure are related to autoimmune oophoritis, which is frequently seen in polyglandular autoimmune syndromes (12). Chronic inflammation causes ovarian destruction and failure. In polyglandular autoimmune syndrome type I (PAS-1), which is characterized by adrenal insufficiency, hypoparathyroidism, and chronic mucocutaneous candidiasis, ovarian failure can occur before menarche and result in primary amenorrhea (13). Autoimmune oophoritis also occurs in females with other autoimmune diseases or can be idiopathic.

Hereditary/genetic features: PAS-1 is an autosomal recessive disease associated with autoimmune regulator (AIRE) gene mutations (14).

Histology: There is folliculotropic lymphoplasmacytic infiltrate, the density of which correlates with the degree of follicular maturation and is most prominent in the theca interna. Primordial follicles are spared.

Neoplasms of the ovary

Approximately half of all childhood ovarian lesions are neoplastic. Approximately 10% of these are malignant, accounting for 1% of all childhood cancer. Germ-cell tumors represent 40%.

Germ-cell tumors

They arise from primitive germ cells of the embryonic gonad.

Immunohistochemistry: Placental alkaline phosphatase (PLAP) is at least focally expressed in all germ-cell tumors. Sal-like protein (SALL4) is a marker for ovarian primitive germ-cell tumors (15).

Dysgerminoma

Dysgerminoma is composed of tumor cells resembling primordial germ cells.

Clinical presentation: The most common malignant germ-cell tumor, accounting for 3–5% of all ovarian cancers (16). It typically occurs in young women (median age of 22 years), but has been reported in infants (17). Serum lactate dehydrogenase is frequently elevated (18). Human chorionic gonadotropin (hCG) is elevated in 3–5% of cases (19). Dysgerminoma is a usually a unilateral, rapidly growing tumor with metastatic potential that responds well to chemo- and radiotherapy. Metastatic spread occurs frequently via the lymphatic route. The prognosis is excellent for unilateral, encapsulated tumors (20,21).

Hereditary/genetic features: C-KIT mutations tend to occur in advanced-stage tumors (16).

Macroscopy: Well-circumscribed, encapsulated tumor with a solid, lobular cut surface. Areas of necrosis, cystic change, and calcification may be present.

Histology: The architectural pattern shows tumor cells arranged in sheets or nests separated by fibrous stroma. The large, polygonal tumor cells have distinct cell membranes, eosinophilic cytoplasm, round nuclei, and prominent nucleoli (Figure 9.1). Mitotic activity is variable; focal hemorrhage and necrosis are common. The stromal septa are infiltrated with lymphocytes. Syncytiotrophoblastic cells can be identified in 5% of tumors. Areas of calcifications or gonadoblastoma should raise concerns for underlying disorders of sex development (DSD). Dysgerminoma is positive for PLAP, octamer-binding protein (OCT) 3/4, C-kit proto-oncogene product (CD117), SALL4, and D2–40. Rare cells can express low-molecular-weight keratins.

Differential diagnosis: Placental alkaline phosphatase can differentiate dysgerminoma from a non-germ-cell tumor such as clear-cell carcinoma or a large-cell lymphoma. OCT3/4 is only positive in dysgerminomas and embryonal carcinoma (EC) and offers more specificity. Low-molecular-weight keratin helps in the differential diagnosis from EC and yolk-sac tumor (YST) where is diffusely positive, vs. dysgerminoma, where it is focally positive; D2–40 is only positive in dysgerminoma. Dysgerminoma is negative for inhibin, distinguishing it from steroid-cell tumors.

303

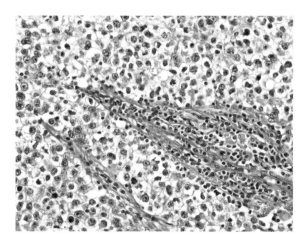

Figure 9.1 Dysgerminoma composed of large, polygonal tumor cells with distinct cell membranes, clear cytoplasm, round nuclei, and prominent nucleoli. Note infiltration by mature lymphocytes.

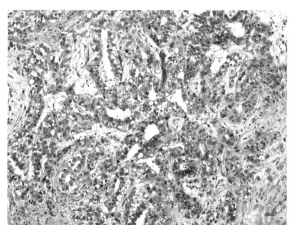

Figure 9.2 Yolk-sac tumor showing a reticular/microcystic pattern composed of a loose myxoid stroma associated with lacunar spaces lined by atypical attenuated epithelium.

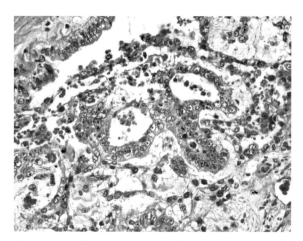

Figure 9.3 Schiller–Duval body in a yolk-sac tumor, including papillary projection with a central vascular core and an outer layer of cuboidal, embryonic cells.

Yolk-sac tumor (YST) (endodermal sinus tumor)

Yolk-sac tumor is a malignant germ-cell tumor assumed to arise from undifferentiated, multipotential embryonal carcinoma, which can selectively differentiate into yolk sac and vitelline elements (22,23).

Clinical presentation: Yolk-sac tumors are the second most common Germ-cell neoplasms of the ovary. The median age of presentation is 18 years (24). They are usually unilateral and present as pelvic masses. Highly elevated levels of serum α-fetoprotein (AFP) are almost pathognomonic of the tumor. The YST is a highly malignant tumor, but since the introduction of multiagent chemotherapy, an overall 80% complete cure rate (25) has been achieved.

Macroscopy: Large, encapsulated masses with gray-yellow, micro- or macrocystic cut surfaces and necrosis.

Histology: These tumors exhibit various architectural patterns. The reticular/microcystic pattern is composed of a loose myxoid stroma associated with lacunar spaces lined by atypical attenuated epithelium with or without periodic acid–Schiff (PAS)-positive hyaline globules, reminiscent of the mesodermal/endodermal pattern encountered in yolk sac (Figure 9.2). Schiller–Duval bodies, papillary projections with central vascular cores and outer layers of cuboidal, embryonic cells, are seen in the endodermal sinus pattern (Figure 9.3). Multiple small vesicles that are lined by flat epithelial cells and surrounded by connective tissue are typical for the polyvesicular vitelline pattern. The solid-type variant reveals clusters of mitotically active small, polygonal epithelial-like cells with clear cytoplasm, large vesicular nuclei, and prominent nucleoli. Nests or cords of large polygonal cells with eosinophilic cytoplasm, which resemble hepatocytes, are separated by fibrous stroma and are characteristic for the hepatoid pattern. The glandular variant can consist of cribriform aggregates of either primitive epithelial endodermal glands, which represent the intestinal type, or glandular structures resembling endometrioid carcinoma, the so-called endometrioid-like type.

Immunohistochemistry: The YST is positive for AFP, glypican-3, SALL4 (15,26,27), alkaline phosphatase (AP), pan-cytokeratin (CK), and sometimes PLAP. It usually does not express OCT3/4, CD117 (28), CK7, and epithelial membrane antigen (EMA) (29).

Differential diagnosis: The solid forms of YST may be mistaken for dysgerminoma. Typical features of dysgerminoma, such as the lymphocytic infiltrate and the expression of CD117 and OCT3/4, aid in the differential diagnosis. In EC, the tumor cells are larger and exhibit more nuclear pleomorphism and granular cytoplasm, and lack the specific pattern of YST. The glandular variant of YST occasionally mimics secretory endometrioid ovarian adenocarcinoma. Estrogen receptor (ER) and progesterone receptor (PR) expression, and squamous metaplasia favor endometrioid adenocarcinoma. Clear-cell carcinoma is diffusely positive for EMA and CK7, but is negative for AFP and SALL4; it is rarely positive for glypican-3 (focally). Inhibin and calretinin distinguish YST from sex-cord–stromal tumors (SCSTs).

Teratoma

Teratomas show elements derived from the three blastodermal layers: ectoderm, mesoderm, and endoderm.

Clinical presentation: Teratomas account for the majority of ovarian germ-cell tumors, over half of which are mature (30).

Subtype: mature teratoma

These consist of two or three mature derivatives of the ectoderm, mesoderm, and endoderm embryonic layers.

Clinical presentation: Mature teratomas present as ovarian masses. They account for 75% of ovarian tumors in patients under the age of 15 years (31) and are benign.

Hereditary/genetic features: Mature teratomas arise from a single germ cell after the first meiotic division, which then develops a diploid karyotype (32).

Macroscopy: Mature teratomas are typically cystic. They consist of a thin-walled cyst with hair and sebum, and may show thickening of the wall with calcification (Rokitansky protuberance).

Histology: The cyst wall is usually lined by skin-like elements, including epidermal adnexa. Other ectodermal derivatives include mature neuroepithelium and ocular structures, such as retinal pigmented epithelium. The mesoderm may be represented by mature cartilage, fat, and smooth and skeletal muscle. Respiratory or intestinal epithelium represents endoderm derivatives. Malignancy arising in mature components is extremely rare in childhood (30).

Subtype: monodermal teratoma

These are mature teratomas derived predominantly from a single germ-cell layer.

Clinical presentation: The most common monodermal teratoma is struma ovarii, which consists entirely of normal or hyperplastic thyroid tissue and is rare in children and adolescents.

Differential diagnosis: Struma ovarii exhibiting a prominent microfollicular adenoma pattern can be confused with a granulosa-cell tumor.

Subtype: immature teratoma (IM)

Immature teratomas contain primitive neuroectodermal tissue.

Clinical presentation: An IM occurs either purely or as part of a malignant germ-cell tumor (MGCT). They typically present in the first two decades as a unilateral palpable mass and are the third most common germ-cell tumor in adolescence. Peritoneal implants are present in 30% of patients at the time of surgery. Serum AFP can be elevated in IM, but AFP levels over 1000 ng/ml (33) should raise concerns for a YST component as part of an MGCT. In addition to tumor grade (34), complete surgical excision is the most important prognostic indicator (35,36). Gliomatosis peritonei, teratoma-induced metaplasia of the submesothelial cells of the peritoneum, can be present (28).

Macroscopy: An IM can range in size from 9–28 cm and reveals solid, gray-white, hemorrhagic cut surfaces with cystic changes.

Histology: In addition to mature elements, IMs contain immature neuroepithelium and mitotically active glial tissue (28). Other forms of immature mesenchymal tissue may be present, but are by themselves insufficient for a diagnosis of immature teratoma (28). Immature neuroectodermal tissue is composed of small blue cells forming rosettes and tubules, and hypercellular glial tissue with brisk mitotic activity (Figure 9.4). The World Health Organization (WHO) grading system is applied to primary tumors and peritoneal deposits. The tumor grade is based on the aggregate amount of immature neuroectodermal tissue counted on low-power fields (40×) on any slide (Table 9.1; 37,38).

Immature mesoderm presents as loose myxoid stroma containing mesenchymal components, such as immature cartilage and rhabdomyoblasts. Less common features include immature endodermal structures, such as embryonic renal tissue resembling Wilms tumor. The immature neuroepithelium is immunoreactive for glial fibrillary acidic protein (GFAP), S100, and neurofilament.

305

Table 9.1 Grading of ovarian immature teratomas (37,38)

Grade 0	Mature teratoma or gliomatosis peritonei
Grade 1	Immature neuroepithelium < 1 lpf/slide
Grade 2	Immature neuroepithelium 1–3 lpf/slide
Grade 3	Immature neuroepithelium > 3 lpf/slide

lpf = low-power field (x40 objective)

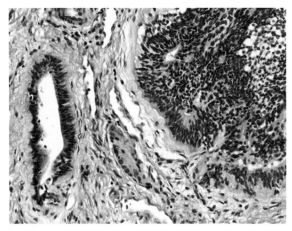

Figure 9.4 Immature teratoma showing neuroectodermal tissue composed of small blue cells forming rosettes and tubules.

Differential diagnosis: In contrast to mature teratoma, the components in IM exhibit different stages of maturation, lack an organized organoid arrangement, and are distributed haphazardly.

Embryonal carcinoma (EC)

Embryonal carcinoma arises from totipotential germ cells with the capability to differentiate towards various somatic or extraembryonal structures.

Clinical presentation: Pure EC is the rarest germ-cell tumor type of the ovaries, (28) and is more frequently seen as part of a malignant mixed germ-cell tumor (MGCT). Embryonal carcinoma presents as a large pelvic mass in young patients, with an average age of 12 years. Levels of AFP can be moderately elevated, even without a YST component. The tumor may contain syncytiotrophoblast with elevation of serum β-hCG (39). Endocrine manifestations such as isosexual pseudoprecocity can be seen in up to 50% of premenarchal patients. Embyonal carcinoma is highly aggressive, with local invasion, and early lymphatic and possibly hematogenous spread, but it responds well to chemotherapy.

Macroscopy: Embryonal carcinomas are gray-white solid tumors with areas of necrosis or hemorrhage.

Histology: In the undifferentiated, primitive form, EC consists of sheets of mitotically active epithelial-like tumor cells with indistinct cell borders, basophilic cytoplasm, anaplastic nuclear features, round vesicular nuclei, and prominent nucleoli. In addition to solid areas, more differentiated ECs have a pseudoglandular appearance, with epithelioid-appearing tumor cells lining clefts and spaces. Embryonal carcinoma is positive for keratin, CD30, and AFP (focally), and is negative for CD117.

Differential diagnosis: The solid component of EC can resemble dysgerminoma. Prominent nuclear pleomorphism and the presence of pseudoglandular spaces favors EC. Reactivity for CK and/or AFP excludes dysgerminoma.

Subtype: Polyembryoma

This is an organoid form of EC with features resembling early embryo (embryonic bodies).

Histology: Embryonic bodies are composed of blastocyst-like formations, formed by embryonic discs, amniotic sacs, and primary yolk sac cavities with focal AFP expression surrounded by mesoblastic loose connective tissue.

Non-gestational choriocarcinoma

This is a germ-cell-derived trophoblastic tumor.

Clinical presentation: A rare neoplasm accounting for < 0.6% of all ovarian neoplasms, far more common as an MGCT component than in its pure form (40). Clinical symptoms include precocious puberty and vaginal bleeding. Serum β-hCG is elevated. This is a highly malignant tumor exhibiting local invasion, and lymphatic and hematogenous dissemination; less responsive to chemotherapy than gestational-type choriocarcinoma.

Hereditary/genetic features: The presence of paternal DNA supports a choriocarcinoma of gestational type and can be used to distinguish it from non-gestational choriocarcinoma.

Macroscopy: Large, solid, gray-white, necrotic, and hemorrhagic tumors.

Histology: Closely intermixed cytotrophoblast and syncytiotrophoblast with very rare or absent intermediate trophoblastic cells. The architectural pattern is predominantly composed of solid sheets of cytotrophoblast with a plexiform or pseudopapillary appearance, surrounded by layers of syncytiotrophoblast.

The cytotrophoblastic cells show well-defined cytoplasmic borders, clear cytoplasm, and round, vesicular nuclei with prominent nucleoli. Mitotic activity may be brisk. Syncytiotrophoblast appear as large, elongated, multinucleated cells with basophilic, vacuolated cytoplasm, and a dense hyperchromatic chromatin pattern in the nuclei. Positive for β-hCG (syncytiotrophoblast) and expresses CK.

Differential diagnosis: In contrast to choriocarcinoma, solid-type EC expresses CD30.

Malignant mixed germ-cell tumors (MGCTs)

Malignant mixed germ-cell tumors are composed of more than one type of malignant germ-cell tumor (41,42).

Clinical presentation: Up to 20% of malignant germ-cell tumors are MGCTs. Hormonal manifestations and serum markers depend on the elements of MGCTs.

Macroscopy: Thorough sampling (at least one section per cm), especially of the solid and heterogeneous areas, is needed in all germ-cell tumors to identify a MGCT.

Sex-cord–stromal tumors (SCSTs)

Sex-cord–stromal tumors are composed of sex-cord derivatives and stromal derivatives.

Immunohistochemistry: Almost all SCSTs express inhibin and calretinin. Eighty percent of SCSTs show nuclear staining for forkhead box (FOX) L2 (43).

Juvenile granulosa-cell tumor (JGCT)

This tumor is composed of neoplastic granulosa cells and stroma.

Clinical presentation: Juvenile granulosa-cell tumors represent 5% of all granulosa-cell tumors (44) and are the most common SCSTs in childhood (45) (average age 17 years). They present with a pelvic mass, isosexual pseudoprecocity related to estrogen production, or menstrual abnormalities. Most JGCTs are diagnosed at stage I and have an excellent prognosis with an overall survival of 93% (44). Recurrences are rare, but can be fatal and tend to occur within the first three years after diagnosis (44).

Hereditary/genetic features: These tumors can be associated with Maffucci syndrome (enchondroma with multiple angiomas) or Ollier's disease (enchondromatosis). They feature the *FOXL2* C134W mutation in 10% of cases (46).

Macroscopy: The cut surface of a JGCT is often gray-yellow with bloody fluid-filled cystic areas.

Histology: Juvenile granulosa-cell tumors are composed of uniform, round to fusiform cells without nuclear grooves. They contain abundant eosinophilic cytoplasm and hyperchromatic nuclei with prominent nucleoli. The cells are arranged in sheets and follicles of varying size and shape, filled with eosinophilic or basophilic fluid. A layer of granulosa cells or theca interna-like cells lines the follicles. Brisk mitotic activity is present, and 15% of cases show bizarre nuclei.

Immunohistochemistry: Juvenile granulosa-cell tumors express inhibin, calretinin, FOXL2, and steroidogenic factor (SF)-1.

Differential diagnosis: A high mitotic index, variable sized and shaped follicles, absence of nuclear grooves, and bizarre nuclei are morphologic features that can help to distinguish JGCTs from adult granulosa cell tumors (AGCTs). Juvenile granulosa-cell tumors may be confused with YST and EC due to patient age, atypia, and mitotic activity. The different immunohistochemical profiles of JGCTs and germ-cell tumors are useful in difficult cases. Another pitfall is small-cell carcinoma of the hypercalcemic type (SCCHT). Expression of calretinin, inhibin, and FOXL2 in JGCTs (absent in SCCHTs), and negativity for EMA and cytokeratin (positive in SCCHTs) can contribute to the differential diagnosis. Although rare in children, clear-cell carcinoma and malignant melanoma need to be excluded.

Adult granulosa cell tumor (AGCT)

Adult granulosa cell tumor is composed of neoplastic granulosa cells and stroma.

Clinical presentation: Adult granulosa-cell tumors represent 80% of the malignant SCST (47,48) and are usually seen in perimenopausal women, but can occur in adolescents and children. Abdominal pain, a pelvic mass, acute hemoperitoneum, and estrogenic manifestation are possible symptoms. Useful serum markers include estradiol and α-inhibin. The most important prognostic factor is stage.

Hereditary/genetic features: The C134W missense somatic mutation, located in the *FOXL2* gene, is present in 97% of AGCT (46).

Macroscopy: Adult granulosa-cell tumors show solid and cystic cut surfaces with frequent necrosis, and cystic, blood-filled areas.

Histology: Uniform tumor cells with scanty cytoplasm, ovoid nuclei and longitudinal grooves. Mitotic activity is usually low. Bizarre or atypical tumor cells are uncommon. Adult granulosa-cell tumors show

307

various architectural patterns. The most characteristic is the microfollicular type, which shows tumor cells with a rosette-like arrangement around a central space, filled with eosinophilic material (Call–Exner body). Other patterns of AGCT include macrofollicular, insular, trabecular, gyriform, watered-silk, or diffuse (sarcomatoid) (49).

Adult granulosa-cell tumors are positive for inhibin, calretinin, SF-1, and FOXL2.

Differential diagnosis: Mainly JGCT and SCCHT. Gonadoblastoma, sex-cord–stromal tumor with annular tubules (SCTAT) and Sertoli–Leydig cell tumor can resemble the microfollicular pattern. The characteristic nuclear grooves are useful for distinguishing AGCT from these entities. The presence of germ cells in gonadoblastoma, of abundant hyaline material in SCTAT, and of Leydig cells in Sertoli–Leydig cell tumor is also helpful in this regard.

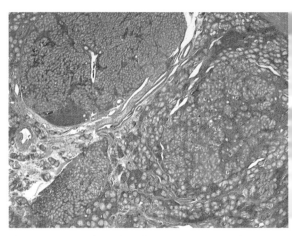

Figure 9.5 A Sertoli–Leydig-cell tumor is composed of mature Sertoli cells arranged in hollow and solid tubules separated by stroma that contains abundant clusters of Leydig cells with eosinophilic granular cytoplasm.

Sertoli–Leydig cell tumor (SLCT)

These are Sertoli-stromal cell tumors.

Clinical presentation: Sertoli–Leydig cell tumor account for 0.5% of all ovarian tumors and occur in young women with an average age of 25 years (50). They present as pelvic masses and with occasional virilization. The prognosis depends on grade and stage: well-differentiated SLCTs are benign, whereas intermediate and poorly differentiated tumors have malignant potential.

Macroscopy: Sertoli–Leydig cell tumors are yellow, solid or cystic, with areas of hemorrhage or necrosis.

Histology: Well-differentiated tumors reveal mature Sertoli cells arranged in hollow and solid tubules, separated by stroma with abundant clusters of Leydig cells of eosinophilic granular cytoplasm (Figure 9.5). In tumors of intermediate differentiation, aggregates of immature, mitotically active Sertoli cells with scant cytoplasm admixed with fibrous stroma and clusters of Leydig cells are seen. Poorly differentiated SLCTs show spindle cells reminiscent of sarcomas with abundant mitotic activity. Leydig cells are scattered and may be difficult to find. The retiform variant of SLCT exhibits irregular slit-like tubules with polypoid structures and papillae, which can show secretions. Endodermal- or mesenchymal-type heterologous elements are found in 20% of SLCTs (51).

Sertoli–Leydig cell tumors are positive for inhibin and calretinin. Melanoma antigen recognized by T-cells (MART)-1 is also positive in Leydig cell tumors (52).

Differential diagnosis: The retiform variant can mimic YST and serous neoplasms.

Sclerosing stromal tumor (SST)

Sclerosing stromal tumor is benign.

Clinical presentation: Sclerosing stromal tumor is an uncommon ovarian SCST that occurs in young women and adolescents (53). It may present with premature menarche, menstrual irregularities, abdominal discomfort, and ascites.

Macroscopy: Sclerosing stromal tumors have an average size of 10 cm and show a yellow, edematous cut surface (49).

Histology: These tumors show a characteristic pseudolobular pattern and are composed of fibroblasts and round, vacuolated cells separated by densely collagenous or markedly edematous hypocellular tissue and prominent vascularity.

Differential diagnosis: Krukenberg tumor can resemble the vacuolated cells of SSTs and be excluded by CK stains.

Sex-cord–stromal tumor with annular tubules (SCTAT)

Sex-cord–stromal tumor with annular tubules is an unclassified SCST.

Clinical presentation: Sex-cord–stromal tumor with annular tubules occurs in young women either sporadically or in 30% of cases in association with Peutz–Jegher's syndrome (PJS) (mucocutaneous pigmentation, hamartomatous polyps, and minimal deviation adenocarcinoma) and can be estrogenic. When associated with PJS, SCTATs are usually benign, whereas sporadic SCTATs behave malignantly in 20% of cases.

Histology: Sex-cord–stromal tumor with annular tubules characteristically shows simple and complex annular tubules, nuclei arranged in an antipodal pattern, abundant hyaline material, and calcifications. In PJS, SCTATs are usually smaller or just microscopic foci.

Differential diagnosis: See AGCT.

Fibroma

Fibroma typically affects postmenopausal women and is rare in children.

Macroscopy: Solid, firm white masses with cystic changes.

Histology: Bland spindle cells are arranged in a storiform or whorled arrangement in a collagenous background. Calcification may be present.

Mixed germ-cell–sex-cord–stromal tumors
Gonadoblastoma (see disorders of sex development)

Surface epithelial tumors
Mucinous and serous neoplasms

These are tumors derived from the surface epithelium of the ovary that are categorized as benign, borderline, or malignant according to the degree of epithelial proliferation observed in the cyst wall lining.

Clinical presentation: Mucinous and serous tumors, especially mucinous or serous cystadenomas (54), account for the majority of epithelial tumors observed in the pediatric population (54). Malignancies are exceedingly rare (55).

Miscellaneous tumors
Small-cell carcinoma, hypercalcemic type (SCCHT)

Definition: An undifferentiated ovarian carcinoma.

Clinical presentation: This type of tumor has been described in females from 2 to 46 years of age (56). Patients usually have advanced-stage disease and present with pelvic masses and hypercalcemia in 60% of cases. It shows an aggressive clinical course with poor prognosis.

Macroscopy: The tumors are solid with areas of necrosis and hemorrhage.

Histology: These carcinomas are composed of small mitotically active tumor cells with scant cytoplasm and hyperchromatic nuclei with prominent nucleoli, arranged in either solid sheets or trabeculae and express CK, EMA, and Wilms tumor (WT1) antigen. They are negative for inhibin, calretinin, and FOXL2.

Differential diagnosis: See JGCT.

Burkitt's lymphoma and metastatic ovarian tumors in children

In endemic areas, Burkitt lymphoma is a common malignant tumor of the ovary. Neuroblastoma and rhabdomyosarcoma can metastasize to the ovaries.

Uterus and cervix, vagina and vulva

Congenital lesions
Anomalies of the Müllerian ducts

The uterus and the upper third of the vagina arise from the paired ducts. Uterine agenesis is caused by the absence of both Müllerian ducts. The presence of just one duct results in a unicornuate uterus, and incomplete formation of the Müllerian ducts causes a hypoplastic uterus. Lateral fusion defects lead to didelphic uterus (double uterus, cervix, and vagina), bicornuate uterus (two uterine horns), and septate uterus (normal external fundus, partial or complete septum) (57).

Clinical presentation: The spectrum ranges from asymptomatic patients to dysmenorrhea, dyspareunia, infertility, and recurrent pregnancy loss.

Mayer–Rokitansky–Kuster–Hauser (MRKH) syndrome

This syndrome presents with absent or severely underdeveloped vagina and uterus due to the lack of Müllerian structure development (57).

Clinical presentation: Mayer–Rokitansky–Kuster–Hauser syndrome affects approximately 1:4500 females. Patients present with primary amenorrhea (57), but have normal external genitalia, ovarian function, and development of secondary sex characteristics.

Transverse vaginal septum (TVS)

Transverse vaginal septum is caused by inadequate cavitation of the vaginal plate, which leads to vertical fusion problems (57).

Clinical presentation: This can be located anywhere in the vagina, varies in thickness, and is often present with hemato- or hydromucocolpos, due to obstruction.

Histology: The upper vagina and cervix reveal endocervical-type epithelium due to the distal obstruction (57). After excision of the TVS, these cells undergo squamous metaplasia.

Benign vaginal lesions
Vaginal adenosis

Vaginal adenosis is the persistence of Müllerian epithelium in the vaginal wall.

Clinical presentation: Vaginal adenosis is associated with DES exposure, but can occur sporadically. The condition has a predilection for the upper third of the vagina and often presents with increased mucinous discharge. Patients with vaginal adenosis are thought to be at higher risk for developing clear-cell carcinoma.

Macroscopy: The vaginal mucosa shows small, granular, red patches.

Histology: The glandular structures are lined by either an endocervical-type mucin-secreting epithelium or a tubo-endometrium with cilia. Metaplastic squamous epithelium can replace adenosis. Special stains for mucin are positive.

Bartholin gland cyst

A cyst that is caused by obstruction of the Bartholin gland duct.

Clinical presentation: Bartholin gland cysts can present as mass lesions at the vaginal introitus. Secondary infection can lead to a Bartholin gland abscess.

Histology: The cyst lining can be composed of squamous, cuboidal mucinous, or transitional-type epithelium.

Müllerian cyst

A cyst originating from Müllerian remnants.

Clinical presentation: A cyst usually < 2 cm in size that can occur in any vaginal location.

Histology: Most frequently, endocervical-type epithelium is seen, but any type of Müllerian epithelium can line the cyst wall. Squamous metaplasia may be present.

Fibroepithelial polyp

Fibroepithelial polyp is a benign mesodermal stromal polyp.

Clinical presentation: Fibroepithelial polyp can occur over a wide age range, from infants to postmenopausal women. Most lesions arise at the lateral wall of the lower third of the vagina and are incidentally found. Fibroepithelial polyps can also occur at the vulva and cervix.

Macroscopy: The condition often presents as either a single papillary or a polypoid, edematous lesion.

Histology: Fibroblastic vascularized stroma lined by stratified squamous epithelium. The stroma shows variable cellularity and can reveal bizarre stromal cells with nuclear pleomorphism, mitotic activity, and

atypical mitosis. The stromal cells are positive for ER and PR.

Differential diagnosis: In contrast to embryonal rhabdomyosarcoma, fibroepithelial polyps lack a cambium layer.

Müllerian papilloma

A papillary neoplasm of mesonephric origin.

Clinical presentation: Müllerian papilloma typically occurs in the vagina or cervix of girls under the age of five years and presents with vaginal bleeding. These neoplasms are generally considered to be benign lesions; however, recurrences and malignant behaviors have been described.

Macroscopy: Müllerian papilloma is an exophytic growing papillary lesion.

Histology: Müllerian papillomas are composed of complex, arborizing papillae with fibrovascular cores. They are covered by bland, low columnar-cuboidal epithelium that can occasionally form solid or glandular areas.

Differential diagnosis: Embryonal rhabdomyosarcoma.

Benign vulvar lesions
Lichen sclerosus (LS)

Lichen sclerosus involves the vulvar skin of prepubertal girls and postmenopausal women. The typical presentation in childhood is vulvar itching, soreness, and dysuria. Lichen sclerosus sometimes resolves with the onset of puberty.

Macroscopy: The skin shows large, hypopigmented patches.

Histology: Thinning of the epithelium, loss or blunting of the rete ridges, homogenous hyalinization of the subepithelial layer, and a band-like chronic inflammatory infiltrate are characteristic.

Gartner duct cyst

Gartner duct cysts are remnants of the mesonephric duct.

Clinical presentation: Gartner duct cysts are located in the lateral vaginal wall.

Histology: The cyst lining is cuboidal and occasionally ciliated.

Mucous cyst

Cyst of possible origin from the urogenital sinus epithelium.

Clinical presentation: Mucinous cysts are commonly seen at the vulvar vestibule.

Histology: The cyst wall is lined by tall, cuboidal mucinous epithelium. The cyst lining is positive for alcian blue and mucicarmine stain.

Cyst of the canal of Nuck

A cyst arising from peritoneal inclusions.

Clinical presentation: These cysts are located in either the inguinal canal or the superior aspect of the labia majora.

Histology: The cyst wall is lined by peritoneum.

Differential diagnosis: These cysts can resemble inguinal hernias.

Childhood asymmetric labium majus enlargement (CALME)

A vulval soft tissue lesion likely representing asymmetric enlargement related to hormonal influences (58). "Prepubertal vulval fibroma" (59) is most likely the same entity as CALME (60).

Clinical presentation: Childhood asymmetric labium majus enlargement usually occurs in prepubertal girls with unilateral expansion of the labium majus, but lacks a distinct palpable lesion (58).

Macroscopy: Childhood asymmetric labium majus enlargement has the appearance of fibro-adipose tissue.

Histology: It exhibits expansion of the fibrous tissue with moderately cellular interconnected bands that surround fat, vessels, or nerves. It consists of plump or round fibroblasts in a pale myxoid matrix with collagen fibers (58). The fibroblasts are ER- and PR-positive.

Superficial angiomyxoma (SAM) (cutaneous myxoma)

Superficial angiomyxoma of the vulvo-perineal region presents in adolescents and young women as a subcutaneous mass lesion < 2.5 cm in size. It is a benign lesion, but has a local recurrence rate of >30% (61).

Hereditary/genetic features: Multifocal SAM can be associated with Carney complex.

Histology: Superficial angiomyxomas show a multinodular growth pattern and contain abundant hyaluronic and myxoid matrix, forming mucin pools (61). Sparse bland, stellate, and spindled cells with smudgy chromatin, occasional pseudoinclusions, or multinucleation are seen in the stroma. Thin-walled, small blood vessels and scattered inflammatory cells are usually present. Entrapped adnexal epithelial components are found in approximately 30% of cases. The

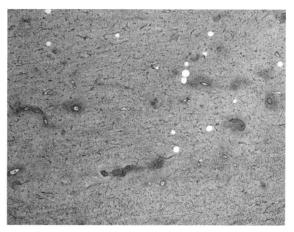

Figure 9.6 Aggressive (deep) angiomyxoma with bland, spindle- or stellate-shaped tumor cells, myxoid stroma changes, and prominent vasculature.

spindled cells express CD34 and vimentin, and are negative for ER and PR.

Aggressive (deep) angiomyxoma (AAM)

Aggressive angiomyxoma usually presents in peri-or postmenopausal women as a slow-growing mass, and is rare in childhood. It is located in the deep soft tissue without involvement of the overlying epithelium and often exceeds 10 cm in size.

Macroscopy: Aggressive angiomyxoma has a lobular, glistening appearance and can entrap other structures.

Histology: Aggressive angiomyxomas show consistent, low-to-moderate cellularity. The bland tumor cells are small, uniform, and of spindle or stellate shape in a background of abundant myxoid stroma and prominent round, medium-to-large vessels (Figure 9.6). Myxoid cells are often found around larger nerves and vascular structures. The spindled cells are positive for ER, PR, and vimentin. Desmin and actin show variable staining. CD34 shows infrequent, focal expression.

Malignancies

Embryonal rhabdomyosarcoma (ERMS) of the vagina and cervix

A malignant soft tissue sarcoma that exhibits skeletal muscle differentiation.

Clinical presentation: Rhabdomyosarcoma is the most common malignant tumor of the female genital tract in childhood. It most commonly presents in the vagina, but can also be seen in the cervix and vulva. Vaginal rhabdomyosarcoma usually occurs in

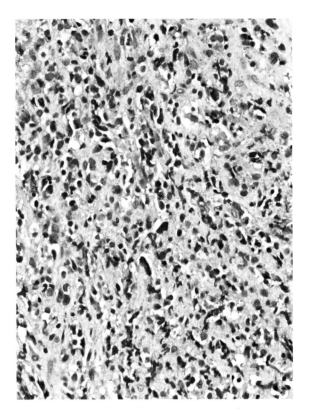

Figure 9.7 Sarcoma botryoides with condensation of primitive rhabdomyoblasts.

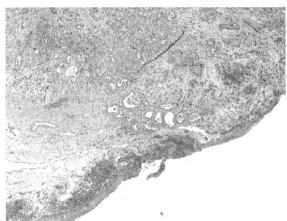

Figure 9.8 Clear-cell carcinoma of the cervix exhibiting cysts and tubules.

children under the age of five years, whereas cervical rhabdomyosarcoma presents at an older age with an average age of 12.4 years (62). Frequent presentations include vaginal bleeding (62,63), a protruding "grape-like" anterior vaginal mass, or a polyp at the cervical os (62). Multiagent chemotherapy followed by surgery, and on occasion radiation therapy, have improved clinical outcomes, with rhabdomyosarcoma of the gynecologic tract having a survival rate of > 90%.

Hereditary/genetic features: Embryonal rhabdomyosarcoma lacks the recurrent reciprocal translocations seen in alveolar rhabdomyosarcoma.

Macroscopy: Sarcoma botryoides, a subtype of ERMS, typically presents as a polypoid lesion with a cluster of "grape-like" masses.

Histology: Sarcoma botryoides (Figure 9.7) is predominantly seen in the vagina and cervix and forms a cambium layer under the vaginal epithelium or around endocervical glands. The cambium layer shows condensation of primitive and differentiated, polyhedral rhabdomyoblasts, which are scattered in a loose, fibromyxomatous, or hypocellular stroma. The tumor cells are round-to-spindle-shaped and have

inconspicuous nucleoli. Cytoplasmic cross-striations may be present. Embryonal rhabdomyosarcoma can show marked differentiation with prominent eosinophilic cytoplasm after neoadjuvant chemotherapy. Small islands of mature cartilage are found in 40% of cervical rhabdomyosarcoma (62) and likely result from metaplasia. Embryonal rhabdomyosarcomas are positive for myoglobin, desmin, muscle-specific actin, and focally to myogenin.

Differential diagnosis: Fibroepithelial polyp and Müllerian papilloma need to be considered.

Clear-cell adenocarcinoma (CCA) of the cervix and vagina

Approximately 60% of CCA cases seen between 1970 and 1990 had a history of *in utero* DES exposure (64). Typically, vaginal CCA involves the anterior or lateral vaginal wall of the upper vagina. It is often seen in association with atypical vaginal adenosis in the tumor periphery. Most patients will present in the second and third decades with spotting or vaginal bleeding (64). The five-year survival rate is higher for CCAs occurring after DES exposure than for sporadic ones (84% vs. 69%, respectively) (65). The tumor may be seen in adolescents (66).

Macroscopy: Clear-cell adenocarcinomas have a nodular or polypoid appearance.

Histology: The histologic findings of CCA in patients exposed to DES are identical to unexposed cases. Architecturally, the tumor shows cysts and tubules (Figure 9.8) alternating with solid areas. Hobnail or flat tumor cells line the tubules (Figure 9.9). Tumor cells can have abundant clear cytoplasm and show variable mitotic activity. The

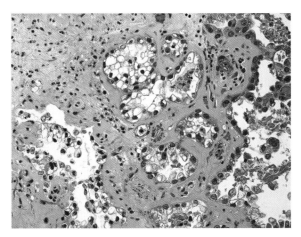

Figure 9.9 Hobnail or flat tumor cells line the tubules in clear-cell carcinoma.

glands in atypical adenosis show stratification and nuclear pleomorphism. Clear-cell adenocarcinoma expresses CK7, CAM 5.2, and vimentin.

Differential diagnosis: Microglandular hyperplasia does not exhibit the hobnail cells and nuclear atypia seen in CCA.

Yolk-sac tumor of the vagina (see also ovarian YST section)

Yolk-sac tumor of the vagina occurs in children less than three years of age and presents with bloody vaginal discharge with a polypoid, vaginal mass.

Histology: The histologic pattern is similar to YST occurring in the ovary. Characteristic features are Schiller–Duval bodies and hyaline droplets, and the architectural pattern may be papillary, reticular, or solid. Anastomosing channels and tubules are lined by cuboidal epithelium with vacuolated cytoplasm and hyperchromatic nuclei.

Tumors of the Ewing family: Ewing's sarcoma/peripheral primitive neuroectodermal tumor (EWS)

This tumor is part of the primitive, small round blue-cell tumors.

Clinical presentation: It may occur as a primary lesion of the vulva, vagina, uterus, or ovaries. Vulvar EWS usually presents as mass lesions in females between 10 and 30 years of age (61).

Hereditary/genetic features: Approximately 90% of cases reveal t(11;22)(q24;q12) translocations (fusions of the *EWS* with the *FLI-1* gene), and 10–15% have variant translocations. Demonstration of the characteristic translocation by fluorescent *in situ* hybridization, is crucial for the diagnosis of EWS in the female reproductive system (66).

Histology: An EWS exhibits monomorphic, small and poorly differentiated cells. Depending on the degree of neuroepithelial differentiation, the tumor cells are round, organized in sheets, and have glycogen-rich cytoplasm or are larger glycogen-negative tumor cells with tapered cytoplasmic processes that can focally form pseudorosettes (61) .The cells are positive for the cluster of differentiation (CD) 99 (MIC2)-, friend leukemia integration-1 transcription factor (FLI-1)-, and vimentin-positive.

Differential diagnosis: Ewing's sarcomas need to be distinguished from ovarian or uterine tumors with central nervous system (CNS)-type neural differentiation (61). These tumors are CD99-negative and lack the characteristic (11:22) translocation.

Male reproductive system

Testis

Non-neoplastic disorders

Congenital/developmental
Monorchidism and polyorchidism
The unilateral absence of a testis (monorchidism) or the presence of a supernumerary testis (polyorchidism).

Clinical presentation: Monorchidism may be accompanied by unilateral renal agenesis, while polyorchidism is associated with testicular torsion, cryptorchidism, and inguinal hernia.

Cystic dysplasia
A rare congenital defect characterized by the presence of irregular cystic spaces within the mediastinum or rete testis.

Clinical presentation: The typical presentation involves unilateral scrotal swelling or testicular enlargement in infancy or adolescence (67). The lesion is often accompanied by other renal abnormalities, most commonly ipsilateral renal agenesis (67).

Macroscopy: The lesion measures up to 7 cm along its greatest dimension and has a white-tan, rubbery, and focally cystic cut surface (67,68). The lesion may compress the surrounding testicular parenchyma.

Histology: Multiple, anastomosing cystic spaces separated by fibrous tissue septa and lined by cuboidal epithelium are present within the rete testis. The lesion extends into and may compress the surrounding testicular parenchyma with resultant atrophy (67,68). The cystic spaces may contain PAS-positive secretions (67).

313

The cuboidal epithelium is reactive with keratin and vimentin and non-reactive with PLAP, carcinoembryonic antigen, and factor VIII (67).

Differential diagnosis: Simple testicular cysts, cysts of the tunica albuginea, cystic teratomas, and epidermoid cysts are known to occur in the testis.

Testicular vascular lesions

Benign and malignant vascular neoplasms and malformations that involve the testis.

Clinical presentation: Patients range in age from the first to the sixth decades and beyond, presenting with testicular discomfort or a palpable mass with or without pain (69).

Classification: These lesions should follow an updated classification system proposed by the International Society for the Study of Vascular Anomalies (ISSVA) (70).

Macroscopy: Depending on the specific type, lesions may feature a more or less well-circumscribed, tan-brown to red, lobulated, and hemorrhagic mass of variable size (69).

Histology: Characterized by the presence of numerous vascular spaces lined by spindled to flattened endothelial cells devoid of atypia (71). The lesion may involve the testicular investing layers and infiltrate between seminiferous tubules or may possess a pseudocapsule with entrapment of adjacent seminiferous tubules (69). Tumor cells react diffusely with CD31 and CD34, and lack reactivity with pancytokeratin (71). Lymphatic endothelial markers (D2–40 and PROX1) are present in mixed vascular malformations with lymphatic elements. In infantile hemangioma, Glut-1 expression is classically present.

Differential diagnosis: Depending on the specific type, treatment may involve enucleation of the lesion and preservation of the testis. Involvement of the testis by syndromic vascular proliferations or malignant endothelial tumors such as angiosarcoma and others may also be seen and require different treatment approaches (72).

Testicular regression syndrome

A congenital condition in which testicular tissue is absent due to complete reabsorption. Testicular regression syndrome may be due to infarction or torsion sustained *in utero* or in the perinatal period (73).

Clinical presentation: Patients present with either unilateral or bilateral absence of a palpable testis at birth or in infancy. Surgical exploration reveals no apparent gonadal tissue. Instead, in the majority of cases, a portion of fibrous tissue is identified in the vicinity of the spermatic cord (73,74).

Macroscopy: A discrete fibrous nodule or nubbin ranging in size from 0.9–2 cm (74).

Histology: Typical histologic features include a vascularized, fibrous nodule with scattered dystrophic calcification and hemosiderin deposition. Spermatic cord ductal structures and epididymis may be identified. Scattered residual seminiferous tubules may be present, although they are uncommon. Germ cells are usually not present (73–75). The risk of malignant degeneration of these lesions is very low (75).

Differential diagnosis: Failure to identify a gonad does not entirely exclude the diagnosis of cryptorchidism. Testicular agenesis should be included in the differential diagnosis.

Cryptorchidism and maldescent

Cryptorchidism is the unilateral or bilateral failure of a testis to descend into the scrotum.

Clinical presentation: Between 1.8 to 4.1% of newborn males greater than 2500 g in weight have an undescended testis (76). Unilateral cryptorchidism is more common; however, bilateral undescended testes occurs in 10–20% of cases (77). While in the vast majority of cases, the testis will descend into the scrotum within one year, in approximately 1% of this subpopulation, the testis remains in an extra-scrotal position. Cryptorchidism is associated with low birth weight and is a major factor in the development of testicular cancer and infertility (76). Patients are treated with orchiopexy, although treatment does not eliminate the risk of testicular cancer.

Classification/subtypes: Undescended testes are classified according to the extra-scrotal position and may be abdominal, inguinal, ectopic, or gliding (77).

Macroscopy: The affected testis demonstrates mild to severe atrophy, and epipidydimal and vascular abnormalities, depending on its location outside the scrotum (78).

Histology: The seminiferous tubules are atrophic with basement membrane thickening, Sertoli-cell hypoplasia, decreased germ-cell numbers, and occasional Sertoli-cell hyperplasia (78,79). These findings tend to increase in severity with patient age and location of the undescended testis (78). Sertoli cell nodules and circumscribed nodules of under-developed Sertoli cells, basement membrane, and spermatogonia may be identified incidentally in cryptorchid testes (80).

Acquired

Testicular and testicular appendage torsion

Torsion of the testis or its appendages may occur at any age from the neonatal period to adulthood. Testicular and appendix testis torsion each characteristically present with sudden-onset diffuse scrotal pain accompanied by abnormal testicular position and lack of a cremasteric reflex. The vast majority of these cases are intravaginal torsion and result from a congenital abnormality of the processus vaginalis. Extravaginal testicular torsion is significantly more common in the newborn or neonatal period, with irreversible testicular damage at presentation in the majority of cases (81,82). Testicular torsion is a well-known complication of cryptorchidism (83).

Macroscopy: The testicle has a dark purple to dusky, smooth, and hemorrhagic external surface. Neonates or infants may present with an atrophic testis (84,85).

Histology: Characteristically include acute hemorrhagic necrosis of the gonad with variable amounts of residual testicular parenchyma. Findings in neonates and infants typically include dystrophic calcification, fibrosis, necrosis, and hemosiderin deposition (84).

Differential diagnosis: Clinically, the differential diagnosis for acute scrotal pain includes testicular torsion and torsion of the appendix testis and epididymitis (82).

Epididymo-orchitis

Inflammation of the epididymis and/or testes.

Clinical presentation: Epididymitis is uncommon in the pediatric population. Patients typically present with a painful, enlarged scrotum, which may be accompanied by painful urination and urethral discharge, or a history of trauma. Infection may be bacterial, viral, or granulomatous (86). The testis is not a frequent site of primary infection. Instead, orchitis often results from the spread of infection from the epididymis or hematogenous spread from another site in children (87). Sexual transmission of *Neisseria gonorrhea* or *Chlamydia trachomatis* is a well-known cause in the adult population. Infection with *Mycobacterium tuberculosis* is also a consideration.

Macroscopy: Epididymitis presents with swelling, prominent vasculature, and a fibrinous exudate (87).

Histology: An acute inflammatory infiltrate of the epididymis and/or testis is present, with abscess formation and necrosis in more severe cases. Chronic epididymo-orchitis is characterized by interstitial fibrosis and chronic inflammatory infiltrate (87). Viral orchitis may mimic a neoplastic process clinically; however, histologic exam reveals normal testicular architecture with a patchy lymphohistiocytic infiltrate, hemorrhage, and edema (88).

Testicular microlithiasis

Idiopathic microcalcifications present in the seminiferous tubules of males of all ages (89).

Clinical presentation: Testicular microlithiasis (TM) is usually a bilateral, incidental finding on scrotal ultrasound or at autopsy. Although TM may be present in any age group, it is rare in prepubertal boys and elderly males (89). It may be associated with cryptorchidism and germ-cell tumors.

Hereditary/genetic features: Mutations in *SLC34A2* may be associated with TM (90).

Histology: Testicular microliths are intratubular, round to ovoid, variably sized microcalcifications with concentric layers of basal lamina-like material external to the calcification. The microliths are generally localized to the central portions of the annular seminiferous tubules, while Sertoli cells and spermatogonia are present at the periphery (91). Microliths may be focal or diffuse, and unilateral or bilateral. Microliths demonstrate strong PAS reactivity, and the surrounding basal lamina-like material stains positively for collagen IV (91).

Toxic injury

Exposure to a therapeutic or environmental toxin, such as phthalates, may result in testicular injury. Chemotherapeutic agents are known to cause azoospermia and testicular atrophy, and may reduce spermatogenesis (92).

Juvenile xanthogranuloma

A benign, usually self-limited, subtype of non-Langerhans histiocytosis.

Clinical presentation: Classically presents as a solitary subcutaneous nodule in young children and infants. The lesions may also be multiple or present as part of a systemic disease. Isolated lesions of the testis occur rarely.

Histology: Juvenile xanthogranuloma limited to the testis (93) presents with cellular infiltrates of mononuclear cells expanding the interstitium. The mononuclear cells have indistinct cellular membranes, pale-staining cytoplasm and ovoid nuclei with delicate chromatin and small nucleoli. Unremarkable seminiferous tubules are randomly distributed. Touton giant cells are usually absent (93).

Testicular tumors

Over 95% of testicular tumors are germ-cell tumors (GCTs). Broadly, prepubertal GCTs can be conservatively managed. Postpubertal tumors follow an adult pattern, the vast majority being malignant and requiring radical treatment (94). Known risk factors are cryptorchidism, disorders of sexual development, and testicular atrophy.

Clinical features: Usually present with painless testicular enlargement. Overall testicular tumors have a good prognosis with 95% five-year survival.

Germ-cell tumors

Yolk-sac tumor (YST)

Malignant GCTs are assumed to arise from undifferentiated, multipotential embryonal carcinoma, which can selectively differentiate into yolk sac and vitelline elements (22,23).

Clinical features: Prepubertal cases constitute the most common prepubertal malignant GCT (95), with peak incidence at 18 months (94,95). These tumors occur in pure form, are usually confined to the testis, and show lower propensity for retroperitoneal nodal spread. Serum AFP is sensitive for detecting residual tumor, occult metastasis, or recurrence. Postpubertal YST usually occurs as part of a mixed GCT and is radically treated (94).

Histology: These tumors are soft and microcystic, and are composed of intermingled epithelial and mesenchymal elements in various patterns: microcystic, glandular-alveolar, or papillary (see Figure 9.2). Epithelial cells are flattened or polygonal. The mesenchymal component appears primitive or may be cellular, resembling smooth muscle. Characteristic findings include Schiller–Duval bodies, a perivascular layer of tumor cells within a space lined by flattened malignant cells (see Figure 9.3), seen in a minority of cases (96), and AFP-positive hyaline globules.

Yolk-sac tumors express AFP, SALL4, and keratin, and are negative for OCT3/4 (28,97).

Teratoma

Subtype: prepubertal mature and immature teratomas

Teratomas are the most common pediatric testicular tumor. These tumors occur from birth to approximately 18 months as solid heterogeneous masses with varying consistency and calcification. Management is conservative.

Cytogenetic features: Prepubertal teratomas are diploid with a normal 46 XY karyotype (28).

Histology: Teratomas show a haphazard, though organoid, mixture of mature tissues, such as skin, respiratory epithelium, and cartilage. Immature components, such as neuroepithelium, occur rarely, but their significance is uncertain; the vast majority of childhood cases with immature elements are benign (32).

Subtype: postpubertal teratoma

Occur predominantly in men between 20 and 40, but sometimes occur in adolescents, usually as components of mixed GCT. Treatment is radical with orchiectomy, retroperitoneal node dissection, and systemic chemotherapy.

Cytogenetic features: These tumors are aneuploid and show 12p amplification, often as i12p. When mixed, the teratomatous elements share cytogenetic abnormalities with the background primitive GCT and are believed to represent differentiation into a malignant GCT (32).

Histology: These tumors are solid and variegated, show variably mature mixed teratomatous elements that lack an organoid pattern, and show widespread atypia and mitotic activity. Adjacent seminiferous tubules show atrophy and intratubular germ-cell neoplasia (IGCN). Immature elements may be seen, but their malignant potential is surpassed by that of the almost invariably present primitive germ-cell elements.

Epidermoid cysts

Clinical presentation: Epidermoid cysts constitute 15% of all pediatric testicular masses (98,99) and are benign.

Histology: Epidermoid cysts are lined by mature stratified squamous epithelium, by definition lacking the pilosebaceous units and hair characteristic of dermoid cysts. No cytological atypia or mitotic activity is observed. The surrounding testis shows normal spermatogenesis, lacking IGCN or testicular atrophy. Provided these adverse features and malignant GCT components are excluded, these lesions are managed conservatively.

Embryonal carcinoma (EC)

Embryonal carcinoma is a frequent component of mixed GCT. Approximately 10% occur in pure form (100).

Histology: These are solid tumors characterized histologically by primitive epithelial cells with markedly pleomorphic nuclei arranged in solid sheets, glands, or papillary structures. They are positive for CD30, EMA, and OCT3/4 (28).

Choriocarcinoma

Choriocarcinoma is one of the rarest of all germ-cell tumors (28). It is seen as part of a mixed germ-cell tumor, or may occur as a pure tumor in the testis. Choriocarcinoma is prone to present as metastasis with a burnt-out primary. Pediatric cases are exceedingly rare.

Malignant mixed germ-cell tumor (MGCT)

Malignant mixed germ-cell tumors constitute approximately one-third of testicular tumors and are more common in the postpubertal testis. All types of primitive GCTs appear to occur with equal frequency and are seen as a random admixture of different components (28,101). These aggressive malignancies are treated radically.

Intratubular germ-cell neoplasia, unclassified type

Refer to the discussion of disorders of sex development.

Seminoma

Clinical presentation: Seminoma, the most common malignant testicular GCT overall, is rare in childhood (102).

Macroscopy: Seminomas are solid, pale yellow, and homogeneous. Hemorrhage and cystic changes should raise suspicions about MGCTs.

Histology: Seminomas show sheets of cells with clear cytoplasm, hyperchromatic nuclei, and prominent nucleoli separated by fibrovascular septa infiltrated by mature lymphocytes, and sometimes granulomas. Cases with microcystic or cribriform architecture may resemble YSTs. Seminoma cells are positive for OCT3/4, and negative for AFP and cytokeratin.

Sex-cord–stromal-cell tumor (SCST)

Sex-cord–stromal-cell tumors of the testes account for 11% of prepubertal testis tumors (103). The age range at first presentation is from infancy to adolescence, depending on tumor type (104). Testicular enlargement in the absence of associated signs or symptoms is the most common clinical presentation, and associated developmental abnormalities of the testis may be present.

Subtypes: The SCSTs that occur in children and adolescents include juvenile granulosa-cell tumors, Sertoli-cell tumors, and Leydig-cell tumors. Inhibin A is useful to differentiate SCSTs from germ-cell tumors of the testis.

Juvenile granulosa cell tumor (JGCT)

This is an uncommon, benign SCST occurring primarily in infancy.

Clinical presentation: Typically present as unilateral testicular masses in children less than one year of age. Juvenile granulosa cell tumors are the most common testicular neoplasms in newborns and infants (105,106). Hormonally active tumors are exceedingly rare (107). Juvenile granulosa cell tumors may occur in cryptorchid testes and in infants with ambiguous genitalia (108).

Hereditary/genetic features: Most cases occur in the setting of a normal karyotype; however, JGCTs may be associated with Y chromosome abnormalities and mosaicism (108).

Macroscopy: The tumors range in size from 1–2 cm and are partially cystic with a gray-white cut surface (109).

Histology: Refer to JGCTs of the ovary. Tumor cells react positively with vimentin and inhibin-α and negatively with PLAP and α-fetoprotein (109, 110).

Differential diagnosis: Juvenile granulosa cell tumors may resemble YSTs. Immunohistochemical staining with inhibin-α, PLAP, and α-fetoprotein will distinguish between these two entities, as will the presence of follicles in JGCTs and the lack of Schiller–Duvall bodies, a characteristic feature of YSTs (111).

Leydig-cell tumor

Rare, mostly benign SCST arising from Leydig cells.

Clinical presentation: Leydig-cell tumors affect prepubertal boys and adult males. Children range in age from three to nine years at diagnosis and typically present with pseudoisosexual precocity as a result of androgen secretion by the neoplasm (112). Tumors may also secrete estrogens and present with feminizing symptoms, such as gynecomastia. A mass may be identified on palpation or ultrasound examination of the testis. Laboratory investigation usually reveals elevation of testosterone in virilizing neoplasms, while α-fetoprotein, placental alkaline phosphatase, and β-human chorionic gonadotropin are typically within normal ranges (113).

Hereditary/genetic features: Activating mutations of the luteinizing hormone receptor gene are associated with the development of some tumors (114).

Macroscopy: A unilateral, sharply circumscribed and distinctly brown-to-yellow nodule embedded within the testicular parenchyma. Bilateral tumors are rare.

Histology: Neoplasm composed of nests, sheets, or trabeculae of tumor cells separated by fine fibrovascular septae. Tumor cells range from large and polygonal with abundant eosinophilic or clear cytoplasm, to small with scant cytoplasm and round-to-oval nuclei with occasional grooves. Reinke crystalloids and lipofuscin pigment may be present. Occasionally, tumor cells are spindled, and foci of ossification and adipose metaplasia are present, although this manifestation is primarily reported in adults (115,116). Inhibin A and vimentin are reactive with tumor cells. Inhibin A is useful to distinguish SCSTs from germ-cell tumors. Another useful marker is MART-1 (52). Leydig-cell tumors do not react with cytokeratins (113).

Sertoli-cell tumor

Rare, generally benign, stromal tumor of the testis.

Clinical presentation: Occurs in children and adolescents typically as a slow-growing, unilateral, painless testicular mass or swelling. Malignant Sertoli-cell tumors may be hormonally active, especially when associated with Peutz–Jegher's syndrome, and, if malignant, tend to metastasize to retroperitoneal lymph nodes (117). In addition, Sertoli-cell tumors are more often bilateral when associated with Carney's and Peutz–Jegher's syndromes (111,118).

Subtypes: Pure Sertoli-cell tumors may be subdivided into Sertoli-cell tumor, not otherwise specified (NOS), large-cell calcifying, and sclerosing subtypes; however, the sclerosing subtype normally occurs in adults.

Macroscopy: Well-circumscribed, focally cystic, firm, and white-tan mass. Tumors typically range in size from 3–4 cm. Hemorrhage may be present; however, necrosis is uncommon (111). Large-cell calcifying Sertoli-cell tumors may have a gritty texture due to the presence of calcifications.

Histology: In general, Sertoli-cell tumor, NOS is characterized by the presence of tubules lined by Sertoli cells. Low-grade tumors are characterized by a nodular pattern with intervening hypocellular fibrous stroma. Tubules may be solid or hollow, and hollow tubules may be dilated. More poorly differentiated neoplasms may lack tubule formation altogether. Vessels, sometimes dilated, may be present within the stroma. Lining tumor cells are polygonal with clear-to-pale or eosinophilic cytoplasm. Cytoplasmic lipid-containing vacuoles may also be present. Nuclei are round to oval with occasional grooves, and mitoses range from rare to numerous. Poorly differentiated tumors may be misdiagnosed as seminoma owing to a more diffuse pattern of growth with little intervening stroma and an inflammatory cell infiltrate (111,119,120).

With the large-cell calcifying Sertoli-cell tumor, various architectural patterns accompany solid tubule formation. Large tumor cells with ample eosinophilic cytoplasm are organized into nests, sheets, ribbons, or cords. Calcification is present, occasionally abundant, and cytologic atypia may be conspicuous (111).

Sertoli-cell tumor, NOS is reactive with inhibin-α and CD99, and non-reactive with PLAP (119,121).

Differential diagnosis: It is important to consider seminoma in less well-differentiated neoplasms and Sertoli-cell nodules.

Metastatic tumors of the testis

General features: Secondary involvement of the testis by leukemia and small round blue-cell tumors is most common in childhood and adolescence (122). Unilateral and solitary lesions may mimic a primary tumor (123).

Metastatic Wilms' tumor

Definition: Wilms' tumor (WT) is a malignant pediatric renal neoplasm arising from nephrogenic blastema (124).

Clinical presentation: Although WT is the most common renal neoplasm occurring in childhood, WT metastatic to the testis or paratesticular tissues, especially as a first presentation of metastatic disease, is exceptionally rare. Fewer than 10 cases have been reported (125).

Metastatic carcinoid tumor

Potentially malignant neoplasm of neuroendocrine cells. Most cases arise from the gastrointestinal tract, while the remainder arise from the lungs, pancreas, biliary tract, and other sites (126).

Clinical presentation: Although carcinoid tumors do occur in children, particularly in the appendix (127), metastasis to the testis is rare.

Involvement by leukemia

Testicular acute lymphoblastic leukemia may present at initial diagnosis or, more commonly, during follow-up as unilateral or bilateral testicular enlargement (128). Approximately 8% of males with acute leukemia will develop testicular involvement, and many will harbor occult metastases, despite complete remission on bone marrow examination and apparent successful treatment with chemotherapy (128,129). Testicular biopsy may be used to diagnose recurrence.

Epididymis, spermatic cord, and paratesticular tissue

Non-neoplastic disorders

Congenital

Abnormalities of the mesonephric duct system (absence of the epididymis, vas deferens, seminal vesicles, and ejaculatory ducts, selective atresia, cysts, diverticula, ectopias, spermatic cord cysts)

Congenital anomalies of the mesonephric duct system are numerous and can be classified as abnormalities of site, number, integrity, fusion, development, and suspension, depending on the structure affected (130).

Clinical presentation: Abnormalities may be asymptomatic, found incidentally on physical exam or present in adulthood as infertility. Unilateral absence of the vas deferens is the most common abnormality of the vas deferens and may accompany agenesis of the epididymis (130).

Hereditary/genetic features: Congenital bilateral absence of the vas deferens is associated with mutations in the cystic fibrosis transmembrane conductance regulator gene (131).

Epididymal cysts (diethylstilbestrol (DES) exposure *in utero*)

Clinical presentation: Typically presents in childhood or adolescence (2 months to 17 years) as an incidental finding on physical exam; however, patients may also present with a scrotal mass with or without pain (132). These lesions have been reported to occur in association with DES exposure (133) and cryptorchidism. Epididymal cysts are not generally clinically significant, except for the risk of torsion (134).

Heterotopic tissue in paratesticular region (adrenal rest)

Extra-adrenal tissue occurring within the paratesticular tissues.

Clinical presentation: Paratesticular adrenal rests are found in 7.5–15% of newborn testes, and most are adjacent to the epididymis or spermatic cord (135). Intratesticular adrenal rests are rare and may present as bilateral testicular masses with concomitant elevations of ACTH. Patients may present with systemic symptoms related to adrenal dysfunction associated with congenital adrenal hyperplasia, Addison's disease, and Cushing's syndrome (135,136).

Histology: Adrenal cortical rests are usually less than 1 mm and are similar in appearance to normal adrenal cortical tissue (135).

Splenogonadal fusion

Fusion of splenic and testicular tissue

Clinical presentation: Splenogonadal fusion may be discovered incidentally at autopsy or may present as a splenic mass lesion in the scrotum or inguinal canal. Fusion may be continuous, with a fibrous connection between the spleen and testis, or discontinuous, with ectopic splenic tissue connected to the testis (136).

Meconium periorchitis

A benign lesion of the paratesticular tissues resulting from bowel perforation and meconium peritonitis associated with cystic fibrosis (CF) (137), bowel abnormalities, or vascular compromise. Spillage of meconium into the abdominal cavity with subsequent leakage into paratesticular soft tissues via a patent processus vaginalis results in a hydrocele. Over time, the lesion calcifies and forms a mass (138,139).

Clinical presentation: The typical presentation is a scrotal mass in infants (age range 3 weeks to 5 months) (140). The lesion should raise concerns for CF. Approximately 7% of neonates with meconium periorchitis have CF (141).

Macroscopy: A 2–3 cm firm, gritty green-brown to yellow mass.

Microscopic features: Histologic exam reveals encapsulated calcified fibrous tissue with rare granulomas, pigment-laden macrophages and multinucleated giant cells (140).

Acquired

Epididymal sarcoidosis

Sarcoidosis is an idiopathic systemic inflammatory disease characterized histologically by the presence of non-caseating granulomas (142,143). Although unknown, the pathogenesis likely involves immune dysregulation.

Clinical presentation: Sarcoidosis most commonly affects the lung, lymphoid tissue, and skin. Other sites of involvement include the liver, eyes, heart, breasts, and joints. Involvement of the testicular and paratesticular structures is uncommon and is present in less than 1% of clinically diagnosed cases (144,145). Patients may be asymptomatic or may present with scrotal complaints or systemic symptoms. Scrotal lesions identified on imaging studies, especially when unilateral, may be confused with malignancy.

Benign tumors of the paratesticular structures

Nodular mesothelial hyperplasia

Nodular mesothelial hyperplasia is a benign reactive process consisting mostly of histiocytes and scattered mesothelial cells.

Clinical presentation: May present as an incidental finding in a hernia sac where there is an associated history of trauma such as incarceration. May also present in the thoracic cavity, including the pericardium and pleura (146). There is no age or sex predilection (147).

Histology: Characterized by a distinct nodular configuration at low-power magnification. The lesion is composed primarily of histiocytes, with mesothelial cells representing a small proportion. Islands of polygonal cells with abundant pale cytoplasm and indistinct cell borders are present throughout. Moderate pleomorphism may be observed; however, mitotic figures are uncommon, and atypical mitotic figures are absent. Nuclei are round to oval and may be grooved (146). The histiocytic population reacts with CD68 immunostaining, while the mesothelial cells will stain positively for calretinin and cytokeratins (146).

Differential diagnosis: The presence of cytologic atypia may lead to concerns regarding neoplastic processes (148).

Adenomatoid tumor

A rare, benign tumor of mesothelial origin with a characteristic glandular architecture.

Clinical presentation: Characteristically presents as a small scrotal mass that may be painful. Adenomatoid tumors are the most common paratesticular neoplasms (149) and may occur in the testis, tunica albuginea, spermatic cord, ejaculatory duct, and most frequently the epididymis (150).

Macroscopy: Typically unilateral and solitary, and ranging in size from 0.3–3.5 cm. Lesions are generally well-circumscribed rounded masses with firm, white-to-gray, and fascicular cut surfaces. Necrosis is uncommon (150).

Histology: Varying proportions of solid, angiomatoid, or adenoid architectural patterns present within fibromatous stroma. Cords, nests, or channels of flattened to cuboidal tumor cells with eosinophilic cytoplasm line pseudoglandular spaces. Thread-like strands of attenuated tumor-cell cytoplasm may bridge these spaces (151). The tumor cells may have an epithelioid appearance or may resemble signet-ring cells due to the presence of cytoplasmic vacuolizations. Lymphoid aggregates and blood vessels commonly occupy the periphery of the lesion. Cytologic atypia, nuclear pleomorphism, and mitoses are not present (150,151). Tumor cells stain positively for cytokeratin, calretinin, and vimentin (149).

Papillary cystadenoma of the epididymis

A rare, benign tumor of mesonephric origin occurring in the epididymis.

Clinical presentation: Papillary cystadenoma of the epididymis (PCE) may be discovered incidentally at autopsy or at physical exam, and typically presents as a slowly enlarging scrotal mass. The lesion may be painful and is usually unilateral.

Hereditary/genetic features: Up to two-thirds of reported cases have occurred in males with von Hippel–Lindau disease, particularly in bilateral cases. Inactivation of the von Hippel–Lindau gene results in increased expression of hypoxia-inducible factor (152,153).

Macroscopy: The tumor arises from the head of the epididymis and is a well-circumscribed 1–5 cm tan-to-yellow mass with varying proportions of solid and cystic components (154,155).

Histology: Papillary cystadenoma of the epididymis is a cystic lesion composed of papillae lined by cuboidal-to-columnar cells with clear cytoplasm. Nuclei are small with inconspicuous nucleoli, and mitoses are rare (155).

Melanotic neuroectodermal tumor (retinal anlage tumor)

A generally benign neoplasm of neural crest origin that most commonly affects the jaw, but may also affect the paratesticular structures in infants and young children (156).

Clinical presentation: A progressive unilateral scrotal swelling involving the epididymis. Recurrence and metastasis of cases occurring in the genitourinary tract are extremely uncommon (157).

Macroscopy: A gray-white to brown mass measuring 1–2 cm.

Histology: The lesion consists of a biphasic population of cells with a pseudoglandular and alveolar architectural pattern. One population is composed of nested, small round cells with little cytoplasm and ovoid, hyperchromatic nuclei, resembling neuroblasts. The second population lines the alveoli and is large with eosinophilic cytoplasm, ovoid nuclei, and cytoplasmic pigmented granules. The tumor stroma is hyalinized and contains frequent blood vessels. Mitoses are uncommon (156,158). Tumor cells react positively with HMB-45, neuron-specific enolase, and synaptophysin. The population of large cells may also react with vimentin (158).

Fibrous hamartoma of infancy

A benign fibroblastic proliferation occurring in young children and infants.

Clinical presentation: Presents primarily in children less than one year of age as a painless nodule with occasional rapid growth. Lesions may occur on the external genitalia, groin, axillae, and upper body. Fibrous hamartoma of infancy (FHI) is more common in boys (159).

Macroscopy: Grossly, FHI is remarkable for a white, fibrous cut surface with the presence of adipose tissue throughout.

Histology: Histologic exam reveals subcutaneous fibrous bands, mature adipose tissue, and nests or nodules of immature mesenchyme (159,160).

Immunohistochemistry: Both the fibrous connective tissue and immature mesenchymal cells stain positively for vimentin (161).

Differential diagnosis: Includes lipofibromatosis and fibromatosis.

Malignant tumors of the paratesticular structures

Rhabdomyosarcoma (spindle-cell variant)

Spindle cell rhabdomyosarcoma (SC-RMS) is a variant of embryonal rhabdomyosarcoma.

Clinical presentation: The spindle-cell variant most commonly affects children and adolescents and primarily occurs in the paratesticular structures.

Macroscopy: A firm, whorled, and white-tan cut surface that may be confused for leiomyosarcoma (162); a pseudosarcomatous fibroblastic reaction post-infarct secondary to testicular torsion should also be discriminated from SC-RMS.

Histology: The tumor is a variably cellular lesion characterized by interwoven bundles of elongated, atypical spindled cells. Nuclei are ovoid and occasionally contain conspicuous nucleoli. Rhabdomyoblasts, cytoplasmic cross-striations, and giant cells are uncommon (163).

Malignant mesothelioma

A rare malignant neoplasm that usually arises from the pleura. Although uncommon, malignant mesothelioma (MME) may also arise from the mesothelial cells lining the tunica vaginalis (164).

Clinical presentation: Malignant mesothelioma of the tunica vaginalis mostly affects men greater than 50 years of age; however, approximately 10% of cases affect males under 25 and there are case reports in adolescents (165). Although exposure to asbestos is commonly associated with the development of this tumor in adults, information on exposure history in this age group is lacking (166). Paratesticular tumors will present with scrotal enlargement or swelling.

Histology: Malignant mesothelioma of the tunica vaginalis is histologically and immunohistochemically similar to mesotheliomas occurring in other sites.

Differential diagnosis: It is important to consider that an adenomatoid tumor can be distinguished from malignant mesothelioma by its lack of nuclear atypia and mitotic figures (166).

Desmoplastic small round-cell tumor

An aggressive malignant round-cell neoplasm occurring predominantly in young males.

Clinical presentation: Presents in older children and adolescents as a scrotal or abdominal mass. Associated systemic symptoms, such as loss of appetite, fever, and fatigue, may be present. Metastatic disease involving the retroperitoneal lymph nodes, lungs, and bones at first presentation is not uncommon (167).

Genetic features: Associated with fusion of the Ewing's sarcoma (EWS) and WT suppressor (WT-1) genes, which is due to a t(11;22)(p13;q12) translocation. The resultant fusion protein activates transcription (168).

Macroscopy: A white-tan, firm, and multinodular mass. Scattered nodules separate from the main mass may be present. Necrosis is generally absent (169,170).

Histology: Characterized by nests, islands, or cords of small, uniform cells separated by bands of collagen with spindled cells and desmoplastic stroma. Tubules, glands, and rosettes may be present within the nests. Tumor cells have scant cytoplasm with indistinct cell

321

boundaries and ovoid nuclei with clumped chromatin and inconspicuous nucleoli. Mitotic figures are common (169,170).

Tumor cells react with desmin, WT1, NSE, AE1/AE3, and CAM 5.2. Desmin reactivity is characterized by a cytoplasmic dot-like pattern of staining (170).

Prostate

Non-neoplastic disorders

Congenital

Cyst of the prostatic utricle (Müllerian cyst)

A rare cyst that arises from the utricle due to failed regression of the Müllerian ducts. The utricle is a midline blind pouch located in the verumontanum towards the base of the prostate and is flanked on either side by the ejaculatory ducts.

Clinical presentation: Cysts of the prostatic utricle may be an incidental finding or may arise secondary to inflammation. These cysts are found in males of all ages. Congenital cysts may be associated with other anomalies of the urinary tract, such as hypospadias, cryptorchidism, and renal agenesis.

Histology: The cyst wall may be lined by squamous, transitional, cuboidal, or columnar epithelium, or may entirely lack lining epithelium. Calcific concretions may be present within the cyst.

Acquired

Periprostatic abscess

Clinical presentation: Presents with urinary retention, fever, bladder distension, and a midline swelling on physical exam. Spread of infection to the genitourinary tract is likely hematogenous, and extension of infection to the adjacent paratesticular structures can occur. Urine cultures may fail to yield an organism.

Malignant tumors of the prostate

Rhabdomyosarcoma

Clinical presentation: Rhabdomyosarcoma (RMS) is a malignant neoplasm of skeletal muscle differentiation and is the most common primary malignant neoplasm arising in the genitourinary tract in infants and children. Rhabdomyosarcoma of the prostate commonly presents as a solid mass accompanied by increased frequency of urination, urinary retention, and/or hematuria (171).

Classification/subtypes of the condition: Embryonal rhabdomyosarcoma comprises the vast majority of cases occurring in children and is subtyped as botryoid, spindled cell, or not otherwise specified, according to the histologic pattern observed.

Histology: See embryonal RMS of the vagina and cervix.

Malignant rhabdoid tumor

A rare and aggressive malignant neoplasm that mainly occurs in the kidney, but also affects other sites, such as the liver, bladder, heart, and chest wall. Only a handful of cases involving the prostate have been reported (172).

Clinical presentation: Malignant rhabdoid tumor of the kidney typically presents in young children and infants, and has a dismal prognosis.

Macroscopy: Tumors are only rarely encapsulated and are grossly remarkable for a pink to gray-tan cut surface with foci of hemorrhage and necrosis and range in size from 1.3–18 cm (172,173).

Histology: The tumor displays a predominantly solid architecture. Tumor cells are uniform, polygonal, large, and discohesive with abundant eosinophilic or basophilic cytoplasm. Intracytoplasmic inclusions may be present. Nuclei are large with a single conspicuous nucleolus. Mitoses are numerous; however, atypical mitoses are uncommon. The interstitium may be focally edematous or myxoid (172,173). Tumor cells invariably react with vimentin, however, the most important feature is the loss of INI-1 nuclear expression by tumor cells (174).

Penis

Non-neoplastic disorders

Congenital

Hypospadias

Definition: A congenital midline fusion defect of the penis characterized by a ventrally located urethral opening, and an incompletely formed prepuce and excess dorsal hood (175,176).

Epispadias

A congenital abnormality of the penis characterized by localization of the urethral opening to the dorsal aspect of the penis. It is usually accompanied by dorsal curvature.

Clinical presentation: Presents at birth in isolation or as part of the bladder exstrophy-epispadias-complex.

Acquired

Balanitis xerotica obliterans

A chronic dermatitis and variant of lichen sclerosus that involves the glans and prepuce, and occasionally the urethra (177).

Clinical presentation: The median age at diagnosis in male children is 10.6 years, with a range of 8 to 13 years, although the condition also occurs in adolescents and adults. Patients may present with phimosis due to tightening of the foreskin, pain, changes in sensation and urinary symptoms. The clinical course is variable, and recurrences are common (177,178). Balanitis xerotica obliterans is associated with penile squamous cell carcinoma in adult males (179).

Hereditary/genetic features: Strongly linked to HLA DQ7 (178).

Histology: The epidermis is hyperkeratotic, atrophic, and displays basal cell vacuolization. The upper dermis is edematous and hypocellular and overlies a chronic lymphocytic infiltrate.

Malignant tumors of the penis

Yolk-sac tumor

Yolk-sac tumor (YST) is the most common germ-cell tumor in prepubertal children.

Clinical presentation: Primary YST of the penis has been reported (180,181), although it is very uncommon.

Disorders of sex development (DSD)

Disorders of sex development comprise congenital conditions with atypical development of the chromosomal, gonadal, or anatomical sex (182). DSD form a complex group of conditions with a diverse etiology. The four different aspects affected are genetic, gonadal, phenotypic, and behavioral sex (183).

Hereditary/genetic features: Known etiologies of DSD include aberrations of the sex chromosomes, such as 45, X0 karyotype in Turner syndrome, or a 46 XX/XY karyotype that can be found in some cases of ovotesticular DSD. Other causes of DSD are mutations in genes involved in gonadal differentiation, for example WT-1, which has a regulatory function in urogenital development and is essential for male sex determination. Point mutations in the WT-1 gene lead to Frasier syndrome (52) and Denys–Drash syndrome.

In patients with 46, XX or 46, XY karyotypes and normally developed gonads, defects in steroid synthesis, end-organ defects, or endogenous or exogenous hormone effects can lead to DSDs. Examples include StAR deficiency, androgenital syndrome (21 α-hydroxylase deficiency), maternal virilizing tumors, and complete androgen insensitivity syndrome (CAIS), respectively.

Classification systems and nomenclature: Multiple classification systems and nomenclatures have been proposed for DSD. The 2006 Chicago consensus guideline (184) is mostly based on the karyotype (46, XY DSD; 46, XX DSD; ovotesticular DSD; 46, XX testicular DSD; 46, XY complete gonadal dysgenesis) rather than on gonadal morphology. Another classification system proposed by Aaronson (185) in 2010 focuses mostly on gonadal histology and, although somewhat simple, it is useful from a pathology perspective. Based on morphologic features of the gonads, the classification system categorizes four subtypes of DSD: ovarian DSD, testicular DSD, ovotesticular DSD, and dysgenetic DSD.

Ovarian and testicular DSD

Ovarian and testicular DSD are characterized by the presence of normal ovarian and testicular tissue, respectively. Leydig cells may be prominent in the testicular tissue.

Ovotesticular DSD (ovotestis)

Ovotesticular DSD is characterized by the presence of ovarian and testicular tissue, which may be separate or admixed, in the same gonad (Figure 9.10). At least one well-developed follicle must be seen in the ovarian tissue, and the testicular tissue must contain organized cords/tubules (185).

Dysgenetic DSD (dysgenetic gonad)

Dysgenetic DSD is characterized by gonadal dysgenesis, i.e. impaired development of the gonads due to abnormal migration and/or organization of the germ cells and surrounding stroma within the fetal urogenital ridge (185).

Subtype: streak gonad

Histology: Streak gonads show variable amounts of dense fibrous tissue and ovarian-type stroma. Wavy, elongated cells are seen in a background of bands of connective tissue. Streak gonads lack germ cells and are devoid of tunica albuginea. Sex-cord–stromal

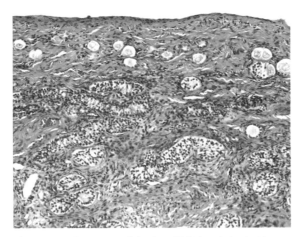

Figure 9.10 Ovotestis: well-developed follicles admixed with organized tubules.

derivatives may be present as cord-like structures in the stroma (184). Thickened hilar vessels and Leydig (hilar)-cell hyperplasia can be frequently seen.

Subtype: undifferentiated gonadal tissue

Histology: Characterized by single or aligned clusters of germ cells, admixed with sex-cord cells in fibrous stroma (184).

Subtype: dysgenetic testicular tissue

Histology: Dysgenetic testes usually show abnormal collagenization of the tunica albuginea, which features ectopic and misshapen testicular cords within its structure.

Subtype: mixed gonadal dysgenesis (MGD)

Definition: In MGD, both Müllerian and Wolffian structures can be found in variable amounts. Usually there is a streak gonad on one side and a dysgenetic testis on the other.

In situ neoplastic lesion arising in dysgenetic DSD

Clinical presentation: The development of invasive germ-cell tumors is always preceded by *in situ* neoplastic lesions, either gonadoblastoma (186–188) or intratubular germ-cell neoplasia (188), which are now considered a continuum (189). Both *in situ* lesions arise from primordial germ cells and gonocytes (190) and give rise to identical spectra of germ-cell tumors. Differences in microenvironment, particularly the lack of functional Sertoli cells, are proposed to lead to female differentiation and subsequent gonadoblastoma, whereas for the development of

intratubular germ-cell neoplasia, a certain level of testicular development is required (189).

Subtype: Gonadoblastoma

Gonadoblastoma is a mixed germ-cell–sex-cord–stromal tumor.

Clinical presentation: The most common neoplastic lesion seen in dysgenetic gonads is gonadoblastoma (183), which is bilateral in 35% of cases. The patients are usually phenotypically female. Approximately 30% of gonadoblastomas are found before 15 years of age. Gonadoblastoma itself is a benign lesion (186); however, it is a known precursor lesion for malignant germ-cell tumors. Gonadoblastomas are overgrown by dysgerminoma in 50% of cases and contain variable amounts of other malignant germ-cell components (immature teratoma, EC, YST, and choriocarcinoma) in an additional 10% of cases (186,191,192).

Hereditary/genetic features: Patients with Y-chromosome fragments on karyotypic or molecular analysis are at risk for development of gonadoblastoma and other subsequent germ-cell neoplasms, likely due to the testis-specific protein-Y-encoded (*TSPY*) gene (193).

Macroscopy: Gonadoblastomas can range from a microscopic focus to a mass lesion measuring several centimeters. They are gray or yellow-brown and exhibit variable amounts of calcifications.

Histology: Gonadoblastomas are composed of immature germ cells similar to the cells observed in dysgerminoma/seminoma and sex-cord–stromal cells of granulosa-cell lineage (192). The sex-cord–stromal cells may surround germ-cell aggregates as a peripheral palisade, may be arranged in a coronal pattern around individual germ cells or germ-cell clusters, or may radially surround small round deposits containing amorphous hyaline, eosinophilic, PAS-positive material (Figures 9.11 and 9.12). The radial pattern can resemble Call–Exner bodies. Leydig-like cells, devoid of Reinke crystals, are observed in two-thirds of gonadoblastomas (186,187). Stromal hyalinization and calcification presenting as laminated plaques or in a characteristic mulberry-like pattern are frequently encountered (186,187). Calcification and hyalinization can eventually result in "burnt-out" gonadoblastoma, with no or only very scattered tumor cells.

Immunohistochemistry: The germ cells are immunoreactive for PLAP, CD117, and OCT 3/4. The sex-cord–stromal derivatives express inhibin and FOXL2,

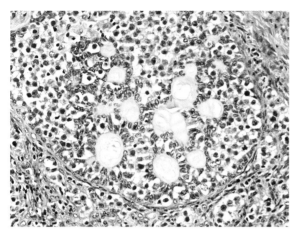

Figure 9.11 Radial pattern of gonadoblastoma resembling Call–Exner bodies and mulberry-like calcification (left).

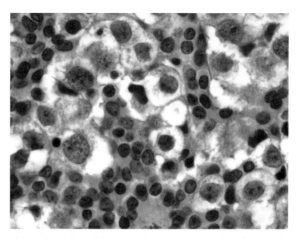

Figure 9.12 Gonadoblastoma: immature germ cells and sex-cord–stromal cells of granulosa cell lineage.

and are negative for sex-determining region Y-box (SOX) 9 (194).

Differential diagnosis: Gonadoblastoma can resemble SCTAT, SLCT, and AGCT, microfollicular type (see also AGCT section).

Subtype: intratubular germ-cell neoplasia of unclassified type (ITGN)

Also known as carcinoma *in situ*, this is a proliferation of neoplastic germ cells confined to the seminiferous tubules.

Histology: This neoplasia reveals large tumor cells with clear-to-eosinophilic cytoplasm and enlarged vesicular nuclei scattered within the seminiferous epithelium. The cells are distributed along the periphery of the seminiferous tubules and are either admixed with non-neoplastic Sertoli cells or fill up the entire lumen. The tubular basement membrane may be thickened. The germ cells are positive for PLAP, CD117, and OCT 3/4. Inhibin and SOX 9 are expressed in the Sertoli cells, which are negative for FOXL2 (192).

Prophylactic gonadectomy

Clinical presentation: Prophylactic bilateral gonadectomy is recommended at an early age for females with dysgenetic DSD and evidence of Y-chromosome material (195,196).

Estimates of the prevalence of germ-cell tumors arising in dysgenetic DSD range from 15% (183) to 30%, (197), and the risk is strongly influenced by the underlying DSD and the patient's age at the time of prophylactic gonadectomy (183,195).

Maturation delay of germ cells

Germ cells in dysgenetic gonads, lacking normal maturation and exhibiting morphological and immunohistochemical features of gonocytes.

Clinical presentation: Maturation delay is more frequently encountered in DSD associated with under-virilization (198) and can be difficult to differentiate from neoplastic transformation.

Histology: Immature germ cells resemble gonocytes. The distribution of OCT3/4-positive germ cells in the tubule, their relationship to the basal lamina, and consideration of the patient's age have been described as useful aids for distinguishing immature germ cells from maturation delay (198).

Gonadal findings in androgen insensitivity syndrome (AIS)

Androgen insensitivity syndrome (testicular feminization) is an end-organ failure to respond to androgens caused by mutations in the *androgen receptor (AR)* gene.

Clinical presentation: Patients with complete androgen insensitivity syndrome (CAIS) are phenotypically female, and often present in childhood with an inguinal hernia containing testicular gonadal tissue or during adolescence with primary amenorrhea. In contrast, patients with partial androgen insensitivity syndrome (PAIS) frequently show ambiguous genitalia.

Hereditary/genetic features: Androgen insensitivity syndrome is an X-linked XY DSD due to various mutations causing abnormalities of the AR. Most patients harbor a 46, XY karyotype, but mosaic forms can occasionally be found (199).

325

Macroscopy: Three typical gross findings have been reported: multiple yellow-tan or white nodules within the testis/gonad; a hyalinized, white, firm nodule of smooth muscle attached to the medial pole (AIS) of the testis; and lateral adnexal cysts (199).

Histology: Testes removed from adult AIS patients resemble immature, infantile, or cryptorchidic testes. Leydig cells are frequently devoid of Reinke's crystals (199) and may reveal the presence of lipid droplets in the cytoplasm, or an undifferentiated appearance (200). Sertoli-cell hamartomas and adenomas are frequently present. Sertoli-cell hamartomas are composed of seminiferous tubules lined by immature Sertoli cells and Leydig cells that can be hyper- or hypoplastic (199). The spindle-cell stroma has been traditionally referred to as "ovarian-like." Small tubules filled with immature Sertoli cells and scant Leydig cells are seen in Sertoli-cell adenomas (199). In prepubertal patients with AIS, the testicular tissue shows only diffuse changes, including Leydig cell hyperplasia and decreased germ-cell numbers (200). No definitive morphologic differences are noted between CAIS and PAIS (199).

Differential diagnosis: Sertoli cell adenoma/hamartoma needs to be distinguished from Sertoli and SLCT tumors. In addition, the clinical history, orderly arranged tubules without lumina, and lack of endocrine activity favor Sertoli-cell adenoma/hamartoma over the other two entities.

References

1. Eustace DL, Congenital absence of fallopian tube and ovary. Eur. J. Obstet. Gynecol. Reprod. Biol. 1992;**46**:157–9.

2. DeCherney AH, Cholst I, Naftolin F, Structure and function of the fallopian tubes following exposure to diethylstilbestrol (DES) during gestation. Fertil. Steril. 1981;**36**:741–5.

3. Anthony E. Y., Caserta MP, Singh J, Chen MY. Adnexal masses in female pediatric patients, AJR 2012;**198**: w426–37.

4. Foster CM, Feuillan P, Padmanabhan V, *et al.* Ovarian function in girls with McCune-Albright syndrome. Pediatr. Res. 1986;**20**:859–63.

5. Dumitrescu CE, Collins MT, McCune-Albright syndrome. Orphanet. J. Rare Dis. 2008;**3**:12.

6. Bremer AA, Polycystic ovary syndrome in the pediatric population. Metab. Syndr. Relat. Disord. 2010;**8**:375–94.

7. Revised 2003 consensus on diagnostic criteria and long-term health risks related to polycystic ovary syndrome (PCOS). Hum. Reprod. 2004;**19**:41–7.

8. Franks S, Polycystic ovary syndrome in adolescents. Int. J. Obes. (Lond) 2008;**32**:1035–41.

9. Moon RJ, Mears A, Kitteringham LJ, *et al.* Davies, Massive ovarian oedema: An unusual abdominal mass in infancy. Pediatr. Blood Cancer 2009;**53**:217–19.

10. Natarajan A, Wales JK, Marven SS, Wright NP, Precocious puberty secondary to massive ovarian oedema in a 6-month-old girl. Eur. J. Endocrinol. 2004;**150**:119–23.

11. Young RH, Scully RE, Fibromatosis and massive edema of the ovary, possibly related entities: A report of 14 cases of fibromatosis and 11 cases of massive edema. Int. J. Gynecol. Pathol. 1984;**3**:153–78.

12. Kauffman RP, Castracane VD, Premature ovarian failure associated with autoimmune polyglandular syndrome: pathophysiological mechanisms and future fertility. J. Womens Health (Larchmt.) 2003;**12**:513–20.

13. Maclaren N, Chen QY, Kukreja A, *et al.* Autoimmune hypogonadism as part of an autoimmune polyglandular syndrome. J. Soc. Gynecol. Investig. 2001;**8**:S52–4.

14. Proust-Lemoine E, Saugier-Veber P, Wemeau JL, Polyglandular autoimmune syndrome type I. Presse Med. 2012;**41**: e651–62.

15. Cao D, Humphrey PA, Allan RW, SALL4 is a novel sensitive and specific marker for metastatic germ cell tumors, with particular utility in detection of metastatic yolk sac tumors. Cancer 2009;**115**:2640–51.

16. Cheng L, Roth LM, Zhang S, *et al.* KIT gene mutation and amplification in dysgerminoma of the ovary. Cancer 2011;**117**:2096–103.

17. Mueller CW, Topkins P, Lapp WA, Dysgerminoma of the ovary; an analysis of 427 cases. Am. J. Obstet. Gynecol. 1950;**60**:153–9.

18. Pressley RH, Muntz HG, Falkenberry S, Rice LW, Serum lactic dehydrogenase as a tumor marker in dysgerminoma. Gynecol. Oncol. 1992;**44**:281–3.

19. Zaloudek CJ, Tavassoli FA, Norris HJ, Dysgerminoma with syncytiotrophoblastic giant cells. A histologically and clinically distinctive subtype of dysgerminoma. Am. J. Surg. Pathol. 1981;**5**:361–7.

20. De Palo G, Lattuada A, Kenda R, *et al.* Germ cell tumors of the ovary: the experience of the National Cancer Institute of Milan. I. Dysgerminoma. Int. J. Radiat. Oncol. Biol. Phys. 1987;**13**:853–60.

21. De Palo G, Pilotti S, Kenda R, *et al.* Natural history of dysgerminoma. Am. J. Obstet. Gynecol. 1982;**143**:799–807.

22. Srigley JR, Mackay B, Toth P, Ayala A, The ultrastructure and histogenesis of male germ neoplasia

with emphasis on seminoma with early carcinomatous features. Ultrastruct. Pathol. 1988;**12**:67–86.

23. Talerman AV, R, Germ cell tumors of the ovary. In R.E. Kurman, L. Ronnett, B., editors, *Blausteins's Pathology of the Female Genital Tract*, New York: Springer; 2011.

24. Fujita M, Inoue M, Tanizawa O, *et al.* Retrospective review of 41 patients with endodermal sinus tumor of the ovary. Int. J. Gynecol. Cancer 1993;**3**:329–35.

25. Peccatori F, Bonazzi C, Chiari S, *et al.* Surgical management of malignant ovarian germ-cell tumors: 10 years' experience of 129 patients. Obstet. Gynecol. 1995;**86**:367–72.

26. Chang MC, Vargas SO, Hornick JL, *et al.* Embryonic stem cell transcription factors and D2–40 (podoplanin) as diagnostic immunohistochemical markers in ovarian germ cell tumors. Int. J. Gynecol. Pathol. 2009;**28**:347–55.

27. Esheba GE, Pate LL, Longacre TA, Oncofetal protein glypican-3 distinguishes yolk sac tumor from clear cell carcinoma of the ovary. Am. J. Surg. Pathol. 2008;**32**:600–607.

28. Ulbright TM, Germ cell tumors of the gonads: A selective review emphasizing problems in differential diagnosis, newly appreciated, and controversial issues. Mod. Pathol. 2005;**18** Suppl 2:S61–79.

29. Ramalingam P, Malpica A, Silva EG, *et al.* The use of cytokeratin 7 and EMA in differentiating ovarian yolk sac tumors from endometrioid and clear cell carcinomas. Am. J. Surg. Pathol. 2004;**28**:1499–505.

30. Harms D, Zahn S, Gobel U, Schneider DT, Pathology and molecular biology of teratomas in childhood and adolescence. Klin. Padiatr. 2006;**218**:296–302.

31. Koonings PP, Campbell K, Mishell DR, Jr., Grimes DA, Relative frequency of primary ovarian neoplasms: A 10-year review. Obstet. Gynecol. 1989;**74**: 921–6.

32. Ulbright TM, Gonadal teratomas: A review and speculation. Adv. Anat. Pathol. 2004;**11**:10–23.

33. Kawai M, Kano T, Kikkawa F, *et al.* Seven tumor markers in benign and malignant germ cell tumors of the ovary. Gynecol. Oncol. 1992;**45**:248–53.

34. Heifetz SA, Cushing B, Giller R, *et al.* Immature teratomas in children: pathologic considerations: A report from the combined Pediatric Oncology Group/Children's Cancer Group. Am. J. Surg. Pathol. 1998;**22**:1115–24.

35. Gobel U, Calaminus G, Schneider DT, *et al.* The malignant potential of teratomas in infancy and childhood: the MAKEI experiences in non-testicular teratoma and implications for a new protocol. Klin. Padiatr. 2006;**218**:309–14.

36. Tapper D, Lack EE, Teratomas in infancy and childhood. A 54-year experience at the Children's Hospital Medical Center. Ann. Surg. 1983;**198**:398–410.

37. Norris HJ, Zirkin HJ, Benson WL, Immature (malignant) teratoma of the ovary: A clinical and pathologic study of 58 cases. Cancer 1976;**37**:2359–2372.

38. O'Connor DM, Norris HJ, The influence of grade on the outcome of stage I ovarian immature (malignant) teratomas and the reproducibility of grading. Int. J. Gynecol. Pathol. 1994;**13**:283–9.

39. Kurman RJ, Norris HJ, Embryonal carcinoma of the ovary: A clinicopathologic entity distinct from endodermal sinus tumor resembling embryonal carcinoma of the adult testis. Cancer 1976;**38**:2420–33.

40. Jacobs AJ, Newland JR, Green RK, Pure choriocarcinoma of the ovary. Obstet. Gynecol. Surv. 1982;**37**:603–9.

41. Gershenson DM, Del Junco G, Copeland LJ, Rutledge FN, Mixed germ cell tumors of the ovary. Obstet. Gynecol. 1984;**64**:200–6.

42. Kurman RJ, Norris HJ, Malignant mixed germ cell tumors of the ovary. A clinical and pathologic analysis of 30 cases. Obstet. Gynecol. 1976;**48**:579–589.

43. Al-Agha OM, Huwait HF, Chow C, *et al.* FOXL2 is a sensitive and specific marker for sex cord-stromal tumors of the ovary. Am. J. Surg. Pathol. 2011;**35**:484–94.

44. Young RH, Dickersin GR, Scully RE, Juvenile granulosa cell tumor of the ovary. A clinicopathological analysis of 125 cases. Am. J. Surg. Pathol. 1984;**8**:575–96.

45. Cecchetto G, Ferrari A, Bernini G, *et al.* Sex cord stromal tumors of the ovary in children: A clinicopathological report from the Italian TREP project. Pediatr. Blood Cancer 2011;**56**:1062–7.

46. Shah SP, Kobel M, Senz J, *et al.* Mutation of FOXL2 in granulosa-cell tumors of the ovary. N. Engl. J. Med. 2009;**360**:2719–29.

47. Bjorkholm E, Silfversward C, Prognostic factors in granulosa-cell tumors. Gynecol. Oncol. 1981;**11**:261–74.

48. Stenwig JT, Hazekamp JT, Beecham JB, Granulosa cell tumors of the ovary. A clinicopathological study of 118 cases with long-term follow-up. Gynecol. Oncol. 1979;**7**:136–52.

49. Prat J, Sex cord-stromal tumors. In Prat J, editor, *Pathology of the Ovary*. Philadelphia, PA: Saunders; 2004.

50. Tavassoli FA, Devilee P, *Pathology and Genetics of Tumours of the Breast and Female Genital Tract*. Lyons: IARC Press; 2003.

51. Prat J, Young RH, Scully RE, Ovarian Sertoli-Leydig cell tumors with heterologous elements. II. Cartilage and skeletal muscle: A clinicopathologic analysis of twelve cases. Cancer 1982;**50**:2465–75.

52. Zhao C, Vinh TN, McManus K, *et al*. Identification of the most sensitive and robust immunohistochemical markers in different categories of ovarian sex cord-stromal tumors. Am. J. Surg. Pathol. 2009;**33**:354–66.

53. Gwin K, Marino-Enriquez A, Martel M, Reyes-Mugica M, Sclerosing stromal tumor: An important differential diagnosis of ovarian neoplasms in childhood and adolescence. Pediatr. Dev. Pathol. 2009;**12**:366–70.

54. Morowitz M, Huff D, von Allmen D, Epithelial ovarian tumors in children: A retrospective analysis, J. Pediatr. Surg. 2003;**38**:331–5.

55. Morris HB, La Vecchia C, Draper GJ, Malignant epithelial tumors of the ovary in childhood: A clinicopathological study of 13 cases in Great Britain 1962–1978. Gynecol. Oncol. 1984;**19**:290–7.

56. Young RH, Oliva E, Scully RE, Small cell carcinoma of the ovary, hypercalcemic type. A clinicopathological analysis of 150 cases. Am. J. Surg. Pathol. 1994;**18**:1102–16.

57. Gell JS, Mullerian anomalies, *Semin Reprod Med* 2003;**21**:375–388.

58. Vargas SO, Kozakewich HP, Boyd TK, *et al*. Childhood asymmetric labium majus enlargement: mimicking a neoplasm. *Am. J. Surg. Pathol.* 2005;**29**.1007–16.

59. Iwasa Y, Fletcher CD, Distinctive prepubertal vulval fibroma: A hitherto unrecognized mesenchymal tumor of prepubertal girls: Analysis of 11 cases. Am. J. Surg. Pathol. 2004;**28**:1601–8.

60. Vargas SO,: Pediatric pathology case 1: Childhood asymmetric labium majus enlargement. USCAP Specialty Conference, 2006.

61. Fetch JL, Soft tissue lesions involving female reproductive organs. In Kurman RJ, Hedrick Ellenson L, Ronnett BM, editors, *Blaustein's Pathology of the Female Genital Tract*, New York: Springer; 2011.

62. Dehner LP, Jarzembowski JA, Hill DA, Embryonal rhabdomyosarcoma of the uterine cervix: A report of 14 cases and a discussion of its unusual clinicopathological associations. Mod. Pathol. 2012;**25**:602–14.

63. Copeland DM, Gerhenson PB, Saul N, *et al*. Sarcoma botyoides of the female geintal tract. *Obstet gynecol* 1985,**66**:262–66.

64. Melnick S, Cole P, Anderson D, Herbst A, Rates and risks of diethylstilbestrol-related clear-cell adenocarcinoma of the vagina and cervix. An update, N. Engl. J. Med. 1987;**316**:514–16.

65. Waggoner SE, Mittendorf R, Biney N, Anderson D, Herbst AL, Influence of in utero diethylstilbestrol exposure on the prognosis and biologic behavior of vaginal clear-cell adenocarcinoma. Gynecol.Oncol. 1994;**55**:238–44.

66. McCluggage WG, Sumathi VP, Nucci MR, *et al*. Ewing family of tumours involving the vulva and vagina: report of a series of four cases. J. Clin. Pathol. 2007;**60**:674–80.

67. Glantz, Hansen K, Caldamone A, Medeiros LJ, Cystic dysplasia of the testis, Hum. Pathol. 1993;**24**:1142–5.

68. Cho CS, Kosek J, Cystic dysplasia of the testis: sonographic and pathologic findings. Radiology 1985;**156**:777–8.

69. Kryvenko ON, Epstein JI, Testicular hemangioma: A series of 8 cases. Am. J. Surg. Pathol. 2013;**37**:860–6.

70. Al-Adnani M, Williams S, Rampling D, *et al*. Histopathological reporting of paediatric cutaneous vascular anomalies in relation to proposed multidisciplinary classification system. J. Clin. Pathol. 2006;**59**:1278–82.

71. Mazal PR, Kratzik C, Kain R, Susani M, Capillary haemangioma of the testis. J. Clin. Pathol. 2000;**53**:641–2.

72. Bruder E, Alaggio R, Kozakewich HP, *et al*. Vascular and perivascular lesions of skin and soft tissues in children and adolescents. Pediatr. Dev. Pathol. 2012;**15**:26–61.

73. Law H, Mushtaq I, Wingrove K, Malone M, Sebire NJ, Histopathological features of testicular regression syndrome: relation to patient age and implications for management. Fetal Pediatr. Pathol. 2006;**25**:119–29.

74. Spires SE, Woolums CS, Pulito AR, Spires SM, Testicular regression syndrome: A clinical and pathologic study of 11 cases. Arch. Pathol. Lab. Med. 2000;**124**:694–8.

75. Emir H, Ayik B, Elicevik M, *et al*. Histological evaluation of the testicular nubbins in patients with nonpalpable testis: Assessment of etiology and surgical approach. Pediatr. Surg. Int. 2007;**23**:41–4.

76. Thorup J, McLachlan R, Cortes D, *et al*. What is new in cryptorchidism and hypospadias – a critical review on the testicular dysgenesis hypothesis. J. Pediatr. Surg. 2010;**45**:2074–86.

77. Taran I, Elder JS, Results of orchiopexy for the undescended testis. World J. Urol. 2006;**24**:231–9.

78. Miliaras D, Vlahakis-Miliaras E, Anagnostopoulos D, *et al*. Gross morphologic variations and histologic changes in cryptorchid testes. Pediatr. Surg. Int. 1997;**12**:158–62.

79. Nistal M, Paniagua R, Diez-Pardo JA, Histologic classification of undescended testes. Hum. Pathol. 1980;**11**:666–74.

80. Vallangeon BD, Eble JN, Ulbright TM, Macroscopic sertoli cell nodule: A study of 6 cases that presented as testicular masses. Am. J. Surg. Pathol. 2010;**34**:1874–80.

81. Arce JD, Cortes M, Vargas JC, Sonographic diagnosis of acute spermatic cord torsion. Rotation of the cord: A key to the diagnosis. Pediatr. Radiol. 2002;**32**:485–91.

82. Karmazyn B, Steinberg R, Kornreich L, *et al.* Clinical and sonographic criteria of acute scrotum in children: A retrospective study of 172 boys. Pediatr. Radiol. 2005;**35**:302–10.

83. Saxena AK, Castellani C, Ruttenstock EM, Hollwarth ME, Testicular torsion: A 15-year single-centre clinical and histological analysis. Acta Paediatr. 2012;**101**:e282–6.

84. Mneimneh WS, Nazeer T, Jennings TA, Torsion of the gonad in the pediatric population: spectrum of histologic findings with focus on aspects specific to neonates and infants. Pediatr. Dev. Pathol. 2013;**16**:74–9.

85. Hajji F, Janane A, Images in clinical medicine. Torsion of undescended testis. N. Engl. J. Med. 2012;**366**:1625.

86. Perimenis P, Athanasopoulos A, Venetsanou-Petrochilou C, Barbalias G, Idiopathic granulomatous orchitis. Eur. Urol. 1991;**19**:118–20.

87. Krieger JN, Epididymitis, orchitis, and related conditions Sex. Transm. Dis. 1984;**11**:173–81.

88. Braaten KM, Young RH, Ferry JA, Viral-type orchitis: A potential mimic of testicular neoplasia. Am. J. Surg. Pathol. 2009;**33**:1477–84.

89. Shanmugasundaram R, Singh JC, Kekre NS, Testicular microlithiasis: Is there an agreed protocol? Indian J. Urol. 2007;**23**:234–9.

90. Corut A, Senyigit A, Ugur SA, *et al.* Mutations in SLC34A2 cause pulmonary alveolar microlithiasis and are possibly associated with testicular microlithiasis. Am. J. Hum. Genet. 2006;**79**:650–6.

91. Drut R, Drut RM, Testicular microlithiasis: histologic and immunohistochemical findings in 11 pediatric cases. Pediatr. Dev. Pathol. 2002;**5**:544–50.

92. Boekelheide K, Mechanisms of toxic damage to spermatogenesis, J. Natl. Cancer Inst. Monogr. 2005;6–8.

93. Suson K, Mathews R, Goldstein JD, Dehner LP, Juvenile xanthogranuloma presenting as a testicular mass in infancy: A clinical and pathologic study of three cases. Pediatr. Dev. Pathol. 2010;**13**:39–45.

94. Ahmed HU, Arya M, Muneer A, Mushtaq I, Sebire NJ, Testicular and paratesticular tumours in the prepubertal population. Lancet Oncol. 2010;**11**:476–83.

95. Pohl HG, Shukla AR, Metcalf PD, *et al.* Prepubertal testis tumors: Actual prevalence rate of histological types, J. Urol. 2004;**172**:2370–2.

96. Ulbright TM, Roth LM, Recent developments in the pathology of germ cell tumors. Semin. Diagn. Pathol. 1987;**4**:304–19.

97. Emerson RE, Ulbright TM, The use of immunohistochemistry in the differential diagnosis of tumors of the testis and paratestis. Semin. Diagn. Pathol. 2005;**22**:33–50.

98. Marulaiah M, Gilhotra A, Moore L, Boucaut H, Goh DW, Testicular and paratesticular pathology in children: A 12-year histopathological review. World J. Surg. 2010;**34**:969–74.

99. Murphy FL, Law H, Mushtaq I, Sebire NJ, Testicular and paratesticular pathology in infants and children: the histopathological experience of a tertiary paediatric unit over a 17 year period. Pediatr. Surg. Int. 2007;**23**:867–72.

100. Holbrook CT, Crist WM, Cain W, Bueschen A, Successful chemotherapy for childhood metastatic embryonal cell carcinoma of the testicle: A preliminary report. Med. Pediatr. Oncol. 1980;**8**:75–81.

101. Mosharafa AA, Foster RS, Leibovich BC, *et al.* Histology in mixed germ cell tumors. Is there a favorite pairing? J. Urol. 2004;**171**:1471–3.

102. Perry C, Servadio C, Seminoma in childhood. J. Urol. 1980;**124**:932–3.

103. Ross JH, Rybicki L, Kay R, Clinical behavior and a contemporary management algorithm for prepubertal testis tumors: A summary of the Prepubertal Testis Tumor Registry. J. Urol. 2002;**168**:1675–8; discussion 1678–9.

104. Schultz KA, Schneider DT, Pashankar F, Ross J, Frazier L, Management of ovarian and testicular sex cord-stromal tumors in children and adolescents. J. Pediatr. Hematol. Oncol. 2012;**34** Suppl 2:S55–63.

105. Lawrence WD, Young RH, Scully RE, Juvenile granulosa cell tumor of the infantile testis. A report of 14 cases. Am. J. Surg. Pathol. 1985;**9**:87–94.

106. Dudani R, Giordano L, Sultania P, *et al.* Juvenile granulosa cell tumor of testis: case report and review of literature. Am. J. Perinatol. 2008;**25**:229–31.

107. Fidda N, Weeks DA, Juvenile granulosa cell tumor of the testis: A case presenting as a small round-cell tumor of childhood, Ultrastruct. Pathol. 2003;**27**:451–5.

108. Young RH, Lawrence WD, Scully RE, Juvenile granulosa cell tumor – another neoplasm associated with abnormal chromosomes and ambiguous genitalia. A report of three cases. Am. J. Surg. Pathol. 1985;**9**:737–43.

109. Harms D, Kock LR, Testicular juvenile granulosa cell and Sertoli cell tumours: A clinicopathological study of 29 cases from the Kiel Paediatric Tumour Registry. Virchows Arch. 1997;**430**:301–9.

110. Partalis N, Tzardi M, Barbagadakis S, Sakellaris G, Juvenile granulosa cell tumor arising from intra-abdominal testis in newborn: case report and review of the literature. Urology 2012;**79**:1152–4.

111. Young RH, Sex cord-stromal tumors of the ovary and testis: their similarities and differences with consideration of selected problems. Mod. Pathol. 2005;**18** Suppl 2: S81–98.

112. Olivier P, Simoneau-Roy J, Francoeur D, *et al.* Leydig cell tumors in children: contrasting clinical, hormonal, anatomical, and molecular characteristics in boys and girls. J. Pediatr. 2012;**161**:1147–52.

113. Al-Agha OM, Axiotis CA, An in-depth look at Leydig cell tumor of the testis. Arch. Pathol. Lab. Med. 2007;**131**:311–17.

114. Liu G, Duranteau L, Carel JC, *et al.* Leydig-cell tumors caused by an activating mutation of the gene encoding the luteinizing hormone receptor. N. Engl. J. Med. 1999;**341**:1731–6.

115. Santonja C, Varona C, Burgos FJ, Nistal M, Leydig cell tumor of testis with adipose metaplasia. Appl. Pathol. 1989;**7**:201–4.

116. Ulbright TM, Srigley JR, Hatzianastassiou DK, Young RH, Leydig cell tumors of the testis with unusual features: Adipose differentiation, calcification with ossification, and spindle-shaped tumor cells. Am. J. Surg. Pathol. 2002;**26**:1424–33.

117. Sharma S, Seam RK, Kapoor HL, Malignant sertoli cell tumour of the testis in a child. J. Surg. Oncol. 1990;**44**:129–31.

118. Wilson DM, Pitts WC, Hintz RL, Rosenfeld RG, Testicular tumors with Peutz-Jeghers syndrome. Cancer 1986;**57**:2238–40.

119. Henley JD, Young RH, Ulbright TM, Malignant Sertoli cell tumors of the testis: A study of 13 examples of a neoplasm frequently misinterpreted as seminoma. Am. J. Surg. Pathol. 2002;**26**:541–50.

120. Kolon TF, Hochman HI, Malignant Sertoli cell tumor in a prepubescent boy. J. Urol. 1997;**158**:608–9.

121. Gordon MD, Corless C, Renshaw AA, Beckstead J, CD99, keratin, and vimentin staining of sex cord-stromal tumors, normal ovary, and testis, Mod. Pathol. 1998;**11**:769–73.

122. Zuk RJ, Trotter SE, Baithun SI, 'Krukenberg' tumour of the testis. Histopathology 1989;**14**:214–16.

123. Ulbright TM, Young RH, Metastatic carcinoma to the testis: A clinicopathologic analysis of 26 nonincidental cases with emphasis on deceptive features. Am. J. Surg. Pathol. 2008;**32**:1683–93.

124. Sebire NJ, Vujanic GM, Paediatric renal tumours: recent developments, new entities and pathological features. Histopathology 2009;**54**:516–28.

125. Kajbafzadeh AM, Javan-Farazmand N, Baghayee A, Hedayat Z, Paratesticular metastasis from Wilms tumor: the possible routs of metastasis and literature review. J. Pediatr. Hematol. Oncol. 2011;**33**:e347–9.

126. Stroosma OB, Delaere KP, Carcinoid tumours of the testis. BJU Int. 2008;**101**:1101–5.

127. Doede T, Foss HD, Waldschmidt J, Carcinoid tumors of the appendix in children: epidemiology, clinical aspects and procedure. Eur. J. Pediatr. Surg. 2000;**10**:372–7.

128. Gutjahr P, Humpl T, Testicular lymphoblastic leukemia/lymphoma. World J. Urol. 1995;**13**:230–2.

129. Stoffel TJ, Nesbit ME, Levitt SH, Extramedullary involvement of the testes in childhood leukemia. Cancer 1975;**35**:1203–11.

130. Vohra S, Morgentaler A, Congenital anomalies of the vas deferens, epididymis, and seminal vesicles. Urology 1997;**49**:313–21.

131. Steiner B, Rosendahl J, Witt H, *et al.* Common CFTR haplotypes and susceptibility to chronic pancreatitis and congenital bilateral absence of the vas deferens. Hum. Mutat. 2011;**32**:912–20.

132. Homayoon K, Suhre CD, Steinhardt GF, Epididymal cysts in children: natural history. J. Urol. 2004;**171**:1274–6.

133. Whitehead ED, Leiter E, Genital abnormalities and abnormal semen analyses in male patients exposed to diethylstilbestrol in utero. J. Urol. 1981;**125**:47–50.

134. Yilmaz E, Batislam E, Bozdogan O, Basar H, Basar MM, Torsion of an epididymal cyst. Int. J. Urol. 2004;**11**:182–3.

135. Rutgers JL, Young RH, Scully RE, The testicular "tumor" of the adrenogenital syndrome. A report of six cases and review of the literature on testicular masses in patients with adrenocortical disorders. Am. J. Surg. Pathol. 1988;**12**:503–13

136. Rubenstein RA, Dogra VS, Seftel AD, Resnick MI, Benign intrascrotal lesions. J. Urol. 2004;**171**:1765–72.

137. Wax JR, Pinette MG, Cartin A, Blackstone J, Prenatal sonographic diagnosis of meconium periorchitis. J. Ultrasound Med. 2007;**26**:415–17.

138. Alanbuki AH, Bandi A, Blackford N, Meconium periorchitis: A case report and literature review. Can. Urol. Assoc. J. 2013;**7**: E495–8.

139. Kalra P, Radhakrishnan J, Meconium periorchitis. Urology 2006;**68**:202.

140. Dehner LP, Scott D, Stocker JT, Meconium periorchitis: A clinicopathologic study of four cases with a review of the literature. Hum. Pathol. 1986;**17**:807–12.

141. Casaccia G, Trucchi A, Nahom A, *et al.* The impact of cystic fibrosis on neonatal intestinal obstruction: the need for prenatal/neonatal screening. Pediatr. Surg. Int. 2003;**19**:75–8.

142. Baughman RP, Culver DA, Judson MA, A concise review of pulmonary sarcoidosis. Am. J. Respir. Crit. Care Med. 2011;**183**:573–81.

143. Smyth LG, Long RM, Lennon G, A case of epididymal sarcoidosis. Can. Urol. Assoc. J. 2011;**5**:E90–1.

144. Turk CO, Schacht M, Ross L, Diagnosis and management of testicular sarcoidosis. J. Urol. 1986;**135**:380–1.

145. Kodama K, Hasegawa T, Egawa M, *et al.* Bilateral epididymal sarcoidosis presenting without radiographic evidence of intrathoracic lesion: Review of sarcoidosis involving the male reproductive tract. Int. J. Urol. 2004;**11**:345–8.

146. Chikkamuniyappa S, Herrick J, Jagirdar JS, Nodular histiocytic/mesothelial hyperplasia: A potential pitfall. Ann. Diagn. Pathol. 2004;**8**:115–20.

147. Rosai J, Dehner LP, Nodular mesothelial hyperplasia in hernia sacs: A benign reactive condition simulating a neoplastic process. Cancer 1975;**35**:165–75.

148. Chan JK, Loo KT, Yau BK, Lam SY, Nodular histiocytic/mesothelial hyperplasia: A lesion potentially mistaken for a neoplasm in transbronchial biopsy. Am. J. Surg. Pathol. 1997;**21**:658–63.

149. Liu YQ, Zhang HX, Wang GL, Ma LL, Huang Y, A giant cystic adenomatoid tumor of the adrenal gland: A case report. Chin. Med. J. (Engl.) 2010;**123**:372–4.

150. Gonzalez Resina R, Carranza A, Congregado Cordoba J, *et al.* (Paratesticular adenomatoid tumor: A report of nine cases) Actas Urol. Esp. 2010;**34**:95–100.

151. Hes O, Perez-Montiel DM, Alvarado Cabrero I, *et al.* Thread-like bridging strands: A morphologic feature present in all adenomatoid tumors. Ann. Diagn. Pathol. 2003;**7**:273–7.

152. Odrzywolski KJ, Mukhopadhyay S, Papillary cystadenoma of the epididymis. Arch. Pathol. Lab. Med. 2010;**134**:630–3.

153. Glasker S, Tran MG, Shively SB, *et al.* Epididymal cystadenomas and epithelial tumourlets: effects of VHL deficiency on the human epididymis. J. Pathol. 2006;**210**:32–41.

154. Uppuluri S, Bhatt S, Tang P, Dogra VS, Clear cell papillary cystadenoma with sonographic and histopathologic correlation. J. Ultrasound Med. 2006;**25**:1451–53.

155. Aydin H, Young RH, Ronnett BM, Epstein JI, Clear cell papillary cystadenoma of the epididymis and mesosalpinx: Immunohistochemical differentiation from metastatic clear cell renal cell carcinoma. Am. J. Surg. Pathol. 2005;**29**:520–3.

156. Calabrese F, Danieli D, Valente M, Melanotic neuroectodermal tumor of the epididymis in infancy: Case report and review of the literature. Urology 1995;**46**:415–18.

157. Johnson RE, Scheithauer BW, Dahlin DC, Melanotic neuroectodermal tumor of infancy. A review of seven cases. Cancer 1983;**52**:661–6.

158. Pettinato G, Manivel JC, d'Amore ES, Jaszcz W, Gorlin RJ, Melanotic neuroectodermal tumor of infancy. A reexamination of a histogenetic problem based on immunohistochemical, flow cytometric, and ultrastructural study of 10 cases. Am. J. Surg. Pathol. 1991;**15**:233–45.

159. Dickey GE, Sotelo-Avila C, Fibrous hamartoma of infancy: Current review. Pediatr. Dev. Pathol. 1999;**2**:236–43.

160. Sotelo-Avila C, Bale PM, Subdermal fibrous hamartoma of infancy: pathology of 40 cases and differential diagnosis. Pediatr. Pathol. 1994;**14**:39–52.

161. Popek EJ, Montgomery EA, Fourcroy JL, Fibrous hamartoma of infancy in the genital region: Findings in 15 cases. J. Urol. 1994;**152**:990–3.

162. Carroll SJ, Nodit L, Spindle cell rhabdomyosarcoma: A brief diagnostic review and differential diagnosis. Arch. Pathol. Lab. Med. 2013;**137**:1155–8.

163. Leuschner I, Newton WA, Jr., Schmidt D, *et al.* Spindle cell variants of embryonal rhabdomyosarcoma in the paratesticular region. A report of the Intergroup Rhabdomyosarcoma Study. Am. J. Surg. Pathol. 1993;**17**:221–30.

164. Plas F, Riedl CR, Pfluger H, Malignant mesothelioma of the tunica vaginalis testis: review of the literature and assessment of prognostic parameters. Cancer 1998;**83**:2437–46.

165. de Lima GR, de Oliveria VP, Reis PH, *et al.* A rare case of malignant hydrocele in a young patient. Pediatr. Urol. 2009;**5**(30):243–5.

166. Antman K, Hassan R, Eisner M, Ries LA, Edwards BK, Update on malignant mesothelioma. Oncology (Williston Park) 2005;**19**:1301–9; discussion 1309–10, 1313–16.

167. Bisogno G, Roganovich J, Sotti G, *et al.* Desmoplastic small round cell tumour in children and adolescents. Med. Pediatr. Oncol. 2000;**34**:338–42.

168. Benjamin LE, Fredericks WJ, Barr FG, Rauscher FJ, 3rd, Fusion of the EWS1 and WT1 genes as a result of the t(11;22)(p13;q12) translocation in desmoplastic small round-cell tumors. Med. Pediatr. Oncol. 1996;**27**:434–9.

169. Cummings OW, Ulbright TM, Young RH, *et al.* Desmoplastic small round-cell tumors of the paratesticular region. A report of six cases. Am. J. Surg. Pathol. 1997;**21**:219–25.

170. Lae ME, Roche PC, Jin L, Lloyd RV, Nascimento AG, Desmoplastic small round-cell tumor: A clinicopathologic, immunohistochemical, and molecular study of 32 tumors. Am. J. Surg. Pathol. 2002;**26**:823–35.

171. Grimsby GM, Ritchey ML, Pediatric urologic oncology. Pediatr. Clin. North Am. 2012;**59**:947–59.

172. Kodet R, Newton WA, Jr., Sachs N, *et al.* Rhabdoid tumors of soft tissues: A clinicopathologic study of 26 cases enrolled on the Intergroup Rhabdomyosarcoma Study. Hum. Pathol. 1991;**22**:674–84.

173. Weeks DA, Beckwith JB, Mierau GW, Luckey DW, Rhabdoid tumor of kidney. A report of 111 cases from the National Wilms' Tumor Study Pathology Center. Am. J. Surg. Pathol. 1989;**13**:439–58.

174. Versteege I, Sevenet N, Lange J, *et al.* Truncating mutations of hSNF5/INI1 in aggressive paediatric cancer. Nature 1998;**394**:203–6.

175. Utsch B, Albers N, Ludwig M, Genetic and molecular aspects of hypospadias. Eur. J. Pediatr. Surg. 2004;**14**:297–302.

176. Baskin LS, Hypospadias and urethral development. J. Urol. 2000;**163**:951–6.

177. Gargollo PC, Kozakewich HP, Bauer SB, *et al.* Balanitis xerotica obliterans in boys. J. Urol. 2005;**174**:1409–12.

178. Tasker GL, Wojnarowska F, Lichen sclerosus. Clin. Exp. Dermatol. 2003;**28**:128–33.

179. Powell J, Robson A, Cranston D, Wojnarowska F, Turner R, High incidence of lichen sclerosus in patients with squamous cell carcinoma of the penis. Br. J. Dermatol. 2001;**145**:85–9.

180. Alurkar SS, Dhabhar BN, Jambhekar NA, Kulkarni JN, Advani SH, Primary endodermal sinus tumor of the penis: A case report. J. Urol. 1992;**148**:131–3.

181. Kennedy R, Lacson A, Congenital endodermal sinus tumor of the penis. J. Pediatr. Surg. 1987;**22**:791–2.

182. Suarez-Quian CA, Martinez-Garcia F, Nistal M, Regadera J, Androgen receptor distribution in adult human testis. J. Clin. Endocrinol. Metab. 1999;**84**:350–8.

183. Cools M, Drop SL, Wolffenbuttel KP, Oosterhuis JW, Looijenga LH, Germ cell tumors in the intersex gonad: old paths, new directions, moving frontiers. Endocr. Rev. 2006;**27**:468–84.

184. Hughes IA, Disorders of sex development: A new definition and classification. Best Pract. Res. Clin. Endocrinol. Metab. 2008;**22**:119–34.

185. Aaronson IA, Aaronson AJ, How should we classify intersex disorders? J. Pediatr. Urol. 2010;**6**:443–6.

186. Scully RE, Gonadoblastoma. A review of 74 cases. Cancer 1970;**25**:1340–56.

187. Scully RE, Gonadoblastoma; a gonadal tumor related to the dysgerminoma (seminoma) and capable of sex-hormone production. Cancer 1953;**6**:455–63.

188. Gondos B, Berthelsen JG, Skakkebaek NE, Intratubular germ cell neoplasia (carcinoma in situ): A preinvasive lesion of the testis. Ann. Clin. Lab. Sci. 1983;**13**:185–92.

189. Hersmus R, de Leeuw BH, Wolffenbuttel KP, *et al.* New insights into type II germ cell tumor pathogenesis based on studies of patients with various forms of disorders of sex development (DSD). Mol. Cell Endocrinol. 2008;**291**:1–10.

190. Oosterhuis JW, Looijenga LH, Testicular germ-cell tumours in a broader perspective. Nat. Rev. Cancer 2005;**5**:210–22.

191. Hart WR, Burkons DM, Germ cell neoplasms arising in gonadoblastomas. Cancer 1979;**43**:669–78.

192. Looijenga LH, Stoop H, de Leeuw HP, *et al.* POU5F1 (OCT3/4) identifies cells with pluripotent potential in human germ cell tumors. Cancer Res. 2003;**63**:2244–50.

193. Lau YF, Li Y, Kido T, Gonadoblastoma locus and the TSPY gene on the human Y chromosome. Birth Defects Res. C Embryo. Today 2009;**87**:114–22.

194. Buell-Gutbrod R, Ivanovic M, Montag A, *et al.* FOXL2 and SOX9 distinguish the lineage of the sex cord-stromal cells in gonadoblastomas. Pediatr. Dev. Pathol. 2011;**14**:391–5.

195. Hughes IA, Houk C, Ahmed SF, Lee PA, Consensus statement on management of intersex disorders. J. Pediatr. Urol. 2006;**2**:148–62.

196. Auber F, Lortat-Jacob S, Sarnacki S, *et al.* Surgical management and genotype/phenotype correlations in WT1 gene-related diseases (Drash, Frasier syndromes). J. Pediatr. Surg. 2003;**38**:124–9.

197. Manuel M, Katayama PK, Jones HW, Jr., The age of occurrence of gonadal tumors in intersex patients with a Y chromosome. Am. J. Obstet. Gynecol. 1976;**124**:293–300.

198. Cools M, van Aerde K, Kersemaekers AM, *et al.* Morphological and immunohistochemical differences between gonadal maturation delay and early germ cell neoplasia in patients with undervirilization syndromes. J. Clin. Endocrinol. Metab. 2005;**90**:5295–303.

199. Rutgers JL, Scully RE, The androgen insensitivity syndrome (testicular feminization): A clinicopathologic study of 43 cases. Int. J. Gynecol. Pathol. 1991;**10**:126–44.

200. Regadera J, Martinez-Garcia F, Paniagua R, Nistal M, Androgen insensitivity syndrome: An immunohistochemical, ultrastructural, and morphometric study. Arch. Pathol. Lab. Med. 1999;**123**:225–34.

Chapter 10

Breast

Pamela Lyle, Jane E. Dahlstrom, and Melinda E. Sanders

Introduction

Breast lesions in childhood and adolescence are rare (1) and more than 95% of all breast lesions occurring in this age group are benign. Table 10.1 provides a summary of their frequencies in this population.

The management of breast lesions in the pediatric and adolescent populations differs from that of adults in that sonography is the initial imaging study, and mammography is reserved for select cases of suspicious discrete masses in older adolescents or for the evaluation of microcalcifications (2). Computed tomography is avoided because of the risks of ionizing radiation in this population. Magnetic resonance imaging may be of value for patients with masses involving deeper structures, such as the chest wall (2). Additionally, immature breasts are at risk of abnormal development if perturbed by medical intervention. Given the extremely low prevalence of malignant breast tumors in the pediatric and adolescent populations, a conservative clinical, radiologic, and pathologic approach is recommended to avoid iatrogenic complications of overtreatment (3).

The most common lesions are fibroadenomas in females (2–5) and gynecomastia in males (2,4,5). This chapter will discuss breast lesions in the pediatric and adolescent populations, aiming to aid the reader in reaching the correct diagnosis, and to discuss their significance.

Fibroepithelial lesions

Fibroepithelial lesions are a group of biphasic tumors that consists of fibroadenomas, phyllodes tumors, and hamartomas. The fibroadenoma variants, tubular adenoma and lactating adenoma, are also considered with this group. Stromal changes that resemble fibroadenomas, but blend with the surrounding fibrous stroma rather than forming a well-circumscribed lesion are referred to as a fibroadenomatoid change.

Fibroadenoma

Fibroadenomas are the most common pediatric breast lesions, representing approximately 68% of lesions reported in females (see Table 10.1). Most fibroadenomas in adolescents are solitary; however, multiple and bilateral lesions have been reported (6,7). When multiple tumors with myxomatous histology occur, the possibility of Carney syndrome should be considered (8,9).

Most fibroadenomas are slow-growing and present as non-tender, firm, well-defined, mobile nodules. Grossly, they usually range from 2 to 5 cm in diameter, are well delineated from the surrounding breast tissue and demonstrate a lobulated, bulging white-gray cut surface with a few slit-like spaces. Some tumors contain myxoid areas. Histologically, fibroadenomas demonstrate two classic patterns, *pericanalicular* and *intracanalicular*, or a mixture thereof. The *pericanalicular* pattern develops from a circumferential stromal proliferation around open ductal structures (Figure 10.1). The intracanalicular pattern results from proliferation of stromal cells leading to collapsed slit-like ductal structures (Figure 10.2). Distinction of the two patterns is not clinically important; however, a prominent intracanalicular pattern can occasionally create a focally leaf-like pattern that may mimic a benign phyllodes tumor. *Cellular fibroadenomas* are defined by increased stromal cellularity, approximately twice that of the typical fibroadenoma (10), but limited mitotic activity (usually < 3 per 10 HPF) and an absence of stromal atypia or overgrowth (Figure 10.3). A greater number of mitoses may even

Table 10.1 Frequency of breast lesions in children and adolescents

	Coffin and Dehner (5)	Bower et al. (4)	Stone et al. (135)	Farrow and Ashikari (22)	Simpson and Barson (136)	West et al. (137)	Elsheikh et al. (138)	Total	Percentage
Fibroadenoma	66	84	104	181	5	19	172	702	68
Gynecomastia	18	23	0	0	0	7	0	48	5
Inflammation	9	9	4	2	0	5	0	40	4
Fibrosis	7	0	2	0	0	0	0	9	1
Pubertal hypertrophy	6	4	0	0	0	0	0	10	1
Cyst	5	1	0	8	0	2	6	31	3
Fat necrosis	3	1	0	5	0	1	0	10	1
Phyllodes tumor	3	0	2	0	0	0	1	8	<1
Fibrocystic disease	2	2	9	25	0	2	58	98	9
Hyperplasia	2	0	17	0	0	0	0	19	2
Rhabdomyosarcoma	2	1	0	2	0	2	2	9	1
Granular cell tumor	2	0	1	0	0	0	0	3	<0.5
Intraductal papillomatosis	1	1	4	13	1	0	0	20	2
Fibromatosis	1	0	0	0	0	0	0	1	<0.1
Duct ectasia	1	0	0	0	0	0	0	1	<0.1
Adenocarcinoma	0	0	1	1	1	0	1	4	<0.5
Other	1	8	1	0	2	4	2	20	2
Total	129	134	145	237	9	42	242	1033	100

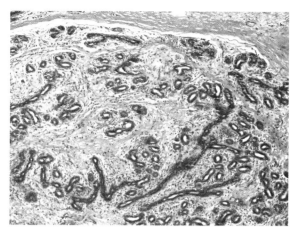

Figure 10.1 Fibroadenoma from a 13-year-old girl with a pericanalicular growth pattern, as characterized by circumferential stromal proliferation around ductal structures (H&E × 20).

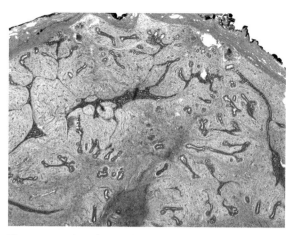

Figure 10.2 Fibroadenoma from a 12-year-old girl with an intracanalicular growth pattern resulting from compression of the ductal spaces by the proliferating stromal cells (H&E × 10).

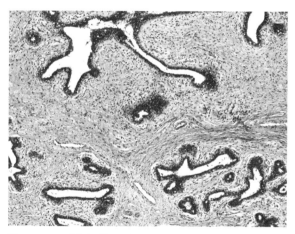

Figure 10.3 Cellular fibroadenoma showing mildly increased stromal cellularity and a regular epithelial to stromal ratio (H&E × 20).

be permissible if accompanied by a similarly proliferative epithelial component. Furthermore, cellular fibroadenomas lack the cleft-like spaces and leafy projections characteristic of benign phyllodes tumors. Another lacking feature is periductal stromal condensation, which is seen in many benign phyllodes tumors. While most fibroadenomas are clearly delineated from the adjacent normal breast parenchyma, occasional lesions may have focally irregular margins (11). Such foci should not be of concern in the absence of other diagnostic features of phyllodes tumor. A summary of the features that help facilitate distinction of cellular fibroadenoma from benign phyllodes tumor and other benign breast lesions presenting as clinical masses in adolescents is provided in Table 10.2.

The clinical entity "giant" or "juvenile" fibroadenoma is defined by a history of rapid growth (2,11,12). These lesions are typically cellular and may show focal areas with branching, elongated clefts reminiscent of benign phyllodes tumor. However, in the absence of other diagnostic features of benign phyllodes tumors (Tables 10.2 and 10.3), these lesions are best diagnosed as cellular fibroadenomas.

Regardless of the architectural pattern, the stroma of fibroadenomas may exhibit multinucleated giant cells, myxoid change, pseudoangiomatous stromal hyperplasia (PASH), hyalinization with or without calcification, and, rarely, ossification. Lipomatous, smooth muscle, and osteochondroid metaplasia may rarely occur (11,13). The epithelial component often shows varying degrees of usual hyperplasia, which is frequently mitotically active. Rare examples of atypical ductal hyperplasia (ADH) occurring in fibroadenomas in adolescents have been reported (14). Although the significance of ADH in this specific context has not been systematically studied in adolescents, limited follow-up studies of ADH in this age group have shown no risk implication (15,16). In addition, ADH, when confined to a fibroadenoma in adult women has no prognostic significance (17,18). Extensive myoepithelial proliferation can also be seen, and care should be taken to avoid its misinterpretation as ADH. Smooth-muscle actin (SMA) and p63 immunohistochemistry can be used to confirm the myoepithelial nature of this proliferation. Ductal carcinoma *in situ* (DCIS) is occasionally associated with fibroadenomas in adult women, and is even less often seen in the adolescent population (19).

Table 10.2 Benign breast lesions presenting as clinical masses in adolescents

	Cellular fibroadenoma	Benign phyllodes tumor	Hamartoma	Pseudoangiomatous stromal hyperplasia (PASH)	Localized fibrocystic changes (juvenile papillomatosis)
Stromal component	Present, varying degrees of stromal expansion (mild to moderate) but with maintenance of a regular stromal epithelial ratio	Present, uniformly expanded (moderate to markedly), regular stromal epithelial ratio (greater than cellular fibroadenoma)	Absent or sclerotic	Collagenous, often with keloid-like fibrosis	Absent, sclerotic, or myofibroblastic
Stromal cellularity	Uniform, mildly increased	Uniform, mild to moderately increased, +/–periductal condensation	N/A	Low	Minimally increased
Stromal atypia	Absent	Mild	N/A	Absent	Absent
Stromal mitoses	Absent to few, usually < 3/10 HPF	Few (< 5/HPF)	N/A	Absent	Absent
Architectural growth pattern	Often intracanalicular	Floridly leaf-like	Often simulates normal breast	Densely fibrous, may contain entrapped benign epithelial elements	Haphazard mixture of fibrocystic changes
Usual/florid epithelial hyperplasia	May be present	May be present	Absent	Absent	Present, often abundant +/– apocrine change
Micropapillomas	Absent	Absent	Absent	Absent	Present, usually multiple
Lesion border (Macroscopic & Microscopic)	Well-defined	Well-defined	Well-defined	May be well-defined or merge with surrounding breast tissue	Ill-defined, merging with surrounding breast tissue
Ultrasound Imaging	Well-circumscribed, round, oval, or macrolobulated mass with fairly uniform hypoechogenicity; +/- slender, fluid-filled clefts. Rarely heterogeneous echotexture representing dystrophic calcifications or necrosis (2)	Well-circumscribed, round, ovoid or macrolobulated hypoechoic mass, often with posterior acoustic enhancement; internal echotexture frequently heterogenous; anechoic cysts or clefts are suggestive; significant overlap with cellular fibroadenoma (2)	Well-circumscribed, solid, oval tumors without microcalcifications; internal hyperechoic or mixed echogenicity	Variable features, but most are solid, hypoechoic ovoid masses with long-axis parallel to chest wall; +/– circumscribed margins (2)	Ill-defined, mass with multiple small cysts, especially at periphery; +/– microcalcification (2)

Table 10.3 Histological features distinguishing benign, borderline, and malignant phyllodes tumors

	Benign	Borderline	Malignant
Stromal Hypercellularity	Mild	Moderate	Marked
Cellular Pleomorphism	Mild	Moderate	Marked
Mitoses (per 10 HPF)	Few (focally <5)	5 – 9	>10 (with atypical forms)
Margins	Well circumscribed; pushing	Circumscribed to some infiltration	Circumscribed to extensive infiltration
Stromal Pattern	Uniform distribution	Heterogeneous stromal expansion	Marked stromal overgrowth
Stromal Overgrowth	No	No	Yes
Heterologous Elements	Rare	Rare	Somewhat common (10–65%) (27)

The term "complex fibroadenoma" is used for lesions containing foci of sclerosing adenosis, apocrine change, or cysts larger than 3 mm. The lesion was originally recognized because it was associated with a slightly increased relative risk for later carcinoma development, while fibroadenomas without these features have no increase in relative risk (17,18).

Tubular variant of fibroadenoma and nodular gestational hyperplasia

The terms "tubular adenoma" and "lactating adenoma" are best considered as variants of fibroadenoma given that they behave in a benign fashion. Thus, the terms tubular variant of fibroadenoma and nodular gestational hyperplasia, respectively, are preferable. Both entities are clinically and macroscopically well circumscribed with a homogeneous white-tan cut surface in the tubular variant and a somewhat softer tan-yellow surface in nodular gestational hyperplasia. Histologically, the tubular variant displays compact uniform tubules, with the normal dual-cell population composed of an inner layer of cuboidal-to-columnar epithelial cells and an outer layer of myoepithelial cells with minimal intervening stroma (Figure 10.4). Nodular gestational hyperplasia occurs during pregnancy or the postpartum period. The clinically detectable mass usually demonstrates coalescence of several large lobular units histologically or, alternatively, shows the architecture of the tubular variant with superimposed secretory change characterized by luminal epithelial cells with large nuclei and abundant

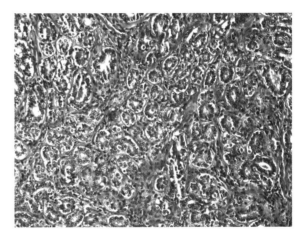

Figure 10.4 Tubular adenoma from a 12-year-old girl featuring compact uniform tubules with minimal intervening stroma. Secretions are frequently present in the lumina (H&E × 20).

vacuolated cytoplasm (Figure 10.5). Of importance and particularly during pregnancy, nodular gestational hyperplasia may infarct and should not be taken as evidence of malignancy based on the presence of necrosis (20).

Phyllodes tumor

Phyllodes tumors in children are extremely rare, and combined data from several large series suggest that they represent approximately 1% of all pediatric breast lesions (Table 10.1; 4,5,12,21,22), with benign phyllodes tumors comprising the majority of pediatric cases (2,23,24).

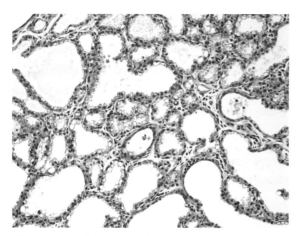

Figure 10.5 Nodular gestational hyperplasia ("Lactating adenoma") with compact glandular elements and vacuolated cytoplasm resembling lactating breast, and sparse stromal component (H&E × 20).

The usual clinical presentation is a solitary, firm, painless breast mass, and there may be a history of rapid growth (24–26). Multifocality and bilaterality are rare. Imaging studies demonstrate a round to lobulated, sharply delineated mass with clefts and occasionally coarse calcifications.

Grossly, phyllodes tumors are well circumscribed, bulging masses, averaging 4–5 cm in greatest dimension, with a tan to pink-gray cut surface that may be myxoid. Tumors up to 30 cm have been reported (27). Smaller lesions are often homogenous with an appearance akin to fibroadenoma, but larger lesions usually show an alternating pattern of whorled leaf-like protrusions within curved cystic clefts, that are usually filled with serous or occasionally serosanguinous fluid (28). The tumors are often described as having been surgically "shelled out" from the uninvolved parenchyma, due to their sharp circumscription (5).

Collectively, phyllodes tumors can be described as a group of biphasic tumors characterized by hypercellular stromal fronds covered by an epithelial component composed of epithelial and myoepithelial cells. These leaf-like projections protrude into cystic, cleft-like spaces, creating an enhanced intracanalicular pattern (Figure 10.6A). Not infrequently, phyllodes tumors contain regions that may resemble an otherwise typical fibroadenoma. This finding highlights the fact that phyllodes tumors exhibit a wide morphologic spectrum, from lesions resembling cellular fibroadenoma to those composed almost exclusively of high-grade sarcoma. Therefore, to facilitate appropriate clinical management, phyllodes tumors are divided into benign, borderline, and malignant

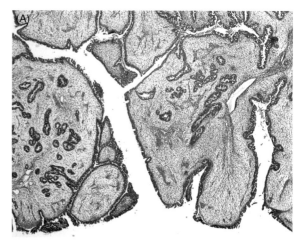

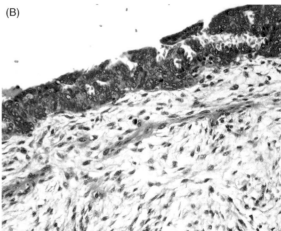

Figure 10.6 Benign phyllodes tumor from a 13-year-old girl. (A) Exaggerated leaf-like stromal fronds lined by epithelium (H&E × 10). (B) Modest cellular expansion with uniform cellularity and minimal pleomorphism. (H&E × 20).

categories based on a combination of histologic features, including the degree of stromal hypercellularity, stromal cytologic atypia and mitoses, stromal overgrowth and the character of the interface with the adjacent normal breast (see Table 10.3; 29). The epithelial component may show usual hyperplasia and occasionally areas of adenosis, apocrine change, or squamous metaplasia (28). Cartilaginous and osseous metaplasia can be seen in all subtypes of phyllodes tumor (12).

Sixty to seventy-five percent of phyllodes tumors fall into the benign category, regardless of age. Benign phyllodes tumors are almost always well circumscribed, exhibit an increased stroma-to-epithelial ratio, a mildly to moderately cellular spindle-cell stroma with mild pleomorphism, few if any mitoses, and no stromal overgrowth (see Table 10.3, Figures 10.6A,B). In some benign phyllodes tumors the stromal cellularity is increased uniformly, while others demonstrate periductal stromal condensation, which can be a helpful distinguishing feature from fibroadenomas, when present. Scattered bizarre stromal giant cells can be seen and should not raise concern in an otherwise benign phyllodes tumor (30). The definitive distinction of a benign phyllodes tumor from a fibroadenoma with a pronounced intracanalicular growth pattern is occasionally difficult. A diagnosis of fibroadenoma is preferable in ambiguous cases to avoid potential overtreatment. This approach is justified by studies showing that these lesions can be managed similarly with respect to continued local growth or recurrence (27,31–34).

Malignant phyllodes tumors show marked stromal cellularity and pleomorphism, and contain frank areas of intermediate-to-high-grade sarcoma, which usually dominate the histologic picture (Figure 10.7). There is usually some combination of stromal overgrowth, necrosis, a high mitotic index (usually >10 per 10 HPF), and infiltrative borders. Stromal overgrowth is defined as the absence of epithelium within one low-power field (4×). The sarcomatous elements are most commonly fibrosarcoma, followed by liposarcoma (Figure 10.7); however, heterologous chondrosarcoma, osteosarcoma, and rhabdomyosarcoma may also be seen (35–39). In the presence of extreme stromal overgrowth of sarcomatous components, the epithelial component may only be identified after extensively sampling of the tumor. Pure mammary sarcomas are extremely rare in the pediatric and adolescent populations (40,41) and should only be diagnosed after thorough sampling has excluded a phyllodes tumor.

As implied by the name, borderline tumors show features between benign and malignant: moderate stromal cellularity, cellular pleomorphism, and mitotic activity without frank sarcoma or stromal overgrowth (see Table 10.3, Figures 10.8A,B). The borders are predominantly pushing, but may show focally permeative areas. Borderline phyllodes have the capacity for local recurrence only.

Most phyllodes tumors exhibit benign behavior, with local recurrences occurring on average in 20% of cases, specifically 15% for benign, 20% for

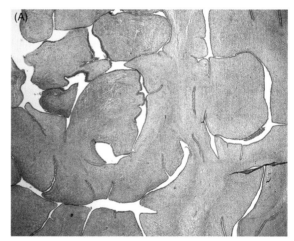

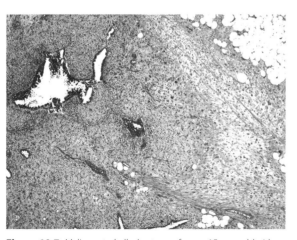

Figure 10.7 Malignant phyllodes tumor from a 15-year-old girl, characterized by stromal overgrowth, marked cellular pleomorphism, and conspicuous, often atypical, mitoses. A well-differentiated liposarcoma component is present in the upper right of the image (H&E × 10).

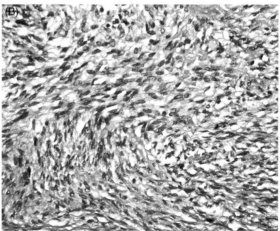

Figure 10.8 Borderline phyllodes tumor from a 17-year-old girl. (A) Exaggerated leaf-like stromal fronds lined by benign epithelium (H&E × 10). (B) Easily identifiable mitoses, uniformly hypercellular spindle-cell stroma and moderate pleomorphism (H&E × 40).

339

borderline, and 27% for malignant (42). The best histologic predictor of local recurrence is the presence of infiltrative borders and positive margins (35,42). Histologic parameters with independent predictive power for recurrence are stromal overgrowth, atypia, and mitotic activity (34). Approximately 2% of phyllodes tumors metastasize; almost exclusively in the setting of a malignant phyllodes tumor (42). The lungs (27,35) and bones are the most common distant sites (35).

Hamartoma

Mammary hamartomas most often present in pre- and perimenopausal women, but may be seen in adolescence (5), although much less commonly than fibroadenomas (43). They have a presentation similar to fibroadenoma: a clinically detected, mobile nodule usually measuring 1 to 4 cm in diameter.

Grossly, hamartomas are always circumscribed and demonstrate a gray-yellow, rubbery, cut surface. Microscopically, they are composed of benign ducts and lobules, hyalinized stroma, and adipose tissue haphazardly arranged in a circumscribed, but unencapsulated nodule (Figure 10.9). A proportion of the lesion may resemble normal breast tissue. Smooth muscle can also be present, and when dominant, the lesion is termed myoid hamartoma. Immunohistochemistry for SMA or desmin may be used to confirm a myogenic immunophenotype (44). Foci of PASH may also be present (45). Hamartomas are distinguished from fibroadenomas and phyllodes tumor by the lack of a regular stromal-to-epithelial relationship, as well as lack of cleft-like spaces (Table 10.2). Given that hamartomas may have areas with the architectural pattern of the normal breast or breast tissue with non-specific benign findings, it may not be possible to diagnose hamartoma on core needle biopsy (46), especially if the clinical and radiologic findings are not available.

Epithelial lesions

Proliferative disease without atypia and non-proliferative changes

The term proliferative disease without atypia encompasses usual and florid epithelial hyperplasia, intraductal papillomas, micropapillomas, and sclerosing adenosis (28). Non-proliferative epithelial changes include micro- and macrocysts, apocrine change, fibrosis, and chronic inflammation. All these lesions fall within the spectrum of the more generic term fibrocystic change. Approximately 10% of breast specimens from girls in mid-to-late adolescence show some combination of these proliferative and non-proliferative changes; however, they are virtually never seen in girls younger than 10 years of age (5).

Usual epithelial hyperplasia or usual hyperplasia without atypia involves the terminal duct lobular unit. In adolescents, usual hyperplasia has the same histologic features as in adult women. The diagnosis is based on the presence of cellular variability, and swirling, uneven cell placement and slit-like intercellular spaces, which are usually peripherally distributed (Figure 10.10). Varying degrees of epithelial

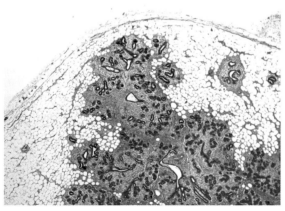

Figure 10.9 Hamartoma composed of a circumscribed nodule of mature adipose tissue containing islands of benign epithelial elements architecturally resembling normal breast tissue (H&E × 10).

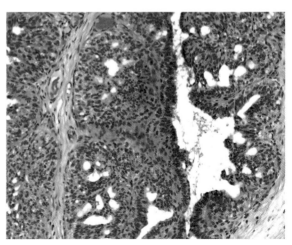

Figure 10.10 Epithelial hyperplasia without atypia from a 17-year-old girl. The hyperplastic epithelium fills the duct space and is characterized by prominent cell-to-cell variability and the formation of slit-like intercellular lumina (H&E × 20).

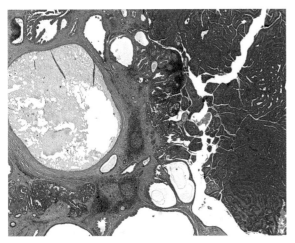

Figure 10.11 Localized fibrocystic changes dominated by clustered papillomas, epithelial hyperplasia without atypia and apocrine cysts presenting as a clinical mass in a 17-year-old girl (H&E × 10).

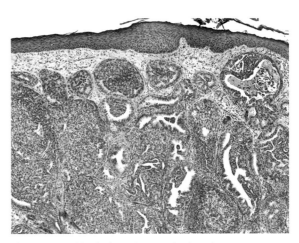

Figure 10.12 Nipple duct adenoma. A subareolar conglomeration of multiple papillomas also containing florid hyperplasia (H&E × 10).

hyperplasia may also be present in fibroglandular lesions (11,17).

Intraductal papillomas occur in ducts near the nipple, while micropapillomas arise from the terminal duct–lobular unit. Intraductal papillomas infrequently occur in adolescent and young adult breasts. They may be associated with bloody nipple discharge (47). Both types of papillomas are microscopically characterized by true papillae, defined by the presence of fibrovascular cores lined by ductal epithelium. The epithelial lining may be columnar or stratified, but importantly remains polarized with respect to the basement membrane and shows cellular variability. Papillomas may also become sclerotic or adenotic. Occasionally, the proliferative epithelium shows a pattern identical to that seen in gynecomastia, characterized by "pinched"-appearing (Figure 10.11), diminutive papillary projections, with apical pyknotic nuclei that should not be mistaken for micropapillary ADH.

Occasionally, localized fibrocystic changes dominated by clustered papillomas, epithelial hyperplasia without atypia and apocrine cysts can present as a clinical mass. Historically, this presentation has been called juvenile papillomatosis (12,48). Despite theorization that this process may pose a risk for subsequent carcinoma (49–52), no link has been established. Following the diagnostic excision, clinical follow-up is all that is required.

Nipple duct adenoma

Nipple duct adenoma, also called florid papillomatosis or subareolar sclerosis duct hyperplasia of the nipple, has rarely been reported in children (5). The usual presentation is a rapidly enlarging subareolar mass with associated nipple discharge and erosion of overlying skin. The lesions are usually less 1 cm in greatest extent and histologically characterized by one or several large, partially sclerosed papillomas that may contain areas of adenosis and florid epithelial hyperplasia (Figure 10.12). Carcinoma and ADH have not been reported in association with nipple duct adenoma in children.

Atypical ductal hyperplasia (ADH)

Formal patterns of ADH are rare in the pediatric population and should be diagnosed with caution (53–54). Very limited follow-up studies of ADH in this age group have shown no risk implication (15,16). However, given the small number of cases and limited follow-up data, the true significance of the diagnosis in this age group is unknown, as there are no longitudinal studies to adequately address a relative risk and time frame for development of a subsequent invasive carcinoma, such as exist for adult women (55). In female adolescents, close clinical follow-up is usually adequate and avoids cosmetic issues and compromise of subsequent normal lactation. In male adolescents, ADH occurs almost

341

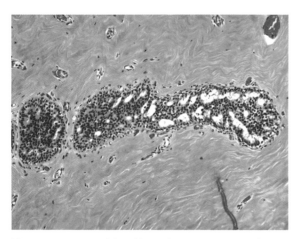

Figure 10.13 Atypical ductal hyperplasia occurring in an obese 15-year-old male with long-standing gynecomastia characterized by partial involvement of a duct by monotonous cuboidal cells forming solid aggregates and a few microlumina. Note the presence of residual polarized, epithelial cells along the basement membrane lining peripherally distributed slit-like spaces characteristic of usual hyperplasia (H&E × 20).

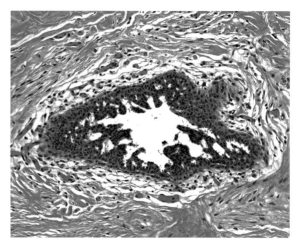

Figure 10.14 Gynecomastia, proliferative phase, with characteristic diminutive intraluminal projections with "pinched-appearing" tips in a 17-year-old boy (H&E × 20).

exclusively in the setting of gynecomastia (53,54; Figure 10.13), and the usual treatment is complete mastectomy (see subsequent section).

Gynecomastia

Gynecomastia is a hormonally driven, non-neoplastic, and often reversible, proliferation of the stromal and ductal components of the male breast that clinically presents as female appearing breast development. It constitutes the most common mammary lesion in adolescent boys and is usually bilateral, although often more prominent in one breast (56,57). The process is always driven by absolute or relative endogenous or exogenous estrogen excess (56,57). Consequently, there are three typical age peaks: in neonates, adolescents, and elderly males, with the highest incidence in 14-year-old boys. While the vast majority of cases are idiopathic, the lesion has been reported in association with many conditions: type-1 neurofibromatosis (58–60), adrenal cortical neoplasms (61,62), congenital adrenal hyperplasia (63), prolactinoma (64), hepatoblastoma, Kleinfelter syndrome, hermaphroditism syndromes (65,66), hypergonadotrophic hypogonadism (67), growth hormone therapy (68), and drugs such as metaclopromide (69) and antipsychotics (70). An inversion at the p450 aromatase gene promoter locus leading to extraglandular aromatization has been demonstrated in two large kindreds with autosomal dominant prepubertal gynecomastia (71). Of note,

neurofibromatosis type-1-associated cases of gynecomastia have additionally shown features of PASH and multinucleated giant cells (58,59,72).

Grossly, gynecomastia presents as a firm and circumscribed mass with a gray-white nodular cut surface. Histologically, the pattern ranges from florid to fibrous, depending on whether the lesion is in the proliferative (early), intermediate, or inactive phase of development (late) (Figures 10.14, 10.15). By definition, gynecomastia is a ductal process, as lobular development is absent in males. In the early and intermediate phases, the ductal epithelium usually shows a characteristic pattern, with attenuated micropapillae with a "pinched" appearance (Figure 10.14). The apical nuclei are small and pyknotic-appearing, while the cells at the base are the size of typical ductal epithelial cells. Usual epithelial hyperplasia is also commonly present (Figure 10.14). In the early and intermediate phases, the periductal stroma is cellular with an admixture of fibroblasts, myofibroblasts, lymphocytes, and plasma cells. Sometimes the stroma exhibits myxoid change. In the inactive, or fibrous phase, the ducts are typically lined by a single layer of epithelial cells and surrounded by hyalinized stroma (Figure 10.15). Both ADH (Figure 10.13) and DCIS may rarely occur in association with gynecomastia in adolescents (53,54,73–76). The same stringent cytologic and extent criteria used to diagnose these lesions in the adult population need be applied; however, given that mastectomy is the recommended treatment for both ADH and DCIS in

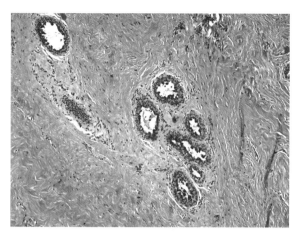

Figure 10.15 Gynecomastia, fibrotic phase, in a 13-year-old male, characterized by non-edematous, collagenized stroma surrounding ducts with less conspicuous epithelial hyperplasia than seen in the proliferative phase (H&E × 20).

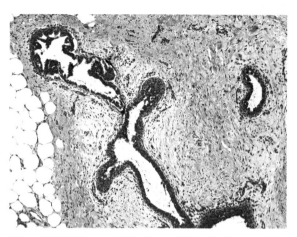

Figure 10.16 Macromastia in a 9-year-old female characterized by gynecomastia-like epithelial hyperplasia, and periductal edema with mild chronic inflammation, which is indistinguishable from proliferative gynecomastia in males (see Figure 10.13) (H&E × 20).

adult males, only extensive lesions or those with inter-mediate- to high-grade histology truly warrant a diag-nosis of DCIS.

Macromastia

Macromastia (juvenile, pubertal, or virginal hypertro-phy) is the diffuse firm enlargement of one or both breasts without nodularity. It occurs in adolescent females beginning at or shortly after menarche and can histologically resemble gynecomastia (5,12; Figure 10.16), so much so that the distinction can be difficult without the clinical history. Other cases vary minimally from normal female breast tissue of similar age (11,12).

Stromal lesions

Pseudoangiomatous stromal hyperplasia (PASH)

Pseudoangiomatous stromal hyperplasia is a benign hormone-dependent myofibroblastic stromal prolifer-ation that histologically resembles a vascular lesion due to the formation of small slit-like spaces (77–79). Pseudoangiomatous stromal hyperplasia can be seen in children, adolescents, and adults (80,81).

Cases warranting the subsequent diagnosis of PASH present as a palpable mass. The typical PASH lesion is characterized by a proliferation of myofibro-blasts forming slit-shaped, pseudovascular spaces within a dense keloid-like stroma (Figure 10.17). These spaces

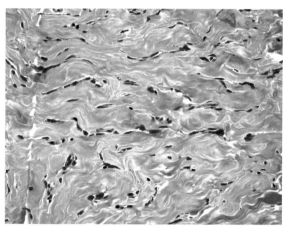

Figure 10.17 Pseudoangiomatous stromal hyperplasia (PASH). Myofibroblasts form the defining pseudoangiomatous spaces within the collagenized stroma (H&E × 40).

do not contain red blood cells. The spindle-shaped myofibroblasts resemble endothelial cells, but lack expression of specific endothelial (factor VIII, CD31, D2–40) and epithelial markers. In the overwhelming majority of cases, the histologic features on hematoxylin and eosin (H&E) are defining, making immunohisto-chemistry unnecessary. However, the myofibroblastic origin of the defining cells can be confirmed by CD34 positivity and specific endothelial markers (82). These myofibroblasts also express desmin, SMA, calponin, and BCL-2 (82). The hormonal basis of this process is evidenced by expression of progesterone receptor by the myofibroblasts (83). The hyalinized stroma may be sharply demarcated from the surrounding

343

breast or ill-defined, blending imperceptibly with the surrounding normal stroma. Pseudoangiomatous stromal hyperplasia does not exhibit mitotic activity, nuclear atypia, necrosis, or calcifications. Microscopic foci of PASH are often incidentally noted as a component of other lesions, such as fibroadenoma, but do not require specific comment.

Occasionally, well-differentiated angiosarcoma, adult fibrosarcoma, and biphasic tumors with dense cellular stroma are considered in the differential diagnosis. Angiosarcoma is extremely rare in children (84) and can be easily excluded by the lack of cytologic atypia, infiltrating and anastomosing vascular spaces, and expression of specific endothelial markers by immunohistochemistry (85). Adult fibrosarcomas are characterized by a monotonous spindle-cell proliferation that infiltrates the surrounding breast parenchyma and adipose tissues. In contrast to PASH, their nuclei are atypical, larger, and show mitotic activity (86).

Fibromatosis

Fibromatosis is a benign lesion histologically identical to lesions of the same name located elsewhere in the body and described elsewhere in this book. Approximately 20% of mammary fibromatosis occurs in the second decade, and rarely in infants (87). The typical presentation is a firm, discrete mass that may involve the chest wall or cause distortion of the overlying skin. The infiltrative process can be locally aggressive. The lesion is usually sporadic, but can be associated with APC gene mutation syndromes, such as familial adenomatous polyposis, Gardner syndrome, or hereditary desmoid syndrome (88–90).

On gross examination, fibromatosis demonstrates a gray-white fibrous cut surface and ranges in size from 1 to 10 cm, with ill-defined or rarely well-circumscribed borders. Microscopically, the bland spindle cells are arranged in long broad fascicles, of varying cellularity and amounts of collagen, that infiltrate the surrounding stroma, often entrapping lobular units and ducts (Figure 10.18A). When abundant, the dense collagen can impart a keloid-like appearance. The cells display oval to spindled nuclei with poorly defined cell borders (Figure 10.18B). Myxoid areas, calcification, and lymphoid aggregates may also be present. The cellularity is often increased at the periphery of the tumor and may be mitotically active, but mitoses generally do not exceed 3 per 10 high-power fields and are never atypical. It is worth

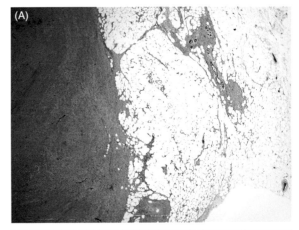

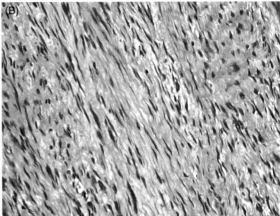

Figure 10.18 Fibromatosis is characterized by: (A) well-demarcated spindle-cell tumor with stellate extensions into adjacent fat (H&E × 10). (B) Broad sweeping fascicles of bland uniform spindle cells in collagenous stroma (H&E × 40).

recognizing that the cellularity and mitotic activity observed in fibromatosis in children and women of child-bearing age is typically greater than that observed in older women and adult men (87).

Immunohistochemistry can be helpful in confirming the diagnosis and distinguishing the lesion from a scar. A fibromatosis demonstrates cytoplasmic staining for actin and nuclear staining for β-catenin in 80% of cases (91), and occasionally may show focal keratin positivity, while p63, BCL-2, CD34, and sex steroid receptors are typically negative. Nodular fasciitis and spindle-cell sarcomas are lesser considerations that can generally be excluded on histologic examination alone. Fibromatosis lacks the short fascicles of plump fibroblasts with prominent nucleoli and conspicuous mitotic activity that characterize nodular fasciitis, and the obvious pleomorphism and numerous, often atypical, mitoses that are the hallmark of many sarcomas.

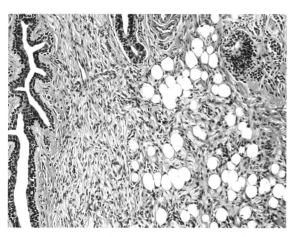

Figure 10.19 Dermatofibrosarcoma protruberans (DFSP) in a three-year-old male. This deep-seated DFSP had no skin involvement and was found to have the characteristic translocation t(17,22) and fusion of COL1A1 and PDGFB by cytogenetics and FISH, respectively (H&E × 20).

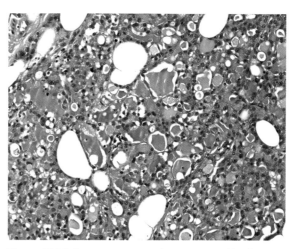

Figure 10.20 Secretory carcinoma from a 21-year-old male, characterized by microcystic spaces lined by apocrine-like cells, and containing abundant secretions (H&E × 20).

Other soft-tissue stromal lesions

Uncommonly, the breast can be the primary site of mesenchymal tumors such as granular-cell tumor, leiomyoma, nerve-sheath tumors, myxomas, nodular fasciitis, and dermatofibrosarcoma protruberans (DFSP). All of these lesions are histologically and immunophenotypically identical to their counterparts in other locations (described elsewhere in this textbook). Breast leiomyomas arise nearly exclusively in the nipple region. We have seen a deep genetically confirmed DFSP of the breast, without skin involvement, in a male toddler (Figure 10.19).

Carcinoma

A recent epidemiologic study of 75 pediatric breast malignancies revealed that 55% of cases were carcinomas (92). Twenty-seven percent were invasive ductal carcinomas of no specific type, followed by DCIS and secretory carcinoma in roughly equal numbers (92). Invasive lobular carcinoma is exceedingly rare in the pediatric population (92,93). A diagnosis of breast carcinoma in young patients should call into question the possibility of a BRCA-1/2 or p53 mutation (94–98). The histologic features of DCIS and invasive carcinomas are identical to their adult counterparts and should be graded, typed, and staged according to the American Joint Committee on Cancer guidelines (99).

Secretory carcinoma was first termed juvenile carcinoma (100) because the original cases were identified in children; however, it is now recognized that less than half of all cases present in patients less than 20 years (101). In children, these tumors have indolent behavior and an excellent prognosis, even with axillary nodal involvement (12,22,102–104).

Secretory carcinoma usually presents as an asymptomatic firm subareolar mass. Grossly, secretory carcinomas are well-circumscribed, mobile lesions, distinct from the nipple, measuring 1–2.5 cm in diameter, and displaying a gray-white firm cut surface, which may mimic fibroadenomas grossly. Microscopically, the lesion consists of one or several tumor lobules separated by prominent bands of densely sclerotic collagen. Microscopically, the tumor consists of small nests or large circumscribed islands of acini and microcysts containing abundant secretions that impart an overall microcystic appearance (Figure 10.20). Individual tumor cells show mild to moderate cytologic atypia. The cytoplasm may be finely granular or clear as a result of vacuolization. Secretory carcinomas express epithelial membrane antigen (EMA) and S100, but are always negative for estrogen receptor, progesterone receptor, and Her2. The intra- and intercellular secretions are positive for alcian blue and periodic acid–Schiff (diastase-resistant) (28). Interestingly, 12 of 13 cases of secretory carcinoma tested showed the same recurrent translocation, t(12;15)(p12;q26.1), that is seen in congenital fibrosarcoma/mesoblastic nephroma (105–109). The resulting ETV6-NTRK3 fusion gene encodes a chimeric tyrosine kinase oncoprotein (110,111).

Hematopoietic neoplasms

Primary lymphoma of the breast is rare in children (112,113). Intermediate- and high-grade non-Hodgkin's B-cell lymphomas (114), especially Burkitt's lymphoma (115,116), are the most common hematopoietic neoplasms with mammary involvement in the pediatric and adolescent populations. Burkitt's lymphoma has a predilection for breast involvement of young pregnant or lactating women (117,118). Primary mammary Hodgkin's disease has also been reported (119). Rarely, the breast may be the site of initial presentation of acute myelogenous leukemia, but is more commonly seen in the setting of relapse (112,120–128).

Metastases

Metastatic tumors to the breast include a variety of more common pediatric malignancies. Of these, alveolar rhabdomyosarcomas comprise the majority of cases (129,130). Approximately 7% of all rhabdomyosarcomas are associated with breast metastases, which can manifest as a single tumor, multiple tumors in the same breast, or bilateral disease. Other reported metastases include Ewing's sarcoma, giant-cell fibroblastoma, liposarcoma, alveolar soft-parts sarcoma, malignant melanoma, and renal-cell carcinoma (12,21,119,120,131–134).

References

1. Ciftci AO, Tanyel FC, Buyukpamukcu N, Hicsonmez A. Female breast masses during childhood: A 25-year review. Eur. J. Pediatr. Surg. 1998;**8**:67–70.

2. Chung EM, Cube R, Hall GJ, *et al*. From the archives of the AFIP: breast masses in children and adolescents: radiologic-pathologic correlation. Radiographics 2009;**29**:907–31.

3. Goldstein DP, Miler V. Breast masses in adolescent females. Clin. Pediatr. (Phila.) 1982;**21**:17–19.

4. Bower R, Bell MJ, Ternberg JL. Management of breast lesions in children and adolescents. J. Pediatr. Surg. 1976;**11**:337–46.

5. Coffin CM, Dehner LP. The breast. In: Stocker JT, Dehner LP, editors, *Pediatric Pathology*, second edn. Philadelphia, PA: Lippencott Williams & Wilkins; 2001:993–1015.

6. Lee KC, Chan JK, Ho LC. Histologic changes in the breast after fine-needle aspiration. Am. J. Surg. Pathol. 1994;**18**:1039–47.

7. Moore RL, Mungara A, Shayan K, Wallace AM. Bilaterally symmetric juvenile fibroadenomas and tubular breast deformity in a prepubescent girl. J. Pediatr. Surg. 2007;**42**:1133–6.

8. Carney JA, Toorkey BC. Myxoid fibroadenoma and allied conditions (myxomatosis) of the breast. A heritable disorder with special associations including cardiac and cutaneous myxomas. Am. J. Surg. Pathol. 1991;**15**:713–21.

9. Courcoutsakis NA, Chow CK, Shawker TH, Carney JA, Stratakis CA. Syndrome of spotty skin pigmentation, myxomas, endocrine overactivity, and schwannomas (Carney complex): breast imaging findings. Radiology 1997;**205**:221–7.

10. Jacobs TW, Chen YY, Guinee DG, Jr., *et al*. Fibroepithelial lesions with cellular stroma on breast core needle biopsy: Are there predictors of outcome on surgical excision? Am. J. Clin. Pathol. 2005;**124**:342–54.

11. Sanders M, Boulos F. The Breast. In: Gilbert-Barness E, editor, *Potter's Pathology of the Fetus, Infant and Child*, second edn. Philadelphia, PA: Mosby Elsevier; 2007:2093–114.

12. Dehner LP, Hill DA, Deschryver K. Pathology of the breast in children, adolescents, and young adults. Semin. Diagn. Pathol. 1999;**16**:235–47.

13. Spagnolo DV, Shilkin KB. Breast neoplasms containing bone and cartilage. Virchows Arch. A Pathol. Anat. Histopathol. 1983;**400**:287–95.

14. Mies C, Rosen PP. Juvenile fibroadenoma with atypical epithelial hyperplasia. Am. J. Surg. Pathol. 1987;**11**:184–90.

15. Eliasen CA. Letter to the editor: Aytpical duct hyperplasia in young females. Am. J. Surg. Path. 1992;**16**:1.

16. Eliasen CA, Cranor ML, Rosen PP. Atypical duct hyperplasia of the breast in young females. Am. J. Surg. Pathol. 1992;**16**:246–51.

17. Carter BA, Page DL, Schuyler P, *et al*. No elevation in long-term breast carcinoma risk for women with fibroadenomas that contain atypical hyperplasia. Cancer 2001;**92**:30–6.

18. Dupont WD, Page DL, Parl FF, *et al*. Long-term risk of breast cancer in women with fibroadenoma. N. Engl. J. Med. 1994;**331**:10–5.

19. Tea MK, Asseryanis E, Kroiss R, Kubista E, Wagner T. Surgical breast lesions in adolescent females. Pediatr. Surg. Int. 2009;**25**:73–5.

20. Majmudar B, Rosales-Quintana S. Infarction of breast fibroadenomas during pregnancy. JAMA 1975;**231**:963–4.

21. Pettinato G, Manivel JC, Kelly DR, Wold LE, Dehner LP. Lesions of the breast in children exclusive of typical fibroadenoma and gynecomastia. A clinicopathologic study of 113 cases. Pathol. Annu. 1989;**24** Pt 2:296–328.

22. Farrow JH, Ashikari H. Breast lesions in young girls. Surg. Clin. North. Am. 1969;**49**:261–9.

23. Rajan PB, Cranor ML, Rosen PP. Cystosarcoma phyllodes in adolescent girls and young women: A study of 45 patients. Am. J. Surg. Pathol. 1998;**22**:64–9.

24. Mollitt DL, Golladay ES, Gloster ES, Jimenez JF. Cystosarcoma phylloides in the adolescent female. J. Pediatr. Surg. 1987;**22**:907–10.

25. Bernstein L, Deapen D, Ross RK. The descriptive epidemiology of malignant cystosarcoma phyllodes tumors of the breast. Cancer 1993;**71**:3020–4.

26. Keelan PA, Myers JL, Wold LE, Katzmann JA, Gibney DJ. Phyllodes tumor: clinicopathologic review of 60 patients and flow cytometric analysis in 30 patients. Hum. Pathol. 1992;**23**:1048–54.

27. Chen WH, Cheng SP, Tzen CY, *et al.* Surgical treatment of phyllodes tumors of the breast: retrospective review of 172 cases. J. Surg. Oncol. 2005;**91**:185–94.

28. Page DL, Anderson TJ. *Diagnostic Histopathology of the Breast.* Edinburgh: Churchill Livingstone; 1987.

29. Tan PH, Tse G, Lee A, Simpson JF, Hanby AM. Fibroepithelial tumors. In: Lakhani SR, Ellis IO, Schnitt SJ, Tan PH, vandeVijver MJ, editors, *WHO Classification of Tumor of the Breast.* Lyon: IARC; 2012:141–7.

30. Powell CM, Cranor ML, Rosen PP. Multinucleated stromal giant cells in mammary fibroepithelial neoplasms. A study of 11 patients. Arch. Pathol. Lab. Med. 1994;**118**:912–6.

31. Grady I, Gorsuch H, Wilburn-Bailey S. Long-term outcome of benign fibroadenomas treated by ultrasound-guided percutaneous excision. Breast J. 2008;**14**:275–8.

32. Nigro DM, Organ CH, Jr. Fibroadenoma of the female breast. Some epidemiologic surprises. Postgrad. Med. 1976;**59**:113–7.

33. Organ CH, Jr., Organ BC. Fibroadenoma of the female breast: A critical clinical assessment. J. Natl. Med. Assoc. 1983;**75**:701–4.

34. Tan PH, Thike AA, Tan WJ, *et al.* Predicting clinical behavior of breast phyllodes tumours: A nomogram based on histological criteria and surgical margins. J. Clin. Pathol. 2012;**65**:69–76.

35. Moffat CJ, Pinder SE, Dixon AR, *et al.* Phyllodes tumours of the breast: A clinicopathological review of thirty-two cases. Histopathology 1995;**27**:205–18.

36. Cohn-Cedermark G, Rutqvist LE, Rosendahl I, Silfversward C. Prognostic factors in cystosarcoma phyllodes. A clinicopathologic study of 77 patients. Cancer 1991;**68**:2017–22.

37. Hawkins RE, Schofield JB, Fisher C, Wiltshaw E, McKinna JA. The clinical and histologic criteria that predict metastases from cystosarcoma phyllodes. Cancer 1992;**69**:141–7.

38. Norris HJ, Taylor HB. Relationship of histologic features to behavior of cystosarcoma phyllodes. Analysis of ninety-four cases. Cancer 1967;**20**:2090–9.

39. Pietruszka M, Barnes L. Cystosarcoma phyllodes: A clinicopathologic analysis of 42 cases. Cancer 1978;**41**:1974–83.

40. Adem C, Reynolds C, Ingle JN, Nascimento AG. Primary breast sarcoma: clinicopathologic series from the Mayo Clinic and review of the literature. Br. J. Cancer 2004;**91**:237–41.

41. Callery CD, Rosen PP, Kinne DW. Sarcoma of the breast. A study of 32 patients with reappraisal of classification and therapy. Ann. Surg. 1985;**201**:527–32.

42. Tan PH, Jayabaskar T, Chuah KL, *et al.* Phyllodes tumors of the breast: the role of pathologic parameters. Am. J. Clin. Pathol. 2005;**123**:529–40.

43. Chang HL, Lerwill MF, Goldstein AM. Breast hamartomas in adolescent females. Breast J. 2009;**15**:515–20.

44. Di Tommaso L, Pasquinelli G, Damiani S. Smooth muscle cell differentiation in mammary stromo-epithelial lesions with evidence of a dual origin: stromal myofibroblasts and myoepithelial cells. Histopathology 2003;**42**:448–56.

45. Chiacchio R, Panico L, D'Antonio A, *et al.* Mammary hamartomas: An immunohistochemical study of ten cases. Pathol. Res. Pract. 1999;**195**:231–6.

46. Tse GM, Law BK, Ma TK, *et al.* Hamartoma of the breast: A clinicopathological review. J. Clin. Pathol. 2002;**55**:951–4.

47. Wilson M, Cranor ML, Rosen PP. Papillary duct hyperplasia of the breast in children and young women. Mod. Pathol. 1993;**6**:570–4.

48. Rosen PP, Cantrell B, Mullen DL, DePalo A. Juvenile papillomatosis (Swiss cheese disease) of the breast. Am. J. Surg. Pathol. 1980;**4**:3–12.

49. Rosen PP, Holmes G, Lesser ML, Kinne DW, Beattie EJ. Juvenile papillomatosis and breast carcinoma. Cancer 1985;**55**:1345–52.

50. Bazzocchi F, Santini D, Martinelli G, *et al.* Juvenile papillomatosis (epitheliosis) of the breast. A clinical and pathologic study of 13 cases. Am. J. Clin. Pathol. 1986;**86**:745–8.

51. Ferguson TB, Jr., McCarty KS, Jr., Filston HC. Juvenile secretory carcinoma and juvenile papillomatosis: diagnosis and treatment. J. Pediatr. Surg. 1987;**22**:637–9.

52. Nonomura A, Kimura A, Mizukami Y, *et al.* Secretory carcinoma of the breast associated with juvenile papillomatosis in a 12-year-old girl. A case report. Acta Cytol. 1995;**39**:569–76.

53. Hamady ZZ, Carder PJ, Brennan TG. Atypical ductal hyperplasia in male breast tissue with gynaecomastia. Histopathology 2005;**47**:111–2.

54. Prasad V, J MK, McLeay W, Raymond W, Cooter RD. Bilateral atypical ductal hyperplasia, an incidental finding in gynaecomastia – case report and literature review. Breast 2005;**14**:317–21.

55. Page DL, Dupont WD, Rogers LW, Rados MS. Atypical hyperplastic lesions of the female breast. A long-term follow-up study. Cancer 1985;**55**:2698–708.

56. Braunstein GD. Gynecomastia. N. Engl. J. Med. 1993;**328**:490–5.

57. Braunstein GD. Clinical practice. Gynecomastia. N. Engl. J. Med. 2007;**357**:1229–37.

58. Damiani S, Eusebi V. Gynecomastia in type-1 neurofibromatosis with features of pseudoangiomatous stromal hyperplasia with giant cells. Report of two cases. Virchows Arch. 2001;**438**:513–6.

59. Kimura S, Tanimoto A, Shimajiri S, *et al.* Unilateral gynecomastia and pseudoangiomatous stromal hyperplasia in neurofibromatosis: case report and review of the literature. Pathol. Res. Pract. 2012;**208**:318–22.

60. Zamecnik M, Michal M, Gogora M, *et al.* Gynecomastia with pseudoangiomatous stromal hyperplasia and multinucleated giant cells. Association with neurofibromatosis type 1. Virchows Arch. 2002;**441**:85–7.

61. Balakumar T, Perry LA, Savage MO. Adrenocortical adenoma – an unusual presentation with hypersecretion of oestradiol, androgens and cortisol. J. Pediatr. Endocrinol. Metab. 1997;**10**:227–9.

62. Ghazi AA, Mofid D, Rahimi F, Marandi H, Nasri H, Afghah S. Oestrogen and cortisol producing adrenal tumour. Arch. Dis. Child. 1994;**71**:358–9.

63. Ajlouni KM, Arnaout MA, Qoussous Y. Congenital adrenal hyperplasia due to 11-beta-hydroxylase deficiency with skeletal abnormalities. J. Endocrinol. Invest. 1996;**19**:316–9.

64. Tyson D, Reggiardo D, Sklar C, David R. Prolactin-secreting macroadenomas in adolescents. Response to bromocriptine therapy. Am. J. Dis. Child. 1993;**147**:1057–61.

65. Ouhilal S, Turco J, Nangia A, Stotland M, Manganiello PD. True hermaphroditism presenting as bilateral gynecomastia in an adolescent phenotypic male. Fertil. Steril. 2005;**83**:1041.

66. Sinnecker GH, Hiort O, Dibbelt L, *et al.* Phenotypic classification of male pseudohermaphroditism due to steroid 5 α-reductase 2 deficiency. Am. J. Med. Genet. 1996;**63**:223–30.

67. Castro-Magana M, Angulo M, Uy J. Male hypogonadism with gynecomastia caused by late-onset deficiency of testicular 17-ketosteroid reductase. N. Engl. J. Med. 1993;**328**:1297–301.

68. Malozowski S, Stadel BV. Prepubertal gynecomastia during growth hormone therapy. J. Pediatr. 1995;**126**:659–61.

69. Madani S, Tolia V. Gynecomastia with metoclopramide use in pediatric patients. J. Clin. Gastroenterol. 1997;**24**:79–81.

70. Pappagallo M, Silva R. The effect of atypical antipsychotic agents on prolactin levels in children and adolescents. J. Child. Adolesc. Psychopharmacol. 2004;**14**:359–71.

71. Binder G, Iliev DI, Dufke A, *et al.* Dominant transmission of prepubertal gynecomastia due to serum estrone excess: hormonal, biochemical, and genetic analysis in a large kindred. J. Clin. Endocrinol. Metab. 2005;**90**:484–92.

72. Zamecnik M, Dubac V. Pseudoangiomatous stromal hyperplasia with giant cells in the female breast. No association with neurofibromatosis? Cesk Patol. 2011;**47**:59–61.

73. Chang HL, Kish JB, Smith BL, Goldstein AM. A 16-year-old male with gynecomastia and ductal carcinoma in situ. Pediatr. Surg. Int. 2008;**24**:1251–3.

74. Corroppolo M, Erculiani E, Zampieri N, *et al.* Ductal carcinoma in situ in a 15-year-old boy with gynaecomastia: A case report. Pediatr. Surg. Int. 2008;**24**:943–5.

75. Lemoine C, Mayer SK, Beaunoyer M, Mongeau C, Ouimet A. Incidental finding of synchronous bilateral ductal carcinoma in situ associated with gynecomastia in a 15-year-old obese boy: case report and review of the literature. J. Pediatr. Surg. 2011;**46**:e17–20.

76. Wadie GM, Banever GT, Moriarty KP, Courtney RA, Boyd T. Ductal carcinoma in situ in a 16-year-old adolescent boy with gynecomastia: A case report. J. Pediatr. Surg. 2005;**40**:1349–53.

77. AbdullGaffar B. Pseudoangiomatous stromal hyperplasia of the breast. Arch. Pathol. Lab. Med. 2009;**133**:1335–8.

78. Ferreira M, Albarracin CT, Resetkova E. Pseudoangiomatous stromal hyperplasia tumor: A clinical, radiologic and pathologic study of 26 cases. Mod. Pathol. 2008;**21**:201–7.

79. Powell CM, Cranor ML, Rosen PP. Pseudoangiomatous stromal hyperplasia (PASH). A mammary stromal tumor with myofibroblastic differentiation. Am. J. Surg. Pathol. 1995;**19**:270–7.

80. Baker M, Chen H, Latchaw L, Memoli V, Ornvold K. Pseudoangiomatous stromal hyperplasia of the breast in a 10-year-old girl. J. Pediatr. Surg. 2011;**46**:e27–31.

81. Shehata BM, Fishman I, Collings MH, *et al.* Pseudoangiomatous stromal hyperplasia of the breast in pediatric patients: An underrecognized entity. Pediatr. Dev. Pathol. 2009;**12**:450–4.

82. Sanders MP, Brooks JS, Palazzo JP. Mesenchymal Lesions of the Breast. In: Palazzo JP, editor, *Difficult Diagnoses in Breast Pathology*, first edn. New York: Demos Medical; 2011:172–95.

83. Virk RK, Khan A. Pseudoangiomatous stromal hyperplasia: An overview. Arch. Pathol. Lab. Med. 2010;**134**:1070–4.

84. van Geel AN, den Bakker MA. Bilateral angiosarcoma of the breast in a fourteen-year-old child. Rare Tumors 2009;**1**:e38:2.

85. Deyrup AT, Miettinen M, North PE, *et al.* Angiosarcomas arising in the viscera and soft tissue of children and young adults: A clinicopathologic study of 15 cases. Am. J. Surg. Pathol. 2009;**33**:264–9.

86. Fisher C, Berg Evd, Molenaar WM. Adult fibrosarcoma. In: Fletcher CDM, Unni KK, Mertens F, editors, *WHO Classification of Tumours of Soft Tissue and Bone*, first edn. Lyon: IARC; 2002:100–1.

87. Devouassoux-Shisheboran M, Schammel MD, Man YG, Tavassoli FA. Fibromatosis of the breast: Age-correlated morphofunctional features of 33 cases. Arch. Pathol. Lab. Med. 2000;**124**:276–80.

88. McMenamin ME, DeSchryver K, Fletcher CD. Fibrous Lesions of the Breast: A Review. Int. J. Surg. Pathol. 2000;**8**:99–108.

89. Rosen PP, Ernsberger D. Mammary fibromatosis. A benign spindle-cell tumor with significant risk for local recurrence. Cancer 1989;**63**:1363–9.

90. Wargotz ES, Norris HJ, Austin RM, Enzinger FM. Fibromatosis of the breast. A clinical and pathological study of 28 cases. Am. J. Surg. Pathol. 1987;**11**:38–45.

91. Carlson JW, Fletcher CD. Immunohistochemistry for beta-catenin in the differential diagnosis of spindle cell lesions: Analysis of a series and review of the literature. Histopathology 2007;**51**:509–14.

92. Gutierrez JC, Housri N, Koniaris LG, Fischer AC, Sola JE. Malignant breast cancer in children: A review of 75 patients. J. Surg. Res. 2008;**147**:182–8.

93. Corpron CA, Black CT, Singletary SE, Andrassy RJ. Breast cancer in adolescent females. J. Pediatr. Surg. 1995;**30**:322–4.

94. Claus EB, Risch N, Thompson WD. Autosomal dominant inheritance of early-onset breast cancer. Implications for risk prediction. Cancer 1994;**73**:643–51.

95. Elger BS, Harding TW. Testing adolescents for a hereditary breast cancer gene (BRCA1): respecting their autonomy is in their best interest. Arch. Pediatr. Adolesc. Med. 2000;**154**:113–9.

96. Malone KE, Daling JR, Thompson JD, *et al.* BRCA1 mutations and breast cancer in the general population: Analyses in women before age 35 years and in women before age 45 years with first-degree family history. JAMA 1998;**279**:922–9.

97. Sidransky D, Tokino T, Helzlsouer K, *et al.* Inherited p53 gene mutations in breast cancer. Cancer Res. 1992;**52**:2984–6.

98. Thompson WD. Genetic epidemiology of breast cancer. Cancer 1994;**74**:279–87.

99. Simpson JF. Breast. In: Edge SB, Byrd DR, Compton CC *et al.*, editors, *AJCC Cancer Staging Manual*, seventh edn. New York: Springer; 2010:347–76.

100. Masse SR, Rioux A, Beauchesne C. Juvenile carcinoma of the breast. Hum. Pathol. 1981;**12**:1044–6.

101. Horowitz DP, Sharma CS, Connolly E, Gidea-Addeo D, Deutsch I. Secretory carcinoma of the breast: results from the survival, epidemiology and end results database. Breast 2012;**21**:350–3.

102. Tanimura A, Konaka K. Carcinoma of the breast in a 5 years old girl. Acta Pathol. Jpn. 1980;**30**:157–60.

103. Tavassoli FA, Norris HJ. Secretory carcinoma of the breast. Cancer 1980;**45**:2404–13.

104. Oberman HA, Stephens PJ. Carcinoma of the breast in childhood. Cancer 1972;**30**:470–4.

105. Eguchi M, Eguchi-Ishimae M, Tojo A, *et al.* Fusion of ETV6 to neurotrophin-3 receptor TRKC in acute myeloid leukemia with t(12;15)(p13;q25). Blood 1999;**93**:1355–63.

106. Knezevich SR, Garnett MJ, Pysher TJ, *et al.* ETV6-NTRK3 gene fusions and trisomy 11 establish a histogenetic link between mesoblastic nephroma and congenital fibrosarcoma. Cancer Res. 1998;**58**:5046–8.

107. Knezevich SR, McFadden DE, Tao W, Lim JF, Sorensen PH. A novel ETV6-NTRK3 gene fusion in congenital fibrosarcoma. Nat. Genet. 1998;**18**:184–7.

108. Rubin BP, Chen CJ, Morgan TW, *et al.* Congenital mesoblastic nephroma t(12;15) is associated with ETV6-NTRK3 gene fusion: cytogenetic and molecular relationship to congenital (infantile) fibrosarcoma. Am. J. Pathol. 1998;**153**:1451–8.

109. Tognon C, Knezevich SR, Huntsman D, *et al.* Expression of the ETV6-NTRK3 gene fusion as a primary event in human secretory breast carcinoma. Cancer Cell 2002;**2**:367–76.

110. Liu Q, Schwaller J, Kutok J, *et al.* Signal transduction and transforming properties of the TEL-TRKC fusions

associated with t(12;15)(p13;q25) in congenital fibrosarcoma and acute myelogenous leukemia. EMBO J. 2000;**19**:1827–38.

111. Wai DH, Knezevich SR, Lucas T, *et al.* The ETV6-NTRK3 gene fusion encodes a chimeric protein tyrosine kinase that transforms NIH3T3 cells. Oncogene 2000;**19**:906–15.

112. Lin Y, Govindan R, Hess JL. Malignant hematopoietic breast tumors. Am. J. Clin. Pathol. 1997;**107**:177–86.

113. Meis JM, Butler JJ, Osborne BM. Hodgkin's disease involving the breast and chest wall. Cancer 1986;**57**:1859–65.

114. Lin P, Jones D, Dorfman DM, Medeiros LJ. Precursor B-cell lymphoblastic lymphoma: A predominantly extranodal tumor with low propensity for leukemic involvement. Am. J. Surg. Pathol. 2000;**24**:1480–90.

115. Fahmy JL, Wood BP, Miller JH. Bilateral breast involvement in a teenage girl with Burkitt lymphoma. Pediatr. Radiol. 1995;**25**:56–7.

116. Hubner KF, Littlefield LG. Burkitt lymphoma in three American children. Clinical and cytogenetic observations. Am. J. Dis. Child. 1975;**129**:1219–23.

117. Arber DA, Simpson JF, Weiss LM, Rappaport H. Non-Hodgkin's lymphoma involving the breast. Am. J. Surg. Pathol. 1994;**18**:288–95.

118. Fadiora SO, Mabayoje VO, Aderoumu AO, *et al.* Generalised Burkitt's lymphoma involving both breasts: A case report. West Afr. J. Med. 2005;**24**:280–2.

119. Rogers DA, Lobe TE, Rao BN, *et al.* Breast malignancy in children. J. Pediatr. Surg. 1994;**29**:48–51.

120. van Hoeven KH, Hibbard CA, Flax H, Jones JG, Suhrland MJ. Metastatic malignant neoplasms and secondary lymphomatous involvement of the breast: A study of 43 cases. Pathol. Annu. 1993;**28** Pt 2:221–41.

121. Ahrar K, McLeary MS, Young LW, Masotto M, Rouse GA. Granulocytic sarcoma (chloroma) of the breast in an adolescent patient: ultrasonographic findings. J. Ultrasound Med. 1998;**17**:383–4.

122. Au WY, Ma SK, Kwong YL, *et al.* Acute myeloid leukemia relapsing as gynecomastia. Leuk. Lymphoma 1999;**36**:191–4.

123. Barker TH. Granulocytic sarcoma of the breast diagnosed by fine needle aspiration (FNA) cytology. Cytopathology 1998;**9**:135–7.

124. Dufour C, Garaventa A, Brisigotti M, Rosanda C, Mori PG. Massively diffuse multifocal granulocytic

sarcoma in a child with acute myeloid leukemia. Tumori 1995;**81**:222–4.

125. Gartenhaus WS, Mir R, Pliskin A, *et al.* Granulocytic sarcoma of breast: Aleukemic bilateral metachronous presentation and literature review. Med. Pediatr. Oncol. 1985;**13**:22–9.

126. Domanic N, Akman N, Muftuoglu AU. Massive breast involvement in acute leukemia. Case report. Helv. Paediatr. Acta 1972;**27**:601–5.

127. Farah RA, Timmons CF, Aquino VM. Relapsed childhood acute lymphoblastic leukemia presenting as an isolated breast mass. Clin. Pediatr. (Phila.) 1999;**38**:545–6.

128. Soyupak SK, Sire D, Inal M, Celiktas M, Akgul E. Secondary involvement of breast with non-Hodgkin's lymphoma in a paediatric patient presenting as bilateral breast masses. Eur. Radiol. 2000;**10**:519–20.

129. Herrera LJ, Lugo-Vicente H. Primary embryonal rhabdomyosarcoma of the breast in an adolescent female: A case report. J. Pediatr. Surg. 1998;**33**:1582–4.

130. Reale D, Guarino M, Sgroi G, *et al.* (Primary embryonal rhabdomyosarcoma of the breast. Description of a case). Pathologica 1994;**86**:98–101.

131. Hanna NN, O'Donnell K, Wolfe GR. Alveolar soft parts sarcoma metastatic to the breast. J. Surg Oncol. 1996;**61**:159–62.

132. Pursner M, Petchprapa C, Haller JO, Orentlicher RJ. Renal carcinoma: bilateral breast metastases in a child. Pediatr. Radiol. 1997;**27**:242–3.

133. Vergier B, Trojani M, de Mascarel I, Coindre JM, Le Treut A. Metastases to the breast: differential diagnosis from primary breast carcinoma. J. Surg. Oncol. 1991;**48**:112–6.

134. Boothroyd A, Carty H. Breast masses in childhood and adolescence. A presentation of 17 cases and a review of the literature. Pediatr. Radiol. 1994;**24**:81–4.

135. Stone AM, Shenker IR, McCarthy K. Adolescent breast masses. Am. J. Surg. 1977;**134**:275–7.

136. Simpson JS, Barson AJ. Breast tumours in infants and children: A 40-year review of cases at a children's hospital. Can. Med. Assoc. J. 1969;**101**:100–2.

137. West KW, Rescorla FJ, Scherer LR, 3rd, Grosfeld JL. Diagnosis and treatment of symptomatic breast masses in the pediatric population. J. Pediatr. Surg. 1995;**30**:182–6; discussion 6–7.

138. Elsheikh A, Keramopoulos A, Lazaris D, Ambela C, Louvrou N, Michalas S. Breast tumors during adolescence. Eur. J. Gynaecol. Oncol. 2000;**21**:408–10.

Soft-tissue tumors in young patients

Cheryl M. Coffin, Mariana M. Cajaiba, Justin M. M. Cates, and Rita Alaggio

Introduction

Neoplasms of soft tissues are relatively common in children and adolescents compared with adults, and most are benign or represent tumor-like malformations, overgrowths, reactive processes, or masses that are difficult to categorize in terms of pathogenesis, whereas sarcomas account for approximately 7% of malignancies in young patients (1–3). This chapter provides an approach to diagnosis for different types of soft-tissue tumors during the first two decades of life.

The approach to diagnosis

Significant advances in diagnosis and treatment of malignant soft-tissue neoplasms in children and adolescents have occurred in recent decades (2,4–6). The anatomic distribution is wide, with nearly half originating within an organ or axial site (1). In the USA, nearly 900 soft-tissue sarcomas per year are diagnosed in the first two decades of life, with nearly half being rhabdomyosarcomas (1,2,6). The specific types of sarcomas vary in relative frequency with age (Table 11.1).

Rhabdomyosarcoma (45%) is most common in the first five years of life and is gradually superceded in later childhood and adolescence by Ewing's sarcoma (23%) and other non-rhabdomyosarcomas (32%) (4,5,7–11). Soft-tissue tumors in children, especially rhabdomyosarcoma, can arise in the setting of a malformation syndrome or genetic disorder (Table 11.2; 1,12).

Since 2002, morphologic and molecular genetic classifications have been codified in the World Health Organization (WHO) *Pathology and Genetics of Tumors of Soft Tissue and Bone* and a new classification has recently been published (13). Several

clinicopathologic categories of soft-tissue neoplasms are now defined: benign, locally recurrent, rarely metastasizing, and malignant. Although the current classification is based on the similarity of a neoplasm to a recognizable type of mature mesenchymal tissue, the pathologist who encounters a soft-tissue neoplasm initially separates the tumor into the broad morphologic categories of spindle-cell, round-cell, epithelioid, myxoid, or vascular proliferations (Table 11.3).

Superficial masses are often excised, while deeper masses are generally assessed by an initial incisional or core needle biopsy rather than primary excision (1,14). The main objectives for the pathologist are to establish the pathologic diagnosis, assess margins if relevant, and obtain relevant pathologic–prognostic–genetic information. Frozen section examination can confirm the presence of lesional tissue, aid in decisions about tissue triage for diagnostic adjuncts and research, and guide further surgical management of the patient (1,14). Specific report guidelines are available for soft-tissue sarcomas in general and for specific sarcomas in young patients, such as ES and rhabdomyosarcoma (15–19). A report template is shown in Table 11.4.

These guidelines have in common the requirements to document the specimen type and whether it is fresh or fixed, the size in three dimensions, the assessment of margins, including distance between the tumor and the margin, the anatomic structures present (such as peripheral nerve and lymph node), and the presence of hemorrhage and necrosis within the mass. A general principle is to sample one tissue block of tumor per centimeter of tumor diameter, in addition to histologically evaluating the surgical margins, neural or vascular margins, lymph nodes, previous biopsy site, and adjacent non-neoplastic tissue. It is best to harvest tissue

Table 11.1 Relative frequencies of soft-tissue sarcomas in children, adolescents and young adults, and older adults

Tumor type	Newborn–15 years	15–30 years	> 30 years
Rhabdomyosarcoma	+++	+	Rare
Ewing's sarcoma	++	++	Rare
Synovial sarcoma	++	++	+
MPNST	++	++	++
Liposarcoma	Rare	+	+++
Kaposi sarcoma	Rare	++	+++
Undifferentiated plemorphic sarcoma	Rare	+	+++
Leiomyosarcoma	Rare	+	+++
Epithelioid sarcoma	Rare	+	+
Gastrointestinal stromal tumor	Rare	Rare	+++
Angiosarcoma	Rare	Rare	+++
Dermatofibrosarcoma protuberans	Rare	Rare	++

Table 11.2 Syndromic and genetic disorders associated with soft-tissue tumors in children

Disorder/Syndrome	Chromosome (Genes)	Tumor(s)
Adenomatous polyposis coli	5q21–22 (APC)	RMS, GAF, DES
Beckwith–Wiedemann	11p15(IGF2, CDKAIC, H19, LIT1)	RMS
Bloom	15q26.1 (RECQL3)	RMS
Constitutional mismatch repair/deficiency	7p22.1 (PSM2)	RMS
Costello	12p12.1 (H-RAS)	RMS
Familial pleuropulmonary blastoma	14q23.13 (DICER)	PPB, RMS
Familial rhabdoid predisposition	22q11.33 (SMARC1B1)	MRT
Gorlin–Goltz (basal cell nevus)	Xp11.23 (PTCH)	FRM, RMS
Hereditary retinoblastoma	13q14.2 (RB1)	RMS, OS
Leiomyomatosis–Alport	Xq22.3 (COL4A6)	LM
Li–Fraumeni	17p13.1 (TP53)	RMS, UPS, PLPS

Table 11.2 (cont.)

Disorder/Syndrome	Chromosome (Genes)	Tumor(s)
Mosaic variegated aneuploidy	15q15.1 (BUB1B)	RMS
Neurofibromatosis type 1	17q11.2 (NF1)	NF, RMS, MPNST
Nijmegen breakage	8q21.3 (NBS1)	RMS
Noonan	12q24 (PTPN11)	RMS, LYM
Roberts	8p21.1 (ESC02)	RMS
Rubinstein–Taybi	16p13.1 (CREBBP)	RMS
Schwannomatosis	22q11.2 (NF2)	SCHW, MRT, RMS
Tuberous sclerosis	9q34 (TSC1), 16p13.3 (TSC2), 12q22-q24.1 (TSC3)	RMS, CRM, CHOR
Werner	8p12-p11.2 (RECOL2)	RMS

Abbreviations: RMS = rhabdomyosarcoma, GAF = Gardner fibroma, DES = desmoid-type fibromatosis, PPB = pleuropulmonary blastoma, MRT = malignant rhabdoid tumor, FRM = fetal rhabdomyoma, LM = leiomyoma, OS = osteosarcoma, UPS = undifferentiated pleomorphic sarcoma, PLPS = pleomorphic liposarcoma, NF = neurofibroma, MPNST = malignant peripheral nerve-sheath tumor, LYM = lymphatic malformation (lymphangioma), SCHW = Schwannoma, CRM = cardiac rhabdomyoma, CHOR = chordoma

from the fresh specimen to use for conventional cytogenetics, fresh tissue, fluorescence *in-situ* hybridization (FISH), or molecular tests when a fresh specimen is received. Immunohistochemistry is an established diagnostic tool to determine the line of differentiation, as well as potential prognostic and genomic markers. Electron microscopy has a potential role for assessing primitive tumors that are difficult to classify with histology and immunohistochemistry. Cytogenetic and molecular diagnostic tests have become essential for evaluation of certain types of soft-tissue tumors (Tables 11.5 and 11.6), although the diagnosis can usually be established with morphology and immunohistochemistry (1,14,15,20–26).

Non-rhabdomyosarcoma soft-tissue sarcomas are graded using either the Pediatric Oncology Group or the French Federation of Cancer Centers (FNCLCC) grading systems, the latter of which is now the preferred system for grading soft-tissue sarcomas in adults (6,13,27–29). Benign, locally aggressive, and rarely metastasizing tumors are not graded. Several caveats are important in determining grade, including

Table 11.3 Morphologic pattern, tumor types, and immunohistochemical profiles of selected soft-tissue tumors in children and adolescents

Morphology	Tumor type	Immunohistochemical Profile
Round cell	Rhabdomyosarcoma	MyoD1, myogenin, desmin, muscle-specific actin
	Ewing sarcoma	CD99, vimentin, synaptophysin
	Desmoplastic small round-cell tumor	Desmin, WT1, EMA, cytokeratins, CD99, NSE
	Clear-cell sarcoma	S100, HMB-45, MelanA, MITF
	Malignant rhabdoid tumor	INI1 loss, EMA, cytokeratins, CD99, Leu7, NSE, synaptophysin
	Synovial sarcoma, poorly differentiated	CD99, EMA, cytokeratins, TLE1, Bcl-2, SOX9
	Extraskeletal mesenchymal chondrosarcoma	SOX9, CD99, Bcl-2
Spindle cell	Nodular fasciitis	Smooth-muscle actin, muscle-specific actin
	Fibromatosis (non-desmoid)	Smooth-muscle actin, muscle-specific actin
	Desmoid-type fibromatosis	β-catenin (nuclear), smooth-muscle actin, and muscle-specific actin
	Inflammatory myofibroblastic tumor	ALK, smooth-muscle actin, muscle-specific actin
	Dermatofibrosarcoma protuberans	CD34
	Low-grade fibromyxoid sarcoma	MUC4, EMA (focal)
	Myofibroma	Smooth-muscle actin, CD34
	Myofibroblastic sarcoma	Smooth-muscle actin, muscle-specific actin, calponin, CD34
	Neurofibroma	CD34, S100 (focal)
	Schwannoma	S100 (diffuse)
	Malignant peripheral nerve-sheath tumor	S100 (<50%), Leu7, CD34
	Smooth-muscle tumors	Smooth-muscle actin, desmin, h-caldesmon
	Rhabdomyosarcoma	MyoD1, myogenin, desmin, muscle-specific actin
	Synovial sarcoma	EMA, cytokeratins, TLE1, Bcl2, SOX9
	Kaposiform hemangioendothelioma	Prox1, LYVE1, D2–40, VEGFR3, CD31, CD34
Epithelioid	Epithelioid sarcoma	Cytokeratins, EMA, INI1 loss
	Alveolar soft-part sarcoma	TFE3
	Epithelioid vascular neoplasms	CD31, CD34, ERG, cytokeratins
	Epithelioid nerve-sheath tumors	S100, keratin
	Epithelioid rhabdomyosarcoma	MyoD1, myogenin, desmin
	Perivascular epithelioid cell tumor (PEComa)	HMB45, melanA, MITF, calponin, smooth-muscle actin
	Myoepithelioma	Keratins, S100, calponin, EMA, GFAP, p63, smooth-muscle actin
Myxoid	Lipoblastoma	S100, CD34
	Myxoid liposarcoma	S100
	Myxoinflammatory fibroblastic sarcoma	CD68, CD34, smooth-muscle actin

sampling limitations of fine-needle aspiration cytology or core needle biopsy specimens that may cause undergrading due to intratumoral heterogeneity and the inability to grade tumors that have been previously treated with chemotherapy or radiation (1,29). A single staging system has not been validated for pediatric soft-tissue sarcomas; different staging definitions are used for rhabdomyosarcomas and non-rhabdomyosarcomas.

From a therapeutic point of view, sarcomas in children can be divided into three broad categories, the first two of which are rhabdomyosarcoma and

Table 11.4 Key elements of the soft tissue tumor pathology report

Diagnosis:
- Soft tissue, specific site
- Procedure type
- Pathologic diagnosis (histologic type)

Other information:
- Tumor size, cm (greatest diameter or all three dimensions)
- Macroscopic extent of tumor
- Mitotic rate per 10 high-power fields
- Necrosis (if present, estimate percent)
- Tumor grade (if applicable)
- Margin status (for excisional biopsy or resection)
- Pathologic staging
- Results of ancillary studies
- Treatment effects (if relevant)

Table 11.5 Genetic abnormalities in round cell, epithelioid, and myxoid soft-tissue tumors in children and adolescents

Tumor	Cytogenetics	Genes involved
Ewing's sarcoma family:		
ES	t(11;22)(q24; q12)	EWSR1-FLI1
	t(21;22)(q22; q12)	EWSR1-ERG
	t(7;22)(p22;q12)	ETV1-EWSR1
	t(17;22)(q12; q12)	E1AF-EWSR1
	t(2;22)	EWSR1-FEV
Desmoplastic small round-cell tumor	t(11;22)(p13; q12)	EWSR1-WT1
Clear-cell sarcoma	t(12;22)(q13; q12)	ATF1-EWSR1
	t(2;22)(q32.3; q12)	CREB1-EWSR1
Extraskeletal myxoid chondrosarcoma	t(9;22)(q22–23; q11–12)	EWSR1-NR4A3
	t(9;17)(q22; q11.2)	NR4A3-RBP56
	t(9;15)(q22;q21)	NR4A3-TCF12
Extraskeletal mesenchymal chondrosarcoma	t(11;22)(q24; q12)	Unknown
Angiomatoid fibrous histiocytoma	t(12;22)(q13; q12)	ATF1-EWSR1
	t(12;16)(q13; q11)	ATF1-FUS

Table 11.5 (cont.)

Tumor	Cytogenetics	Genes involved
Myoepithelioma	t(6;22)(p21;q12)	EWSR1-POU51
	t(1;22)(q23;q12)	EWSR1-PBX1
Other round-cell tumors:		
Ewing-like sarcomas	t(4;19)(q35;q13)	CIC-DUX4
	t(10;19)(q26; q13)	CIC-DUX4
	Inversion of X chromosome	BCOR-CCNB3
Alveolar rhabdomyosarcoma	t(2;13)(q35;q14)	PAX3-FOXO1
	t(1;13)(p36;q14)	PAX7-FOXO1
Malignant rhabdoid tumor	22q11 deletion, mutation	SMARCB1
Epithelioid tumors:		
Epithelioid sarcoma	22q11–12 alterations	SMARCB1
Alveolar soft-part sarcoma	t(X;17)(p11;q25)	ASPSCR1-TFE3
Myxoid tumors:		
Angiofibroma of soft tissue	t(5;8)(p15;q12)	Unknown
Lipoblastoma	8q13 alterations	PLAG1
Myxoid liposarcoma	t(12;16)(q13; p11)	FUS-DDIT3
	t(12;22)(q13; p12)	DDIT3-EWSR1

ES, which are highly chemosensitive, and a third group which includes most other sarcomas that are generally also found in adults and are less responsive to chemotherapy (6,15,30,31). However, despite a current trend to assess histologic response to treatment, the utility of grading treatment effects has not yet been proven for soft-tissue sarcomas, with the possible exception of ES (30,32). Ongoing Children's Oncology Group studies will assess the significance and grading of treatment effect in non-rhabdomyosarcomatous soft-tissue sarcoma.

Another important consideration in children and adolescents is whether a soft-tissue neoplasm may be a manifestation of a syndrome or hereditary condition,

Table 11.6 Genetic abnormalities in spindle-cell tumors

Tumor	Cytogenetics	Genes involved
Benign:		
Nodular fasciitis		MYH9-USP6
Fibroma of tendon sheath	t(2;11)(q31–32; q12)	Unknown
Desmoplastic fibroblastoma	t(2;11)(q31;q12)	Unknown
	t(11;17)(q12; p11.2)	Unknown
Schwannoma	22q12 loss	NF2 loss
Spindle-cell lipoma	16q13-qter rearrangement	Unknown
	Monosomy 13	Unknown
	Partial deletion (13q)	Unknown
Intermediate:		
Desmoid fibromatosis	+8,+20	Unknown
	5q21–22 loss	APC loss or mutation
	β-catenin mutation	CTNNB1
Aggressive angiomyxoma	12q15 rearrangement	HMGA2
Dermatofibrosarcoma protuberans and giant-cell fibroblastoma	t(17;22)(q21; q13)	COL1A1-PDGFB
	Ring chromosome (DFSP)	COL1A1-PDGFB
Angiomatoid fibrous histiocytoma	t(12;22)(q13; q12)	EWSR1-ATF1
	t(2;22)(q33;q12)	EWSR1-CREB1
	t(12;16)(q13; p11)	FUS-ATF1
Infantile fibrosarcoma	t(12;15)(p13; q25)*	ETV6-NTRK3
	Trisomies 8, 11, 17, 20	
Inflammatory myofibroblastic tumor	t(1;2)(q22;p23)	TPM3-ALK
	t(2;19)(p23;p13)	TPM4-ALK
	t(2;17)(p23;q23)	CLTC-ALK
	t(2;2)(p23;q13)	RANBP2-ALK
	t(2;2)(p23;q35)	ATIC-ALK
	t(2;11)(p23;p15)	CARS-ALK
	t(2;4)(p23;q21)	SEC31A-ALK

Table 11.6 (cont.)

Tumor	Cytogenetics	Genes involved
	inv(2)(p23;q35)	ATIC-ALK
Malignant:		
Embryonal rhabdomyosarcoma	LOH at 11p15; +2, +7, +8, +11, +12, +20, +21, +13q21; -1p35 −36, −3, −6, −7, −9q22, −14q21 −32, −17	Various pathways
Synovial sarcoma**	t(X;18)(p11.2; q11.2)	SS18–SSX2
	t(X;18)(p11.2; q11.2)	SS18–SSX4
	t(X;18)(p11.2; q11.2)	SS18–SSX1
	t(X;20)	SS18L1–SSX1
Malignant peripheral nerve- sheath tumor	Complex	–
Leiomyosarcoma	Deletion of 1p	Unknown
Low-grade fibromyxoid sarcoma	t(7;16)(q33;p11)	FUS-CREB3L2
	t(11;16)(p13; p11)	FUS-CREB3L1
Myxoinflammatory fibroblastic sarcoma	t(1;10)(p22–31; q24–25)	Deregulation of FGF8 and TGFBR3

* Also found in cellular mesoblastic nephroma, acute myeloid leukemia, and secretory carcinoma of breast.
** Monophasic variant harbors SS18-SSX1 or SS18-SSX2; biphasic variant mainly displays SS18-SSX1. SS18-SSX2 may be associated with a better outcome.

or a complication of immunosuppression, environmental exposures, or previous treatment for a first malignant neoplasm (1,33,34).

Vascular and perivascular tumors (see also Chapter 1)

Approximately 25% of soft-tissue tumors in children and adolescents have a vascular phenotype and more than 90% are benign. Both the WHO classification and the International Society for the Study of Vascular Anomalies (ISSVA) classification are currently used, and both are based on the resemblance to normal blood or lymphatic vessels (35–41). Vascular masses include reactive, malformative, neoplastic, and

355

nosologically indeterminate lesions, such as soft-tissue angiomatosis and multifocal lymphangioendotheliomatosis with thrombocytopenia (35). Malformations are beyond the scope of this chapter.

Several presumably reactive proliferations simulate vascular neoplasms (35,36). Lobular capillary hemangioma (pyogenic granuloma) is a cutaneous or mucosal, sessile, polypoid, or nodular mass that often bleeds or ulcerates. Intravenous variants also occur. The bland endothelial cells are arranged in lobules and form compact clusters around arborizing blood vessels. The mitotic rate varies. Acute inflammation, edema, and ulceration may be prominent. Papillary endothelial hyperplasia (Masson lesion) occurs in children as a distinct lesion or as a reactive component within a vascular malformation or neoplasm. The circumscribed proliferation is composed of plump hyperplastic endothelial cells supported by delicate fibrous stalks containing a central vessel or a hyalinized zone. Papillary endothelial hyperplasia simulates angiosarcoma, but is distinguished by its lack of cellular atypia and pleomorphism, relatively low mitotic rate, and circumscribed growth pattern. Bacillary angiomatosis is a reactive lesion associated with infection and resembles lobular capillary hemangioma, but is rare in children.

Many vascular malformations and neoplasms have been referred to as "hemangioma" over the years, and the current preference is to reserve this term for neoplasms with specific diagnostic criteria, and to classify malformations according to their specific histologic components.

Infantile hemangioma affects nearly 40% of all infants as a solitary or multifocal mass (35,36,42). It occurs in the skin, subcutaneous tissue, and soft tissue throughout the body, but especially in the head and neck. The clinical and histopathologic features of infantile hemangioma reflect the proliferative and involutional growth phases (38,43). With immunohistochemistry, the endothelial cells show distinctive reactivity for glucose transporter-1 protein (GLUT1), which is a sensitive and specific marker, and the reactivity persists through the proliferative, involutional, and end stage of infantile hemangioma. Other endothelial markers, including CD31 and CD34, are also expressed. Diffuse neonatal angiomatosis, with cutaneous and visceral lesions, is histologically identical to infantile hemangioma.

Congenital hemangiomas have a lobular architecture, and the endothelial proliferation is similar to

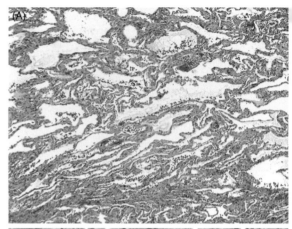

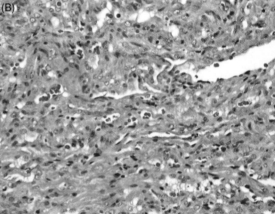

Figure 11.1 Spindle-cell hemangioma. (A) Cavernous thin-walled blood vessels have an infiltrative pattern with variably cellular tissue between the vascular spaces (H&E × 100). (B) Solid spindled foci consist of fibroblasts, pericytes, and endothelial cells with occasional prominent clear cytoplasmic vacuoles (H&E × 400).

infantile hemangioma, but is non-reactive for GLUT1. *Spindle-cell hemangioma* is a benign lesion, possibly a malformation, which presents in the skin of a distal extremity as a bluish nodule (35,44). It is associated with Maffucci or Klippel–Trenaunay syndrome and other hereditary conditions. Solid spindled foci with slit-like spaces and cavernous thin-walled vascular channels devoid of smooth muscle have an infiltrative pattern and may be accompanied by organizing thrombi, papillary endothelial hyperplasia, and intraluminal calcifications (Figure 11.1a). The solid component consists of fibroblasts, pericytes, and endothelial cells. Sometimes the endothelial cells contain prominent clear cytoplasmic vacuoles (Figure 11.1b). The endothelial cells express CD31, CD34, and focal D2–40.

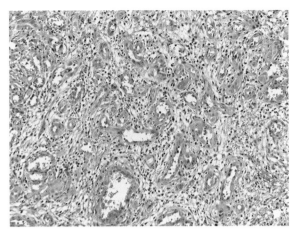

Figure 11.2 Epithelioid hemangioma displays vessels lined by plump and cuboidal endothelial cells with abundant eosinophilic cytoplasm, a myxoid and fibrous stroma, and lymphoplasmacytic and eosinophilic inflammation (H &E × 20).

Epithelioid hemangioma is a well-circumscribed lobular tumor composed of vessels lined with plump, round, or cuboidal endothelial cells with folded nuclei, prominent nucleoli, abundant eosinophilic, and sometimes vacuolated cytoplasm in a myxoid or fibrous stroma (45,46). Prominent inflammation with eosinophils, lymphocytes, plasma cells, and mast cells may be present (Figure 11.2). The tumor may be associated with lymphadenopathy and peripheral eosinophilia. It is related morphologically to angiolymphoid hyperplasia with eosinophilia.

Other types of cutaneous and soft-tissue hemangiomas are relatively uncommon in children and adolescents, and include giant-cell angioblastoma (47), synovial hemangioma, microvenular hemangioma, and cherry hemangioma.

Vascular lesions with a tendency for local recurrence or rare incidence of metastasis are typified by kaposiform hemangioendothelioma and papillary intravascular hemangioendothelioma. *Kaposiform hemangioendothelioma* is a locally aggressive, superficial, subcutaneous, or deep soft-tissue mass with infiltrative growth and is typically accompanied by the Kasabach–Merritt phenomenon (35,38,48,49). The vascular lobules vary in size and coalesce to form nodules and sheets. Some are well-canalized with round or elongated capillaries, and others are solid and composed of spindle cells with slit-like spaces (Figure 11.3). *Tufted angioma* may be closely related to kaposiform hemangioendothelioma, both clinically and pathologically (35,38,50). It is a cutaneous lesion that may be accompanied by hypertrichosis,

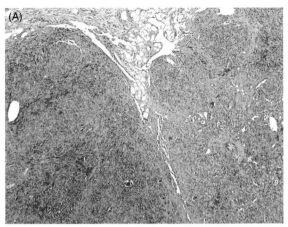

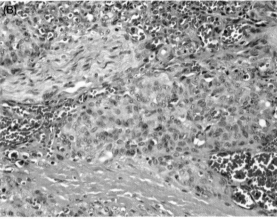

Figure 11.3 Kaposiform hemangioendothelioma. (A) The multilobular soft-tissue mass has an infiltrative growth pattern with irregular lymphatic channels between cellular lobules (H&E × 100). (B) Cellular areas are composed of clustered polygonal and spindle cells with slit-like vascular spaces (H&E × 40).

hyperhidrosis, or the Kasabach–Merritt phenomenon. Tightly aggregated endothelial cells form concentric whirls and have a peripheral semilunar cleft. Like kaposiform hemangioendothelioma, tufted angioma is reactive for D2–40 in a distinctive pattern in the peripheral dilated vessels around the tufts of endothelial cells. Another lymphatic endothelial marker, PROX-1, is expressed in both kaposiform hemangioendothelioma and tufted angioma (51,52).

Papillary intralymphatic angioendothelioma (Dabska tumor) is a rare cutaneous or soft-tissue tumor in children (35,53). It is composed of thin-walled intercommunicating blood vessels lined by cuboidal endothelial cells that form intraluminal papillae. Occasionally, a rosetting pattern and hyaline stromal cores are present.

Other locally recurring or rarely metastasizing vascular neoplasms such as retiform hemangioendothelioma, pseudomyogenic hemangioendothelioma, and composite hemangioendothelioma, are rare in young patients.

Malignant vascular neoplasms of any type are very uncommon in children and adolescents (7,35,41). *Epithelioid hemangioendothelioma* is a low-grade angiocentric vascular tumor that rarely metastasizes. It is composed of epithelioid endothelial cells arranged in cords and nests in a myxohyaline stroma. The endothelial cells have eosinophilic cytoplasm and may display intracytoplasmic vacuoles containing one or several erythrocytes. The infiltrative growth pattern simulates angiosarcoma (35,54). Atypical features of prominent spindling, cellular atypia, pleomorphism, necrosis, and a mitotic rate greater than one per ten high power fields raise a concern about epithelioid angiosarcoma. Angiosarcoma is exceptionally rare in childhood and may occur in the context of a variety of syndromes or as a second malignant neoplasm. A majority of angiosarcomas in children arise in the mediastinum or heart, but may also involve skin, viscera, breast, or deep soft tissues of the abdomen and pelvis (55,56). The ill-defined mass has a soft, spongy, or firm consistency with blood-filled cavities and focal necrosis. Histologically, well-differentiated and poorly differentiated areas alternate and are composed of anastomosing blood vessels lined by atypical endothelial cells, solid spindled areas, or papillary heaped-up foci. The range of morphological features from well to poorly differentiated angiosarcoma encompasses increasing nuclear and cytologic atypia, papillary or solid architecture, progressively less obvious lumen formation, and increasing mitoses. The epithelioid variant of angiosarcoma is composed of large round cells with abundant cytoplasm and cytoplasmic vacuoles. Angiosarcoma shows immunohistochemical reactivity with CD31 and CD34, and occasionally D2–40.

Kaposi sarcoma may be encountered in children with a primary or secondary immunodeficiency (35,57,58). Early flat patchy lesions are composed of small vessels around large ectatic blood vessels. As the lesion develops into the plaque stage, loosely ramifying networks of irregular blood vessels and spindle cells develop. Nodular Kaposi sarcoma is composed of densely cellular, mitotically active spindle cells with nuclear pleomorphism and variable cytoplasmic hyaline globules (59,60). Immunoreactivity is present for CD31, D2–40, and human herpes virus 8, the last of which is very useful in differential diagnosis.

Perivascular tumors currently include glomus tumors, myopericytoma, and myofibroma (discussed

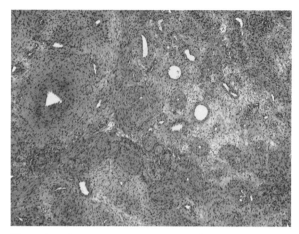

Figure 11.4 Myopericytoma is composed of blood vessels surrounded by concentric arrangements of plump oval to fusiform cells in a myxoid background (H&E × 20).

separately with the fibroblastic-myofibroblastic tumors). Glomus-cell lesions are currently divided into glomus tumor and glomuvenous malformations, although clinical and genetic features, including *glomulin* gene (*GLMN*) mutations, suggest that they form a continuum (35,61–63). *Glomuvenous malformations*, formerly designated as glomangioma, consist of infiltrative multinodular proliferations of large dilated veins, surrounded by one or more layers of cuboidal glomus cells in the vessel wall. *Glomus tumor* is composed of vascular spaces surrounded by rows of bland round cells in layers two to three cells thick, typically reactive for smooth-muscle actin (61). *Myopericytoma* is a well-demarcated mass with short oval or fusiform cells concentrically arranged around blood vessels; the cells are reactive for smooth-muscle actin and h-caldesmon (64; Figure 11.4). Some myopericytomas have a translocation t(7;12)(p22;q13) with an *ACTB* and *GLI1* gene fusion (65).

Smooth- and skeletal-muscle tumors

Neoplasms with the phenotype of smooth or skeletal muscle can arise throughout the body, regardless of whether muscle would normally be found in the site (12). The most common of these neoplasms is rhabdomyosarcoma. Benign striated-muscle tumors and smooth-muscle tumors are relatively infrequent in children and adolescents.

Rhabdomyomas account for less than 2% of striated-muscle tumors and include cardiac, fetal, adult, and genital subtypes (12,66). *Cardiac rhabdomyoma* is often associated with tuberous sclerosis, but

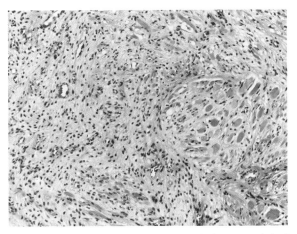

Figure 11.5 Fetal rhabdomyoma is composed of immature skeletal muscle cells with a range of differentiation and cellularity, in a myxoid background without atypia or mitotic activity (H&E × 20).

may also be seen in patients with trisomy 13, trisomy 21, or structural anomalies of the heart. It is considered a hamartomatous proliferation rather than a neoplasm, and it may spontaneously regress. The cardiac myocytes form clusters or nodules and have abundant vacuolated clear cytoplasm traversed by strands of pink material and small nuclei. Immunohistochemistry demonstrates reactivity for muscle-specific actin, desmin, hamartin, tuberin, and HMB45. *Fetal rhabdomyoma* most frequently occurs in the first three years of life, especially in the subcutaneous tissues of the head and neck, although the anatomic distribution is wide and includes a cutaneous form (12,67,68; Figure 11.5). Some are associated with the nevoid basal-cell carcinoma syndrome (Gorlin–Goltz syndrome) and have a PTCH1 gene mutation. The soft circumscribed mass has a mucoid cut surface; the skeletal muscle cells display a range of differentiation and cellularity in a variably myxoid background. The classic myxoid type consists of undifferentiated mesenchymal cells, immature muscle cells, and larger strap cells with cross striations, all of which lack atypia and significant mitotic activity. Spindled rhabdomyoblasts in bundles are the predominant feature of cellular rhabdomyoma. Immunohistochemistry demonstrates a striated muscle phenotype. Rhabdomyoma can simulate rhabdomyosarcoma, but is distinguished by its circumscription, superficial location, cellular maturation, and lack of severe nuclear atypia and mitotic activity. Genital rhabdomyomas occur in adolescents, and adult rhabdomyomas are very rare in young patients

(12,69). Focal myositis is a mass-forming inflammatory non-neoplastic lesion of skeletal muscle and simulates other tumors with myopathic changes, chronic inflammation, and fibrosis (70, 71).

Rhabdomyosarcoma is the most common soft-tissue sarcoma of children and adolescents, and has the phenotype of immature skeletal muscle (12,72–76). One third of cases are diagnosed in the first three years of life, and it can occur in infancy and as a congenital tumor (77). The two major subtypes in children and adolescents are embryonal rhabdomyosarcoma, including the botryoid variant, and alveolar rhabdomyosarcoma (12,78–80). Other subtypes, such as sclerosing, epithelioid, and pleomorphic rhabdomyosarcoma can occur in the young, but are quite rare (81,82; Figure 11.6). Rhabdomyosarcomas in adults generally have a more unfavorable outcome (83–86). Rhabdomyosarcomas are associated with a variety of genetic disorders and tumor predisposition syndromes (12,87–90).

Embryonal rhabdomyosarcoma shares morphologic, immunohistologic, and biological features with embryofetal skeletal muscle. The fleshy, tan mass is poorly circumscribed. The botryoid variant has a multinodular or polypoid, soft or myxoid appearance and involves mucosa-lined surfaces.

Spindle-cell rhabdomyosarcoma is firm and pale-tan, and the dense solid-cut surface resembles a smooth muscle or fibrous tumor. Spindled rhabdomyosarcoma is composed of fascicles and sheets of spindled, elongated rhabdomyoblasts with eosinophilic cytoplasm. Histologically, embryonal rhabdomyosarcoma displays a morphologic spectrum, ranging from primitive round or angulated cells in a pale or myxoid stroma, to a proliferation of rhabdomyoblasts, strap cells, multinucleated cells, and elongated cells with progressively increasing eosinophilic cytoplasm and occasional cytoplasmic cross striations (12,91). *Botryoid embryonal rhabdomyosarcoma* is characterized by a condensed layer of subepithelial tumor cells called the cambium layer; this can vary in thickness and may be discontinuous beneath the mucosa. Heterologous differentiation in the form of cartilage, neuroectodermal tissue, and bone may be seen, especially in genital botryoid embryonal rhabdomyosarcoma (92). Anaplasia, characterized by atypical cells with nuclear enlargement, hyperchromasia, and atypical mitoses, is present in a subset of rhabdomyosarcomas, especially embryonal rhabdomyosarcoma (91).

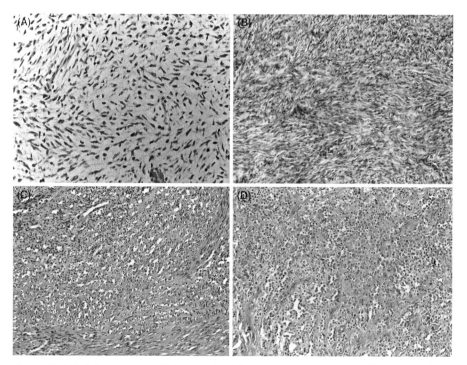

Figure 11.6 Rhabdomyosarcoma. (A) Embryonal rhabdomyosarcoma consists of spindled and round cells with a primitive appearance in a myxoid background (H&E × 40). (B) Spindle-cell rhabdomyosarcoma displays interlacing bundles of spindle cells with variable amounts of eosinophilic cytoplasm (H&E × 20). (C) Sclerosing rhabdomyosarcoma has abundant collagen in the background and may display a pseudoglandular or pseudoalveolar architecture in addition to spindle cells (H&E × 20). (D) Alveolar rhabdomyosarcoma is composed of nests of round tumor cells aligned along fibrous septa (H&E × 20).

Alveolar rhabdomyosarcoma is the most aggressive type of rhabdomyosarcoma in children and adolescents, and is more common in older children and teenagers (12,80). The extremities are the most common site. The fleshy, expansile mass may be soft or fibrous. Histologically, classic alveolar rhabdomyosarcoma displays round, relatively uniform tumor cells distributed along fibrous septa, with a nesting or glandular pattern, and clear spaces with discohesive tumor cells, including multinucleated tumor cells with eosinophilic cytoplasm, floating in the spaces. Strap cells and rhabdomyoblasts may be encountered in some examples of alveolar rhabdomyosarcoma.

Immunohistochemistry is very useful for establishing the skeletal muscle phenotype, especially in less-differentiated embryonal rhabdomyosarcomas and in alveolar rhabdomyosarcomas. Myogenin and MyoD1 show nuclear reactivity, usually in a focal distribution in embryonal rhabdomyosarcoma (88,93–95). Diffuse strong myogenin staining may predict poor survival (93,96). Muscle-specific actin and desmin show cytoplasmic reactivity in most cases. Expression of CD99, synaptophysin, smooth muscle actin, cytokeratin, S100 protein, CD99, neurofilament, and a variety of lymphoid markers represent potential diagnostic pitfalls in rhabdomyosarcoma (12).

A variety of cytogenetic aberrations, including chromosomal gains and losses, occur in embryonal rhabdomyosarcoma, and loss of heterozygosity of chromosomal region 11p15.5 is frequent, but as yet lacks diagnostic specificity (12).

Most alveolar rhabdomyosarcomas harbor a gene fusion between *PAX3* or *PAX7* and *FOXO1*, but a subset lacks this fusion and is similar to embryonal rhabdomyosarcoma in clinical behavior and response to treatment (12,97–102). The *PAX3-FOXO1* fusion in particular seems to portend more aggressive biologic potential, while rhabdomyosarcomas with alveolar morphology in the absence of a gene fusion are similar to embryonal rhabdomyosarcoma in biologic behavior.

Treatment effects in rhabdomyosarcomas include cytodifferentiation and a variety of reactive changes such as chronic inflammation, hemosiderin-laden macrophages, myxoid degeneration, and fibrosis. These have no clear prognostic significance (30,103,104).

Ectomesenchymoma is a rare tumor composed of rhabdomyosarcoma and variable neural, neuronal, or neuroectodermal components. In the future, it may be regarded as a subtype of rhabdomyosarcoma because of its clinicopathologic and molecular similarities (105).

Smooth-muscle tumors are much rarer in children and adolescents than in adults and are mostly hamartomas, or benign or low-grade neoplasms, with a relative paucity of leiomyosarcoma and an absence of gynecologic leiomyoma (12,106). Immunohistochemistry is useful in the phenotypic characterization with reactivity for smooth-muscle actin, muscle-specific actin, desmin, calponin, and h-caldesmon (107). h-Caldesmon is particularly useful because it does not typically stain fibrous, myofibroblastic, or myoepithelial proliferations. Smooth-muscle hamartoma is a nodular plaque that involves skin or submucosa with disorganized fascicles of mature smooth muscle. Leiomyomatosis is a diffusely infiltrative proliferation of mature smooth muscle associated with Alport syndrome (108).

Leiomyoma occurs throughout childhood and adolescence at a low frequency and in different sites in young patients, with approximately 25% originating in soft tissue and skin. With the exception of cases associated with Carney triad, Alport syndrome, and immunodeficiency, most pediatric leiomyomas are solitary. The mature smooth-muscle cells are arranged in whorls and bundles accompanied by collagen, without mitoses or atypia. Deep tumors may have dystrophic calcification.

Leiomyosarcomas in children and adolescents are histologically identical but prognostically superior to the adult counterpart and account for less than 5% of pediatric sarcomas (12,109–113). The skin, superficial and deep soft tissue, and viscera are sites of origin. In addition to classic leiomyosarcoma, myxoid, epithelioid, pleomorphic, and inflammatory variants can occur in young patients.

Smooth-muscle tumors of uncertain malignant potential can occur in immunocompromised children and adolescents with primary or secondary immunodeficiency, the latter related to chemotherapy, transplantation, or HIV infection (12,114–118). Often multifocal, these unusual tumors involve viscera, soft tissue, skin, brain, and bones, and are typically associated with Epstein–Barr virus infection (119). A perivascular growth pattern is characteristic, and the tumor may contain a prominent lymphocytic infiltrate. The spindle-cell proliferation has only mild or moderate atypia, variable mitoses, and occasional foci of myxoid change or round-cell morphology. In addition to smooth muscle immunohistochemical markers, they are positive for *in situ* hybridization for Epstein–Barr virus-encoded small RNA (EBER). Smooth muscle tumors of uncertain malignant potential in immunocompromised patients are less aggressive than conventional leiomyosarcoma and may respond to cessation of immunosuppression, in addition to other types of chemotherapy.

Fibroblastic, myofibroblastic, and myopericytic tumors

Fibroblastic and myofibroblastic tumors account for more than 10% of pediatric soft-tissue tumors, and most are benign (1,120). Many of these tumors share striking morphologic and immunohistochemical similarities, but have different clinical, biologic, and genetic features. They are composed of fibroblasts and myofibroblasts, which represent "activated fibroblasts," with variable degrees of contractile ability.

At the reactive end of the spectrum, keloids and hypertrophic scars are manifestations of abnormal wound healing with exuberant proliferation of fibroblasts and variable collagenization. *Nodular fasciitis* and its variant cranial fasciitis, along with other types of fasciitis (proliferative, ischemic) and *myositis* (focal, proliferative, myositis ossificans), are benign proliferations that simulate malignancy due to rapid growth, cellularity, atypia, and mitotic activity. Among these, *nodular fasciitis* is relatively frequent in the first two decades of life, and cranial fasciitis occurs almost exclusively in infancy and early childhood (120–122). The nodule is composed of densely cellular short fascicles and less cellular sheets of spindle cells in a myxoid matrix, accompanied by ganglion-like myofibroblasts, mucoid microcysts, focal hemorrhage, variable inflammation with histiocytes and lymphocytes, and scattered osteoclast-like giant cells (Figure 11.7). The spindled myofibroblasts express smooth-muscle actin. Nodular fasciitis harbors a *MYH9-USP6* gene fusion and is regarded as a benign lesion in the category of "transient neoplasia" (123). Cranial fasciitis is histologically similar, but typically occurs on the posterior scalp of infants and is more uniform in its microscopic appearance than nodular fasciitis. It can closely resemble desmoid fibromatosis.

Myositis ossificans can be solitary or multifocal and involves skeletal muscle or parosteal soft tissue as a

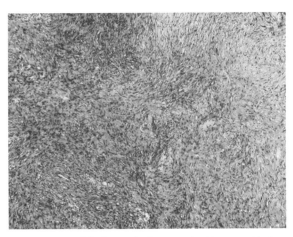

Figure 11.7 Nodular fasciitis displays a zonal architecture with short interlacing bundles of spindle cells, mucoid microcysts, a patchy mononuclear inflammatory infiltrate, and clear clefts between tumor cells (H&E × 20).

circumscribed nodule with a zonal pattern of peripheral bone, and osteoid and central myofibroblasts, histiocytes, and blood vessels. In the early phase, prior to ossification, myositis ossificans simulates nodular fasciitis. Fibroosseous pseudotumor of the digits is a form of myositis ossificans, which occurs on fingers and toes and is more common in adults (124).

Fibrous umbilical polyp is a benign nodular proliferation of fibroblasts in the umbilical region of infants and may be a reactive lesion related to fasciitis (125).

Calcifying fibrous tumor is a hyalinized fibrous mass with scattered dystrophic and psammomatous calcifications and a patchy lymphocytic infiltrate with or without lymphoid aggregates (126,127).

Soft-tissue fibromas are a group of benign fibroblastic proliferations, which may occur sporadically or as a manifestation of a syndrome or genetic disorder (121). Superficial, hypocellular, abundantly collagenized fibrous masses can occur in patients with adenomatous polyposis coli/Gardner syndrome (Gardner fibroma), Proteus syndrome, tuberous sclerosis, and phenylketonuria (121). *Gardner fibroma* is particularly significant because of its association with desmoid-type fibromatosis and *APC* mutation and may be the sentinel event for recognition of an *APC* mutation in the child and the family (128,129). It consists of a diffuse patternless proliferation of coarse collagen fibers accompanied by inconspicuous bland spindle cells, with the collagen fibers separated by clear cracks. Entrapped normal tissues such as fat nerves and vessels with a sparse mast-cell infiltrate are typical. Fibroma of tendon sheath and desmoplastic

fibroblastoma may occur in children, but are much more common in adults.

The fibromatoses are the largest group of fibroblastic-myofibroblastic tumors in children and include a spectrum of lesions with or without the capacity for spontaneous regression or local recurrence (120,121,130).

Infantile myofibroma, or myofibromatosis, has been classified with fibromatoses in the past, but is now regarded as a lesion with a combination of myofibroblasts and myopericytes, which are specialized myofibroblasts located around blood vessels (121,131–133). There are two major clinical-prognostic groups. The poor prognostic group has visceral involvement, and the favorable group presents as either a solitary mass or multicentric masses in varying combinations of skin, subcutaneous tissue, deep soft tissue, and bone without visceral involvement (125,134–136). Solitary and multicentric myofibromas without visceral involvement are the most common subtypes. The nodular mass has a firm consistency and white or tan cut surface with variable red softening, central necrosis, hemorrhage, and cystic change. Calcifications frequently accompany zonal necrosis. Histologically, whorled bundles of spindle cells with eosinophilic cytoplasm and uniform oval nuclei are present (Figure 11.8). Some examples are partly or almost entirely composed of more immature-appearing hemangiopericytoma-like areas composed of primitive, round, or slightly elongated cells with scant cytoplasm and irregular thin-walled branching blood vessels. Such cases can display small foci of spindle cell differentiation at the periphery and often display peripheral satellite nodules that bulge into or fill adjacent blood vessels with both spindled and primitive rounded mesenchymal cells. The immunohistochemical profile includes reactivity for smooth muscle actin in the spindled, myofibroblastic cells, and endothelial reactivity for CD34 in the primitive hemangiopericytoma-like foci. Non-specific cytogenetic abnormalities involving chromosomes 6 and 8 have been reported, and cases with an autosomal dominant pattern of inheritance may be seen (137,138). Apoptosis is the proposed mechanism for spontaneous regression in both solitary and multicentric myofibromas, and occasional patients with visceral involvement may have a prolonged clinical course, with waxing and waning of lesions. Genetic studies on tumor tissue can be useful for the distinction of more cellular variants of myofibroma from infantile fibrosarcoma, which has a characteristic gene rearrangement (139).

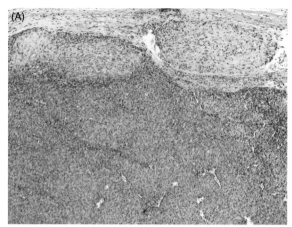

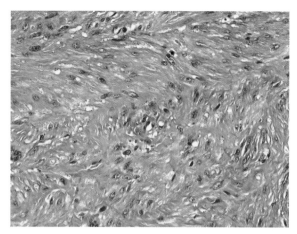

Figure 11.9 Inclusion-bearing fibromatosis consists of bland spindle cells with small round eosinophilic cytoplasmic inclusions in a collagenized background (H&E × 40).

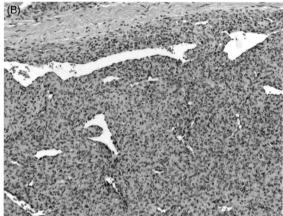

Figure 11.8 Myofibroma. (A) Sheets and fascicles of spindle cells focally bulge into vascular spaces and form a whorled pattern (H&E × 10). (B) An area with a hemangiopericytoma-like vascular pattern is composed of spindled, round, and polygonal primitive cells (H&E × 20).

Fibromatosis colli is a spontaneously regressing mass composed of fascicles of fibroblasts with focal hypercellularity, a collagenized stoma, and peripheral entrapment of skeletal muscle fibers (121).

Inclusion-bearing fibromatosis, also known as *infantile digital fibroma*, typically displays spindle cells with characteristic round eosinophilic cytoplasmic inclusions and most often occurs on the digits of infants and young children. Because of the recognition of histologically identical tumors in older patients and in locations away from the hands and feet, the preferred name is now inclusion-bearing fibromatosis. The firm superficial nodule has a fibrous cut surface. Bland fibroblasts form whorled bundles, fascicles, or storiform sheets with an abundantly collagenized stroma (121,140–142). The small round eosinophilic cytoplasmic inclusions may be difficult to identify, but are highlighted by the Masson trichrome or phosphotungstic acid hematoxylin stain. With time, fibrosis increases and inclusions become sparse to non-existent. With immunohistochemistry, the tumor cells express smooth-muscle actin, calponin, and desmin (Figure 11.9).

Fibrous hamartoma of infancy presents at birth or within the first two years of life as a poorly circumscribed mass in superficial soft tissue (121,143,144). The characteristic triphasic organoid histologic pattern consists of immature, myxoid, or basophilic mesenchymal tissue composed of primitive, small, or stellate cells arranged in sheets, whirls, and nests, mature bands of fibrous tissue, and mature adipose tissue without lipoblasts (Figure 11.10). The fibroblastic areas show immunoreactivity for smooth-muscle actin, and the mature adipose tissue stains for S100 protein, but the primitive mesenchymal cells are nonreactive for all markers except vimentin. Some cases show a prominent central or dominant area of abundant collagen and pseudoangiectoid spaces lined by angulated or multilobulated cells, and these areas typically stain for CD34. Identification of the triphasic organoid pattern at the periphery of the lesion aids in diagnosis. Translocations have been reported in rare cases (121,145).

Calcifying aponeurotic fibroma, or *juvenile aponeurotic fibroma*, has a predilection for the distal extremities (121,146). In the early stages, it contains cartilage intermingled with bands and sheets of bland fibrous tissue. Cellularity varies and may be high in lesions occurring in young children. With maturation, the immature cartilaginous foci give way to granular

363

(A)

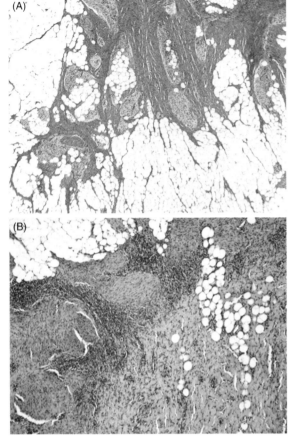

(B)

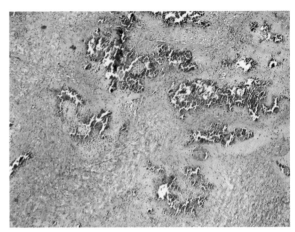

Figure 11.11 Calcifying aponeurotic fibroma characteristically displays granular areas of calcification surrounded by a bland proliferation of spindle cells in a collagenized background; some myxoid areas have a chondroid appearance (H&E × 10).

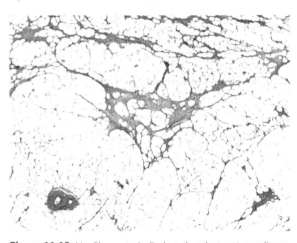

Figure 11.10 Fibrous hamartoma of infancy. (A) The classic triphasic organoid architecture is composed of fascicles of fibroblastic cells, mature adipose tissue, and immature myxoid mesenchymal tissue (H&E × 10). (B). The mesenchymal tissue in this case has a more basophilic appearance, and collagenized areas with a pseudoangiectoid clefting pattern are present (H&E × 20).

Figure 11.12 Lipofibromatosis displays abundant mature adipose tissue traversed by variably thick or delicate bundles of mature fibrous tissue with a focal interlacing architecture (H&E × 10).

calcifications or necrobiotic areas surrounded by plump epithelioid fibroblasts and multinucleated giant cells. With further maturation, the cellular fibroblastic component diminishes, and the mass becomes hypocellular and calcified, with only occasional fascicles of spindled fibroblasts (Figure 11.11). Rare cases have developed fibrosarcoma.

Lipofibromatosis is an uncommon neoplasm of fibroblasts and mature adipose tissue with a high likelihood of local recurrence (121,147–149). Sheets of mature adipose tissue are traversed by well-defined fascicles of fibroblasts with variable myxoid change and collagen in the background. The spindle cells display immunoreactivity for smooth-muscle actin. Rare cases contain pigmented cells, which express melanocytic markers such as S100 protein, HMB45, Melan-A, and tyrosinase. A single case with a complex translocation has been reported (150;

Figure 11.12). The recurrence rate of 75% may reflect persistent growth following incomplete excision, because the margins of the lesion are difficult to identify (121,147). Some authors consider lipofibromatosis to be a form of infantile fibromatosis.

Juvenile nasopharyngeal fibroma (angiofibroma) occurs in the posterior nasal cavity of adolescent males and presents with nosebleeds and nasal obstruction. The firm, spongy, gray tumor shows focal areas of hemorrhage. The fibrous and myxoid stroma with bland spindled fibroblasts contains numerous evenly arranged, irregularly shaped blood vessels without atypia. Chromosomal gains or deletions may be seen, and nasopharyngeal angiofibroma may be associated with *APC* mutations (151).

(A)

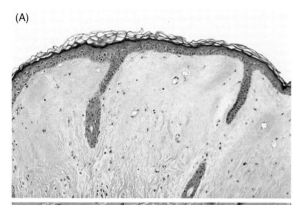

(B)

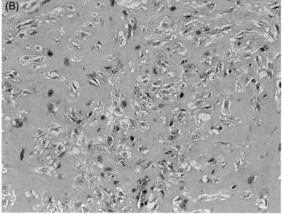

Figure 11.13 Juvenile hyaline fibromatosis. (A) The dermis contains a nodular proliferation of cells in an abundant hyaline eosinophilic matrix (H&E × 10). (B) Plump and elongated spindle cells are embedded in the eosinophilic matrix (H&E × 40).

Juvenile and infantile hyaline fibromatosis result from mutations in the *capillary morphogenesis gene 2 (CMG2)* and represent variants of the same disorder with different presentations based on age of onset. The nodular proliferation of elongated spindle cells in fascicles and cords is embedded in an abundant eosinophilic matrix with occasional calcospherites (121,152,153; Figure 11.13).

Palmar and plantar fibromatoses are usually considered adult fibromatoses, but palmar fibromatosis in particular can occur in young patients and has an autosomal dominance inheritance pattern (121,154,155). In the early phase, plump myofibroblasts and fibroblasts form nodules and cellular fascicles with a basophilic matrix. As the lesion matures, it becomes less cellular, and fusiform fibroblasts are arranged in parallel bundles with a central area of hemorrhage. In the end phase, the lesion is hypocellular and densely collagenized. The recurrence rate is greater than 80%.

Desmoid-type fibromatosis accounts for up to 60% of fibrous tumors in childhood, and up to 30% of childhood desmoids occur in the first year of life (120,121,156,157). Risk factors include *APC* mutation, Gardner fibroma, trauma, irradiation, and prior surgery. It involves superficial or deep soft tissue and, in children, is most frequently located on the extremities and trunk. Although it may appear to be well-circumscribed, bundles of fibrous tissue radiate into surrounding soft tissue as extensions of the tumor and are difficult to recognize surgically at the time of excision or at frozen section. Histologically, the uniform spindle cells are arranged in long fascicles or sheets with parallel thin-walled vessels aligned along the fascicles. The stroma is focally or diffusely collagenized or myxoid with scattered mucoid microcysts. The tumor cells are bland, and the mitotic rate is usually low, although it has no bearing on recurrence risk. A sparse mast-cell infiltrate is present (Figure 11.14). With immunohistochemistry, the tumor cells show variable combinations of reactivity for smooth-muscle actin, muscle-specific actin, and desmin, but no reactivity for CD34. Nuclear β-catenin positivity is seen in most but not all desmoids (158). Genetically, desmoids harbor mutations of *APC* and *β-catenin* and may have trisomies of chromosomes 8 and 20. Some data suggest that a specific *β-catenin* mutation, *CTNNB1-45F*, indicates a higher risk of local recurrence (159,160). Evaluation of surgical margins is important because of the tendency for recurrence. Postirradiation fibrosarcoma has been reported in patients whose desmoids were treated with radiation therapy (161).

Fibroblastic-myofibroblastic tumors with a very low risk of metastasis include inflammatory myofibroblastic tumor (IMT), infantile fibrosarcoma, primitive myxoid mesenchymal tumor of infancy, solitary fibrous tumor, giant-cell fibroblastoma, dermatofibrosarcoma protuberans, and other rare entities.

Inflammatory myofibroblastic tumor (IMT) is a neoplasm composed of spindle cells accompanied by a lymphoplasmacytic inflammatory infiltrate with variable eosinophils. More than half have an *ALK* gene rearrangement with a variety of fusion partners (121,162–164). Although the age range is wide, IMT is most frequent in the first three decades of life and occurs most often in the abdominal cavity, pelvis, retroperitoneum, and thoracic cavity. Some are accompanied by a syndrome of fever, weight loss, malaise, anemia, thrombocytosis, and polyclonal hyperglobulinemia. The circumscribed or multinodular mass has a

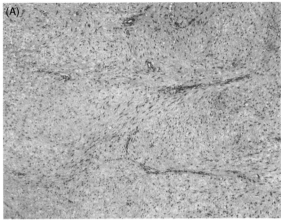

Figure 11.15 Inflammatory myofibroblastic tumor is composed of spindled and plump polygonal ganglion-like cells accompanied by a lymphoplasmacytic inflammatory infiltrate and occasional eosinophils (H&E × 20).

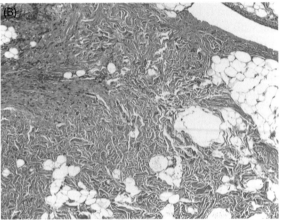

Figure 11.14 Desmoid-type fibromatosis. (A) Sweeping fascicles of bland spindle cells are separated by delicate elongated blood vessels (H&E × 10). (B) Desmoid fibromatosis in the top left portion of the figure merges with an area of Gardner fibroma characterized by formless sheets of coarse collagen fibers separated by clear cracks and entrapping benign adipose tissue (H&E × 20).

fleshy and myxoid texture. The myofibroblastic proliferation displays several morphologic patterns with varying degrees of cellularity, inflammation, and a myxoid or collagenized stroma. The most characteristic histologic pattern consists of compact cellular bundles or sheets of spindled and plump polygonal ganglion-like myofibroblasts accompanied by abundant plasma cells with fewer eosinophils and lymphocytes. The myxoid-vascular pattern displays more widely dispersed spindled and ganglion-like cells in an abundant myxoid stroma with small blood vessels. The collagenized pattern contains abundant collagen with sparse spindle and inflammatory cells and occasional calcifications (Figure 11.15). Some cases, especially those with the *ALK-RANBP2* gene rearrangement, are composed of round or polygonal epithelioid cells with vesicular

nuclei, prominent nucleoli, and eosinophilic cytoplasm (165,166). Immunohistochemistry demonstrates variable reactivity for smooth-muscle actin, muscle-specific actin, and desmin, and up to one-third also shows focal reactivity for cytokeratin (162,163). The *ALK* gene on chromosome 2p23 is associated with immunohistochemical reactivity for ALK protein in a cytoplasmic pattern. Extrapulmonary IMT has a 25% recurrence rate, and metastasis occurs in less than 2% of patients. The frequency of metastasis appears to be greater in ALK-negative IMT (162).

Infantile fibrosarcoma is a rarely metastasizing neoplasm that affects infants and children less than two years of age and characteristically harbors an *ETV6-NTRK3* gene fusion (121,167–169) in addition to a variety of extra chromosomes. The primitive cellular tumor is composed of spindle, polygonal, and round cells in varying proportions, with zonal necrosis and a prominent hemangiopericytoma-like vascular pattern in some areas. Mitoses are not prognostically significant. Collagen bundles, extramedullary hematopoiesis, and chronic inflammation may be seen. The immunohistochemical profile is nonspecific (Figure 11.16). The histologic and cytogenetic features are similar to cellular congenital mesoblastic nephroma.

Giant-cell fibroblastoma and *dermatofibrosarcoma protuberans* share similar biologic potential and cytogenetic abnormalities, and some cases display combined histologic features (170–172). Consequently they can be considered a single entity with a clinical

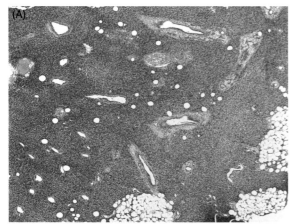

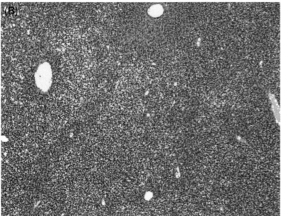

Figure 11.16 Infantile fibrosarcoma. (A) The tumor is composed of sheets and sweeping fascicles of primitive cells with a focal hemangiopericytoma-like vascular pattern and infiltration of adjacent benign adipose tissue (H&E × 10). (B) The tumor cells form sheets and vague fascicles, and range from round to polygonal to spindled (H&E × 20).

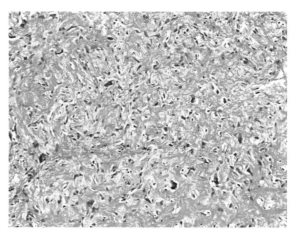

Figure 11.17 Giant-cell fibroblastoma displays abundant collagen in the background, with clear clefts lined by spindled cells and cells with a multilobulated or multinucleated appearance (H&E × 20).

and morphologic spectrum (173,174). Both can present as congenital tumors. Giant-cell fibroblastoma is a plaque-like or nodular mass with a tan cut surface and infiltrative margins. Spindled, plump, and multinucleated cells are dispersed in a collagenized or myxoid background with clefted sinusoidal spaces lined by the tumor cells. The stroma contains patchy chronic inflammation and mast cells (Figure 11.17). Strands of tumor cells infiltrate and entrap adjacent non-neoplastic tissues in the dermis, subcutaneous tissue, and skeletal muscle. The overlying epidermis may be hyperplastic. In some cases, more compact cellular areas merge with storiform bundles of dermatofibrosarcoma protuberans. In contrast to giant-cell fibroblastoma, dermatofibrosarcoma protuberans characteristically has a storiform pattern with uniform

spindle cells, variable stromal fibrosis and myxoid change, and honeycomb-like infiltration of subcutaneous adipose tissue (175–179). Myoid nodules are an unusual morphologic variant and are composed of nodules and bundles of smooth-muscle actin-positive perivascular smooth-muscle cells. The tumor may also display palisading and Verocay-like bodies that simulate a nerve-sheath tumor. The rare *Bednar tumor variant* contains pigmented cells. Both giant-cell fibroblastoma and dermatofibrosarcoma protuberans display immunohistochemical reactivity for CD34 (170,180). Factor 13A may be present and is typically focal in giant-cell fibroblastoma and diffuse in dermatofibrosarcoma protuberans. Both tumors harbor t(17;22)(q22;q13), a *COL1A1-PDGFB* fusion gene, with a balanced or unbalanced t(17;12)(q22;q13), or a supernumerary ring chromosome (181,182). Combined pattern tumors have the same tendency for local recurrence (181). Recurrent giant-cell fibroblastoma can display a pattern of dermatofibrosarcoma protuberans with or without the original features of giant-cell fibroblastoma; this is most easily identified at the periphery of the mass. A subset also develops foci of fibrosarcoma (183). Recurrence is less likely if giant-cell fibroblastoma and dermatofibrosarcoma protuberans are excised with clear surgical margins (184,185).

Other locally recurrent, rarely metastasizing fibroblastic-myofibroblastic tumors that can occur in childhood include primitive myxoid mesenchymal tumor of infancy (186), solitary fibrous tumor (187,188), and myxoinflammatory fibroblastic sarcoma (121,189).

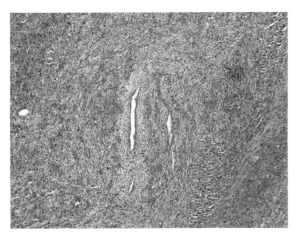

Figure 11.18 Low-grade fibromyxoid sarcoma displays variable myxoid and collagenized areas with swirling fascicles of spindle cells and curving blood vessels (H&E × 10).

Among the fibroblastic-myofibroblastic sarcomas, low-grade fibromyxoid sarcoma and myofibrosarcoma occur more often in young patients than other fibrosarcoma subtypes, although all are rare (121). *Low-grade fibromyxoid sarcoma* arises in superficial or deep soft tissue, and in children it has a predilection for the superficial soft tissues of the head and neck (190). The nodular mass has several histologic patterns with varying combinations in individual cases. Characteristically, a biphasic proliferation of fibrous collagenized spindle cells blends with loose myxoid areas containing uniform spindle cells with swirling fascicles or storiform bundles with arcading vessels (Figure 11.18). The variant of hyalinizing spindle-cell tumor with giant collagen rosettes displays eosinophilic collagen aggregates surrounded by concentric spindled and epithelioid cells. Immunohistochemistry demonstrates reactivity for MUC4 and epithelial membrane antigen (191,192). A recurrent translocation involving the *FUS* gene is characteristic, and most cases harbor a *FUS-CREB3L2* gene fusion (191,193). *Myofibrosarcoma* in children has a predilection for the head and neck and tends to be low grade (194,195). The circumscribed, focally infiltrative mass consists of fascicles or sheets of spindle cells with mild atypia, variable mitoses, and rare necrosis. The tumor cells are reactive for smooth-muscle actin and calponin. *Infantile rhabdomyofibrosarcoma* is an exceedingly rare tumor with aggressive clinical behavior and overlapping morphologic features with infantile fibrosarcoma and rhabdomyosarcoma (196,197).

Fibrohistiocytic tumors

Fibrohistiocytic tumors encompass a heterogenous group of cutaneous, subcutaneous, and deep soft-tissue masses, many of which are benign or have a tendency for local recurrence and very low likelihood of metastasis (170,198,199). The cellular constituents include fibroblasts, myofibroblasts, histiocytes, and a variety of other inflammatory cells. *Benign fibrous histiocytoma* is the prototypic lesion, and it is relatively common, although much more frequent in adults, occurring in the superficial and deep soft tissues, with a number of histologic variants. The dermal benign fibrous histiocytoma (dermatofibroma), cellular fibrous histiocytoma, and deep fibrous histiocytoma are the most likely of these to be encountered in children (200,201). *Dermatofibroma* presents as a solitary or clustered group of papules or nodules with slow growth on the extremity or trunk. Spindled fibroblastic and myofibroblastic cells intermingle with histiocytes, hemosiderin-laden macrophages, multinucleated giant cells, and plasma cells form a nodule with a pushing border. A focal storiform architecture may be present. The lesional cells are immunoreactive for CD68, factor 13A, and D2–40 (202). CD34 positivity may be seen at the periphery or advancing border, but is not present centrally within dermatofibroma. In later stages, a fibrotic dermatofibroma mimics a scar or fibromatosis. *Cellular fibrous histiocytoma* is a more monomorphic or storiform hypercellular fibroblastic lesion with an arborizing vascular background with an immunohistochemical profile similar to benign fibrous histiocytoma and a higher risk of local recurrence (203). *Deep fibrous histiocytoma* occurs in soft tissue throughout the body and has histologic features similar to benign or cellular fibrous histiocytoma and also can display a focal hemangiopericytoma-like pattern (204). The immunohistochemical profile is similar to other types of fibrous histiocytoma. Deep fibrous histiocytoma can recur locally or rarely metastasizes to regional or distant locations.

Tenosynovial giant-cell tumor includes both the localized nodular giant-cell tumor of tendon sheath (nodular tenosynovitis) and diffusely infiltrative giant-cell tumor (16,170,205,206). Tenosynovial giant-cell tumor is subdivided according to its location in soft tissues or synovium, and its growth pattern as a localized or diffuse mass. The diffuse form is more likely to recur. When it occurs in the joint space, tenosynovial giant-cell tumor is also known as pigmented

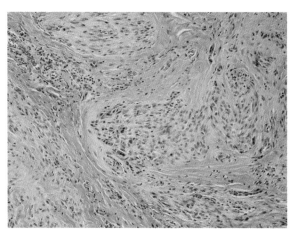

Figure 11.19 Plexiform fibrohistiocytic tumor is composed of nodules of mononuclear histiocytes intermingled with giant cells and separated by bundles of fibrous tissue with abundant collagen (H&E × 40).

villonodular synovitis (207). Histologically round and polygonal epithelioid mononuclear cells form sheets or lobules and are accompanied by lipid or hemosiderin-laden macrophages, multinucleated osteoclast-like giant cells, fibroblasts, and lymphocytes. The diffusely infiltrative subtype may display chondroid metaplasia. Immunohistochemistry demonstrates reactivity for CD68, CD163, CD145, and clusterin (16,205,208,209). A subpopulation of cells may be reactive for desmin and D2–40. Cytogenetically, tenosynovial giant-cell tumor harbors a chromosomal rearrangement of 1p21-p13 with a translocation involving the *CSF1* gene (210).

Locally recurring and rarely metastasizing fibrohistiocytic tumors with a predilection for children and adolescents include plexiform fibrohistiocytic tumor; atypical fibroxanthoma and giant-cell tumor of soft tissue are very rare in young patients.

Plexiform fibrohistiocytic tumor is a poorly circumscribed dermal or subcutaneous tumor with a predilection for the shoulder or arm, although it can occur anywhere on the body (211). Histologic subtypes include fibrohistiocytic, fibroblastic, and mixed forms. The fibrohistiocytic variant is composed of nodules of mononuclear histiocytes and multinucleated cells separated by fascicles of fibrous tissue (Figure 11.19). The fibroblast-predominant form is composed of bundles of spindle cells intermingled with plexiform nodules or clusters of histiocytes, which may be accompanied by osteoclast-like giant cells and chronic inflammation. The mixed type

demonstrates both patterns. The histiocytes in plexiform fibrohistiocytic tumor are polygonal to oval with fine chromatin and occasional nucleoli. Both the histiocytes and multinucleated giant cells are CD68 positive, and the spindle fibroblasts demonstrate reactivity for smooth-muscle actin. The lesion may also express D2–40.

Malignant fibrous histiocytoma, now known as *undifferentiated pleomorphic sarcoma*, is relatively uncommon in children and adolescents (72,170,212). In some cases, it may be a pleomorphic form of fibrosarcoma or other defined type of sarcoma, and immunohistochemistry is critical in the distinction from pleomorphic rhabdomyosarcoma, pleomorphic liposarcoma, dedifferentiated liposarcoma, leiomyosarcoma, malignant peripheral nerve-sheath tumor, and myxofibrosarcoma (170,212,213). When these possibilities are excluded, undifferentiated pleomorphic sarcoma accounts for much less than 5% of soft-tissue sarcomas in children. The outcome seems to be better in young patients, and approximately 20% recur or metastasize following complete excision (212).

Histiocytic and dendritic neoplasms may contain spindle cells intermingled with histiocytes and other inflammatory cells and thus resemble fibrohistiocytic tumors. Langerhans-cell histiocytosis, juvenile xanthogranuloma, follicular dendritic-cell neoplasms, interdigitating dendritic-cell tumor, dendritic-cell sarcoma, and histiocytic sarcoma are distinguished by a combination of clinicopathologic and immunohistochemical features (170). *Juvenile xanthogranuloma*, a non-Langerhans cell histiocytic- and dendritic-cell proliferation, is most common in young children, and up to 75% are diagnosed before one year of age, including congenital cases. Solitary lesions are much more common than multifocal or systemic juvenile xanthogranuloma. Sites include skin, soft tissue including the skeletal muscle, and rarely organs or the cranial cavity (170,214–217). The cut surface is characteristically yellow or reddish brown. Early juvenile xanthogranuloma may display a predominance of foamy or xanthomatized cells, with or without a storiform architecture. The classic histology displays sheets of mononuclear histiocytes accompanied by multinucleated giant cells, including Touton cells with a peripheral wreath of nuclei, vacuolated xanthomatized cells, and an inflammatory infiltrate of eosinophils and lymphocytes (215,218,219; Figure 11.20). Mitoses and atypia vary and have no prognostic significance. In the late phase, spindled fibroblastic cells are prominent.

369

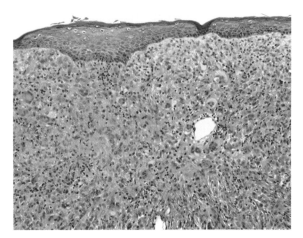

Figure 11.20 Juvenile xanthogranuloma forms a nodule composed of histiocytes, variable lymphocytic, and eosinophilic inflammation, and vacuolated xanthomatized cells (H&E × 40).

With immunohistochemistry, the lesion expresses CD68 and factor 13A, but not CD1a, and S100 protein reactivity is variable.

Peripheral-nerve and other neurogenic tumors

Peripheral-nerve and other neurogenic tumors are an important group of soft-tissue neoplasms in children and adolescents, with relatively frequent familial, genetic, and syndromic implications (220–223). A variety of reactive, hamartomatous, and malformative lesions also form masses; traumatic neuroma, neuromuscular choristoma (hamartoma), neural lipofibroma (perineural lipoma), heterotopic meningeal nodules, and heterotopic neuroglial tissue have been reviewed in detail elsewhere (220). While they can originate in or involve soft tissue, neoplasms such as melanotic neuroectodermal tumor of infancy, neuroblastoma, paraganglioma, myxopapillary ependymoma, and unusual mesenchymal proliferations that arise in congenital melanocytic nevi are not generally classified among soft-tissue tumors, and are not covered in further detail here. The extended family of Ewing's sarcoma and other tumors with an *EWS* gene rearrangement are covered in a separate section.

Neurofibroma is the most common nerve-sheath tumor in children and adolescents and may be solitary, multiple, or plexiform (220,224,225). The latter two subtypes signify a high likelihood of neurofibromatosis type 1, an autosomal dominant disorder that affects 1 in 3500 individuals (226–230). Diffuse and plexiform neurofibromas can involve the dermis, subcutaneous tissue, or deep soft tissue (231,232). Plexiform neurofibromas can manifest before five years of age and may be congenital and multiple, while cutaneous neurofibromas tend to appear later in childhood and adolescence (226,230). Neurofibromas are composed of Schwann cells accompanied by CD34-positive fibroblasts, perineurial cells, and mast cells. Diffuse neurofibroma displays a monotonous proliferation of fusiform spindle cells with wavy nuclei and inconspicuous cytoplasm, in a pale myxoid background with coarse collagen fibers. *Diffuse neurofibroma* expands the dermis and extends into subcutaneous tissue. *Plexiform neurofibroma* consists of similar nodules of spindle cells demarcated by fibrous tissue and may accompany a diffuse neurofibroma. The associated peripheral nerves in plexiform neurofibroma may be thickened or multinodular. Mitotic figures, hypercellularity, and nuclear enlargement and hyperchromasia in neurofibroma are harbingers of transformation to malignant peripheral nerve-sheath tumor. Immunoreactivity for p53 may be useful in the further recognition of malignant peripheral nerve sheath tumor arising in the background of neurofibroma (233,234). Cellular atypia in the absence of mitoses is associated with *CDKN2A/B* gene deletion, which supports the concept of atypical neurofibroma as a premalignant lesion. With immunohistochemistry, neurofibroma is reactive for S100 protein, CD34, SOX10, collagen type 4, and neurofilament, but their presence to varying degrees in other nerve-sheath tumors such as schwannoma and malignant peripheral nerve-sheath tumor limits diagnostic utility (220,221).

Schwannoma is a benign neoplasm that is sporadic or associated with neurofibromatosis type 2 (220,221,235). The cutaneous or soft-tissue mass is well-circumscribed and encapsulated, with variable hemorrhage, fibrosis, and cystic change. The spindle cells form two basic patterns. Fusiform cellular foci, with or without parallel bundles of nuclei or Verocay bodies, define the Antoni A pattern. Myxoid, less-cellular areas define the Antoni B pattern. Mast cells, lymphocytes, and aggregates of foamy histiocytes may be seen. Mitoses have no diagnostic or prognostic significance. Variants include cellular, multinodular, plexiform, and melanotic schwannoma (220,221,236,237). Immunohistochemical stains in schwannoma demonstrate strong diffuse reactivity for S100 protein; calretinin expression may be useful

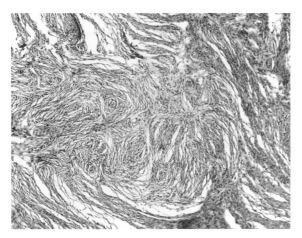

Figure 11.21 Perineurioma displays whirls and storiform bundles of spindle cells in a fibromyxoid background (H&E × 10).

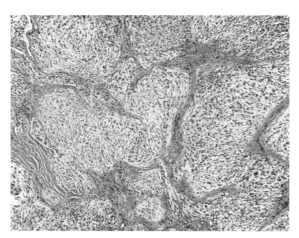

Figure 11.22 Neurothekeoma displays nodules of spindled and epithelioid cells in a myxoid background (H&E × 20).

in the distinction from malignant peripheral nerve-sheath tumor and neurofibroma (238). Schwannomas may also be positive for CD57, glial fibrillary acidic protein, and AE1/AE3 cytokeratin.

Schwannomatosis consists of multiple schwanno-mas in the absence of vestibular nerve involvement (239). It can be familial and associated with mutations in *SMARCB1* and *NF2* (240, 241). Some have patchy loss of nuclear expression of INI-1 protein and may also be associated with familial malignant rhabdoid tumor (242).

Other benign peripheral nerve-sheath tumors that can affect young patients include perineurioma, neu-rothekeoma, and nerve-sheath myxoma. *Intraneural perineurioma* is more frequent in children than extra-neural, which is typically found in adults (220,221,243–246). Spindle or epithelioid cells form whorls and storiform bundles in a fibrous background; the intraneural perineurioma originates in a nerve and may have a plexiform appearance (Figure 11.21). Sclerosing perineurioma displays strands or cords of spindled or epithelioid cells in a collagenized stroma (247). Immunoreactivity for epithelial membrane antigen, claudin 1, GLUT-1, and CD34 are present, but S100 protein is absent. Rare cases are associated with neurofibromatosis type 1, neurofibromatosis type 2, and Beckwith–Wiedemann syndrome (248–250). Tumors with hybrid features of schwannoma and perineurioma can occur in children (251). *Nerve-sheath myxoma* is a superficial solitary or multinodu-lar mass in the dermis and consists of cords and nests of epithelioid schwannian cells in an abundant myxoid matrix, surrounded by a fibrous border. The lesion is

reactive for S100 protein, glial fibrillary acidic protein, and CD57 (252). *Neurothekeoma* involves skin or mucosa and has cellular, myxoid, and mixed subtypes, with nodules of spindled and epithelioid cells, and multinucleated osteoclast-like giant cells in a variably myxoid background (220,253–255; Figure 11.22). Neurothekeomas are immunoreactive for NKI-C3, neuron-specific enolase, CD10, and CD68, but not for S100 protein (254).

Granular cell tumors of neural origin, which are S100-positive, are uncommon in children (220) and are distinct from the S100-negative congenital epulis (256) and the dermal non-neural granular-cell tumor (257). The S100-positive *granular-cell tumor* is a small, poorly circumscribed plaque or nodule composed of uniform, large, pale, polygonal, or spindle cells with granular cytoplasm, round uniform dark nuclei, in a dense stroma. Mitoses, necrosis, and atypia are usually absent. Granular cell tumors may contain multi-nucleated cells and peripheral lymphoid aggregates, and the plexiform perineural granular-cell tumor is a morphologic variant. In addition to positivity for S100 protein, reactivity is variable for CD56, CD57, myelin basic protein, and other nerve-sheath markers (220,258).

Malignant peripheral nerve-sheath tumor (MPNST) is one of the more frequent non-rhabdomyosarcomatous soft-tissue sarcomas in chil-dren and adolescents, and up to 20% are diagnosed in the first two decades of life, mostly in later childhood and adolescence, either sporadically or in association with neurofibromatosis type 1 (8,72,259,260). Several series have focused on the clinicopathologic features of

371

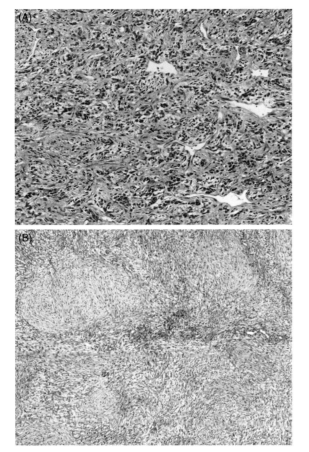

Figure 11.23 Malignant peripheral nerve-sheath tumor. (A) High-grade peripheral nerve-sheath tumor is composed of a cellular proliferation of atypical polygonal and spindle cells with a whirling pattern and hemangiopericytoma-like blood vessels (H&E × 20). (B) Low-grade malignant peripheral nerve-sheath tumor displays lower cellularity and less atypia (H&E × 20).

elongated or wavy nuclei, and occasional nuclear pseudoinclusions. Variations include a storiform or herringbone pattern, whorling, and perivascular condensations of tumor cells (Figure 11.23). Although spindle cells are most characteristic, epithelioid, round, and rhabdoid cells may be encountered. There is a capacity for heterologous differentiation with rhabdomyosarcomatous, chondrosarcomatous, osteosarcomatous, or primitive neuroectodermal tumor-like elements, as well as glandular epithelial differentiation. Epithelioid MPNST is not associated with NF1, but can arise within a pre-existing schwannoma (269). The immunohistochemical profile is variable, with reactivity in up to 50% of cases for S100 protein, which is generally weak and focal, except in epithelioid MPNST, and CD57; occasionally other markers are identified (220). The expression of p53 protein appears to be a poor prognostic indicator, as well as a marker of malignant transformation in plexiform neurofibroma with evolution to MPNST (234,270). *MDM2* amplification occurs in a subset of cases (271). Cytogenetic and molecular genetic studies have demonstrated aneuploidy with a variety of cytogenetic and molecular abnormalities (272,273). Evaluation of margins is critical for the pathologic workup, since involvement of resection margins is a poor prognostic indicator. Although MPNST may be graded using either the Pediatric Oncology Group or FNCLCC grading systems, there is controversy as to whether this is useful and whether all MPNSTs should simply be regarded as high-grade malignancies (29,220,274). Better-defined prognostic indicators include anatomic site, tumor size, and extensive necrosis.

Gastrointestinal stromal tumor in childhood

Although relatively common among adult mesenchymal tumors, gastrointestinal stromal tumor (GIST) is rare in children and adolescents, with a mean age of 13 years in pediatric series (275–282). Most lack *CKIT* or *PDGFRA* mutations (283). In young patients, GIST may be associated with tumor syndromes such as neurofibromatosis type 1, Carney triad, and Carney–Stratakis dyad. Gastrointestinal stromal tumor in the young has a predilection for females, and more than 80% occur in the stomach, are often multifocal, and metastasize to lymph nodes. Histologic types include spindle, epithelioid, and mixed-cell variants, with a predominance of epithelioid GIST in children

MPNST in childhood (261–266). It is important to remember that children with neurofibromatosis type 1 have an increased risk of other sarcomas, especially embryonal rhabdomyosarcoma (267,268). The soft-tissue mass may be associated with a large nerve or a pre-existing neurofibroma and is usually greater than 5 cm in diameter, although smaller tumors have been reported (220,221). The cut surface is myxoid or firm, with or without hemorrhage and necrosis. When MPNST arises within a plexiform neurofibroma or in a patient with neurofibromatosis type 1, it may have a multinodular appearance with multifocal involvement of a nerve or a plexiform neurofibroma. Histologically, fascicles of spindle cells are dispersed in a myxoid background or packed together closely. The tumor cells have indistinct cytoplasm, hyperchromatic and

(284,285). The tumors center on the myenteric plexus and may be associated with hyperplasia of interstitial cells of Cajal. Immunohistochemistry reveals reactivity for CD117 (KIT) in 71% of pediatric GIST. CD117-negative GIST is positive for DOG1 (ANO1) (286). CD34 and smooth-muscle actin reactivity may be present, and S100 protein and desmin are rarely expressed. Gastrointestinal stromal tumor associated with the Carney triad and the Carney–Stratakis dyad are CD117-negative and lack expression of mitochondrial protein succinate dehydrogenase (SDHB) (287–290). Histologic-prognostic criteria used in adult GIST are not reliable in young patients. Even GIST with a low proliferative index or mitotic rate, small size, or other low-risk features may metastasize in children and adolescents.

Adipocytic tumors

Although frequent in adults, the circumscribed *solitary lipoma* is rare in childhood, and various overgrowths of adipose tissue or lipomatoses as a manifestation of a syndrome, developmental abnormality, or malformation are more frequent (291). Lipoblastoma with maturation is another mimic of lipoma in young patients. The intraspinal "lipoma," or lumbosacral lipoma, is typically associated with a neural-tube defect (292), and perineural lipoma is associated with macrodactyly. Both the classic lipoma and the lipomatoses are composed of mature adipocytes. Lipomas in children, as well as in adults, display a constellation of morphologic subtypes based on the presence of tissues other than fat, the most common of which is *angiolipoma*, with abundant small blood vessels. *Hibernoma*, a benign tumor of brown-fat origin, is also rare in young patients and may be associated with neural-tube defects, Turner syndrome, and pheochromocytoma. The combination of round cells with granular eosinophilic and vacuolated cytoplasm, multivacuolated lipoblasts, and mature fat, is characteristic for hibernoma, which also has a cytogenetic abnormality at 11q13 (293).

Lipoblastoma is the prototypical fatty neoplasm of childhood and is closely related to embryonic white fat (291,294,295). More than 90% are diagnosed before the age of three years, although the age range extends into and beyond adolescence. The circumscribed or infiltrative mass can exceed 15 cm, and the most frequent sites are the trunk and extremities. Some patients with lipoblastoma have associated developmental delay or other developmental abnormalities, seizures, or malformations (294,296). Histologically,

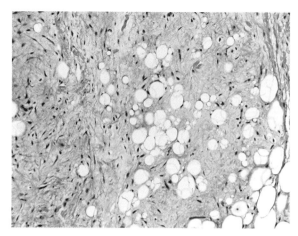

Figure 11.24 Lipoblastoma displays lobules of primitive spindle mesenchymal cells in a myxoid background, multivacuolated lipoblasts, small signet-ring-shaped lipoblasts, and mature adipocytes (H&E × 40).

lipoblastoma has a characteristic lobular architecture with well-demarcated lobules of hypocellular myxoid and adipose tissue separated by bands of collagenized fibrous tissue. The lobules contain a combination of primitive mesenchymal cells in a myxoid stroma, accompanied by delicate plexiform blood vessels in the myxoid areas, multivacuolated lipoblasts, signet-ring cells, and mature adipocytes. Multinucleated floret cells and sparse mast cells are frequently seen. The myxoid material may form diffuse sheets, cystic spaces, or pools. There is no cellular atypia, and mitoses are unusual (Figure 11.24). With immunohistochemistry, lipoblastomas typically display reactivity for S100 protein and CD34, and recently PLAG1 protein has been demonstrated (294,297). The primitive mesenchymal cells in myxoid areas express desmin. Many lipoblastomas have a rearrangement or amplification of the *PLAG1* oncogene at chromosome 8q11–13 (298,299). Lipoblastoma can undergo spontaneous maturation, and the most extensively differentiated examples resemble ordinary lipoma or fibrolipoma and may be distinguishable only by detection of the *PLAG1* abnormalities or histologically by a residual lobular architecture or small foci of myxoid differentiation. The local recurrence rate of up to 50% is probably due to incomplete excision (294).

Liposarcoma accounts for less than 3% of soft-tissue sarcomas in children and adolescents (199,291). More than 90% occur in the second decade, and most of these are myxoid liposarcomas with a variable hypercellular component (300–303). The soft multilobulated mass has a myxoid matrix with a delicate branching vascular network similar to the myxoid foci in lipoblastoma.

However, *myxoid liposarcoma* lacks a well-defined lobular architecture. The tumor is composed of a combination of primitive spindle cells, monovacuolated signet-ring cells, multivacuolated lipoblasts, and scattered mature adipocytes. The myxoid material may form small cysts or pools. Mitoses are present, but the mitotic rate is typically low, and nuclear atypia is mild. Hypercellular areas consist of closely packed cells with scant cytoplasm and overlapping nuclei; this round cell is very rare in childhood myxoid liposarcoma. Myxoid liposarcoma has a characteristic translocation, t(12;16) (q13;p11) with a *FUS-DDIT3* gene fusion and can also have a variant translocation with a *DDIT3-EWSR1* gene fusion (304).

Two distinct variants of liposarcoma with a myxoid component have a predilection for childhood. The *spindle-myxoid liposarcoma* contains areas of classic myxoid liposarcoma intermingled with well-defined fascicles of spindle cells (302). The *pleomorphic-myxoid liposarcoma* contains areas identical to myxoid liposarcoma plus a pleomorphic neoplasm with increased cellularity, large pleomorphic and hyperchromatic lipoblasts, undifferentiated tumor cells, atypical mitoses, and necrosis. The pleomorphic-myxoid subtype is highly aggressive and has a predilection for the mediastinum. Both myxoid-spindle-cell and myxoid-pleomorphic liposarcoma lack the rearrangements of classic myxoid liposarcoma.

Other conventional subtypes also occur rarely in young patients, including well-differentiated liposarcoma, dedifferentiated liposarcoma, and pleomorphic liposarcoma, the last of which may be associated with Li– Fraumeni syndrome (302,305,306). Cytogenetics is useful in distinguishing among the different types of adipose tumors, regardless of age (307,308).

Extraskeletal osseous, cartilaginous, and chordoid tumors

Cartilage-forming, bone-forming, and chordoid tumors are rare in the soft tissues of children, with the possible exception of soft-tissue chondroma (309–311). The hands and the feet are the most frequent sites for soft-tissue chondroma, although pulmonary chondroma may occur in children with Carney triad. Familial multiple cutaneous chondromas have also been reported. The well-circumscribed nodule is usually less than 3 cm and consists of lobules of mature cartilage surrounded by fibrous tissue. Histologic variations include hypercellularity, nuclear

hyperchromasia, binucleation, occasional mitoses, ossification, mineralization, myxoid change, an infiltrate of macrophages, and multinucleated osteoclast-like giant cells. Occasional soft-tissue chondromas have an abnormality on chromosome 12q13–15, with disruption of the *HMGA2* gene (312).

Extraskeletal chondrosarcoma is rare at any age. Extraskeletal myxoid chondrosarcoma is discussed below in the section on tumors of uncertain differentiation. *Extraskeletal mesenchymal chondrosarcoma* has a predilection for the first three decades of life and may be congenital. It typically arises in the lower extremity, head and neck, and central nervous system (309,313–316). The fleshy tumor may contain grossly visible or microscopically detectable chondroid nodules with or without mineralization and ossification. Sheets of undifferentiated round and spindle cells form a highly cellular tumor with a hemangiopericytoma-like vascular pattern (Figure 11.25). The well-differentiated cartilaginous nodules are irregularly dispersed within the neoplasm and are S100-positive; they may not be present on a small biopsy. Demonstration of immunohistochemical reactivity for SOX-9 may be useful in distinguishing mesenchymal chondrosarcoma from other spindle-cell sarcomas, except for synovial sarcoma. CD57, CD99, and Bcl-2-expression are frequent, but not specific (317–319). Several cases of extraskeletal mesenchymal chondrosarcoma with a cytogenetic abnormality have been reported.

Extraskeletal osteosarcoma is exceptionally rare in childhood, and the pathologic findings are identical to the osseous counterpart (320,321). It can occur as a second malignant neoplasm or in association with hereditary retinoblastoma.

Chordoma is rare in children and even rarer as an extraosseous soft-tissue neoplasm (322). Sites include the sacrococcygeal region and buttocks (323,324). In young children, chordoma may be associated with the tuberous sclerosis complex (325). Histologic types in soft tissue are similar to those in bone, including conventional chordoma with a lobular architecture, abundant myxoid matrix, and characteristic physaliferous cells, chondroid chordoma with a varying chondroid matrix, and atypical or poorly differentiated chordoma with hypercellularity, atypia, and frequent mitoses. Dedifferentiated chordoma is a high-grade spindle cell sarcoma (322,323; Figure 11.26). T-brachyury expression is a sensitive and specific immunohistochemical marker for chordoma (324); cytokeratin, epithelial membrane antigen, and S100 protein are frequently

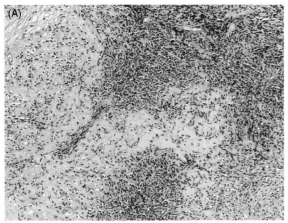

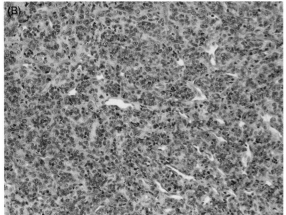

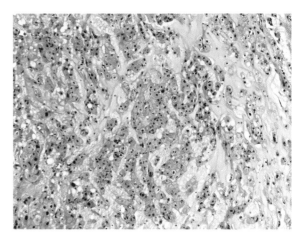

Figure 11.26 Chordoma is composed of nests and cords of large epithelioid multivacuolated cells with round nuclei in a myxoid background (H&E × 20).

Figure 11.25 Mesenchymal chondrosarcoma. (A) Well-differentiated cartilaginous nodules are separated by a primitive highly cellular proliferation of atypical cells (H&E × 20). (B) The primitive cells may be round and have a prominent hemangiopericytoma-like appearance, which may be the dominant component in extraskeletal mesenchymal chondrosarcoma (H&E × 40).

expressed, and nuclear INI-1 protein expression may be lost (322,326). Proliferative activity with Ki-67 does not predict outcome (322). Young children and infants with atypical chordoma seem to have an increased rate of recurrence and metastasis, and a decreased survival compared to older patients (322,323). Benign notochordal cell tumor, which typically occurs in bone, and notochordal vestiges, which typically occur in intervertebral discs, are histologic mimics and potential precursor legions (327).

Mesenchymal tumors with *EWS* gene rearrangements

The extended family of tumors with *EWS* gene rearrangements includes ES, desmoplastic small round-cell tumor, clear-cell sarcoma of soft parts,

extraskeletal myxoid chondrosarcoma, angiomatoid fibrohistiocytoma, extraskeletal mesenchymal chondrosarcoma, and myoepithelioma. In addition, a variety of "Ewing-like" sarcomas have recently been reported with novel translocations that do not involve the *EWS* gene, although the tumors share similar histologic and immunohistochemical profiles, and responses to ES treatment protocols. The extended family of *EWS*-related tumors is summarized in Table 11.5 (275,328–330).

Ewing's sarcoma/primitive neuroectodermal tumor (ES/PNET), although rare, is one of the more common soft-tissue sarcomas in children and adolescents, and 20 to 40% originate in soft tissue, especially in the trunk and extremities, but also in the head and neck, retroperitoneum, and solid organs; ES may also be superficial or disseminated without an obvious primary site at the initial presentation (331). Although most extraosseous ES occur in adolescence or later, some arise in early childhood, some occur as a second malignant neoplasm, and rare cases are familial (332). There is a male predilection, and ES is rare in the African-American population. The white or tan focally hemorrhagic or necrotic mass may be circumscribed or multinodular and infiltrative. Histologically, classic ES displays formless sheets and lobules of uniform, round, and oval cells, with fine chromatin and small nucleoli, scant, clear, or amphophilic cytoplasm, and variable mitoses. The aggregates or lobules of cells may be surrounded by bands of fibrous tissue. In some cases, the tumor cells form

375

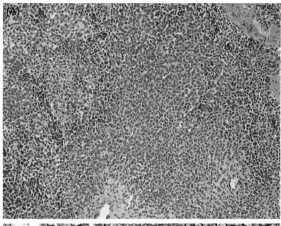

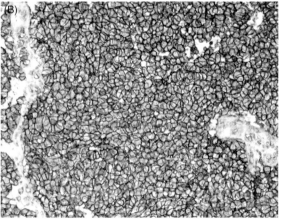

Figure 11.27 Ewing's sarcoma/PNET. (A) Sheets of primitive round cells are the classic appearance of Ewing's sarcoma (H&E × 10). (B) Diffuse membranous positivity for CD99 is characteristic (immunohistochemistry, × 40).

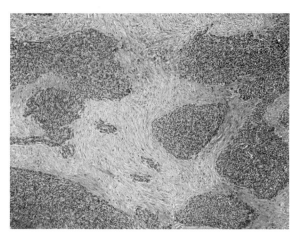

Figure 11.28 Desmoplastic small-cell tumor displays a geographic pattern of irregular nests of primitive round tumor cells separated by broad bands of densely collagenized fibrous tissue (H&E × 20).

Table 11.3) and can be detected with FISH or reverse transcriptase polymerase chain reaction, as well as by conventional cytogenetics (337). Many other genetic changes have been reported in ES and do not have diagnostic utility, although *p53* mutation and *p16* alterations, including *CDKN2A* deletion, appear to be poor prognostic indicators. Fli1 nuclear protein is expressed, especially in cases with an *EWS-Fli1* gene fusion, but lacks specificity (338–340).

Desmoplastic small round-cell tumor is an aggressive neoplasm with a predilection for body cavities, viscera, and soft tissue (341–344). It has overlapping histologic, immunohistochemical, and cytogenetic and molecular genetic features with ES, and also has a male predilection. Multifocal masses simulate implants, and a dominant solitary tumor is unusual. Histologically, nests and large lobules of cells are demarcated by a dense fibrous stroma in a geographic pattern. The tumor cells are round or ovoid with angulated nuclei, scant cytoplasm, and occasional rhabdoid or signet-ring morphology. Rare tumors show focal gland formation, trabecular profiles, or formless sheets of cells without an abundant stroma (Figure 11.28). Polyphenotypic immunohistochemical expression of cytokeratins, epithelial membrane antigen, desmin, and CD57 are typical. CD99 displays a diffuse membranous pattern in up to half of desmoplastic small round-cell tumors. WT1 is also positive when antibodies directed toward the carboxy-terminus of the protein are used. The characteristic genetic abnormality is a translocation t(11;22) (p13;q12) with an *EWSR1-WT1* gene fusion, found in more than 90% of cases. Variant translocations have also

rosettes. Histologic variations include filigree, atypical or large-cell, adamantinoma-like, pseudovascular, pelioid or sclerosing variants (333,334). Following treatment, ES typically shows extensive necrosis and can display rare ganglion-like cells or develop an alveolar pattern with tumor cells arranged around spaces and accompanied by fibrosis and hemosiderin-laden macrophages (335). Immunohistochemistry is useful to support the diagnosis and to exclude other round-cell neoplasms, with reactivity in ES for CD99, synaptophysin, and occasionally S100 protein and cytokeratin. The CD99 pattern is typically diffuse and membranous (Figure 11.27). Cytokeratins either displays a dot-like or membranous cytoplasmic pattern. Muscle markers are seldom expressed (336), and, if present, should prompt consideration of rhabdomyosarcoma or ectomesenchymoma. The translocations associated with ES involve the *EWS* gene on chromosome 22 (see been reported. FISH and RT-PCR are useful to support the diagnosis.

Clear-cell sarcoma of tendons and aponeuroses occurs on the distal extremities and in other sites (345–348). The firm white-gray mass can reach a large size. Uniform fascicles and nests of spindled or epithelioid cells have pale or eosinophilic cytoplasm and round nuclei with prominent nucleoli. The cytoplasm contains melanin in less than half of cases. Morphologic variants include myxoid, clear, and rhabdoid cells, nuclear pseudoinclusions, and multinucleated giant cells. Immunohistochemically, expression of S100 protein, HMB45, micro-ophthalmia transcription factor, and melanin are characteristic. The translocation t(12;22)(q13;q12) generates an *EWSR1-ATF1* gene fusion in about 75% of clear-cell sarcomas, and a variant translocation with an *EWSR1-CREB1* fusion has been reported (349,350). So-called "clear-cell sarcoma" of the gastrointestinal tract in very young children has some similarities with clear-cell sarcoma of tendons and aponeuroses, but tends to have less expression of melanocytic markers and more frequently displays the *EWSR1-CREB1* gene fusion (351). Whether it is a variant of soft-tissue clear-cell sarcoma or a unique entity has not been resolved.

Extraskeletal myxoid chondrosarcoma is rare in children and is a round-cell tumor with a myxoid background and without cartilage (352–355). There are no characteristic immunophenotypic changes, and the immunohistochemical profile is variable. Up to 75% harbor a translocation t(9;17)(q22;q11) with an *EWSR1-NR4A3* gene fusion, although other cytogenetic abnormalities have been reported (356).

Angiomatoid fibrous histiocytoma originates most often in the extremities, especially in the dermis or subcutaneous tissue, but may also arise in deep soft tissue or within organs, such as the lung. It may be associated with B-type symptoms (170,357,358). Grossly, the mass may resemble a lymph node, and hemorrhage may be visible on the cut surface. Histologically, angiomatoid fibrous histiocytoma is surrounded by a fibrous pseudocapsule accompanied by an infiltrate of lymphocytes and plasma cells, with or without focal lymphoid nodules. Centrally, compact, uniform, ovoid, or spindle cells with rounded nuclei and variable mitoses form sheets and may contain angiomatoid blood-filled spaces, hemosiderin-laden macrophages, nuclear pleomorphism, and nuclear atypia (Figure 11.29). The mitotic rate varies and has no prognostic significance. Reactivity for

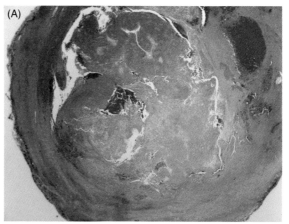

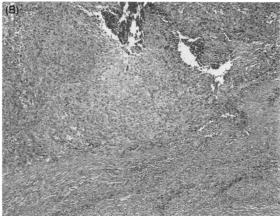

Figure 11.29 Angiomatoid fibrous histiocytoma. (A) The tumor nodule is surrounded by a fibrous pseudocapsule with lymphoplasmacytic inflammation and a central proliferation of compact cells with irregular blood-filled spaces (H &E × 40). (B) The tumor cells are closely packed and blood-filled spaces lack an endothelial lining (H&E × 20).

CD68 is typical, but non-specific, and up to 50% of cases also have reactivity for desmin and CD99, but do not express other muscle or myofibroblastic markers. Angiomatoid fibrous histiocytoma has a variety of translocations involving the, *FUS* and *ATF1* genes. The most common translocation is t(2;22) (q33, q12) with an EWSR1-CREB1 fusion. The t(12;16) (q13; q11) with FUS-ATF, or t(12;22) (q13;q12) with EWSRI-ATF1 are rarer (359–361).

Recently, several groups of *"Ewing-like sarcomas"* with unique translocations, round-cell morphology, and variable CD99 immunohistochemical reactivity, have been described. One group is characterized by a *CIC-DUX4* translocation and is currently treated on Ewing's sarcoma protocols (362,363). Another group

377

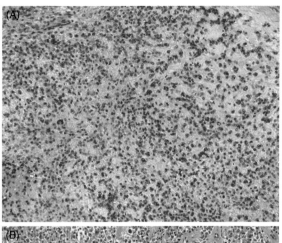

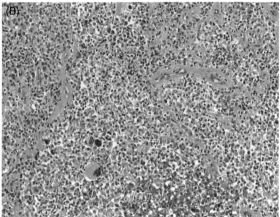

Figure 11.30 Myoepithelioma. (A) Epithelioid and round cells are embedded in a myxoid background (H&E × 20). (B) In myoepithelial carcinoma, the tumor cells are more pleomorphic with large hyperchromatic tumor cells and occasional prominent nucleoli (H&E × 40).

mainly involves bone and is characterized by a *BCOR-CCNB3* gene fusion (330).

Myoepithelial neoplasms, including myoepithelioma and myoepithelial carcinoma, are poorly differentiated tumors with myoepithelial cell differentiation, and approximately 20% occur in patients less than 20 years of age (364–366). The extremities are the most common location, although other sites may be affected. Histologically, a lobulated or reticulated proliferation of epithelioid, round, and spindle cells occurs in a myxoid or hyaline background. Variations include solid, trabecular, nodular, myxoid, pseudoglandular, and reticulated patterns, and round, stellate, clear, plasmacytoid, spindled, rhabdoid, or oncocytic cytomorphology (Figure 11.30). The term myoepithelial carcinoma refers to tumors in which aggressive behavior is

anticipated, based on the presence of large pleomorphic nuclei, prominent nucleoli, and an increased nuclear-to-cytoplasmic ratio. With immunohistochemistry, myoepitheliomas are reactive for keratins, p63, epithelial membrane antigen, S100 protein, glial fibrillary acidic protein, calponin, smooth-muscle actin, and desmin in various combinations. The genetic changes are variable, but a significant subset have translocations involving the *EWSR1* gene with various partners, including *POU5F1*, *ZNF444*, *PBX1*, and other unidentified fusion genes (367). Some other cases also have loss of SMARCB1/INI1 protein.

Other mesenchymal tumors of uncertain differentiation

The prototypical spindle-cell sarcoma of uncertain differentiation in children and adolescents is *synovial sarcoma*, which represents the most common non-rhabdomyosarcomatous soft-tissue sarcoma in children and adolescents (275,368–370). Synovial sarcoma has a wide range of biologic behavior and histopathologic features. Although it increases in frequency during the second decade, younger children and even infants may be affected. A few studies have addressed synovial sarcoma in children and adolescents in some detail, and approximately 15 to 30% occur in the first two decades of life. The painless mass has a predilection for soft tissue around large joints, especially the knee and ankle, but it can also occur in soft tissue throughout the body, in body cavities, in solid organs, or in the dermis. Minute tumors less than 1 cm in diameter occasionally arise on the distal extremities (371). The tumor may be extensively calcified in rare cases. Histologically, biphasic or monophasic patterns are encountered. A variegated proliferation of hypercellular and hypocellular zones is seen with epithelioid and spindle-cell foci in biphasic synovial sarcoma. The epithelioid areas form primitive glands, solid clusters, or papillary structures with a whirling or stranding architecture. The spindle-cell foci in monophasic synovial sarcoma consist of uniform elongated spindle cells arranged in fascicles and with a widely variable mitotic rate. Calcifying synovial sarcoma contains massive stromal calcifications and mitochondrial calcifications in addition to occasional metaplastic ossification, and this variant appears to have a more favorable prognosis. Poorly differentiated synovial sarcoma includes a round-cell proliferation resembling ES rhabdoid

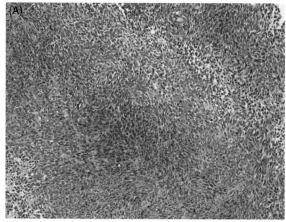

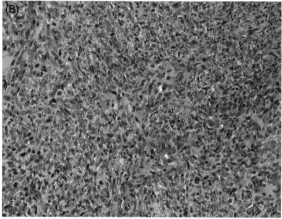

Figure 11.31 (A) Synovial sarcoma is composed of sheets and fascicles of spindled and plump cells with focal epithelioid clusters and rare primitive gland-like structures (H&E × 20). (B) Monophasic synovial sarcoma may consist of primitive round cells that resemble Ewing's sarcoma (H &E × 40).

cells, or plump tumor cells with prominent nuclear atypia. In the absence of an epithelial component, a swirling or lobular architectural pattern, hemangiopericytoma-like vasculature, keloidal collagen bundles, myxoid zones, and small calcifications point toward a diagnosis of synovial sarcoma. Following chemotherapy, some synovial sarcomas display more prominent glandular differentiation than in the primary tumor (Figure 11.31). The immunohistochemical profile includes expression of cytokeratins and epithelial membrane antigen. Although Bcl-2 expression is non-specific, it typically shows a diffuse, sharply membranous pattern of staining. Many other markers may be expressed by synovial sarcoma, including CD57, CD99 with a membranous pattern, CD56, neurofilament, S100 protein, and actins. Nuclear TLE1 is a sensitive marker that may not be entirely specific, although the TLE1 protein may reflect the presence of a translocation (372). Synovial sarcoma nearly always has a balanced reciprocal translocation t(X;18) with fusion of the *SYT* and *SSX* genes (373). There is a correlation between the translocation subtype and the histology in that epithelial differentiation in biphasic synovial sarcoma is more frequently associated with the *SYT-SSX1* fusion and monophasic histologic features with *SYT-SSX2*. However, there are exceptions in both directions. Pathologic prognostic indicators for synovial sarcoma include tumor diameter greater than 5 cm, mitotic rate greater than five per ten high-power fields, and high grade (374,375). Younger patients have a more favorable prognosis.

Other spindle-cell tumors of uncertain origin, such as ossifying fibromyxoid tumor of soft parts, are rare in children and adolescents, and its existence has been questioned for patients younger than ten years of age.

Sarcomas with an epithelioid morphologic pattern and uncertain histogenesis include alveolar soft-part sarcoma, epithelioid sarcoma, and perivascular epithelioid cell neoplasms. *Alveolar soft-part sarcoma* is typically a tumor of adolescence and early adulthood, with a mass in skeletal muscle or deep soft tissue (376–379). Organoid clusters of tumor cells are separated by thin bands of fibrous tissue or form diffuse sheets with only a focal nesting pattern. Histologic variations include a glomeruloid arrangement of tumor cells and focal necrosis and calcification. Although the nuclei are usually bland, occasional cases have hyperchromatic nuclei with pleomorphism and frequent mitoses. The cytoplasm contains PAS-positive, diastase-resistant crystalline material that represents accumulation of monocarboxylate transporter 1 and CD147 (Figure 11.32). Alveolar soft-part sarcoma has an unbalanced translocation der (17)(X;17)(p11;q25) with fusion of the *TFE3* gene to the *ASPL* gene or a variant fusion, accompanied by overexpression of the TFE3 protein (380–383). Careful pathologic evaluation of the surgical resection margins is important because of the risk of late metastases to lung, lymph nodes, brain, bone, and liver.

Epithelioid sarcoma accounts for less than 10% of non-rhabdomyosarcomas in children, with males more often affected than females (384–387). The painless dermal or subcutaneous nodule arises on the extremities, head and neck, or genital region. Single or multiple tumor nodules are composed of large polygonal cells with eosinophilic cytoplasm that merge with more elongated spindle cells and may

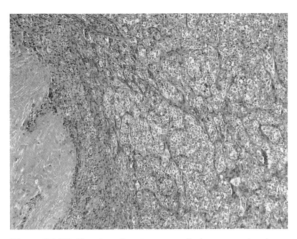

Figure 11.32 Alveolar soft-part sarcoma displays a prominent nesting pattern of plump polygonal cells with pale eosinophilic cytoplasm and uniform round nuclei (H&E × 20).

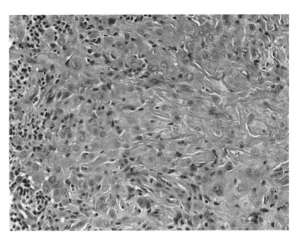

Figure 11.33 Epithelioid sarcoma is composed of large plump cells with round nuclei, prominent nucleoli, and abundant pale to eosinophilic cytoplasm with variable mitoses (H&E × 40).

display central necrosis and calcification. Although some cases have cellular pleomorphism, in most the tumor cells are bland. Discohesive areas filled with blood mimic a vascular tumor. In the proximal type of epithelioid sarcoma, large polygonal cells have pleomorphic nuclei, rhabdoid cytology, frequent necrosis, and mitoses (Figure 11.33). Both classic and proximal epithelioid sarcomas display immunohistochemical reactivity for cytokeratins, epithelial membrane antigen, and vimentin. Loss of nuclear INI-1 protein is detected in up to 90% of cases, although *SMARC1/INI1* gene alterations are less frequent than in malignant rhabdoid tumor (388, 389). *NUT*-rearranged carcinoma may be a differential diagnostic consideration for a high-grade, clinically aggressive neoplasm with epithelioid morphology.

Malignant rhabdoid tumor in soft tissue occurs mainly in deep sites, including the extremities, head and neck, abdominal cavity, retroperitoneum, and trunk. It can also present solitary or multiple skin lesions. Between 20 and 85% of cases are metastatic at initial diagnosis. Congenital disseminated malignant rhabdoid tumor can occur in the absence of an identical primary neoplasm (390). Soft-tissue rhabdoid tumor is sometimes associated with central nervous system rhabdoid tumor or with other malignancies in syndromes such as the familial rhabdoid predisposition syndrome, Goldenhar syndrome, and Phelan–McDermid syndrome. Classic rhabdoid tumor consists of sheets or trabeculae of round or polygonal cells, with large round nuclei, fine chromatin, a prominent eosinophilic nucleolus, and abundant eosinophilic cytoplasm with a perinuclear cytoplasmic

globule (Figure 11.34). Primitive undifferentiated cells with a subtle rim of cytoplasm may also predominate and mimic Ewing's sarcoma or other round-cell malignancies (391). The immunohistochemical profile is polyphenotypic, with staining for vimentin, keratin, epithelial membrane antigen, S100 protein, CD99, synaptophysin, smooth-muscle actin, and muscle-specific actin in varying proportions of cases. Loss of nuclear INI-1 protein is observed in most but not all malignant rhabdoid tumors. Cytogenetically, either germline mutation or biallelic inactivation of the *SMARCB1* gene on chromosome 22q11.2 is present in nearly all malignant rhabdoid tumors (392,393). Absence of the nuclear INI-1 protein may be detected by immunohistochemistry, but is not completely diagnostic of rhabdoid tumor because of its loss in other tumors with rhabdoid morphology, particularly epithelioid sarcoma, schwannomas, familial schwannomatosis, extraskeletal myxoid chondrosarcoma, myoepithelioma, and rare cases of poorly differentiated synovial sarcoma (388,394–397). Recently a series of undifferentiated sarcomas with deletion or mutation of the *SMARCB1* gene and absence of the typical rhabdoid morphology was reported. INI-1-negative small-cell hepatoblastomas reported in the past are now regarded as hepatic malignant rhabdoid tumor. Rare INI-1-positive rhabdoid tumors may harbor other genetic alterations.

Perivascular epithelioid cell tumor or PEComa consists of a group of neoplasms composed of epithelioid or spindle cells with clear-to-eosinophilic cytoplasm and a characteristic arrangement around blood vessels. These are very rare in children and have been summarized in recent reviews (275).

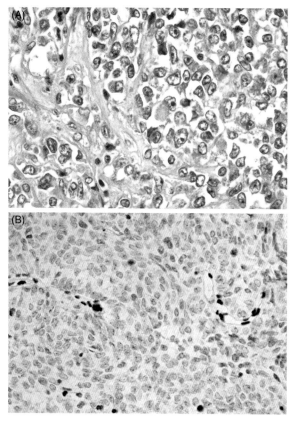

Figure 11.34 Malignant rhabdoid tumor. (A) The tumor cells form sheets and have round nuclei with prominent eosinophilic nucleoli and variable amounts of globular eosinophilic cytoplasm (H&E × 20). (B) An immunohistochemical stain for INI1 shows loss of nuclear INI1 protein expression in the tumor cells of malignant rhabdoid tumor and preservation of expression in non-neoplastic endothelial and stromal cells (immunohistochemistry, × 40).

Myxoid lesions are relatively uncommon in children, except for embryonal and botryoid rhabdomyosarcoma and myxoid variants of other well-defined types of sarcomas such as myxoid synovial sarcoma, low-grade fibromyxoid sarcoma, myxofibrosarcoma, and myxoid liposarcoma (291,398). Myxoma of soft tissue or skeletal muscle is rare, but may be found in children with the Carney complex or fibrous dysplasia. Aggressive angiomyxoma and superficial angiomyxoma rarely affect children and adolescents (399,400).

Although many tumors are classifiable at this point in time with a combination of light microscopy, immunohistochemistry, ultrastructural analysis, and molecular and cytogenetic tests, a substantial proportion of sarcomas in children and adolescents continue to be unclassifiable beyond "undifferentiated sarcoma," "sarcoma not otherwise specified," or "undifferentiated malignant neoplasm" (212,401–405). The recent reports of Ewing-like round cell sarcomas with *SMARCB1* aberrations, *CIC-DUX4* translocations, and *BCOR-CCNB3* gene rearrangements indicate that advances in morphologic-genetic classifications will aid in recognition of new and possibly unique entities (330,362,363,406).

Summary

Tremendous progress in classification, diagnosis, and treatment of soft-tissue tumors has taken place in recent decades, although challenges and opportunities remain for now and well into the future. Classification systems continue to evolve, with increasing integration of morphologic, cytogenetic, and molecular genetic information. Newer modalities on the frontiers of sarcoma include proteomics, lipomics, metabolomics, and epigenetics, and the role of inflammation in neoplasia, and how environmental and individual biologic factors affect the capacity for a child or adolescents to develop a tumor and respond to treatment remain largely unexplored. The next several decades will be an interesting time as old and new challenges are addressed and as efforts are made to improve clinical outcomes.

References

1. Coffin CM, Alaggio R, Dehner LP. Some general considerations about the clinicopathologic aspects of soft tissue tumors in children and adolescents. Pediatr. Dev. Pathol. 2012;**15**:11–25.

2. Siegel R, Naishadham D, Jemal A. Cancer statistics, 2012. CA Cancer J. Clin. 2012;**62**:10–29.

3. Howlader N, Noone AM, Krapcho M, *et al.*, editors. *SEER Cancer Statistics Review, 1975–2008*. Bethesda, MD: National Cancer Institute;2011.

4. Smith MA, Gurney JG, Gloeckler Ries LA. Cancer among adolescents 15–19 years old. In: Ries LAG, Smith MA, Gurney JG, *et al.*, editors, *Cancer Incidence and Survival Among Children and Adolescents: United States SEER Program, 1975–1995*, National Cancer Institute, SEER Program. NIH Pub. No.99–4649. Bethesda: National Institutes of Health; 1999;157–64.

5. Sultan I, Casanova M, Al-Jumaily U, *et al.* Soft tissue sarcomas in the first year of life. Eur. J. Cancer 2010;**46**:2449–56.

6. Spunt SL, Skapek SX, Coffin CM. Pediatric nonrhabdomyosarcoma soft tissue sarcomas. Oncologist 2008;**13**:668–78.

7. Harms D. Soft tissue sarcomas in the Kiel Pediatric Tumor Registry. Curr. Top. Pathol. 1995;**89**:31–45.

381

8. Hayes-Jordan AA, Spunt SL, Poquette CA, *et al.* Nonrhabdomyosarcoma soft tissue sarcomas in children: is age at diagnosis an important variable? J. Pediatr. Surg. 2000;**35**:948–53.

9. Spunt SL, Hill DA, Motosue AM, *et al.* Clinical features and outcome of initially unresected nonmetastatic pediatric nonrhabdomyosarcoma soft tissue sarcoma. J. Clin. Oncol. 2002;**20**:3225–35.

10. Ferrari A, Casanova M, Collini P, *et al.* Adult-type soft tissue sarcomas in pediatric-age patients: experience at the Istituto Nazionale Tumori in Milan. J. Clin. Oncol. 2005;**23**:4021–30.

11. Spunt SL, Pappo AS. Childhood nonrhabdomyosarcoma soft tissue sarcomas are not adult-type tumors. J. Clin. Oncol. 2006;**24**(12):1958–9; author reply 1959–60.

12. Parham DM, Alaggio R, Coffin CM. Myogenic tumors in children and adolescents. Pediatr. Dev. Pathol. 2012;**15**(1):211–38.

13. Fletcher CDM, Bridge JA, Hogendoorn P, Mertens F, editors. *Classification of Tumours of Soft Tissue and Bones. WHO Classification of tumours*, Volume **5**, Lyon: IARC Press; 2013.

14. Coffin CM, Dehner LP. Pathologic evaluation of pediatric soft tissue tumors. Am. J. Clin. Pathol. 1998;**109**:S38–52.

15. Rubin BP, Fletcher CDM, Inwards C, *et al.* Protocol for the examination of specimens from patients with soft tissue tumors if intermediate malignant potential, malignant soft tissue tumors, and benign/locally aggressive and malignant bone tumors. Arch. Pathol. Lab. Med. 2006;**130**:1616–29.

16. Rubin BP, Goldblum JR. Pathology of soft tissue sarcoma. J. Natl. Comp. Cancer Net. 2007;**5**:411–8.

17. Carpentieri DF, Qualman SJ, Bowen J, *et al.* Protocol for the examination of specimens from pediatric and adult patients with osseous and extraosseous Ewing sarcoma family of tumors, including peripheral primitive neuroectodermal tumor and Ewing sarcoma. Arch. Pathol. Lab. Med. 2005;**129**:866–73.

18. Qualman SJ, Bowen J, Parham DM, *et al.* Protocol for the examination of specimens from patients (children and young adults) with rhabdomyosarcoma. Arch. Pathol. Lab. Med. 2003;**127**:1290–7.

19. Goodlad JR, Fletcher CD, Smith MA. Surgical resection of primary soft tissue sarcoma. Incidence of residual tumor in 95 patients needing re-excision after local resection. J. Bone Joint Surg. Br. 1996;**78**:658–61.

20. Slater O, Shipley J. Clinical relevance of molecular genetics to pediatric sarcomas. J. Clin. Pathol. 2007;**60**:1187–94.

21. Bridge JA, Cushman-Vokoun AM. Molecular diagnostics of soft tissue tumors. Arch. Pathol. Lab. Med. 2011;**135**:588–601.

22. Romeo S, Dei Tos AP. Soft tissue tumors associated with EWSR1 translocation. Virchows Arch. 2010;**456**:153–66.

23. Tanas MR, Goldblum JR. Fluorescence in situ hybridization in the diagnosis of soft tissue neoplasms: A review. Adv. Anat. Pathol. 2009;**16**:383–91.

24. Fisher C. Soft tissue sarcomas with non-*EWS* translocations: molecular genetic features and pathologic and clinical correlations. Virchows Arch. 2010;**456**:153–66.

25. Ordóñez JL, Osuna D, García-Domínguez DJ, *et al.* The clinical relevance of molecular genetics in soft tissue sarcomas. Adv. Anat. Pathol. 2010;**17**:162–81.

26. Nishio J, Iwasaki H, Nabeshima K, *et al.* Cytogenetics and molecular genetics of myxoid soft-tissue sarcomas. Genet. Res. Int. 2011;**2011**:497148.

27. Parham DM, Webber BL, Jenkins JJ III, *et al.* Nonrhabdomyosarcomatous soft tissue sarcomas of childhood: formulation of a simplified system for grading. Mod. Pathol. 1995;**8**:705–10.

28. Khoury JD, Coffin CM, Spunt SL, *et al.* Grading of nonrhabdomyosarcoma soft tissue sarcoma in children and adolescents: A comparison of parameters used for the Fédération Nationale des Centers de Lutte Contre le Cancer and Pediatric Oncology Group Systems. Cancer 2010;**116**:2266–74.

29. Coindre JM, Terrier P, Guillou L, *et al.* Predictive value of grade for metastasis development in the main histologic types of adult soft tissue sarcomas: A study of 1240 patients from the French Federation of Cancer Centers Sarcoma Group. Cancer 2001;**91**:1914–26.

30. Coffin CM, Lowichik A, Zhou H. Treatment effects in pediatric soft tissue and bone tumors: practical considerations for the pathologist. Am. J. Clin. Pathol. 2005;**123**:75–90.

31. Lucas DR, Kshirsagar MP, Biermann JS, *et al.* Histologic alterations from neoadjuvant chemotherapy in high-grade extremity soft tissue sarcoma: clinicopathologic correlation. Oncologist 2008;**13**:451–8.

32. Ferrari S, Bertoni F, Palmerini E, *et al.* Predictive factors of histologic response to primary chemotherapy in patients with Ewing sarcoma. J. Pediatr. Hematol. Oncol. 2007;**29**:364–8.

33. Bisogno G, Sotti G, Ferrari A, *et al.* Soft tissue sarcoma as a second malignant neoplasm in the pediatric age group. Cancer 2004;**100**:1758–65.

34. Merks JHM, Caron HN, Hennekam RCM. High incidence of malformation syndromes in a series of 1,073 children with cancer. Am. J. Med. Gen. 2005;**13A**:132–43.

35. Bruder E, Alaggio R, Kozakewich HP, *et al.* Vascular and perivascular lesions of skin and soft tissues in

children and adolescents. Pediatr. Dev. Pathol. 2012;**15**:26–61.

36. North PE, Waner M, Buckmiller L, *et al.* Vascular tumors of infancy and childhood: beyond capillary hemangioma. Cardiovasc. Pathol. 2006;**15**:303–17.

37. Mulliken JB. Classification of vascular birthmarks. In: Mulliken JB, Young AE, editors, *Vascular Birthmarks, Hemangiomas, and Malformations.* Philadelphia, PA: WB Saunders;1988:24–37.

38. North PE. Vascular tumors and malformations of infancy and childhood. Pathol. Case Rev. 2008;**13**:213–35.

39. Gupta A, Kozakewich H. Histopathology of vascular anomalies. Clin. Plast. Surg. 2011;**38**:31–44.

40. Coffin CM, Dehner LP. Soft tissue tumors in first year of life: A report of 190 cases. Pediatr. Pathol. 1990;**10**:509–26.

41. Coffin CM, Dehner LP. Vascular tumors in children and adolescents: A clinicopathologic study of 228 tumors in 222 patients. Pathol. Annu. 1993;**1**:97–120.

42. Coffin CM, Vanderhooft S. The conundrum of angiomatosis. Pathol. Case Rev. 2009;**14**:93–9.

43. Mulliken JB. Diagnosis and natural history of hemangioma. In: Mulliken JB, Young AE, editors, *Vascular Birthmarks, Hemangiomas, and Malformations.* Philadelphia, PA: WB Saunders;1988:41–62.

44. Perkins P, Weiss SW. Spindle cell hemangioendothelioma: An analysis of 78 cases with reassessment of its pathogenesis and biologic behavior. Am. J. Surg. Pathol. 1996;**20**:1196–204.

45. Rosai J, Gold J, Landy R. The histiocytoid hemangiomas: A unifying concept embracing several previously described entities of skin, soft tissue, large vessels, bone, and heart. Hum. Pathol. 1979;**10**:707–30.

46. Fetsch JF, Weiss SW. Observations concerning the pathogenesis of epithelioid hemangioma (angiolymphoid hyperplasia). Mod. Pathol. 1991;**4**:449–55.

47. Vargas SO, Perez-Atayde AR, González-Crussi F, *et al.* Giant cell angioblastoma: three additional occurrences of a distinct pathologic entity. Am. J. Surg. Pathol. 2001;**25**:185–96.

48. Lyons LL, North PE, Mac-Moune Lai F, *et al.* Kaposiform hemangioendothelioma: A study of 33 cases emphasizing its pathologic, immunophenotypic, and biologic uniqueness from juvenile hemangioma. Am. J. Surg. Pathol. 2004;**28**:559–68.

49. Enjolras O, Mulliken JB, Wassef M, *et al.* Residual lesions after Kasabach-Merritt phenomenon in 41 patients. J. Am. Acad. Dermatol. 2000;**42**:225–35.

50. Osio A, Fraitag S, Hadj-Rabia S, *et al.* Clinical spectrum of tufted angiomas in childhood. Arch. Dermatol. 2010;**146**:758–63.

51. Arai E, Kuramochi A, Tsuchida T, *et al.* Usefulness of D2–40 immunohistochemistry for differentiation between kaposiform hemangioendothelioma and tufted angioma. J. Cutan. Pathol. 2006;**33**:492–7.

52. Le Huu AR, Jokinen CH, Rubin BP, *et al.* Expression of PROX-1 lymphatic endothelial nuclear transcription factor in kaposiform hemangioendothelioma and tufted angioma. Am. J. Surg. Pathol. 2010;**34**:1563–73.

53. Fanburg-Smith JC, Michal M, Partanen TA, *et al.* Papillary intralymphatic angioendothelioma (PILA): A report of twelve cases of a distinctive vascular tumor with phenotypic features of lymphatic vessels. Am. J. Surg. Pathol. 1999;**23**:1004–10.

54. Mentzel T, Beham A, Calonje E, *et al.* Epithelioid hemangioendothelioma of skin and soft tissues: clinicopathologic and immunohistochemical study of 30 cases. Am. J. Surg. Pathol. 1997;**21**:363–74.

55. Deyrup AT, Miettinen M, North PE, *et al.* Angiosarcomas arising in the viscera and soft tissue of children and young adults. Am. J. Surg. Pathol. 2009;**33**:264–9.

56. Deyrup AT, Miettinen M, North PE, *et al.* Pediatric cutaneous angiosarcomas: A clinicopathologic study of 10 cases. Am. J. Surg. Pathol. 2011;**35**:70–5.

57. Cairncross LL, Davidson A, Millar AJ, *et al.* Kaposi sarcoma in children with HIV: A clinical series from Red Cross Children's Hospital. J. Pediatr. Surg. 2009;**44**:373–6.

58. Arkin LM, Cox CM, Kovarik CL. Kaposi's sarcoma in the pediatric population: the critical need for a tissue diagnosis. Pediatr. Infect. Dis. J. 2009;**28**:426–8.

59. Wada DA, Perkins SL, Tripp S, *et al.* Human herpesvirus 8 and iron staining are useful in differentiating Kaposi sarcoma from interstitial granuloma annulare. Am. J. Clin. Pathol. 2007;**127**:1–8.

60. Cheuk W, Wong KOY, Wong CSC, *et al.* Immunostaining for human herpesvirus 8: latent nuclear antigen-1 helps distinguish Kaposi sarcoma from its mimickers. Am. J. Clin. Pathol. 2004;**121**:335–42.

61. Gombos Z, Zhang PJ. Glomus tumor. Arch. Pathol. Lab. Med. 2008;**132**:1448–52.

62. Brouillard P, Ghassibé M, Penington A, *et al.* Four common *glomulin* mutations cause two thirds of glomuvenous malformations ('familial glomangiomas'): evidence for a founder effect. J. Med. Genet. 2005;**42**:e13.

63. Brouillard P, Vikkula M. Genetic causes of vascular malformations. Hum. Mol. Genet. 2007;**16**:R140–9.

64. Mentzel T, Dei Tos AP, Sapi Z, *et al.* Myopericytoma of skin and soft tissues: clinicopathologic and immunohistochemical study of 54 cases. Am. J. Surg. Pathol. 2006;**30**:104–13.

65. Dahlén A, Mertens F, Mandahl N, *et al.* Molecular genetic characterization of the genomic *ACTB-GLI* fusion in pericytoma with t(7;12). Biochem. Biophys. Res. Commun. 2004;**325**:1318–23.

66. Burke A, Virmani R. Pediatric heart tumors. Cardiovasc. Pathol. 2008;**17**(4):193–8.

67. Kapadia SB, Meis JM, Frisman DM, *et al.* Fetal rhabdomyoma of the head and neck: A clinicopathologic and immunophenotypic study of 24 cases. Hum. Pathol. 1993;**24**:754–65.

68. Walsh SN, Hurt MA. Cutaneous fetal rhabdomyoma: A case report and historical review of the literature. Am. J. Surg. Pathol. 2008;**32**:485–91.

69. Koutsimpelas D, Weber A, Lippert BM, *et al.* Multifocal adult rhabdomyoma of the head and neck: A cause report and literature review. Auris Nasus Larynx 2008;**35**:313–7.

70. Auerbach A, Fanburg-Smith JC, Wang G, *et al.* Focal myositis: A clinicopathologic study of 115 cases of an intramuscular mass-like reactive process. Am. J. Surg. Pathol. 2009;**33**:1016–24.

71. Gaeta M, Mazziotti S, Minutoli F, *et al.* MR imaging findings of focal myositis: A pseudotumor that may mimic muscle neoplasm. Skeletal Radiol. 2009;**38**(6):571–8.

72. Harms D. Soft tissue malignancies in childhood and adolescence. Pathology and clinical relevance based on data from the Kiel Pediatric Tumor Registry. Handchir. Mikrochir. Plast. Chir. 2004;**36**:268 74.

73. McDowell HP. Update on childhood rhabdomyosarcoma. Arch. Dis. Child. 2003;**88**:354–7.

74. Bisogno G, Compostella A, Ferrari A, *et al.* Rhabdomyosarcoma in adolescents: A report from the AIEOP soft tissue sarcoma committee. Cancer 2012;**118**(3):821–7.

75. Saab R, Spunt SL, Skapek SX. Myogenesis and rhabdomyosarcoma the Jekyll and Hyde of skeletal muscle. Curr. Top. Dev. Biol. 2011;**94**:197–234.

76. Perez EA, Kassira N, Cheung MC, *et al.* Rhabdomyosarcoma in children: A SEER population based study. J. Surg. Res. 2011;**170**:e243–51.

77. Malempati S, Rodeberg DA, Donaldson SS, *et al.* Rhabdomyosarcoma in infants younger than 1 year: A report from the Children's Oncology Group. Cancer 2011;**117**:3493–501.

78. Asmar L, Gehan EA, Newton WA, *et al.* Agreement among and within groups of pathologists in the classification of rhabdomyosarcoma and related childhood sarcomas. Report of an international study of four pathology classifications. Cancer 1994;**74**:2579–88.

79. Cavazzana AO, Schmidt D, Ninfo V, *et al.* Spindle cell rhabdomyosarcoma: A prognostically favorable variant of rhabdomyosarcoma. Am. J. Surg. Pathol. 1992;**16**:229–35.

80. Newton WA Jr, Gehan EA, Webber BL, *et al.* Classification of rhabdomyosarcomas and related sarcomas. Pathologic aspects and proposal for a new classification – an Intergroup Rhabdomyosarcoma Study. Cancer 1995;**76**:1073–85.

81. Furlong MA, Mentzel T, Fanburg-Smith JC. Pleomorphic rhabdomyosarcoma in adults: A clinicopathologic study of 38 cases with emphasis on morphologic variants and recent skeletal muscle-specific markers. Mod. Pathol. 2001;**14**:595–603.

82. Jo VY, Mariño-Enriquez A, Fletcher CDM. Epithelioid rhabdomyosarcoma: clinicopathologic analysis of 16 cases of a morphologically distinct variant of rhabdomyosarcoma. Am. J. Surg. Pathol. 2011;**35**(:1523–39.

83. van Gaal JC, Flucke UE, Roeffen MH, *et al.* Anaplastic lymphoma kinase aberrations in rhabdomyosarcoma: clinical and prognostic implications. J. Clin. Oncol. 2012;**30**:308–15.

84. Ferrari A, Sultan I, Huang TT, *et al.* Soft tissue sarcoma across the age spectrum: A population-based study from the Surveillance Epidemiology and End Results database. Pediatr. Blood Cancer 2011;**57**:943–9.

85. Nascimento AF, Fletcher CD. Spindle cell rhabdomyosarcoma in adults. Am. J. Surg. Pathol. 2005;**29**:1106–13.

86. Sultan I, Qaddoumi I, Yaser S, *et al.* Comparing adult and pediatric rhabdomyosarcoma in the Surveillance, Epidemiology and End Results program, 1973 to 2005: An analysis of 2,600 patients. J. Clin. Oncol. 2009;**27**:3391–7.

87. Yang P, Grufferman S, Khoury MJ, *et al.* Association of childhood rhabdomyosarcoma with neurofibromatosis type 1 and birth defects. Genet. Epidemiol. 1995;**12**:467–74.

88. Parham DM, Ellison DA. Rhabdomyosarcomas in adults and children: An update. Arch. Pathol. Lab. Med. 2006;**130**(10):1454–65.

89. Doros L, Yang J, Dehner L, *et al. DICER1* mutations in embryonal rhabdomyosarcomas from children with and without familial PPB-tumor predisposition syndrome. Pediatr. Blood Cancer 2012;**59**:558–60.

90. Malempati S, Hawkins DS. Rhabdomyosarcoma: review of the Children's Oncology Group (COG) soft-tissue sarcoma committee experience and rationale for current COG studies. Pediatr. Blood Cancer 2012;**59**:5–10.

91. Qualman S, Lynch J, Bridge J, *et al.* Prevalence and clinical impact of anaplasia in childhood rhabdomyosarcoma: A report from the soft tissue

sarcoma committee of the Children's Oncology Group. Cancer 2008;1133242–7.

92. Dehner LP, Jarzembowski JA, Hill DA. Embryonal rhabdomyosarcoma of the uterine cervix: A report of 14 cases and a discussion of its unusual clinicopathological associations. Mod. Pathol. 2012;**25**:602–14.

93. Cessna MH, Zhou H, Perkins SL, et al. Are myogenin and MyoD1 expression specific for rhabdomyosarcoma? A study of 150 cases, with emphasis on spindle cell mimics. Am. J. Surg. Pathol. 2001;**25**):1150–7.

94. Sebire NJ, Malone M. Myogenin and MyoD1 expression in paediatric rhabdomyosarcomas. J. Clin. Pathol. 2003;**56**:412–6.

95. Morotti RA, Nicol KK, Parham DM, et al. An immunohistochemical algorithm to facilitate diagnosis and subtyping of rhabdomyosarcoma: The Children's Oncology Group experience. Am. J. Surg. Pathol. 2006;**30**:962–8.

96. Heerema-McKenney A, Wijnaendts CD, Pulliam JF, et al. Diffuse myogenin expression by immunohistochemistry is an independent marker of poor survival in pediatric rhabdomyosarcoma: A tissue microarray study of 71 primary tumors including correlation with molecular phenotype. Am. J. Surg. Pathol. 2008;**32**:1513–22.

97. Sorensen PH, Lynch JC, Qualman SJ, et al. *PAX3-FKHR* and *PAX7-FKHR* gene fusions are prognostic indicators in alveolar rhabdomyosarcoma: A report from the Children's Oncology Group. J. Clin. Oncol. 2002;**20**:2672–9.

98. Parham DM, Qualman SJ, Teot L, et al. Correlation between histology and *PAX/FKHR* fusion status in alveolar rhabdomyosarcoma: A report from the Children's Oncology Group. Am. J. Surg. Pathol. 2007;**31**:895–901.

99. Davicioni E, Anderson MJ, Finckenstein FG, et al. Molecular classification of rhabdomyosarcoma – genotypic and phenotypic determinants of diagnosis: A report from the Children's Oncology Group. Am. J. Pathol. 2009;**174**:550–64.

100. Williamson D, Missiaglia E, de Reyniès A, et al. Fusion gene-negative alveolar rhabdomyosarcoma is clinically and molecularly indistinguishable from embryonal rhabdomyosarcoma. J. Clin. Oncol. 2010;**28**:2151–8.

101. Wexler LH, Ladanyi M. Diagnosing alveolar rhabdomyosarcoma: morphology must be coupled with fusion confirmation. J. Clin. Oncol. 2010;**28**:2126–8.

102. Kikuchi K, Rubin BP, Keller C. Developmental origins of fusion-negative rhabdomyosarcomas. Curr. Top. Dev. Biol. 2011;**96**:33–56.

103. Coffin CM, Rulon J, Smith L, et al. Pathologic features of rhabdomyosarcoma before and after treatment: A clinicopathologic and immunohistochemical analysis. Mod. Pathol. 1997;**10**:1175–87.

104. Arndt CAS, Hammond S, Rodeberg D, et al. Significance of persistent mature rhabdomyoblasts in bladder/prostate rhabdomyosarcoma: results from IRS IV. J. Pediatr. Hematol. Oncol. 2006;**28**(9):563–7.

105. Floris G, Debiec-Rychter M, Wozniak A, et al. Malignant ectomesenchymoma: genetic profile reflects rhabdomyosarcomatous differentiation. Diagn. Mol. Pathol. 2007;**16**:243–8.

106. Weiss SW. Smooth muscle tumors of soft tissue. Adv. Anat. Pathol. 2002;**9**:351–9.

107. Ceballos KM, Nielsen GP, Selig MK, et al. Is anti-h-caldesmon useful for distinguishing smooth muscle and myofibroblastic tumors? An immunohistochemical study. Am. J. Clin. Pathol. 2000;**114**:746–53.

108. Garcia-Torres R, Cruz D, Orozco L, et al. Alport syndrome and diffuse leiomyomatosis. Clinical aspects, pathology, molecular biology and extracellular matrix studies. A synthesis. Nephrologie 2000;**21**:9–12.

109. Swanson PE, Wick MR, Dehner LP. Leiomyosarcoma of somatic soft tissues in childhood: An immunohistochemical analysis of six cases with ultrastructural correlation. Hum. Pathol. 1991;**22**:569–77.

110. de Saint Aubain Somerhausen N, Fletcher CDM. Leiomyosarcoma of soft tissue in childhood: clinicopathologic analysis of 20 cases. Am. J. Surg. Pathol. 1999;**23**:755–63.

111. Hwang ES, Gerald W, Wollner N, et al. Leiomyosarcoma in childhood and adolescence. Ann. Surg. Oncol. 1997;**4**:223–7.

112. Ferrari A, Bisogno G, Cassanova M, et al. Childhood leiomyosarcoma: A report from the soft tissue sarcoma Italian Cooperative Group. Ann. Oncol. 2001;**12**:1163–8.

113. Blaise G, Nikkels AF, Quatresooz P, et al. Childhood cutaneous leiomyosarcoma. Pediatr. Dermatol. 2009;**26**:477–9.

114. Jonigk D, Laenger F, Maegel L, et al. Molecular and clinicopathological analysis of Epstein-Barr virus-associated posttransplant smooth muscle tumors. Am. J. Transplant. 2012;**12**:1908–17.

115. Purgina B, Rao UNM, Miettinen M, et al. AIDS-related EBV-associated smooth muscle tumors: A review of 64 published cases. Patholog. Res. Int. 2011;**2011**:561548.

116. Yin X, Wu T, Yan Y, et al. Treatment for leiomyosarcoma and leiomyoma in children with HIV infection. Cochrane Database Syst. Rev. 2010;**5**:1–18.

117. Balarezo FS, Joshi VV. Proliferative and neoplastic disorders in children with acquired immunodeficiency syndrome. Adv. Anat. Pathol. 2002;**9**:360–70.

118. Kumar S, Santi M, Vezina G, et al. Epstein-Barr virus-associated smooth muscle tumor of the basal ganglia in an HIV+ child: case report and review of the literature. Pediatr. Dev. Pathol. 2004;**7**:198–203.

119. Deyrup AT, Lee VK, Hill CE, et al. Epstein-Barr virus-associated smooth muscle tumors are distinctive mesenchymal tumors reflecting multiple infection events: A clinicopathologic and molecular analysis of 29 tumors from 19 patients. Am. J. Surg. Pathol. 2006;**30**:75–82.

120. Coffin CM, Dehner LP. Fibroblastic-myofibroblastic tumors in children and adolescents: A clinicopathologic study of 108 examples in 103 patients. Pediatr. Pathol. 1991;**11**:569–88.

121. Coffin CM, Alaggio R. Fibroblastic and myofibroblastic tumors in children and adolescents. Pediatr. Dev. Pathol. 2012;**15**(1):127–80.

122. Rosenberg AE. Pseudosarcomas of soft tissue. Arch. Pathol. Lab. Med. 2008;**132**:579–86.

123. Erickson-Johnson MR, Chou MM, Evers BR, et al. Nodular fasciitis: A novel model of transient neoplasia induced by *MYH9-USP6* gene fusion. Lab. Invest. 2011;**91**:1427–33.

124. de Silva MV, Reid R. Myositis ossificans and fibroosseous pseudotumor of digits: A clinicopathological review of 64 cases with emphasis on diagnostic pitfalls Int. J. Surg. Pathol. 2003;**11**:187–95.

125. Vargas SO. Fibrous umbilical polyp: A distinct fasciitis-like proliferation of early childhood with a marked male predominance. Am. J. Surg. Pathol. 2001;**25**:1438–42.

126. Fetsch JF, Montgomery EA, Meis JM. Calcifying fibrous pseudotumor. Am. J. Surg. Pathol. 1993;**17**:502–8.

127. Nascimento AF, Ruiz R, Hornick JL, et al. Calcifying fibrous 'pseudotumor': clinicopathologic study of 15 cases and analysis of its relationship to inflammatory myofibroblastic tumor. Int. J. Surg. Pathol. 2002;**10**:189–96.

128. Wehrli BM, Weiss SW, Yandow S, et al. Gardner-associated fibromas (GAF) in young patients: A distinct fibrous lesion that identifies unsuspected Gardner syndrome and risk for fibromatosis. Am. J. Surg. Pathol. 2001;**25**:645–51.

129. Coffin CM, Hornick JL, Zhouu H, et al. Gardner fibroma: A clinicopathologic and immunohistochemical analysis of 45 patients with 57 fibromas. Am. J. Surg. Pathol. 2007;**31**:410–6.

130. Schmidt D. Fibrous tumors and tumor-like lesions of childhood: diagnosis, differential diagnosis, and prognosis. Curr. *Top. Pathol.* 1995;**89**:175–91.

131. Mentzel T, Calonje E, Nascimento AG, et al. Infantile hemangiopericytoma vs. infantile myofibromatosis: study of a series suggesting a continuous spectrum of infantile myofibroblastic lesions. Am. J. Surg. Pathol. 1994;**18**:922–30.

132. Granter SR, Badizadegan K, Fletcher CD. Myofibromatosis in adults, glomangiopericytoma, and myopericytoma: A spectrum of tumors showing perivascular and myoid differentiation. Am. J. Surg. Pathol. 1998;**22**:513–25.

133. Coffin C, Boccon-Gibod L. Fibroblastic-myofibroblastic proliferations of childhood and adolescence. Ann. Pathol. 2004;**24**:605–20.

134. Chung EB, Enzinger FM. Infantile myofibromatosis. Cancer 1981;**48**:1807–18.

135. Coffin CM, Neilson KA, Ingels S, et al. Congenital generalized myofibromatosis: A disseminated angiocentric myofibromatosis. Pediatr. Pathol. Lab. Med. 1995;**15**:571–87.

136. Oudijk L, den Bakker MA, Hop WC, et al. Solitary, multifocal and generalized myofibromas: clinicopathological and immunohistochemical features of 114 cases. Histopathology 2012;**60**(6B):E1–E11.

137. Stenman G, Nadal N, Persson S, et al. del(6)(q12q15) as the sole cytogenetic anomaly in a case of solitary infantile myofibromatosis. Oncol. Rep. 1999;**6**:1101–4.

138. Zand DJ, Huff D, Everman D, et al. Autosomal dominant inheritance of infantile myofibromatosis. Am. J. Med. Genet. A 2004;**126A**:261–6.

139. Alaggio R, Barisani D, Ninfo V, et al. Morphologic overlap between infantile myofibromatosis and infantile fibrosarcoma: A pitfall in diagnosis. Pediatr. Dev. Pathol. 2008;**11**:355–62.

140. Laskin WB, Meittinen M, Fetsch JF. Infantile digital fibroma/fibromatosis: A clinicopathologic and immunohistochemical study of 69 tumors from 57 patients with long-term follow-up. Am. J. Surg. Pathol. 2009;**33**:1–13.

141. Taylor HO, Gellis SE, Schmidt BA, et al. Infantile digital fibromatosis. Ann. Plast. Surg. 2008;**61**:472–6.

142. Grenier N, Liang C, Capaldi L, et al. A range of histologic findings in infantile digital fibromatosis. Pediatr. Dermatol. 2008;**25**:72–5.

143. Enzinger FM. Fibrous hamartoma of infancy. Cancer 1965;**18**:241–8.

144. Fletcher CD, Powell G, van Noordern S, et al. Fibrous hamartoma of infancy: A histochemical and immunohistochemical study. Histopathology 1988;**12**:65–74.

145. Rougemont AL, Fetni R, Murthy S, et al. A complex translocation (6;12;8)(q25;q24.3;q13) in a fibrous hamartoma of infancy. Cancer Genet. Cytogenet. 2006;**171**:115–8.

146. Fetsch JF, Miettinen M. Calcifying aponeurotic fibroma: A clinicopathologic study of 22 cases arising in uncommon sites. Hum. Pathol. 1998;**29**:1504–10.

147. Fetsch JF, Miettinen M, Laskin WB, *et al.* A clinicopathologic study of 45 pediatric soft tissue tumors with an admixture of adipose tissue and fibroblastic elements, and a proposal for classification as lipofibromatosis. Am. J. Surg. Pathol. 2000;**24**:1491–1500.

148. Teo HE, Peh WC, Chan MY, *et al.* Infantile lipofibromatosis of the upper limb. Skeletal Radiol. 2005;**34**:799–802.

149. Ayadi L, Charfi S, Ben Hamed Y, *et al.* Pigmented lipofibromatosis in unusual location: case report and review of the literature. Virchows Arch. 2008;**452**:462–7.

150. Kenney B, Richkind KE, Friedlaender G, *et al.* Chromosomal rearrangements in lipofibromatosis. Cancer Genet. Cytogenet. 2007;**179**:136–9.

151. Coutinho-Camillo CM, Brentani MM, Nagai MA. Genetic alterations in juvenile nasopharyngeal angiofibromas. Head Neck 2008;**30**:390–400.

152. Mayer-da-Silva A, Poiares-Baptista A, Guerra Rodrigo F, *et al.* Juvenile hyaline fibromatosis: A histologic and immunohistochemical study. Arch. Pathol. Lab. Med. 1988;**112**:928–31.

153. Hanks S, Adams S, Douglas J, *et al.* Mutations in the gene encoding capillary morphogenesis protein 2 cause juvenile hyaline fibromatosis and infantile systemic hyalinosis. Am. J. Hum. Genet. 2003;**73**:791–800.

154. Chinyama CN, Roblin P, Watson SJ, *et al.* Fibromatoses and related tumors of the hand in children: A clinicopathologic review. Hand Clin. 2000;**16**:625–35,ix.

155. Fetsch JF, Laskin WB, Miettinen M. Palmar-plantar fibromatosis in children and preadolescents: A clinicopathologic study of 56 cases with newly recognized demographics and extended follow-up information. Am. J. Surg. Pathol. 2005;**29**:1095–105.

156. Coffin CM, Randall RL, Million L, *et al.* Desmoid fibromatosis in childhood and adolescence: An analysis of 65 patients in the first two decades of life. Mod. Pathol. 2010;**23**:394A.

157. Meazza C, Bisogno G, Gronchi A, *et al.* Aggressive fibromatosis in children and adolescents: the Italian experience. Cancer 2010;**116**:233–40.

158. Gebert C, Hardes J, Kersting C, *et al.* Expression of beta-catenin and p53 are prognostic factors in deep aggressive fibromatosis. Histopathology 2007;**50**:491–7.

159. Lazar AJ, Tuvin D, Hajibashi S, *et al.* Specific mutations in the *beta-catenin* gene (*CTNNB1*) correlate with local recurrence in sporadic desmoid tumors. Am. J. Pathol. 2008;**173**:1518–27.

160. Wang WL, Nero C, Pappo A, *et al. CTNNB1* genotyping and APC screening in pediatric desmoid tumors: A proposed algorithm. Pediatr. Dev. Pathol. 2012.

161. Cates JM, Black J, Wolfe CC, *et al.* Morphologic and immunophenotypic analysis of desmoid-type fibromatosis after radiation therapy. Hum. Pathol. 2012;**43**:1418–24.

162. Coffin CM, Hornick JL, Fletcher CD. Inflammatory myofibroblastic tumor: comparison of clinicopathologic, histologic, and immunohistochemical features including ALK expression in atypical and aggressive cases. Am. J. Surg. Pathol. 2007;**31**:509–20.

163. Coffin CM, Watterson J, Priest JR, *et al.* Extrapulmonary inflammatory myofibroblastic tumor (inflammatory pseudotumor): A clinicopathologic and immunohistochemical study of 84 cases. Am. J. Surg. Pathol. 1995;**19**:859–72.

164. Gleason BC, Hornick JL. Inflammatory myofibroblastic tumours: where are we now? J. Clin. Pathol. 2008;**61**:428–37.

165. Chen ST, Lee JC. An inflammatory myofibroblastic tumor in liver with *ALK* and *RANBP2* gene rearrangement: combination of distinct morphologic, immunohistochemical, and genetic features. Hum. Pathol. 2008;**39**:1854–8.

166. Marino-Enriquez A, Wang WL, Roy A, *et al.* Epithelioid inflammatory myofibroblastic sarcoma: An aggressive intraabdominal variant of inflammatory myofibroblastic tumor with nuclear membrane or perinuclear ALK. Am. J. Surg. Pathol. 2011;**35**:135–44.

167. Knezevich SR, Garnett MJ, Pysher TJ, *et al. ETV6-NTRK3* gene fusions and trisomy 11 establish a histogenetic link between mesoblastic nephroma and congenital fibrosarcoma. Cancer Res. 1998;**58**:5046–8.

168. Coffin CM, Jaszez W, O'Shea PA, *et al.* So-called congenital-infantile fibrosarcoma: does it exist and what is it? Pediatr. Pathol. 1994;**14**:133–50.

169. Sheng WQ, Hisaoka M, Okamoto S, *et al.* Congenital-infantile fibrosarcoma: A clinicopathologic study of 10 cases and molecular detection of the *ETV6-NTRK3* fusion transcripts using paraffin embedded tissues. Am. J. Clin. Pathol. 2001;**115**:348–55.

170. Black J, Coffin CM, Dehner LP. Fibrohistiocytic tumors and related neoplasms in children and adolescents. Pediatr. Dev. Pathol. 2012;**15**:181–210.

171. Fletcher CD. Giant cell fibroblastoma of soft tissue: A clinicopathological and immunohistochemical study. Histopathology 1988;**13**:499–508.

172. Jha P, Moosavi C, Fanburg-Smith JC. Giant cell fibroblastoma: An update and addition of 86 new cases from the Armed Forces Institute of Pathology, in honor

of Dr. Enzinger Franz M. Ann. Diagn. Pathol. 2007;**11**:81–8.

173. Terrier-Lacombe MJ, Guillou L, Maire G, *et al.* Dermatofibrosarcoma protuberans, giant cell fibroblastoma, and hybrid lesions in children: clinicopathologic comparative analysis of 28 cases with molecular data – a study from the French Federation of Cancer Centers Sarcoma Group. Am. J. Surg. Pathol. 2003;**27**:27–39.

174. Weinstein JM, Drolet BA, Esterly NB, *et al.* Congenital dermatofibrosarcoma protuberans: variability in presentation. Arch. Dermatol. 2003;**139**:207–11.

175. Jafarian F, McCuaig C, Kokta V, *et al.* Dermatofibrosarcoma protuberans in childhood and adolescence: report of eight patients. Pediatr. Dermatol. 2008;**25**:317–25.

176. Pappo AS, Rao BN, Cain A, *et al.* Dermatofibrosarcoma protuberans: the pediatric experience at St. Jude Children's Research Hospital. Pediatr. Hematol. Oncol. 1997;**14**:563–8.

177. Reimann JD, Fletcher CD. Myxoid dermatofibrosarcoma protuberans: A rare variant analyzed in a series of 23 cases. Am. J. Surg. Pathol. 2007;**31**:1371–7.

178. Calonje E, Fletcher CD. Myoid differentiation in dermatofibrosarcoma protuberans and its fibrosarcomatous variant: clinicopathologic analysis of 5 cases. J. Cutan. Pathol. 1996;**23**:30–6.

179. Llatjós R, Fernández-Figueras MT, Díaz-Cascajo C, *et al.* Palisading and verocay body-prominent dermatofibrosarcoma protuberans: A report of three cases. Histopathology 2000;**37**:452–5.

180. Maire G, Fraitag S, Galmiche L, *et al.* A clinical, histologic, and molecular study of 9 cases of congenital dermatofibrosarcoma protuberans. Arch. Dermatol. 2007;**143**:203–10.

181. Beham A, Fletcher CD. Dermatofibrosarcoma protuberans with areas resembling giant cell fibroblastoma: report of two cases. Histopathology 1990;**17**:165–7.

182. Llombart B, Sanmartín O, López-Guerrero JA, *et al.* Dermatofibrosarcoma protuberans: clinical, pathological, and genetic (*COL1A1-PDGFB*) study with therapeutic implications. Histopathology 2009;**54**:860–72.

183. Abbott JJ, Oliveira AM, Nascimento AG. The prognostic significance of fibrosarcomatous transformation in dermatofibrosarcoma protuberans. Am. J. Surg. Pathol. 2006;**30**:436–43.

184. Farma JM, Ammori JB, Zager JS, *et al.* Dermatofibrosarcoma protuberans: how wide should we resect? Ann. Surg. Oncol. 2010;**17**:2112–8.

185. Najarian DJ, Morrison C, Sait SN, *et al.* Recurrent giant cell fibroblastoma treated with Mohs micrographic surgery. Dermatol. Surg. 2010;**36**:417–21.

186. Alaggio R, Ninfo V, Rosolen A, *et al.* Primitive myxoid mesenchymal tumor of infancy: A clinicopathologic report of 6 cases. Am. J. Surg. Pathol. 2006;**30**:388–94.

187. Hanau CA, Miettinen M. Solitary fibrous tumor: histological and immunohistochemical spectrum of benign and malignant variants presenting at different sites. Hum. Pathol. 1995;**26**:440–9.

188. Lucci LM, Anderson RL, Harrie RP, *et al.* Solitary fibrous tumor of the orbit in a child. Ophthal. Plast. Reconstr. Surg. 2001;**17**:369–73.

189. Alaggio R, Coffin CM, Dall'igna P, *et al.* Myxo-inflammatory fibroblastic tumor – report of a case and review of the literature. Pediatr. Dev. Pathol. 2012;**15**:254–8.

190. Billings SD, Giblen G, Ganburg-Smith JC. Superficial low-grade fibromyxoid sarcoma (Evans tumor): A clinicopathologic analysis of 19 cases with a unique observation in the pediatric population. Am. J. Surg. Pathol. 2005;**29**:204–10.

191. Guillou L, Benhattar J, Gengler C, *et al.* Translocation-positive low-grade fibromyxoid sarcoma: clinicopathologic and molecular analysis of a series expanding the morphologic spectrum and suggesting potential relationship to sclerosing epithelioid fibrosarcoma: A study from the French Sarcoma Group. Am. J. Surg. Pathol. 2007;**31**:1387–402.

192. Doyle LA, Möller E, Dal Cin P, *et al.* MUC4 is a highly sensitive and specific marker for low-grade fibromyxoid sarcoma. Am. J. Surg. Pathol. 2011;**35**:733–41.

193. Mertens F, Fletcher CD, Antonescu CR, *et al.* Clinicopathologic and molecular genetic characterization of low-grade fibromyxoid sarcoma, and cloning of a novel *FUS/CREB3L1* fusion gene. Lab. Invest. 2005;**85**:408–15.

194. Smith DM, Mahmoud HH, Jenkins JJ, 3rd, *et al.* Low-grade myofibrosarcoma of the head and neck: importance of surgical therapy. J. Pediatr. Hematol. Oncol. 2004;**26**:119–20.

195. Keller C, Gibbs CN, Kelly SM, *et al.* Low-grade myofibrosarcoma of the head and neck: importance of surgical therapy. J. Pediatr. Hematol. Oncol. 2004;**26**:119–20.

196. Lundgren L, Angervall L, Stenman G, *et al.* Infantile rhabdomyofibrosarcoma: A high-grade sarcoma distinguishable from infantile fibrosarcoma and rhabdomyosarcoma. Hum. Pathol. 1993;**24**:785–95.

197. Mentzel T, Mentzel HJ, Katenkamp D. Infantile rhabdomyofibrosarcoma: An aggressive tumor in the spectrum of spindle cell tumors in childhood. Pathologe 1996;**17**:296–300.

198. Billings SD, Folpe AL. Cutaneous and subcutaneous fibrohistiocytic tumors of intermediate malignancy: An update. Am. J. Dermatopathol. 2004;**26**:141–55.

199. Coffin CM, Dehner LP, O'Shea PA. *Pediatric Soft Tissue Tumors: A Clinical, Pathological, and Therapeutic Approach*, first edn. Baltimore: Williams & Wilkins, 1997.

200. Gershtenson PC, Krunic AL, Chen HM. Multiple clustered dermatofibroma: case report and review of the literature. J. Cutan. Pathol. 2010;**37**:e42–5.

201. Zelger B, Zelger BG, Burgdorf WH. Dermatofibroma-a critical evaluation. Int. J. Surg. Pathol. 2004;**12**:333–44.

202. Kaddu S, Leinweber B. Podoplanin expression in fibrous histiocytomas and cellular neurothekeomas. Am. J. Dermatopathol. 2009;**31**:137–9.

203. Calonje E, Mentzel T, Fletcher CD. Cellular benign fibrous histiocytoma. Clinicopathologic analysis of 74 cases of a distinctive variant of cutaneous fibrous histiocytoma with frequent recurrence. Am. J. Surg. Pathol. 1994;**18**:668–76.

204. Gleason BC, Fletcher CD. Deep "benign" fibrous histiocytoma: clinicopathologic analysis of 69 cases of a rare tumor indicating occasional metastatic potential. Am. J. Surg. Pathol. 2008;**32**:354–62.

205. Somerhausen NS, Fletcher CD. Diffuse-type giant cell tumor: clinicopathologic and immunohistochemical analysis of 50 cases with extraarticular disease. Am. J. Surg. Pathol. 2000;**24**:479–92.

206. Sciot E, Rosai J, Dal Cin P, *et al.* Analysis of 35 cases of localized and diffuse tenosynovial giant cell tumor: A report from the Chromosomes and Morphology (CHAMP) study group. Mod. Pathol. 1999;**12**:576–9.

207. Murphey MD, Rhee JH, Lewis RB, *et al.* Pigmented villonodular synovitis: radiologic-pathologic correlation. Radiographics 2008;**28**:1493–518.

208. Nguyen TT, Schwartz EJ, West RB, *et al.* Expression of CD163 (hemoglobin scavenger receptor) in normal tissues, lymphomas, carcinomas, and sarcomas is largely restricted to the monocyte/macrophage lineage. Am. J. Surg. Pathol. 2005;**29**:617–24.

209. Boland JM, Folpe AL, Hornick JL, *et al.* Clusterin is expressed in normal synoviocytes and in tenosynovial giant cell tumors of localized and diffuse types: diagnostic and histogenetic implications. Am. J. Surg. Pathol. 2009;**33**:1225–9.

210. West RB, Rubin BP, Miller MA, *et al.* A landscape effect in tenosynovial giant-cell tumor from activation of CSF1 expression by a translocation in a minority of tumor cells. Proc. Natl. Acad. Sci. USA 2006;**103**:690–5.

211. Moosavi C, Jha P, Fanburg-Smith JC. An update on plexiform fibrohistiocytic tumor and addition of 66 new cases from the Armed Forces Institute of Pathology, in honor of Franz M. Enzinger, MD. Ann. Diagn. Pathol. 2007;**11**:313–9.

212. Alaggio R, Collini P, Randall RL, *et al.* Undifferentiated high-grade pleomorphic sarcomas in children: A clinicopathologic study of 10 cases and review of the literature. Pediatr. Dev. Pathol. 2010;**13**:209–17.

213. Dei Tos AP. Classification of pleomorphic sarcomas: where are we now? Histopathology 2006;**48**:51–62.

214. Janssen D, Harms D. Juvenile xanthogranuloma in childhood and adolescence: A clinicopathologic study of 129 patients from the Kiel Pediatric Tumor Registry. Am. J. Surg. Pathol. 2005;**29**:21–8.

215. Dehner LP. Juvenile xanthogranulomas in the first two decades of life: A clinicopathologic study of 174 cases with cutaneous and extracutaneous manifestations. Am. J. Surg. Pathol. 2003;**27**(5):579–93.

216. Suson K, Mathews R, Goldstein JD, *et al.* Juvenile xanthogranuloma presenting as a testicular mass in infancy: A clinical and pathologic study of three cases. Pediatr. Dev. Pathol. 2010;**13**:39–45.

217. Stover DG, Alapati S, Regueira O, *et al.* Treatment of juvenile xanthogranuloma. Pediatr. Blood Cancer 2008;**51**:130–3.

218. Orsey A, Paessler M, Lange BJ, *et al.* Central nervous system juvenile xanthogranuloma with malignant transformation. Pediatr. Blood Cancer 2008;**50**:927–30.

219. Takeuchi M, Nakayama M, Nakano A, *et al.* Congenital systemic juvenile xanthogranuloma with placental lesion. Pediatr. Int. 2009;**51**:833–6.

220. Cates JMM, Coffin CM. Neurogenic tumors of soft tissue. Pediatr. Dev. Pathol. 2012;**15**:62–107.

221. Rodriguez FJ, Folpe AL, Giannini C, *et al.* Pathology of peripheral nerve sheath tumors: diagnostic overview and update on selected diagnostic problems. Acta Neuropathol. 2012;**123**:295–319.

222. Ferner RE. The neurofibromatoses. Pract. Neurol. 2010:**10**:82–93.

223. McClatchey AI. Neurofibromatosis. Annu. Rev. Pathol. 2007;**2**:191–216.

224. Waggoner DJ, Towbin J, Gottesman G, *et al.* Clinic-based study of plexiform neurofibromas in neurofibromatosis 1. Am. J. Med. Genet. 2000;**92**:132–5.

225. Tucker T, Friedman JM, Friedrich RE, *et al.* Longitudinal study of neurofibromatosis 1 associated plexiform neurofibromas. J. Med. Genet. 2009;**46**:81–5.

226. Ferner RE. Neurofibromatosis 1 and neurofibromatosis 2: A twenty first century perspective. Lancet Neurol. 2007;**6**:340–51.

227. Lu-Emerson C, Plotkin SR. The neurofibromatoses. Part 1: NF1. Rev. Neurol. Dis. 2009;**6**:E47–53.

228. Williams VC, Lucas J, Babcock MA, *et al.* Neurofibromatosis type 1 revisited. Pediatrics 2009;**123**:124–33.

229. DeBella K, Szudek J, Friedman JM. Use of the National Institutes of Health criteria for diagnosis of neurofibromatosis 1 in children. Pediatrics 2000;**105**(3 Pt 1):608–14.

230. Boulanger JM, Larbrisseau A. Neurofibromatosis type 1 in a pediatric population: Ste-Justine's experience. Can. J. Neurol. Sci. 2005;**32**:225–31.

231. Ferner RE, Huson SM, Thomas N, *et al.* Guidelines for the diagnosis and management of individuals with neurofibromatosis 1. J. Med. Genet. 2007;**44**:81–8.

232. Rosser T, Packer RJ. Neurofibromas in children with neurofibromatosis 1. J. Child. Neurol. 2002;**17**:585–91.

233. Liapis H, Marley EF, Lin Y, *et al.* p53 and Ki-67 proliferating cell nuclear antigen in benign and malignant peripheral nerve sheath tumors in children. Pediatr. Dev. Pathol. 1999;**2**:377–84.

234. Zhou H, Coffin CM, Perkins SL, *et al.* Malignant peripheral nerve sheath tumor: A comparison of grade, immunophenotype, and cell cycle/growth activation marker expression in sporadic and neurofibromatosis 1-related lesions. Am. J. Surg. Pathol. 2003;**27**:1337–45.

235. Ruggieri M, Iannetti P, Polizzi A, *et al.* Earliest clinical manifestations and natural history of neurofibromatosis type 2 (NF2) in childhood: A study of 24 patients. Neuropediatrics 2005;**36**:21–34.

236. Woodruff JM, Scheithauer BW, Kurtkaya-Yapicier O, *et al.* Congenital and childhood plexiform (multinodular) cellular schwannoma: A troublesome mimic of malignant peripheral nerve sheath tumor. Am. J. Surg. Pathol. 2003;**27**:1321–9.

237. Kurtkaya-Yapicier O, Scheithauer B, Woodruff JM. The pathobiologic spectrum of Schwannomas. Histol. Histopathol. 2003;**18**:925–34.

238. Fine SW, McClain SA, Li M. Immunohistochemical staining for calretinin is useful for differentiating schwannomas from neurofibromas. Am. J. Clin. Pathol. 2004;**122**:552–9.

239. MacCollin M, Chiocca EA, Evans DG, *et al.* Diagnostic criteria for schwannomatosis. Neurology 2005;**64**:1838–45.

240. Smith MJ, Wallace AJ, Bowers NL, *et al.* Frequency of *SMARCB1* mutations in familial and sporadic schwannomatosis. Neurogenetics 2012;**13**(2):141–5.

241. Hadfield KD, Newman WG, Bowers NL, *et al.* Molecular characterisation of *SMARCB1* and *NF2* in familial and sporadic schwannomatosis. J. Med. Genet. 2008;**45**:332–9.

242. Swensen JJ, Keyser J, Coffin CM, *et al.* Familial occurrence of schwannomas and malignant rhabdoid tumour associated with a duplication in SMARCB1. J. Med. Genet. 2009;**46**:68–72.

243. Macarenco RS, Ellinger F, Oliveira AM. Perineurioma: A distinctive and underrecognized peripheral nerve sheath neoplasm. Arch. Pathol. Lab. Med. 2007;**131**:625–36.

244. Boyanton BL Jr, Jones JK, Shenaq SM, *et al.* Intraneural perineurioma: A systematic review with illustrative cases. Arch. Pathol. Lab. Med. 2007;**131**:1382–92.

245. Hornick JL, Fletcher CDM. Soft tissue perineurioma: clinicopathologic analysis of 81 cases including those with atypical histologic features. Am. J. Surg. Pathol. 2005;**29**:845–58.

246. Mauermann ML, Amrami KK, Kuntz NL, *et al.* Longitudinal study of intraneural perineurioma – a benign, focal hypertrophic neuropathy of youth. Brain 2009;**132**(Pt 8):2265–76.

247. Rubin AI, Yassaee M, Johnson W, *et al.* Multiple cutaneous sclerosing perineuriomas: An extensive presentation with involvement of the bilateral upper extremities. J. Cutan. Pathol. 2009;36 Suppl **1**:60–5.

248. Pitchford CW, Schwartz HS, Atkinson JB, *et al.* Soft tissue perineurioma in a patient with neurofibromatosis type 2: A tumor not previously associated with the *NF2* syndrome. Am. J. Surg. Pathol. 2006;**30**:1624–9.

249. Ausmus GG, Piliang MP, Bergfeld WF, *et al.* Soft-tissue perineurioma in a 20-year-old patient with neurofibromatosis type 1 (NF1): report of a case and review of the literature. J. Cutan. Pathol. 2007;**34**:726–30.

250. Chen L, Li Y, Lin JH. Intraneural perineurioma in a child with Beckwith-Wiedemann syndrome. J. Pediatr. Surg. 2005;**40**:e12–4.

251. Hornick JL, Bundock EA, Fletcher CDM. Hybrid schwannoma/perineurioma: clinicopathologic analysis of 42 distinctive benign nerve sheath tumors. Am. J. Surg. Pathol. 2009;**33**:1554–61.

252. Fetsch JF, Laskin WB, Miettinen M. Nerve sheath myxoma: A clinicopathologic and immunohistochemical analysis of 57 morphologically distinctive, S-100 protein- and GFAP-positive, myxoid peripheral nerve sheath tumors with a predilection for the extremities and a high local recurrence rate. Am. J. Surg. Pathol. 2005;**29**:1615–24.

253. Fetsch JF, Laskin WB, Hallman JR, *et al.* Neurothekeoma: An analysis of 178 tumors with detailed immunohistochemical data and long-term patient follow-up information. Am. J. Surg. Pathol. 2007;**31**:1103–14.

254. Hornick JL, Fletcher CD. Cellular neurothekeoma: detailed characterization in a series of 133 cases. Am. J. Surg. Pathol. 2007;**31**:329–40.

255. Jaffer S, Ambrosini-Spaltro A, Mancini AM, *et al.* Neurothekeoma and plexiform fibrohistiocytic tumor: mere histologic resemblance or histogenetic relationship? Am. J. Surg. Pathol. 2009;**33**:905–13.

256. Vered M, Dobriyan A, Buchner A. Congenital granular cell epulis presents an immunohistochemical profile that distinguishes it from the granular cell tumor of the adult. Virchows Arch. 2009;**454**:303–10.

257. Chaudhry IH, Calonje E. Dermal non-neural granular cell tumour (so-called primitive polypoid granular cell tumour): A distinctive entity further delineated in a clinicopathological study of 11 cases. Histopathology 2005;**47**:179–85.

258. Le BH, Boyer PJ, Lewis JE, *et al.* Granular cell tumor: immunohistochemical assessment of inhibin-α, protein gene product 9.5, S100 protein, CD68, and Ki-67 proliferative index with clinical correlation. Arch. Pathol. Lab. Med. 2004;**128**:771–5.

259. Tucker T, Wolkenstein P, Revuz J, *et al.* Association between benign and malignant peripheral nerve sheath tumors in NF1. Neurology 2005;**65**:205–11.

260. Brems H, Beert E, de Ravel T, *et al.* Mechanisms in the pathogenesis of malignant tumours in neurofibromatosis type 1. Lancet Oncol. 2009;**10**:508–15.

261. Ducatman BS, Scheithauer BW, Piepgras DG, *et al.* Malignant peripheral nerve sheath tumors in childhood. J. Neuro-Oncol. 1984;**2**:241–8.

262. Raney B, Schnaufer L, Ziegler M, *et al.* Treatment of children with neurogenic sarcoma. Experience at the Children's Hospital of Philadelphia, 1958–1984. Cancer 1987;**59**:1–5.

263. Meis JM, Enzinger FM, Martz KL, *et al.* Malignant peripheral nerve sheath tumors (malignant schwannomas) in children. Am. J. Surg. Pathol. 1992;**16**:694–707.

264. deCou JM, Rao BN, Parham DM, *et al.* Malignant peripheral nerve sheath tumors: the St. Jude Children's Research Hospital experience. Ann. Surg. Oncol. 1995;**2**(6):524–9.

265. Neville H, Corpron C, Blakely ML, *et al.* Pediatric neurofibrosarcoma. J. Pediatr. Surg. 2003;**38**(3):343–6.

266. Carli M, Ferrari A, Mattke A, *et al.* Pediatric malignant peripheral nerve sheath tumor: the Italian and German soft tissue sarcoma cooperative group. J. Clin. Oncol. 2005;**23**(33):8422–30.

267. Coffin CM, Cassity J, Viskochil D, *et al.* Non-neurogenic sarcomas in four children and young adults with neurofibromatosis type 1. Am. J. Genet. A 2004;**127A**(1):40–3.

268. Ferrari A, Bisogno G, Macaluso A, *et al.* Soft-tissue sarcomas in children and adolescents with neurofibromatosis type 1. Cancer 2007;**109**(7):1406–12.

269. McMenamin ME, Fletcher CD. Expanding the spectrum of malignant change in schwannomas: epithelioid malignant change, epithelioid malignant peripheral nerve sheath tumor, and epithelioid angiosarcoma: A study of 17 cases. Am. J. Surg. Pathol. 2001;**25**(1):13–25.

270. Brekke HR, Kolberg M, Skotheim RI, *et al.* Identification of p53 as a strong predictor of survival for patients with malignant peripheral nerve sheath tumors. Neuro-Oncol. 2009;**11**(5):514–28.

271. Wallander ML, Tripp S, Layfield LJ. *MDM2* amplification in malignant peripheral nerve sheath tumors correlates with p53 protein expression. Arch. Pathol. Lab. Med. 2012;**136**:95–9.

272. Bridge RS Jr, Bridge JA, Neff JR, *et al.* Recurrent chromosomal imbalances and structurally abnormal breakpoints within complex karyotypes of malignant peripheral nerve sheath tumour and malignant triton tumour: A cytogenetic and molecular cytogenetic study. J. Clin. Pathol. 2004;**57**(11):1172–8.

273. Yu J, Deshmukh H, Payton JE, *et al.* Array-based comparative genomic hybridization identifies *CDK4* and *FOXM1* alterations as independent predictors of survival in malignant peripheral nerve sheath tumor. Clin. Cancer Res. 2011;**17**(7):1924–34.

274. Anghileri M, Miceli R, Fiore M, *et al.* Malignant peripheral nerve sheath tumors: prognostic factors and survival in a series of patients treated at a single institution. Cancer 2006;**107**(5):1065–74.

275. Alaggio R, Coffin CM, Vargas SO. Soft tissue tumors of uncertain origin. Pediatr. Dev. Pathol. 2012;**15**(1):267–305.

276. Janeway KA, Weldon CB. Pediatric gastrointestinal stromal tumor. Semin. Pediatr. Surg. 2012;**21**(1):31–43.

277. Pappo AS, Janeway K, Laguaglia M, *et al.* Special considerations in pediatric gastrointestinal tumors. J. Surg. Oncol. 2011;**104**(8):928–32.

278. Benesch M, Leuschner I, Wardelmann E, *et al.* Gastrointestinal stromal tumors in children and young adults: A clinicopathologic series with long-term follow-up from the database of the Cooperative Weichteilsarkom Studiengruppe (CWS). Eur. J. Cancer 2011;**47**(11):1692–8.

279. Benesch M, Wardelmann E, Ferrari A, *et al.* Gastrointestinal stromal tumors (GIST) in children and adolescents: A comprehensive review of the current literature. Pediatr. Blood Cancer 2009;**53**(7):1171–9.

280. Pappo AS, Janeway KA. Pediatric gastrointestinal stromal tumors. Hematol. Oncol. Clin. North Am. 2009;**23**(1):15–34,vii.

281. Price VE, Zielenska M, Chilton-MacNeill S, *et al.* Clinical and molecular characteristics of pediatric

gastrointestinal stromal tumors (GISTs). Pediatr. Blood Cancer 2005;**45**(1):20–4.

282. Prakash S, Sarran L, Socci N, *et al.* Gastrointestinal stromal tumors in children and young adults: A clinicopathologic, molecular, and genomic study of 15 cases and review of the literature. J. Pediatr. Hematol. Oncol. 2005;**27**(4):179–87.

283. Agaram NP, Laguaglia MP, Ustun B, *et al.* Molecular characterization of pediatric gastrointestinal stromal tumors. Clin. Cancer Res. 2008;**14**(10):3204–15.

284. Miettinen M, Lasota J. Gastrointestinal stromal tumors: Review on morphology, molecular pathology, prognosis, and differential diagnosis. Arch. Pathol. Lab. Med. 2006;**130**(10):1466–78.

285. Miettinen M, Lasota J, Sobin LH. Gastrointestinal stromal tumors of the stomach in children and young adults: A clinicopathologic, immunohistochemical, and molecular genetic study of 44 cases with long-term follow-up and review of the literature. Am. J. Surg. Pathol. 2005;**29**(10):1373–81.

286. Liegl B, Hornick JL, Corless CL, *et al.* Monoclonal antibody DOG1.1 shows higher sensitivity than KIT in the diagnosis of gastrointestinal stromal tumors, including unusual subtypes. Am. J. Surg. Pathol. 2009;**33**(3):437–46.

287. Miettinen M, Wang ZF, Sarlomo-Rikala M, *et al.* Succinate dehydrogenase-deficient GISTs: A clinicopathologic, immunohistochemical, and molecular genetic study of 66 gastric GISTs with predilection to young age. Am. J. Surg. Pathol. 2011;**35**(11):1712–21.

288. Gill AJ, Chou A, Vilain R, *et al.* Immunohistochemistry for SDHB divides gastrointestinal stromal tumors (GISTs) into 2 distinct types. Am. J. Surg. Pathol. 2010;**34**(5):636–44.

289. Zhang L, Smyrk TC, Young WF Jr, *et al.* Gastric stromal tumors in Carney triad are different clinically, pathologically, and behaviorally from sporadic gastric gastrointestinal stromal tumors: findings in 104 cases. Am. J. Surg. Pathol. 2010;**34**(1):53–64.

290. Gaal J, Stratakis CA, Carney JA, *et al.* SDHB immunohistochemistry: A useful tool in the diagnosis of Carney-Stratakis and Carney triad gastrointestinal stromal tumors. Mod. Pathol. 2011;**24**(1):147–51.

291. Coffin CM, Alaggio R. Adipose and myxoid tumors of childhood and adolescence. Pediatr. Dev. Pathol. 2012;**15**(1):239–54.

292. Xenos C, Sgouros S, Walsh R, *et al.* Spinal lipomas in children. Pediatr. Neurosurg. 2000;**32**(6):295–307.

293. Maire G, Forus A, Foa C, *et al.* 11q13 alterations in two cases of hibernoma: large heterozygous deletions and rearrangement breakpoints near GARP in 11q13.5. Genes Chromosomes Cancer 2003;**37**(4):389–95.

294. Coffin CM, Lowichik A, Putnam A. Lipoblastoma (LPB): A clinicopathologic and immunohistochemical analysis of 59 cases Am. J. Surg. Pathol. 2009;**33**(11):1705–12.

295. Hicks J, Dilley A, Patel D, *et al.* Lipoblastoma and lipoblastomatosis in infancy and childhood: histopathologic, ultrastructural, and cytogenetic features. Ultrastruct. Pathol. 2001;**25**(4):321–33.

296. Hill S, Rademaker M. A collection of rare anomalies: multiple digital glomuvenous malformations, epidermal naevus, temporal alopecia, heterochromia and abdominal lipoblastoma. Clin. Exp. Dermatol. 2009;**34**(8):e862–4.

297. Matsuyama A, Hisaoka M, Hashimoto H. PLAG1 expression in mesenchymal tumors: An immunohistochemical study with special emphasis on the pathogenetical distinction between soft tissue myoepithelioma and pleomorphic adenoma of the salivary gland. Pathol. Int. 2012;**62**(1):1–7.

298. Brandal P, Bjerkehagen B, Heim S. Rearrangement of chromosomal region 8q11–13 in lipomatous tumours: correlation with lipoblastoma morphology. J. Pathol. 2006;**208**(3):388–94.

299. Bartuma H, Domanski HA, Von Steyern FV, *et al.* Cytogenetic and molecular cytogenetic findings in lipoblastoma. Cancer Genet. Cytogenet. 2008;**183**(1):60–3.

300. Ferrari A, Casanova M, Spreafico F, *et al.* Childhood liposarcoma: A single-institutional twenty-year experience. Pediatr. Hematol. Oncol. 1999;**16**:415–21.

301. La Quaglia MP, Spiro SA, Ghavimi F, *et al.* Liposarcoma in patients younger than or equal to 22 years of age. Cancer 1993;**72**(10):3114–9.

302. Alaggio R, Coffin CM, Weiss SW, *et al.* Liposarcomas in young patients: A study of 82 cases occurring in patients younger than 22 years of age. Am. J. Surg. Pathol. 2009;**33**(5):645–58.

303. Huh WW, Yuen C, Munsell M, *et al.* Liposarcoma in children and young adults: A multi-institutional experience. Pediatr. Blood Cancer 2011;**57**(7):1142–6.

304. Antonescu CR, Elahi A, Healey JH, *et al.* Monoclonality of multifocal myxoid liposarcoma: confirmation by analysis of *TLS-CHOP* or *EWS-CHOP* rearrangements. Clin. Cancer Res. 2000;**6**(7):2788–93.

305. Debelenko LV, Perez-Atayde AR, Dubois SG, *et al. p53+/mdm2*- atypical lipomatous tumor/well-differentiated liposarcoma in young children: An early expression of Li-Fraumeni syndrome. Pediatr. Dev. Pathol. 2009;**13**:218–24.

306. Rudzinski E, Mawn L, Kuttesch J, *et al.* Orbital pleomorphic liposarcoma in an eight-year-old boy. Pediatr. Dev. Pathol. 2011;**14**:339–44.

307. Meis-Kindblom JM, Sjögren H, Kindblom LG, et al. Cytogenetic and molecular genetic analyses of liposarcoma and its soft tissue simulators: recognition of new variants and differential diagnosis. Virchows Arch. 2001;**439**(2):141–51.

308. Tallini G, Akerman M, Dal Cin P, et al. Combined morphologic and karyotypic study of 28 myxoid liposarcomas: implications for a revised morphologic typing (a report from the CHAMP group). Am. J. Surg. Pathol. 1996;**20**(9):1047–55.

309. Cates JMM, Coffin CM. Extraskeletal cartilaginous, osseous, and chordoid tumors in children and adolescents. Pediatr. Dev. Pathol. 2012;**15**(1):255–66.

310. Pollock L, Malone M, Shaw DG. Childhood soft tissue chondroma: A case report. Pediatr. Pathol. Lab. Med. 1995;**15**(3):437–41.

311. Humphreys TR, Herzberg AJ, Elenitsas R, et al. Familial occurrence of multiple cutaneous chondromas. Am. J. Dermatopathol. 1994;**16**(1):56–9.

312. Dahlén A, Mertens F, Rydholm A, et al. Fusion, disruption, and expression of HMGA2 in bone and soft tissue chondromas. Mod. Pathol. 2003;**16**(11):1132–40.

313. Tuncer S, Kebudi R, Peksayar G, et al. Congenital mesenchymal chondrosarcoma of the orbit: case report and review of the literature. Ophthalmology 2004;**111**(5):1016–22.

314. Cesari M, Bertoni F, Bacchini P, et al. Mesenchymal chondrosarcoma. An analysis of patients treated at a single institution. Tumori 2007;**93**(5):423–7.

315. Dantonello TM, Int-Veen C, Leuschner I, et al. Mesenchymal chondrosarcoma of soft tissues and bone in children, adolescents, and young adults: experiences of the CWS and COSS study groups. Cancer 2008;**112**(11):2424–31.

316. De Cecio R, Migliaccio I, Falleti J, et al. Congenital intracranial mesenchymal chondrosarcoma: case report and review of the literature in pediatric patients. Pediatr. Dev. Pathol 2008;**11**(4):309–13.

317. Granter SR, Renshaw AA, Fletcher CD, et al. CD99 reactivity in mesenchymal chondrosarcoma. Hum. Pathol. 1996;**27**(12):1273–6.

318. Fanburg-Smith JC, Auerbach A, Marwaha JS, et al. Reappraisal of mesenchymal chondrosarcoma: novel morphologic observations of the hyaline cartilage and endochondral ossification and beta-catenin, Sox9, and osteocalcin immunostaining of 22 cases. Hum. Pathol. 2010;**41**(5):653–62.

319. Fanburg-Smith JC, Auerbach A, Marwaha JS, et al. Immunoprofile of mesenchymal chondrosarcoma: Aberrant desmin and EMA expression, retention of INI-1, and negative estrogen receptor in 22 female-predominant central nervous system and musculoskeletal cases. Ann. Diagn. Pathol. 2010;**14**(1):8–14.

320. Kauffman SL, Stout AP. Extraskeletal osteogenic sarcomas and chondrosarcomas in children. Cancer 1963;**16**:432–9.

321. Humphrey GM, Brown I, Squire R, et al. Extraosseous osteogenic sarcoma: A rare pediatric malignancy: case report and review of the literature. J. Pediatr. Surg. 1999;**34**(6):1025–8.

322. Ridenour III RV, Ahrens WA, Folpe AL, et al. Clinical and histopathologic features of chordomas in children and young adults. Pediatr. Dev. Pathol. 2010;**13**:9–17.

323. Coffin CM, Swanson PE, Wick MR, et al. Chordoma in childhood and adolescence. A clinicopathologic analysis of 12 cases. Arch. Pathol. Lab. Med. 1993;**117**(9):927–33.

324. Tirabosco R, Mangham DC, Rosenberg AE, et al. Brachyury expression in extra-axial skeletal and soft tissue chordomas: A marker that distinguishes chordoma from mixed tumor/myoepithelioma/parachordoma in soft tissue. Am. J. Surg. Pathol. 2008;**32**(4):572–80.

325. McMaster ML, Goldstein AM, Parry DM. Clinical features distinguish childhood chordoma associated with tuberous sclerosis complex (TSC) from chordoma in the general paediatric population. J. Med. Genet. 2011;**48**(7):444–9.

326. Coffin CM, Swanson PE, Wick MR, et al. An immunohistochemical comparison of chordoma with renal cell carcinoma, colorectal adenocarcinoma, and myxopapillary ependymoma: A potential diagnostic dilemma in the diminutive biopsy. Mod. Pathol. 1993;**6**(5):531–8.

327. Yamaguchi T, Suzuki S, Ishiiwa H, et al. Benign notochordal cell tumors: A comparative histological study of benign notochordal cell tumors, classic chordomas, and notochordal vestiges of fetal intervertebral discs. Am. J. Surg. Pathol. 2004;**28**(6):756–61.

328. Tsokos M, Alaggio RD, Dehner LP, et al. Ewing sarcoma/peripheral primitive neuroectodermal tumor and related tumors. Pediatr. Dev. Pathol. 2012;**15**(1):108–26.

329. Ludwig JA. Ewing sarcoma: historical perspectives, current state-of-the-art, and opportunities for targeted therapy in the future. Curr. Opin. Oncol. 2008;**20**(4):412–8.

330. Pierron G, Tirode F, Lucchesi C, et al. A new subtype of bone sarcoma defined by BCOR-CCNB3 gene fusion. Nat. Genet. 2012;**44**(4):461–6.

331. Terrier-Lacombe MJ, Guillou L, Chibon F, et al. Superficial primitive Ewing's sarcoma: A clinicopathologic and molecular cytogenetic analysis of 14 cases. Mod. Pathol. 2009;**22**:87–94.

332. Spunt SL, Rodriguez-Galindo C, Fuller CE, et al. Ewing sarcoma-family tumors that arise after treatment of primary childhood cancer. Cancer 2006;**107**:201–6.

333. Folpe AL, Goldblum JR, Rubin BP, *et al.* Morphologic and immunophenotypic diversity in Ewing family tumors: A study of 66 genetically confirmed cases. Am. J. Surg. Pathol. 2005;**29**;1025–33.

334. Machado I, Noguera R, Mateos EA, *et al.* The many faces of atypical Ewing's sarcoma. A true entity mimicking sarcomas, carcinomas and lymphomas. Virchows Arch. 2011;**458**:281–90.

335. Bacci G, Ferrari S, Bertoni F, *et al.* Prognostic factors in nonmetastatic Ewing's sarcoma of bone treated with adjuvant chemotherapy: Analysis of 359 patients at the Istituto Ortopedico Rizzoli. J. Clin. Oncol. 2000;**18**:4–11.

336. Barisella M, Collini P, Orsenigo M, *et al.* Unusual myogenic and melanocytic differentiation of soft tissue pPNETS: An immunohistochemical and molecular study of 3 cases. Am. J. Surg. Pathol. 2010;**34**:1002–6. u7. 319.

337. Barr FG, Womer RB. Molecular diagnosis of Ewing family tumors. Too many translocations . . .? J. Mol. Diagn. 2007;**9**:437–40.

338. Folpe AL, Hill CE, Parham DM, *et al.* Immunohistochemical detection of FLI-1 protein expression: A study of 132 round-cell tumors with emphasis on CD99-positive mimics of Ewing's sarcoma/primitive neuroectodermal tumor. Am. J. Surg. Pathol. 2000;**24**:1657–62.

339. Llombart-Bosch A, Navarro S, Immunohistochemical detection of EWS and FLI-1 proteins in Ewing sarcoma and primitive neuroectodermal tumors: comparative analysis with CD99 (MIC-2) expression. Appl. Immunohistochem. Mol. Morphol. 2001;**9**:255–60.

340. Mhawech-Fauceglia P, Herrmann F, Penetrante R, *et al.* Diagnostic utility of FLI-1 monoclonal antibody and dual-colour, break-apart probe fluorescence in situ (FISH) analysis in Ewing's sarcoma/primitive neuroectodermal tumour (EWS/PNET). A comparative study with CD99 and FLI-1 polyclonal antibodies. Histopathology 2006;**49**:569–75.

341. Bisogno G, Roganovich J, Sotti G, *et al.* Desmoplastic small round cell tumour in children and adolescents. Med. Pediatr. Oncol. 2000;**34**(5):338–42.

342. Chang F. Desmoplastic small round-cell tumors: Cytologic, histologic, and immunohistochemical features. Arch. Pathol. Lab. Med. 2006;**130**(5):728–32.

343. Gerald WL, Miller HK, Battifora H, *et al.* Intra-abdominal desmoplastic small round-cell tumor: Report of 19 cases of a distinctive type of high-grade polyphenotypic malignancy affecting young individuals. Am. J. Surg. Pathol. 1991;**15**:499–513.

344. Saab R, Khoury JD, Krasin M, *et al.* Desmoplastic small round-cell tumor in childhood: The St. Jude Children's Research Hospital experience. Pediatr. Blood Cancer 2007;**49**:274–9.

345. Dim DC, Cooley LD, Miranda RN. Clear cell sarcoma of tendons and aponeuroses: A review. Arch. Pathol. Lab. Med. 2007;**131**(1):152–6.

346. Ferrari A, Casanova M, Bisogno G, *et al.* Clear cell sarcoma of tendons and aponeuroses in pediatric patients: A report from the Italian and German Soft Tissue Sarcoma Cooperative Group. Cancer 2002;**12**:3269–76.

347. Hisaoka M, Ishida T, Kuo TT, *et al.* Clear cell sarcoma of soft tissue: A clinicopathologic, immunohistochemical, and molecular analysis of 33 cases. Am. J. Surg. Pathol. 2008;**32**:452–60.

348. Meis-Kindblom JM. Clear cell sarcoma of tendons and aponeuroses: A historical perspective and tribute to the man behind the entity. Adv. Anat. Pathol. 2006;**13** (6):286–92.

349. Coindre JM, Hostein I, Terrier P, *et al.* Diagnosis of clear cell sarcoma by real-time reverse transcriptase-polymerase chain reaction analysis of paraffin embedded tissues: clinicopathologic and molecular analysis of 44 patients from the French sarcoma group. Cancer 2006;**107**:1055–64.

350. Granville L, Hicks J, Popek E, *et al.* Visceral clear cell sarcoma of the soft tissue with confirmation by *EWTS-ATF1* fusion detection. Ultrastruct. Pathol. 2006;**30**:111–8.

351. Joo M, Chang SH, Kim H, *et al.* Primary gastrointestinal clear cell sarcoma: report of 2 cases, one case associated with IgG4-related sclerosing disease, and review of literature. Ann. Diagn. Pathol. 2009;**13** (1):30–5.

352. Antonescu CR, Argani P, Erlandson RA, *et al.* Skeletal and extraskeletal myxoid chondrosarcoma: A comparative clinicopathologic, ultrastructural, and molecular study. Cancer 1998;**83**(8):1504–21.

353. Hachitanda Y, Tsuneyoshi M, Daimaru Y, *et al.* Extraskeletal myxoid chondrosarcoma in young children. Cancer 1988;**61**:2521–6.

354. Meis-Kindblom JM, Bergh P, Gunterberg B, *et al.* Extraskeletal myxoid chondrosarcoma: A reappraisal of its morphologic spectrum and prognostic factors based on 117 cases. Am. J. Surg. Pathol. 1999;**23**:636–50.

355. Okamoto S, Hisaoka M, Ishida T, *et al.* Extraskeletal myxoid chondrosarcoma: A clinicopathologic, immunohistochemical, and molecular analysis of 18 cases. Hum. Pathol. 2001;**32**:1116–24.

356. Panagopoulos I, Mencinger M, Dietrich CU, *et al.* Fusion of the *RBP56* and CHN genes in extraskeletal myxoid chondrosarcomas with translocation t(9;17) (q22;q11). Oncogene 1999;**18**(52):7594–8.

357. Ren L, Guo SP, Zhou XG, *et al.* Angiomatoid fibrous histiocytoma: first report of primary pulmonary origin. Am. J. Surg. Pathol. 2009;**33**(10):1570–4.

358. Fanburg-Smith JC, Miettinen M. Angiomatoid "malignant" fibrous histiocytoma: A clinicopathologic study of 158 cases and further exploration of the myoid phenotype. Hum. Pathol. 1999;30(11):1336–43.

359. Antonescu CR, Dal Cin P, Nafa K, et al. EWSR1-CREB1 is the predominant gene fusion in angiomatoid fibrous histiocytoma. Genes Chromosomes Cancer 2007;46(12):1051–60.

360. Thway K. Angiomatoid fibrous histiocytoma: A review with recent genetic findings. Arch. Pathol. Lab. Med. 2008;132(2):273–7.

361. Shao L, Singh V, Cooley L. Angiomatoid fibrous histiocytoma with t(2;22) (q33;q12.2) and EWSR1 gene rearrangement. Pediatr. Dev. Pathol. 2009;12(2):143–6.

362. Yoshimoto M, Graham C, Chilton-MacNeill S, et al. Detailed cytogenetic and array analysis of pediatric primitive sarcomas reveals a recurrent CIC-DUX4 fusion gene event. Cancer Genet Cytogenet 2009;195:1–11.

363. Italiano A, Sung YS, Zhang L, et al. High prevalence of CIC fusion with Double-Homeobox (DUX4) transcription factors in EWSR1-negative undifferentiated small blue round cell sarcomas. Genes Chromosomes Cancer 2012;51(3):207–18.

364. Gleason BC, Fletcher CD. Myoepithelial carcinoma of soft tissue in children: An aggressive neoplasm analyzed in a series of 29 cases. Am. J. Surg. Pathol. 2007;31:1813–24.

365. Gleason BC, Hornick JL. Myoepithelial tumours of skin and soft tissue: An update. Diagn. Histopathol. 2008;14:552–62.

366. Hornick JL, Fletcher CDM. Myoepithelial tumors of soft tissue. A clinicopathologic and immunohistochemical study of 101 cases with evaluation of prognostic parameters. Am. J. Surg. Pathol. 2003;27(9):1183–96.

367. Antonescu CR, Zhang L, Chang NE, et al. EWSR1-POU5F1 fusion in soft tissue myoepithelial tumors: A molecular analysis of sixty-six cases, including soft tissue, bone, and visceral lesions, showing common involvement of the EWSR1 gene. Genes Chromosomes Cancer 2010;49:1114–24.

368. Amary MF, Berisha F, Bernardi F del C, et al. Detection of SS18-SSX fusion transcripts in formalin-fixed paraffin-embedded neoplasms: Analysis of conventional RT-PCR, qRT-PCR and dual color FISH as diagnostic tools for synovial sarcoma. Mod. Pathol. 2007;20:482–96.

369. Ferrari A, Gronchi A, Casanova M, et al. Synovial sarcoma: A retrospective analysis of 271 patients of all ages treated at a single institution. Cancer 2004;101(3):627–34.

370. Sultan I, Rodriguez-Galindo C, Saab R, et al. Comparing children and adults with synovial sarcoma

371. Michal M, Fanburg-Smith JC, Lasota J, et al. Minute synovial sarcomas of the hands and feet: A clinicopathologic study of 21 tumors less than 1 cm. Am. J. Surg. Pathol. 2006;30:721–6.

372. Jagdis A, Rubin BP, Tubbs RR, et al. Prospective evaluation of TLE1 as a diagnostic immunohistochemical marker in synovial sarcoma. Am. J. Surg. Pathol. 2009;33:1743–51.

373. Pelmus M, Guillou L, Hostein E, et al. Monophasic fibrous and poorly differentiated synovial sarcoma: Immunohistochemical reassessment of 60 t(X;18) (SYT-SSX)-positive cases. Am. J. Surg. Pathol. 2002;26:1434–40.

374. Lewis JJ, Antonescu CR, Leung DH, et al. Synovial sarcoma: A multivariate analysis of prognostic factors in 112 patients with primary localized tumors of the extremity. J. Clin. Oncol. 2000;18(10):2087–94.

375. Okcu MF, Munsell M, Treuner J, et al. Synovial sarcoma of childhood and adolescence: Amulticenter, multivariate analysis of outcome. J. Clin. Oncol. 2003;21:1602–11.

376. Casanova M, Ferrari A, Bisogno G, et al. Alveolar soft part sarcoma in children and adolescents: A report from the Soft-Tissue Sarcoma Italian Cooperative Group. Ann. Oncol. 2000;11(11):1445–9.

377. Fanburg-Smith JC, Miettinen M, Folpe AL, et al. Lingual alveolar soft part sarcoma; 14 cases: novel, clinical, and morphological observations. Histopathology 2004;45:526–37.

378. Folpe AL, Deyrup AT. Alveolar soft-part sarcoma: A review and update. J. Clin. Pathol. 2006;59(11):1127–32.

379. Kayton ML, Meyers P, Wexler LH, et al. Clinical presentation, treatment, and outcome of alveolar soft part sarcoma in children, adolescents, and young adults. J. Pediatr. Surg. 2006;41:187–93.

380. Aulmann S, Longerich T, Schirmacher P, et al. Detection of the ASPSCR1-TFE3 gene fusion in paraffin-embedded alveolar soft part sarcomas. Histopathology 2007;50(7):881–6.

381. Ladanyi M, Lui MY, Antonescu CR, et al. The der (17)t (X;17)(p11;q25) of human alveolar soft part sarcoma fuses the TFE3 transcription factor gene to ASPL, a novel gene at 17q25. Oncogene 2001;20:48–57.

382. Pang LJ, Chang B, Zou H, et al. Alveolar soft part sarcoma: A bimarker diagnostic strategy using TFE3 immunoassay and ASPL-TFE3 fusion transcripts in paraffin-embedded tumor tissues. Diagn. Mol. Pathol. 2008;17(4):245–52.

383. Williams A, Bartle G, Sumathi VP, et al. Detection of ASPL/TFE3 fusion transcripts and the TFE3 antigen in

in the Surveillance, Epidemiology, and End Results program, 1983 to 2005: An analysis of 1268 patients. Cancer 2009;115(15):3537–47.

formalin-fixed, paraffin-embedded tissue in a series of 18 cases of alveolar soft part sarcoma: Useful diagnostic tools in cases with unusual histological features. Virchows Arch. 2011;**458**:291–300.

384. Armah HB, Parwani AV. Epithelioid sarcoma. Arch. Pathol. Lab. Med. 2009;**133**(5):814–9.

385. Casanova M, Ferrari A, Collini P, *et al.* Epithelioid sarcoma in children and adolescents: A report from the Italian Soft Tissue Sarcoma Committee. Cancer 2006;**106**:708–17.

386. Chbani L, Guillou L, Terrier P, *et al.* Epithelioid sarcoma: A clinicopathologic and immunohistochemical analysis of 106 cases from the French sarcoma group. Am. J. Surg. Pathol. 2009;**131**:222–7.

387. Schmidt D, Harms D. Epithelioid sarcoma in children and adolescents: An immunohistochemical study. Virchows Arch. A Pathol. Anat. Histopathol. 1987;**410**:423–31.

388. Hornick JL, Dal Cin P, Fletcher CDM. Loss of INI1 expression is characteristic of both conventional and proximal-type epithelioid sarcoma. Am. J. Surg. Pathol. 2009;**33**(4):542–50.

389. Kohashi K, Izumi T, Oda Y, *et al.* Infrequent *SMARCB1/INI1* gene alteration in epithelioid sarcoma: A useful tool in distinguishing epithelioid sarcoma from malignant rhabdoid tumor. Hum. Pathol. 2009;**40**(3):349 55.

390. White FV, Dehner LP, Belchis DA, *et al.* Congenital disseminated malignant rhabdoid tumor: A distinct clinicopathologic entity demonstrating abnormalities of chromosome 22q11. Am. J. Surg. Pathol. 1999;**23**:249–56.

391. Alaggio R, Boldrini R, di Venosa B, *et al.* Pediatric extrarenal rhabdoid tumors with unusual morphology: A diagnostic pitfall for small biopsies. Pathol. Res. Pract. 2009;**205**:451–7.

392. Bourdeaut F, Lequin D, Brugieres L, *et al.* Frequent *hSNF5/INI1* germline mutations in patients with rhabdoid tumor. Clin. Cancer Res. 2011;**17**:31–8.

393. Oda Y, Tsuneyoshi M. Extrarenal rhabdoid tumors of soft tissue: clinicopathological and molecular genetic review and distinction from other soft tissue sarcomas with rhabdoid features. Pathol. Int. 2006;**56**(6):287–95.

394. Hoot AC, Russo P, Judkins AR, *et al.* Immunohistochemical analysis of hSNF5/INI1 distinguishes renal and extra-renal malignant rhabdoid tumors from other pediatric soft tissue tumors. Am. J. Surg. Pathol. 2004;**28**:1485–91.

395. Judkins AR. Immunohistochemistry of INI1 expression: A new tool for old challenges in CNS and soft tissue pathology. Adv. Anat. Pathol. 2007;**14**(5):335–9.

396. Machado I, Noguera R, Santonja N, *et al.* Immunohistochemical study as a tool in differential diagnosis of pediatric malignant rhabdoid tumor. Appl. Immunohistochem. Mol. Morphol. 2010;**18**:150–8.

397. Sigauke E, Rakheja D, Maddox DL, *et al.* Absence of expression of SMARCB1/INI1 in malignant rhabdoid tumors of the central nervous system, kidneys and soft tissue: An immunohistochemical study with implications for diagnosis. Mod. Pathol. 2006;**19**:717–25.

398. Graadt van Roggen JF, Hogendoorn PCW, Fletcher CDM. Myxoid tumours of soft tissue. Histopathology 1999;**35**:291–312.

399. White J, Chan YF. Aggressive angiomyxoma of the vulva in an 11-year-old girl. Pediatr. Pathol. 1994;**14**:27–37.

400. Calonje E, Guerin D, McCormick D, *et al.* Superficial angiomyxoma: Clinicopathologic analysis of a series of distinctive but poorly recognized cutaneous tumors with tendency for recurrence. Am. J. Surg. Pathol. 1999;**23**:910–79.

401. Alaggio R, Bisogno G, Rosato A, *et al.* Undifferentiated sarcoma: Does it exist? A clinicopathologic study of 7 pediatric cases and review of literature. Hum. Pathol. 2009;**40**(11):1600–10.

402. Pawel BR, Hamoudi AB, Asmar L, *et al.* Undifferentiated sarcomas of children: pathology and clinical behavior. An Intergroup Rhabdomyosarcoma Study. Med. Pediatr. Oncol. 1997;**29**:170–80.

403. Somers GR, Gupta AA, Doria AS, *et al.* Pediatric undifferentiated sarcoma of the soft tissues: A clinicopathologic study. Pediatr. Dev. Pathol. 2006;**9**(2):132–42.

404. Raney RB, Anderson JR, Barr FG, *et al.* Rhabdomyosarcoma and undifferentiated sarcoma in the first two decades of life: A selective review of Intergroup Rhabdomyosarcoma Study Group experience and rationale for Intergroup Rhabdomyosarcoma Study V. J. Pediatr. Hematol. Oncol. 2001;**23**(4):215–220.

405. Alaggio R, Rosolen A, Sartori F, *et al.* Spindle cell tumor with EWS-WT1 transcript and a favorable clinical course: A variant of DSCT, a variant of leiomyosarcoma, or a new entity? Report of 2 pediatric cases. Am. J. Surg. Pathol. 2007;**31**:454–9.

406. Kreiger PA, Judkins AR, Russo PA, *et al.* Loss of INI1 expression defines a unique subset of pediatric undifferentiated soft tissue sarcomas. Mod. Pathol. 2009;**22**(1):142–50.

Chapter 12

Bone and joint lesions

Paul S. Dickman and Julie C. Fanburg-Smith

Introduction

Bone lesions are different from all other specimens. They carry within them a record of their growth history and previous behavior that is detectable by clinical and specimen radiology. The information in radiologic imaging is critical to understanding and interpreting the microscopic findings. It is not necessary to be an expert in radiology, but it is important to utilize the services of a musculoskeletal radiologist. A radiologic review should always be obtained when evaluating the pathology of these lesions, even if the histological, immunohistochemical, and other features are thought to be diagnostic. Clinical radiology becomes the gross pathology. This review often provides information that is not available in any other way. Because of this special role of radiology, including X-ray, CT, and MRI, radiologic findings are listed and referred to for most of the lesions discussed in this chapter.

The brief discussions of the entities in this chapter are intended to be introductions. For more detail the reader is referred to standard textbooks listed under References(1–6).

Bone tumors and tumor-like lesions

Chondrogenic tumors

Osteochondroma (OC)

The most common benign bone tumor, OC is a benign reactive osteocartilaginous external projection occurring on the surface of bone as a displaced fragment of growth plate creating long-bone-like growth. It can be solitary, or multiple in hereditary multiple exostoses (HME)(7).

Clinical presentation: The sporadic (solitary) form of OC is six times more common than the HME

syndrome, which has an incidence of 1:50 000 persons. The age of presentation is usually < 20 years. Patients are generally asymptomatic. Osteochondromas are removed with their overlying periosteum only if causing mechanical or cosmetic issues, or if the lesion has a fracture, non-union, or malignant transformation. Common locations include metaphyseal femur (30%), usually around the knee, tibia (20%), humerus (20%), hand and foot (10%), pelvis (5%), and scapula (4%). Rare malignant transformation may occur in HME.

Genetics: Loss of distal 8q has been described (8). Males are more commonly affected with multiple OC than females, due to incomplete penetrance in females for the *EXT1* and *EXT2* genes, located respectively at 8q24 and 11p11–12.

Macroscopy: Osteochondroma may be sessile or pedunculated and usually points at a 45° angle from the joint. The cartilaginous cap thickness is often visualized by radiologic imaging (Figure 12.1). In children, the benign cartilage cap thickness may be > 3 cm. Continuity of cortex and medullary space with host cortex and marrow is diagnostic. Periosteum overlies the cartilaginous cap.

Histology: Host cortex and marrow are continuous with the lesion, with a cauliflower-like cartilaginous cap of varying thickness and overlying periosteum (Figure 12.2). Growth plate may be present, simulating normal long bone.

Enchondroma (EC)

This is a common benign cartilaginous tumor occurring in trabecular or cortical bone. It can also be periosteal or present in soft tissue (7).

Clinical presentation: Enchondroma is common in small tubular bones and less common in long bones, more common in males, particularly in multiple EC

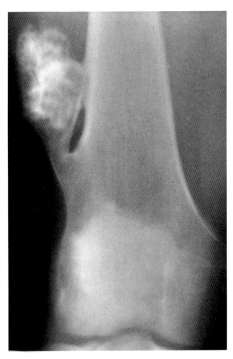

Figure 12.1 Osteochondroma (imaging). Lesion projects from cortical surface with continuity of medulla and cortex.

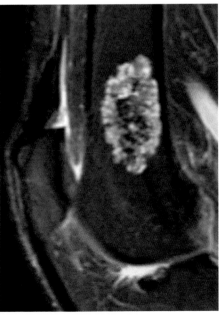

Figure 12.3 Enchondroma (imaging). Lesion is medullary with C- and O-shaped calcifications.

(Maffucci; Ollier). Most ECs remain benign, but up to a third of patients with multiple ECs experience malignant transformation. They rarely cause pain unless associated with a fracture; in the absence of fracture,

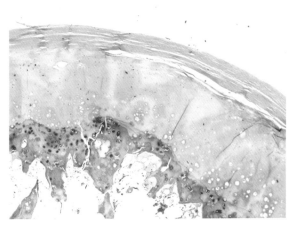

Figure 12.2 Osteochondroma. The cartilage cap thickness is usually no more than 3 cm in children, often excised with overlying periosteum (H&E × 20).

pain is a more ominous sign of malignancy. Patients with multiple ECs may have purely intracortical chondromas. Periosteal chondroma causes saucerization of cortex. Soft-tissue chondroma is most commonly found in the hands and feet (see Chapter 11). So-called pulmonary chondroma, part of the Carney triad, is better considered a hamartoma. Ollier disease is a developmental failure of normal endochondral ossification with multiple metaphyseal cartilaginous tumors. Maffucci syndrome consists of enchondromatosis plus spindle-cell hemangio(endothelio)mas, benign soft-tissue vascular tumors that often overlie bony lesions. On imaging, EC are lytic lesions with popcorn-like and C- and O-shaped calcifications due to peripheral lobular endochondral ossification (Figure 12.3; 9).

Genetics: *IDH1* and *IDH2* mutations are associated with EC in syndromes including Ollier disease, Maffucci syndrome, and D-2-hydroxyglutaric aciduria (10).

Macroscopy: Small tubular bone (finger) lesions can erode cortex, but are still contained within periosteum; long-bone lesions, by definition, do not cause endosteal scalloping of more than two-thirds of the cortical thickness.

Histology: Enchondroma is characterized by lobules of mature hyaline cartilage with pink endochondral ossification at the lobular periphery (Figure 12.4). Binucleation, myxoid change, mild cytologic atypia and increased cellularity may occur, particularly in finger lesions (Figure 12.5). A permeative growth pattern with host bone entrapment or skip lesions involving Haversian canal or cortical breakthrough to soft tissue

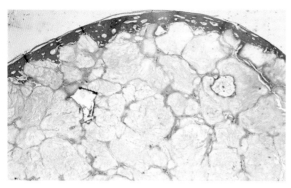

Figure 12.4 Enchondroma. Lesion is composed of hyaline cartilage lobules with endochondral ossification at periphery. Usually no soft tissue involvement is seen unless fracture occurs (H&E × 10).

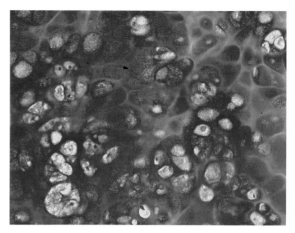

Figure 12.5 Enchondroma. Little cytologic atypia is seen except for myxoid areas in finger lesions. Rare binuceation may be present, but one cell per lacuna and absence of enlarged nuclei are the norm (H&E × 60).

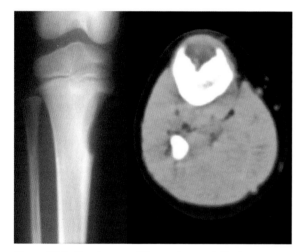

Figure 12.6 Chondromyxoid fibroma (imaging). The lesion is eccentric and metaphyseal.

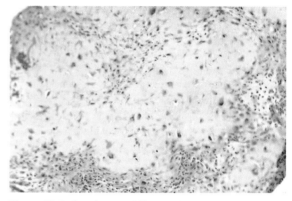

Figure 12.7 Chondromyxoid fibroma. The lesion has a peripheral condensation of cells and central, mildly atypical stellate cells embedded in a chondromyxoid matrix (H&E × 40).

should not be present; the latter may be observed with fracture, still retained within periosteum.

Chondromyxoid fibroma (CMF)

Chondromyxoid fibroma, a benign tumor composed of lobules of stellate cells in a chondromyxoid stroma, is the rarest of cartilage tumors (7).

Clinical presentation: Chondromyxoid fibroma is usually found in the lower extremity with 55% around the knee, most commonly proximal tibia, and 20–25% in the foot. Rib and ilium can also be involved. Most patients are < 30 years old, with male predominance. Pain for several years is the most common symptom. Radiologically, CMF is eccentric, often intracortical, and metaphyseal with a high signal on T2-weighted MRI (Figure 12.6). Rare matrix can be observed. Curettage with bone grafting is the usual treatment.

Genetics: Complex unbalanced rearrangements of chromosome 6q have been described (8,11).

Macroscopy: Chondromyxoid fibroma is multilobular, with scalloped margins and septations, and is fibrous, rather than glistening gray-white like other cartilage tumors.

Histology: Lobules of peripherally cellular and centrally hypocellular stellate cells in a chondromyxoid stroma are characteristic, although varying proportions and arrangements of these features as well as calcification, giant cells, and hyaline cartilage can be present (Figure 12.7). Aneurysmal bone cyst (ABC) may be seen in 10% of cases. S100 protein positivity may be present.

Differential diagnosis: Because of cytologic atypia, CMF can be histologically worrisome for malignancy.

399

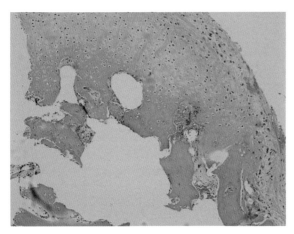

Figure 12.8 Subungual exostosis. The appearance is of osteochondromatous proliferation with areas of enlarged, hyperchromatic nuclei that may suggest malignancy (H&E × 20).

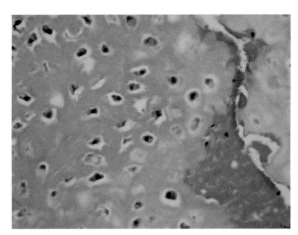

Figure 12.9 Bizarre parosteal osteochondromatous proliferation. Fibrous, cartilaginous, and bony components with cytologic atypia are present (H&E × 60).

Subungual exostosis (SE)

Subungual exostosis is a subungual reactive osteocartilaginous proliferation without cortical or marrow continuity, usually arising in the large toe.

Clinical presentation: Most patients are adolescent or young adults with a few months' symptoms of rapid growth, sometimes after trauma. Radiologically, SE occurs subungually at the dorsal distal tip of the distal phalanx and may not initially appear attached to bone.

Genetics: t(X;6)(q22;q13–14) is unique to the lesion, with deregulation of the insulin receptor substrate 4 (*IRS4*) gene (12).

Macroscopy: Osteocartilaginous surface or soft-tissue proliferation is seen under the nail of the dorsal distal phalanx.

Histology: Subungual exostosis is initially fibrous, with fibrocartilaginous metaplasia that ossifies and progresses to a calcified and cartilaginous osteochondromatous proliferation with no cortical or marrow continuity (Figure 12.8). The lesion can be quite florid and histologically worrisome.

Differential diagnosis: The features may overlap bizarre parosteal osteochondromatous proliferation (BPOP) with blue bizarre cartilage. Osteochondroma, florid reactive periostitis, Turret exostosis, fibroosseous pseudotumor of digit (FOPD), and other subungual lesions may be considered.

Bizarre parosteal osteochondromatous proliferation (BPOP), Nora lesion

This is a rare reactive process of the proximal and middle phalanges on a spectrum with reactive florid periostitis and Turret exostosis. It may be related to subungual exostosis, with histologic overlap with FOPD (13,14).

Clinical presentation: Bizarre parosteal osteochondromatous proliferation is most common in the proximal and mid-phalanges of the hand, but can also be in the feet and long bones. It is a surface process with no continuity with host cortex or marrow. The recurrence rate can be high after excision.

Genetics: t(1;17)(q32;q21) and other translocations involving 1q32 have been described (15).

Macroscopy: The lesion is on the mid- to proximal phalangeal surface, without cortical or marrow continuity.

Histology: Bizarre parosteal osteochondromatous proliferation displays fibrous tissue, cellular bizarre blue bone, and cartilage, with cytologic atypia (Figure 12.9).

Differential diagnosis: Subungual exostosis, reactive periostitis, Turret exostosis, and FOPD may be considered, depending on location and histology.

Synovial chondromatosis (SC)

Primary SC is a multifold cartilaginous proliferation occurring in synovium, joints, bursae, or tendon sheaths. Secondary SC arises in traumatic conditions such as degenerative joint disease (DJD), Charcot joints, and other traumatic lesions (16–18).

Clinical presentation: Pain, painless swelling, or locking of joint may be seen.

Genetics: Trisomy 5 and 12q13–15 abnormalities have been described (8).

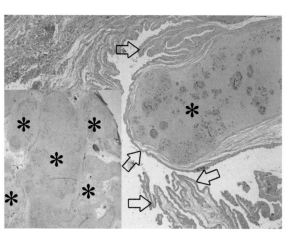

Figure 12.10 Synovial osteochondromatosis. In primary disease, multiple lobules of hyaline cartilage and bone are embedded in synovium (H&E × 20).

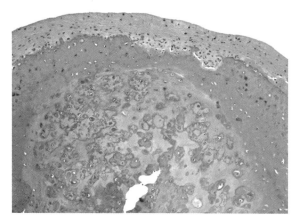

Figure 12.11 Synovial osteochondromatosis. Secondary synovial osteochondromatosis is similar in appearance to primary disease with formation of osteocartilaginous loose bodies (H&E × 10).

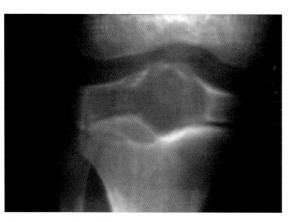

Figure 12.12 Chondroblastoma (imaging). The lesion is characteristically a radiolucent well-circumscribed epiphyseal mass.

Macroscopy: Multiple glistening bluish-white ovoid lobules vary from 0.1 to several cm.

Histology: Lesions consist of multiple hyaline cartilage nodules covered by synovium (Figures 12.10 and 12.11). Peripheral bone may be seen (synovial osteochondromatosis). Chondroblasts can be cellular and atypical, but mitoses, necrosis, and osseous invasion are not observed (19).

Differential diagnosis: Chondroma of soft parts is a solitary nodule usually occurring in hands and feet with no synovial association. Chondrosarcoma (CS) can rarely arise in SC, but shows bony invasion.

Chondroblastoma (CBL)

Chondroblastoma is a benign epiphyseal cartilaginous tumor, usually in skeletally immature patients (7).

Clinical presentation: Chondroblastoma usually occurs between the ages of 5 and 25 years with a male predilection. Aneurysmal bone cyst (ABC) may be a secondary finding in 30%, with fluid-fluid levels on imaging; typical chondroid imaging characteristics are not observed and an intermediate T2 signal may simulate malignancy. Usually extensive surrounding edema is present with joint effusion in half the patients. Chondroblastomas are lytic and often central or eccentric in epiphysis, with minimal secondary metaphyseal extension (Figure 12.12). Proximal femur, followed by distal femur, proximal tibia, and humerus are common sites. It can also occur in acetabulum and ilium and is usually solitary, although two lesions have been reported. Patients may present with pain of long duration. More aggressive clinical and histologic features may indicate resection vs. curettage and grafting.

Genetics: Recurrent breakpoints at 2q35, 3q21–23, and 18q21 have been identified (11).

Macroscopy: Chondroblastomas can have very aggressive growth patterns including so-called "benign metastasizing" features. Tan-white tissue with cyst formation may be seen on curettage.

Histology: Classic features of CBL include chondroblasts with ovoid primitive reniform nuclei and eccentric plump eosinophilic cytoplasm, multinucleated osteoclast-like giant cells with fewer nuclei than giant-cell tumor of bone, and chicken-wire calcification around individual chondroblasts (Figures 12.13 and 12.14). Approximately 30% display secondary ABC. Involvement of joint, normal-appearing mitoses, vascular invasion and soft-tissue involvement (after fracture) all correlate with aggressive behavior. Malignancy

401

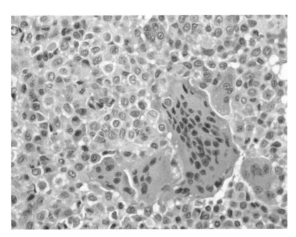

Figure 12.13 Chondroblastoma. The typical appearance demonstrates chondroblasts and osteoclast type giant cells (H&E × 20).

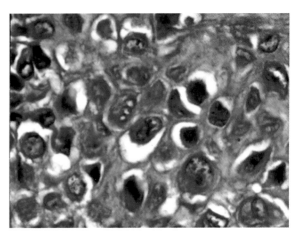

Figure 12.14 Chondroblastoma. Higher magnification shows chicken-wire calcification around and between chondroblasts (H&E × 40).

may be considered with metastasis. Lesions are positive for S100 protein, and negative for langerin and CD1a.

Differential diagnosis: Radiologically, an epiphyseal-centered lesion with sclerotic rim and edema separate CBL from giant-cell tumor of bone (GCTB); the latter is a metaphyseal-centered tumor, extending to the end of bones in adults (closed growth plate). Histologically chondroblasts can resemble Langerhans histiocytes and the giant cells may prompt a diagnosis of GCTB; langerin and CD1a staining in the former, and S100 protein in the latter are helpful for differential diagnosis. Sometimes aggressive CBL can be difficult to distinguish from clear-cell CS, but they are distunguishable by careful attention to morphologic detail.

Chondrosarcoma (CS)

Chondrosarcoma is a malignant tumor of chondroblastic phenotype (20,21).

Clinical presentation: Most CSs occur in older adults with a male predilection. Children may have CS arising secondarily in EC syndromes such as Maffucci or Ollier. Chondrosarcoma can also rarely arise from SC or OC. Conventional (hyaline or myxoid) CS is painful and generally found in an axial central location and sometimes in proximal long bones, occasionally with pathologic fracture. Mesenchymal CS is most common in young adults with female predominance, more frequent in bone than soft tissue. Locations include long bone and axial skeleton, including skull. Rarely myxoid CS can be intraosseous.

Subtypes: Conventional CS, including hyaline, is usually low grade; myxoid CS usually has increased

cellularity and intermediate grade; peripheral spindling indicates high-grade CS. Dedifferentiated CS consists of a low-grade CS adjacent to malignant fibrous histiocytoma (MFH)-like spindle-cell sarcoma. Secondary CS arises in benign cartilage tumors; mesenchymal CS has low-grade hyaline areas of metaplastic cartilage adjacent to small round blue cells with hemangiopericytoma-like vessels. Myxoid CS may be primary in bone.

Genetics: Trisomy 7 has been described (8,11). *EWS* translocation is characteristic of extraskeletal myxoid CS.

Macroscopy: Radiologically, hyaline CS is a destructive axial tumor that involves bone and soft tissue. Cartilaginous areas are white-gray and glistening (Figure 12.15).

Histology: Conventional CS is composed of hyaline cartilage with increased cellularity, enlarged nuclei, binucleation or mulitnucleation (within lacunae), and cell drop-out (necrosis). Growth characteristics of malignant cartilaginous tumor include trabecular entrapment with displacement and engulfment of host trabeculae, so that host trabecular bone is surrounded by tumor (Figures 12.16 and 12.17). Skip involvement of Haversian canals and soft-tissue involvement by intraosseous tumor may be seen. All cartilage tumors are positive for SOX9, a master regulator of chondrogenesis. S100 protein is also positive; CD57 and neuron-specific enolase (NSE) may be positive and keratins are negative.

Differential diagnosis: The most important consideration is EC vs. CS. Chondroblastic osteosarcoma (OS) in patients under 25 vs. CS of

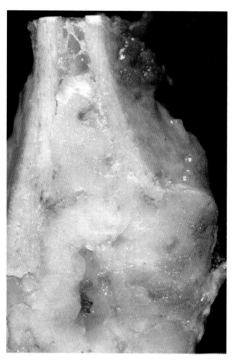

Figure 12.15 Chondrosarcoma. A tumor in a long bone has cortical scalloping and breakthrough.

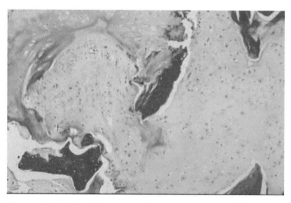

Figure 12.17 Chondrosarcoma. Entrapment consists of breaking off of surrounding host bone by tumor (H&E × 30).

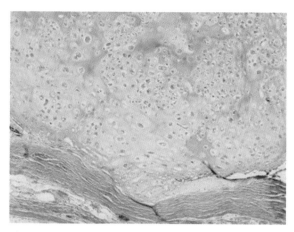

Figure 12.16 Chondrosarcoma. Features of malignancy include enlarged binucleate or multinucleate cells, hypercellularity, high nuclear:cytoplasmic ratio, and cell drop-out (H&E × 20).

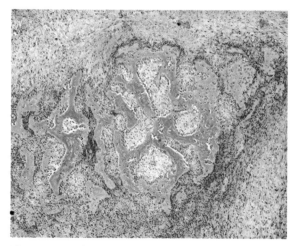

Figure 12.18 Fibro-osseous pseudotumor of digit. Mature woven bone with osteoblastic rimming is seen (H&E × 20).

Osteogenic lesions

Fibroosseous pseudotumor of the digits (FOPD) and myositis ossificans (MO)

These entities are reactive soft-tissue zonal heterotopic bone formations, often in sites of previous trauma (14).

Clinical presentation: Myositis ossificans is a reactive lesion in skeletal muscle of proximal extremities and trunk of young patients that generally matures over several weeks to form a peripheral rim of bone. Fibroosseous pseudotumor of the digits is a similar, less-organized reactive lesion of the digits, most commonly the proximal phalanx of the index digit (Figure 12.18). Both lesions start as reactive worrisome-

axial skeleton, usually pelvis, should be considered. Mesenchymal CS evokes the differential diagnosis of small round blue-cell tumors, such as Ewing sarcoma/primitive neuroectodermal tumor (ES/PNET), rhabdomyosarcoma (RMS), lymphoma, neuroblastoma (NBL), and others; these entities can be distinguished by clinical, radiologic, morphologic, immunohistochemical and molecular genetic features (22,23).

403

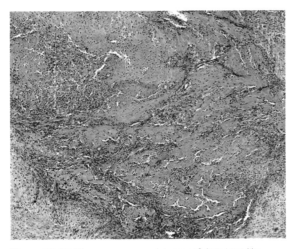

Figure 12.19 Fibro-osseous pseudotumor of digit. Lace-like immature bone is shown (H&E × 20).

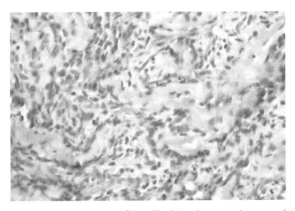

Figure 12.21 Myositis ossificans. The lesion has a zonal pattern of ossification, with central osteoid-like appearance and peripheral osteoblastic rimming (H&E × 30).

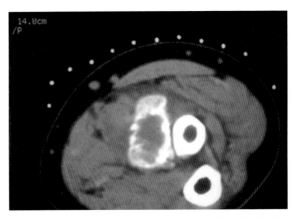

Figure 12.20 Myositis ossificans (imaging). Ovoid peripheral soft tissue ossification is characteristic.

Differential diagnosis: Early and central components can be histologically worrisome for osteosarcoma, but clinical, radiologic, and histologic evidence of zonal organization with maturation are characteristic of MO and FOPD.

Bone island (BI)

A BI is a small incidental developmental process consisting of focal bone with increased cortical-type density within cancellous (trabecular) bone.

Clinical presentation: Bone islands are usually small (0.1–0.2 cm), but can measure up to 1 cm. On extremely rare occasions, a BI may be a nidus for development of secondary malignancy.

Macroscopy: A BI is an island of dense bone in intramedullary spongy bone.

Histology: Bone islands are composed of compact mature lamellar bone with well-developed Haversian and interstitial systems within intramedullary spaces, with a spoke-like pattern in surrounding trabeculae (Figure 12.22). No enchondral ossification or cartilage is observed.

Differential diagnosis: Bone islands can mimic sclerotic OS or osteoid osteoma (OO), but careful attention to radiologic features will identify BI.

Protuberant fibro-osseous lesion of temporal bone (PFOLTB) (Bullough lesion or bump)

This is a benign surface fibroosseous lesion of the calvarium (24,25).

Clinical presentation: Protuberant fibro-osseous lesion of temporal bone occurs on the surface of the temporal bone intimately related to the occipitomastoid suture. It presents as a retroauricular soft-tissue

appearing lesions that mature over two to six weeks to form a peripheral bony shell. Age varies, with children more commonly affected by MO and adults by FOPD. There is a slight male predilection in MO and female in FOPD. In FOPD, most patients have antecedent trauma related to repetitive manual use; FOPD can also present with edema and digital pain. Both lesions can be diagnosed and treated by simple excision, without recurrence.

Macroscopy: Eggshell-like peripheral calcification as lesions mature is characteristic.

Histology: Most MO and half of FOPD have a zonal organization, with mature woven bone peripherally and immature lace-like woven bone centrally; all bone demonstrates osteoblastic rimming (Figures 12.19–12.21). The bone is accompanied by myofibroblastic tissue.

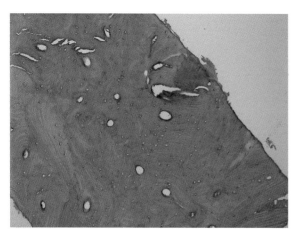

Figure 12.22 Bone island. The appearance is of compact mature lamellar bone (H&E × 20).

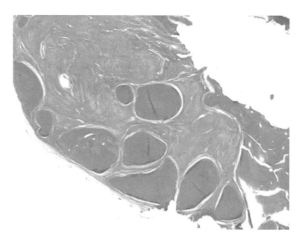

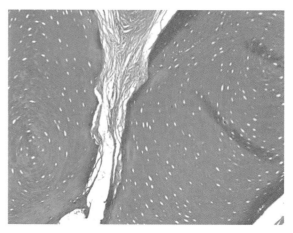

Figures 12.23 and 12.24 Protuberant fibro-osseous lesion of temporal bone (Bullough lesion). This lesion is composed of rounded and ovoid zones of ossification within a bland fibrous stroma. (Images courtesy of Dr. Michael Klein.) (H&E × 20 and × 30).

mass with calcific densities, confined to the soft tissues on the outer table of the skull without intraosseous involvement. It may have a 1–10-year history prior to presentation and is benign without documentation of local recurrence; excision is the treatment of choice.

Macroscopy: This is a protuberant bony lesion of the calvarium.

Histology: Protuberant fibro-osseous lesion of temporal bone is characterized by rounded and ovoid zones of ossification within a bland fibrous stroma (Figures 12.23 and 12.24).

Differential diagnosis: The main consideration is parosteal OS.

Osteoma (OM)

Osteoma is a benign, densely sclerotic localized proliferation of cortical bone.

Clinical presentation: Osteoma frequently involves bones of the paranasal sinuses and skull, and rarely manifests as a long-bone parosteal lesion. The nature is uncertain, but it is not generally regarded as neoplastic. Osteomas are most commonly detected as incidental findings and are a component of Gardner syndrome, a variant of familial adenomatous polyposis (FAP) that includes intestinal polyps and carcinoma, fibromatosis (Gardner fibromas and intra-abdominal desmoid fibromatosis), dental anomalies, and epidermal keratinous cysts (see Chapter 3). Osteoma only rarely occurs in the first and second decades. On radiologic imaging the lesions measure up to 2 cm with a broad base that merges with the surrounding cortex; they are cured by excision.

Genetics: Gardner syndrome is associated with mutations of *APC*, the tumor-suppressor gene at 5q22.2.

β-catenin accumulates in the nucleus in Gardner lesions due to tumor-suppressor gene *APC/Wnt* activation.

Macroscopy: Osteoma is a rounded exophytic nodule of densely calcified bone, often compared to ivory in appearance and consistency.

Histology: It consists of markedly thickened trabeculae of cortical lamellar bone, with or without woven bone. Marrow spaces are inconspicuous. A cancellous variant resembles trabecular bone with fat. Sinus lesions may have central fibrous areas with active osteoblasts and osteoclasts. Surfaces are lined by bland osteoblasts, and lacunae contain small osteocytes (Figure 12.25). β-catenin is located in the nuclei.

Differential diagnosis: Parosteal OS, particularly in long bones, is the most important entity; osteomas lack the proliferating spindle-cell component of this lesion. Osteoma closely resembles melorheostosis

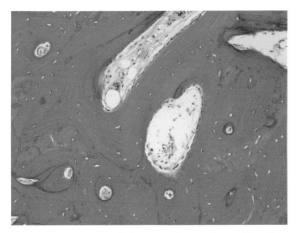

Figure 12.25 Osteoma.The lesion has thickened cortical lamellar bone trabeculae lined by benign osteoblasts with osteocytes in lacunae. Sinus osteomas may have fibrous areas. It is usually protuberant from bone surface (H&E × 40).

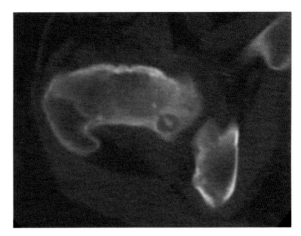

Figure 12.26 Osteoid osteoma (imaging). Note lucent area with sclerotic margin and calcified central nidus.

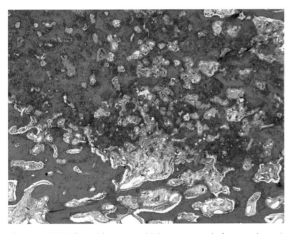

Figure 12.27 Osteoid osteoma. Nidus composed of woven bone is at top, while surrounding dense cortical bone with thickened trabeculae lies at periphery (H&E × 20).

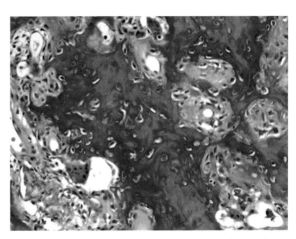

Figure 12.28 Osteoid osteoma. High-power view of woven bone in nidus is shown. Bland fibrovascular tissue is present in marrow spaces (H&E × 40).

(a progressive disorder characterized by hyperostosis of the cortical bone), and the entities may not be distinguishable.

Osteoid osteoma (OO) and osteoblastoma (OBL)

Osteoid osteoma is a benign small, zonal and usually intracortical bone-forming tumor, in proximal extremity or pelvis; OBL is a larger histologically identical process in posterior elements of the spine.

Clinical presentation: Osteoid osteoma occurs in children, with a male predominance. By definition OO measures < 1.0 cm, while OBL measures >1.5 to 2.0 cm. Osteoid osteoma has a classic clinical presentation of pain at night, relieved by aspirin, because of

prostaglandin production by the tumor, whereas OBL can cause pain that is not relieved by aspirin. Osteoid osteoma is found in long bones, such as the femur and tibia, or rarely in the pelvis; it is intracortical with a zonal central radiolucent nidus surrounded by dense cortical sclerosis on X-ray and a targetoid appearance on CT (Figure 12.26). Osteoblastoma is often found in the posterior elements of the spine (Figure 12.27).

Macroscopy: The lesions are red, gritty, and cortical-based, with a granular sclerotic rim.

Histology: Both lesions have a nidus of woven bone rimmed mainly by osteoblasts and occasional osteoclasts, with surrounding hypocellular fibrovascular stroma (Figures 12.28–12.32). Each lesion has associated rimming of bony spicules, often with

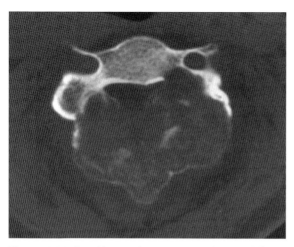

Figure 12.29 Osteoblastoma (imaging). Lucent lesion with focal calcification is present in vertebral body.

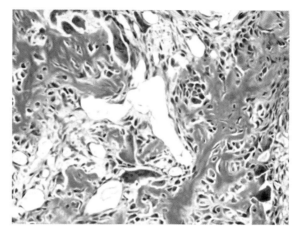

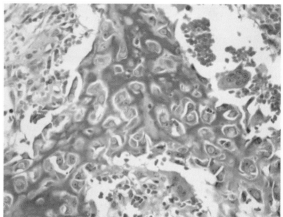

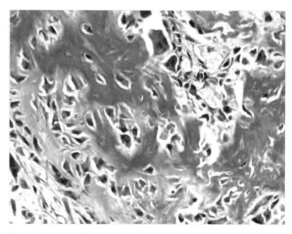

interconnectivity of the central woven bone. The peripheral cortical bone is hypertrophic in OO. Osteoblastic phenotype is best marked by osteocalcin, but immunohistochemistry is not necessary for diagnosis.

Differential diagnosis: Osteosarcoma can be considered when osteoblasts are large and atypical, and the woven bone appears lace-like in the center. However, widespread osteoblastic rimming, with absence of a cellular stroma seen at low power is characteristic of OO and OBL and generally excludes OS.

Osteosarcoma (OS)

Osteosarcoma is a malignant tumor in which atypical tumor cells manufacture osteoid and bone; the tumor cells also often produce cartilage and fibrous tissue (21).

Clinical presentation: Medullary OS constitutes the vast majority of cases. The tumor commonly occurs as a metadiaphyseal lesion of long bones of the extremities, but may involve other bones. The lesion destroys the bone of origin and frequently expands from medulla through cortex into soft tissue. Radiological imaging demonstrates lifting and penetration of the periosteum, forming a Codman angle (triangle) (Figures 12.33 and 12.34). Dense calcification is seen in bone, and areas of soft tissue are calcified, sometimes in a sun-burst pattern (26).

Genetics: Osteosarcoma has complicated genetic changes that often vary from tumor to tumor (27). Rearrangements of chromosomes 8, 17, and 20 have been emphasized (28). In cases of small-cell OS, genetic findings characteristic of ES/PNET will exclude OS.

Figures 12.30–12.32 Osteoblastoma. The lesion is composed of proliferating osteoblasts with surrounding woven osteoid matrix. Lesional cells display mild atypia, but features of osteosarcoma cells (hyperchromaticity, pleomorphism, and abnormal mitoses) are not observed (H&E × 40).

Macroscopy: Lesions resected en bloc are large, metaphyseal, hard, and often gritty when heavily mineralized. When less mineralization is present

407

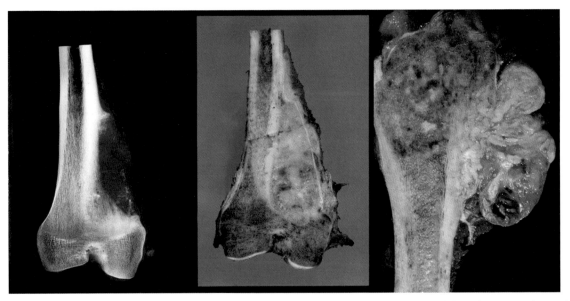

Figures 12.33 and 12.34 Osteosarcoma (imaging and gross specimen). Lesions are metadiaphyseal with bone formation and cortical destruction.

the lesions are myxoid or rubbery (Figures 12.33 and 12.34). Telangiectatic OS resembles bloody vascularized soft tissue with cystic spaces and firm areas of osteoid.

Histology: The tumor displays pleomorphic hyperchromatic nuclei in lesional cells. Tumor cells frequently are surrounded by and manufacture osteoid, often arranged in a lace-like pattern (Figure 12.35). The latter finding is diagnostic. Metastatic lesions have a similar appearance; lung nodules are often densely calcified. Chondroblastic OS produces cartilaginous matrix in addition to osteoid (Figure 12.36). Telangiectatic OS frequently resembles ABC radiologically, but has thicker cyst walls; it is composed of blood-filled cystic spaces lined by atypical mesenchymal cells. Typical areas of OS with osteoid deposition may be difficult to find in a large specimen. The lesion is treated similarly to conventional OS, with a similar outcome. A rarer variant is small-cell OS, in which areas of conventional OS alternate with areas resembling ES/PNET. These lesions may be difficult to diagnose if osteoid is minimal, but can be sorted out by immunohistochemistry and molecular studies. Osteocalcin and osteonectin stains are often positive, but immunohistochemical studies are usually not necessary, except in small-cell OS; the latter must be distinguished from other blue-cell tumors by a battery of stains, including CD99, CD56, NB84, synaptophysin,

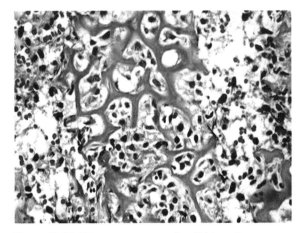

Figure 12.35 Osteosarcoma, conventional high-grade. Pleomorphic tumor cells with hyperchromatic nuclei are surrounded by delicate strands of osteoid made by the cells (H&E ×40).

and tyrosine hydroxylase, or hematolymphoid markers (29–31).

Differential diagnosis: Chondrosarcoma is considered when tumors produce abundant chondroid matrix; the presence of high-grade features in a patient under 25 years favors OS, and identification of osteoid is supportive. The differential diagnosis of small-cell OS includes ES/PNET, metastatic NBL or alveolar RMS, leukemia/lymphoma, and other entities with a similar appearance; immunohistochemistry, and cytogenetic

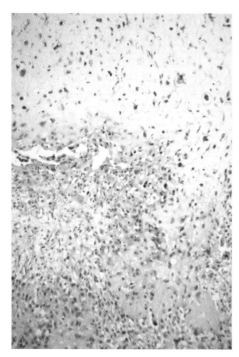

Figure 12.36 Chondroblastic osteosarcoma. A chondroid matrix predominates (H&E × 20).

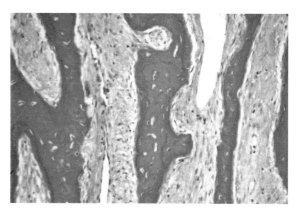

Figure 12.37 Parosteal osteosarcoma. Bland bony trabeculae alternate with stroma composed of mildly atypical spindle cells (H&E × 20).

and molecular genetic studies may be necessary for certain diagnosis.

Low-grade surface OS

The most common surface tumors are periosteal and parosteal OS. Parosteal OS arises from cortex and seldom penetrates into the medulla. The lesion is composed of thickened bony spicules interspersed with spindle-cell islands with mild atypia (Figure 12.37). Periosteal OS is largely composed of proliferating hyaline cartilage and bone, with atypical chondroblasts and osteoblasts, resembling chondroblastic OS. Both are treated with resection, but often require chemotherapy to avoid recurrences. These lesions rarely metastasize. A specific MDM2 molecular involvement is associated with low-grade central and parosteal OS.

Other OS variants

High-grade surface OS arises from the cortex, but resembles conventional OS histologically.

Resection specimen management of malignant bone tumors

The most common pediatric tumors originating in bone are OS and ES/PNET, with CS constituting the

second most common tumor across all ages. Correlation of pathology with radiologic imaging is critically important. Proper management of resection specimens provides information that assists in prognosis. In current practice, following biopsy for diagnosis and neo-adjuvant (preresection) chemotherapy, the bone of the primary site is resected. Previously excision with adequate margins often required amputation, but now limb salvage procedures, with or without placement of an allograft or prosthesis contribute to an improved quality of life.

Following excision, degree of response to chemotherapy is evaluated. The specimen is inspected, oriented, and measured. The bone is sawed longitudinally through the largest tumor diameter, generally using a band saw. The specimen may be frozen prior to sawing. After the first cut, a second parallel cut is made, producing a thin slice of bone and soft tissue. The slice is photographed, fixed, decalcified, and entirely submitted for processing. The photograph is used to create a section diagram (Figure 12.38). The response to chemotherapy (Figure 12.39) is expressed as a percentage of the entire tumor cross-section, using the section diagram with correlated cassette labels. Additional perpendicular sections of tumor are taken to assess the relationship of tumor to soft tissue and resection margins, neurovascular bundle, joint, and prior biopsy site. Grading may be carried out using the French federation grading scheme (FNCLCC), but most subtypes of OS and CS carry a specific grade. For example, by definition, central OS is low grade, as is parosteal OS; chondroblastic OS is usually intermediate grade, and osteoblastic OS is generally

409

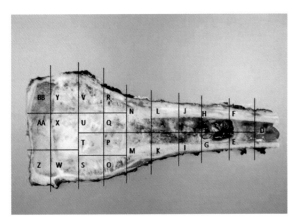

Figure 12.38 Osteosarcoma resection. Treated tumor is sawed through largest dimension, and slice is completely submitted according to map to assess response to chemotherapy.

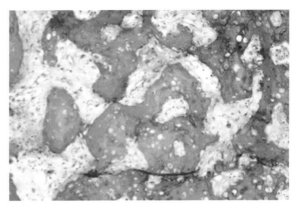

Figure 12.39 Treated osteosarcoma. Response to chemotherapy results in disappearance of most tumor cells and replacement by fibrosis. Tumor osteoid remains intact (H&E × 20).

high grade. Most hyaline cartilage CS are low grade, or intermediate if myxoid. High-grade chondroblastic tumors in patients < 25 years should be considered potential chondroblastic OS and examined for tumor osteoid formation. Ewing sarcoma/ primitive neuroectodermal tumor is invariably high grade. Adjuvant therapy is used according to the tumor grade. In OS, viability of more than 10% of tumor carries a poor prognosis. For ES/PNET, several studies have shown similar correlation of tumor response to prognosis (31,32).

Fibrogenic tumors

Desmoplastic fibroma (DF)

Desmoplastic fibroma is a benign locally aggressive fibroblastic bone tumor; it is the intraosseous equivalent of fibromatosis (desmoid) of soft tissue (33).

Clinical presentation: Desmoplastic fibroma is rare and can be found in any bone. Patients are generally adolescent or young adults with an equal sex predilection, who present with pain, deformity, or loss of function. Desmoplastic fibroma can be locally aggressive and require resection.

Genetics: Trisomies 8 and 20 have been described (34). Unlike fibromatosis of soft tissue, DF does not utilize the *APC/Wnt* pathway. In the jaw, those cases with β-catenin nuclear positivity most likely represent soft-tissue fibromatosis secondarily involving bone.

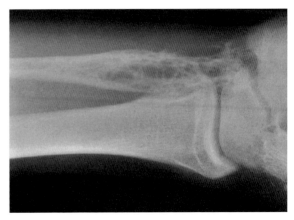

Figure 12.40 Desmoplastic fibroma (imaging). Bubbly fibular lesion expands bone with mild cortical involvement.

Macroscopy: The lesion has a rubbery, firm, creamy-white cut surface and variegated whorled pattern with a scalloped, bony border. It can extend by pushing into soft tissue, usually with retention of overlying periosteum (Figures 12.40 and 12.41).

Histology: Desmoplastic fibroma varies from aggressive to bland myxoid fibroblastic proliferation, sometimes with cartwheel whorls of uniform ovoid cells (Figure 12.42). No cytologic atypia, mitotic activity, or necrosis are present. Elongated vessels may display perivascular hemorrhage. Keloidal collagen may be observed; β-catenin, keratin, desmin, CD34, and S100 protein are negative.

Differential diagnosis: The absence of cytologic atypia excludes sarcoma (MFH) or paucicellular

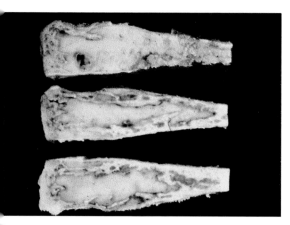

Figure 12.41 Desmoplastic fibroma. Dense fibrous tissue replaces marrow spaces.

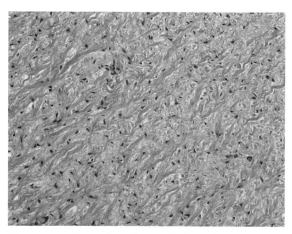

Figure 12.42 Desmoplastic fibroma. The lesion demonstrates typical ovoid bland cells in cartwheel arrangements, keloid-like collagen and absence of bone formation. The lesion is similar to soft tissue aggressive (desmoid) fibromatosis (H&E × 20).

metastatic carcinoma with desmoplasia. Overlap with scant bone in stroma-rich FD may be suggested, and some debate exists that these may be related lesions.

Fibrohistiocytic tumors

Non-ossifying fibroma (NOF)

Non-ossifying fibroma is a benign fibrohistiocytic tumor. It is also known as fibrous cortical defect, metaphyseal fibrous defect, fibrous histiocytoma (FH) of bone, and fibroxanthoma.

Clinical presentation: In children NOF is usually an incidental finding in an eccentric metaphyseal location in femur or tibia, with a geographic margin (Figure 12.43). It is classified as FH if > 5 cm, in an older child, and presenting with pain.

Macroscopy: Non-ossifying fibroma has a pale-cream and rust-brown cut surface, and causes cortical thinning.

Histology: Non-ossifying fibroma is composed of spindled myofibroblasts, scattered osteoclast-type giant cells, and xanthoma cells; inflammation and hemosiderin are often seen (Figures 12.44 and 12.45). Giant cells have few nuclei. The xanthoma cells are a key helpful feature. The lesion is identical to FH of dermis. Actin may accompany histiocytic markers; NOF is negative for keratins, EMA, CD34, S100 protein, and desmin.

Differential diagnosis: Giant-cell tumor of bone (GCTB) can be distinguished from NOF by its back-to-back osteoclast-type giant cells, abundant nuclei per

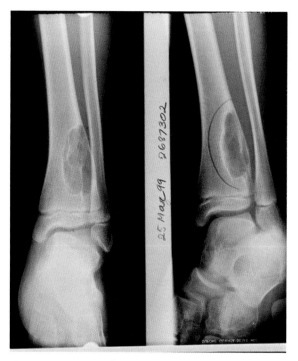

Figure 12.43 Non-ossifiying fibroma (imaging). Metaphyseal lesion has sclerotic margins and lucent subcortical center.

giant cell, identical nuclei in stroma, and absence of xanthoma cells. The clinico-radiological features and morphology can also separate NOF from the brown tumor of hyperparathyroidism.

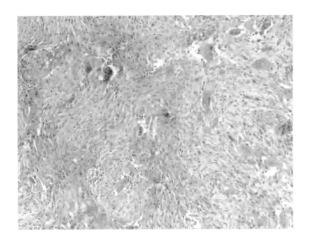

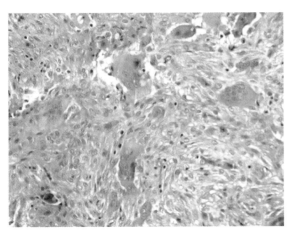

Figures 12.44 and 12.45 Non-ossifying fibroma. Histology displays bland fibroblasts with admixed osteoclast-like multinucleated giant cells (H&E × 20 and × 40).

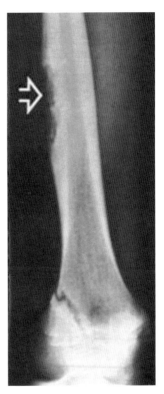

Figure 12.46 Ewing's sarcoma/primitive neuroectodermal tumor (imaging). Permeative diaphyseal lesion with cortical destruction is shown. No bone formation is seen.

Ewing's sarcoma

Ewing's sarcoma/primitive neuroectodermal tumor (ES/PNET)

This is the second most common malignant tumor of bone in the pediatric age group; it is of mesenchymal and neural histogenesis (21,30,31,35). Ewing described a "myeloma" or "endothelioma" of bone that was sensitive to radiation therapy, but always recurred with fatal results (31). Primitive neuroectodermal tumor and ES are considered clinically, radiologically, genetically, and prognostically the same tumor, which occurs predominantly in bone, with 10–20% of cases in soft tissue (see Chapter 11).

Clinical presentation: On imaging, the tumor has a permeative pattern with vague lesional margins and lacks osteoid (Figure 12.46). Large soft-tissue masses may lie between periosteum and cortex. An onion-skin pattern results from cycles of periosteal elevation by intraosseous tumor. Radionuclide and MRI scans are useful in evaluating suspicious lesions. Treatment consists of combination chemotherapy followed by resection. Radiation is used for unresectable or residual tumor. Three-year event-free survival is approximately 65–70%.

Genetics: This was the first pediatric solid tumor identified with a characteristic chromosomal signature. The most common reciprocal translocation, t(11;22)(q24;q12), involves the *Fli-1* gene on chromosome 11q and the *EWS* gene, in the *ETS* family, on chromosome 22q. In other variants, *EWS* is paired with other *ETS* or non-*ETS* genes. Rarely the *EWS* family gene *FUS* is found. Other genetic techniques include cytogenetics on fresh tissue, fluorescence *in situ* hybridization (FISH) or reverse transcriptase polymerase chain reaction (RT-PCR) (36; see Chapter 15).

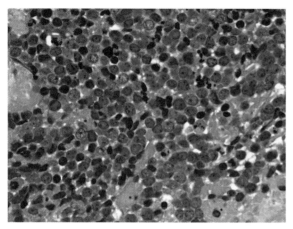

Figure 12.47 Ewing's sarcoma/primitive neuroectodermal tumor. Sheets of tumor cells have bland nuclear chromatin with inconspicuous nucleoli, accompanied by little cytoplasm (H&E × 40).

Macroscopy: Biopsies are soft, whitish-tan or gray-pink, but may be firm or hard depending on the amount of mineralized bone. Following chemotherapy, lesions are often firm due to fibrosis, with periosteal new bone formation and an associated extraosseous mass.

Histology: An ES/PNET is composed of 20 μm round cells with round nuclei surrounded by minimal cytoplasm (Figure 12.47). The nuclei contain fine chromatin and frequent single small nucleoli. Interspersed are cells with darker nuclei and cytoplasm. Tumor cells may contain cytoplasmic glycogen (PAS-positive) and are arranged in sheets with frequent necrosis; viable cells are clustered around blood vessels. Neural differentiation may be recognized by more ovoid nuclei, the presence of Homer–Wright rosettes with neuropil in the center, and focal immunostaining for neural markers. Tumors display distinctive membrane reactivity for MIC2 (CD99), and may express a wide variety of neural-associated antigens, including synaptophysin, NSE, PGP 9.5, CD56, CD57, focal S100, and others. Fli-1 nuclear expression correlates with the presence of t(11;22), but is not consistent. Caveolin-1 is positive in the majority of ES/PNET (37,38); keratin may be focally positive.

Differential diagnosis: This includes other primitive small round-cell tumors, including NBL, alveolar RMS, desmoplastic round-cell tumor, lymphoma, poorly differentiated synovial sarcoma, small-cell OS, mesenchymal CS, NUT carcinoma, and undifferentiated sarcoma (31,39).

Hematopoietic neoplasms

Systemic mastocytosis (SM)

Systemic mastocytosis is a proliferation of mast cells in various sites and organs. The most common lesional site, termed urticaria pigmentosa, is skin, while systemic disease frequently involves skeleton. Lesional mast cells cause disease by degranulation and release of biologic immune mediators, including histamine, heparin, cathepsin G, prostaglandin D2, TNF-α, and others. Mast-cell secretions may be stimulated by trauma, temperature, and multiple drugs (40; see Chapter 1).

Clinical presentation: The immune mediators contribute to pruritus, flushing, headaches, dizziness, and other symptoms, including anaphylaxis. Hepatosplenomegaly, elevated alkaline phosphatase, and non-specific hematologic abnormalities are observed. On imaging, bone lesions may be sclerotic, osteopenic, or both, with indistinct borders, generating a differential diagnosis that includes malignancies and bone infarcts. Systemic mastocytosis is often indolent, and only rarely it is aggressive, associated with anemia, thrombocytopenia, liver-function test abnormalities, and other diseases. Treatment is directed at signs and symptoms associated with mast-cell secretions, including antihistamines, cromolyn, H1 and H2 blockers, and other anti-inflammatory agents (41).

Genetics: In children, lesional mast cells may have somatic mutation of the tyrosine kinase receptor c-kit.

Histology: Lesions demonstrate nodular, diffuse, or granulomatous marrow infiltration by mast cells accompanied by thickened bony trabeculae and fibrosis. Mast cells mimic monocytes or histiocytes, but have granular cytoplasm on Giemsa stain. Mast-cell tryptase, CD117, and markers of histiocytes and granulocytes are positive.

Differential diagnosis: This includes Langerhans-cell histiocytosis (LCH), leukemia/lymphoma, and metastasis.

Osteoclastic giant-cell-rich tumors

Central giant-cell tumor (CGCT) or giant-cell reparative granuloma (GCRG)

These tumors are reparative, spindled fibroblastic, and histiocytic proliferations with hemosiderin.

413

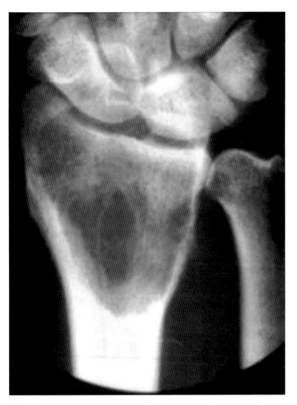

Figure 12.48 Giant-cell tumor of bone (imaging). Lesion is lytic with sclerotic margins.

Clinical presentation: The age range is from childhood to older adults. Most cases are in the jaw, facial bones, and skull. Those in short bones of hands and feet and long bones of the extremities are probably equivalent to solid ABC after GCTB is excluded. The lesions can present with pain, swelling, or pathologic fracture.

Genetics: t(X;4)(q22;q31.3) has been reported (42)

Macroscopy: On imaging, the lesion is lytic without mineralization, and expansile, destroying bone and thinning cortex, with no periosteal reaction.

Histology: Features include reactive granulation tissue, spindled fibroblasts, focal hemorrhage, and scattered small giant cells with few nuclei. The giant cells may cluster around areas of hemorrhage. Irregular bony trabeculae have osteoclastic giant cells on some surfaces.

Differential diagnosis: Because of giant cells and hemorrhage, ABC, GCTB, brown tumor, and pigmented villonodular synovitis (PVNS) may be considered.

Giant-cell tumor of bone (GCTB)

Giant-cell tumor of bone is a benign, but locally aggressive, giant-cell-rich tumor. Accompanying mononuclear cells represent the neoplastic cells that produce receptor activator of a nuclear factor κ-B ligand (RANKL), which stimulates osteoclasts.

Clinical presentation: Giant-cell tumor of bone arises in metaphyses and may be eccentric. In children it stops at the growth plate; however, when the growth plate is closed it extends to the end of the bone. Most lesions occur in skeletally mature patients. Radiology demonstrates a lytic lesion with focally sclerotic margin, presenting eccentrically in metaphysis and extending to the end of the bone (Figure 12.48). Giant-cell tumor of bone is locally aggressive and local recurrence is possible. So-called benign metastasizing or malignant forms usually represent giant-cell-rich MFH or giant-cell-rich OS (43,44). The most common long bone sites are distal femur, proximal tibia, distal radius, and proximal humerus, with the sacrum most common in the axial skeleton.

Genetics: Reduction in telomere length in several chromosomes (11p, 13p, 14p, 15p, 19p, 20p, and 21p) has been identified and is possibly associated with more aggressive behaviour (45).

Macroscopy: Giant cell tumor of bone has a bloody gross appearance; associated secondary ABC is often present.

Histology: Sheets of osteoclast-type giant cells, often packed with 50–100 nuclei, have nuclear features identical to the stromal mononuclear cells (Figures 12.49 and 12.50). Mitoses may be present, but should be minimal and of normal form. Spindled cells with hemosiderin and paucity of giant cells can be present, especially at the tumor periphery. With repeated recurrences and increased mitotic activity, one should look for malignant histologic features. Lace-like osteoid with atypical cells, atypical mitoses, or geographic necrosis should be absent from GCTB and raise the suspicion of OS. Immunohistochemistry is not required for diagnosis. Giant cell tumor of bone cells mark as histiocytes with CD68 and CD163.

Differential diagnosis: This includes NOF, ABC, CBL, brown tumor of hyperparathyroidism, and other giant-cell-rich bone tumors that can resemble GCTB histologically.

Notochordal tumors

Chordoma (CDM)

Chordoma is a slow-growing malignant midline tumor arising in regions of presumed residual notochord elements (21).

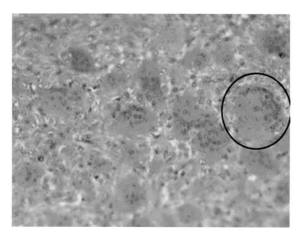

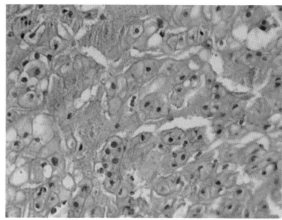

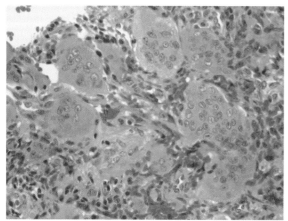

Figures 12.49 and 12.50 Giant-cell tumor of bone. The lesion is composed of sheets of multinucleated giant cells with numerous (50–100) nuclei. The stroma is composed of bland mononuclear cells with nuclei similar to those of the giant cells (H&E × 20 and × 40).

Figures 12.51 and 12.52 Chordoma. Strands of polygonal physaliphorous cells have clear, bubbly cytoplasm. Nuclei vary in size, pleomorphism and chromaticity (H&E × 20 and ×40).

Clinical presentation: Most common sites are skull base and sacrum, but any vertebral level can be involved. Males are affected about twice as often as females. Chordoma occurs predominantly in the fifth and sixth decades, and in childhood in the second decade. Skull base chondroid CDMs are common in children. On imaging, CDMs are midline destructive lesions, often with accompanying soft tissue masses. Both CT and MRI are useful in distinguishing the tumor from adjacent structures. Metastasis occurs in one-third to half of cases. Chordomas are slow-growing, but locally aggressive and require surgical excision, often difficult to achieve because of skull and spinal sites. Radiation is usually required in cranial lesions.

Genetics: Abnormalities include clonal changes such as hypodiploidy, loss of various chromosomes, and deletions. Gains of 5q and 7q have been identified, and loss of heterozygosity at 1p36 has been reported (8).

Macroscopy: The tumors are lobular with firm blue-gray masses divided by fibrous septa.

Histology: Chordomas are composed of clusters and strands of polygonal cells wrapping around one another with pale cytoplasm in a myxoid matrix (Figure 12.51). Tumor cells with bubbly cytoplasm are called physaliphorous cells (Figure 12.52), but are not always present. Nuclei vary from small to enlarged, pleomorphic, and hyperchromatic. Sarcoma-like areas may be present. Skull-base tumors in children may be solid and highly cellular with prominent cartilaginous matrix (chondroid CDM). Tumor cells are positive for cytokeratins (especially CK8, CK18, and CK19), EMA, and S100. Brachyury is a reliable marker.

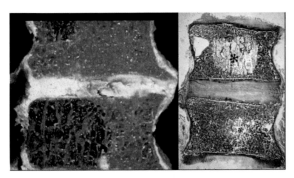

Figure 12.53 Capillary hemangioma. Vertebral lesions appear reddish on gross examination, with somewhat cystic appearance at low power.

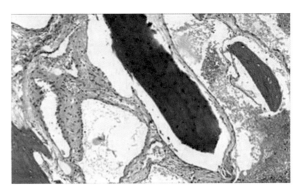

Figure 12.54 Capillary hemangioma. Dilated cavernous vascular spaces with bland endothelial cells are present in the marrow (H&E × 20).

Differential diagnosis: The differential diagnosis includes CS, but CS lacks keratin, EMA, and brachyury expression. Metastatic adenocarcinoma is extremely rare in children. Giant notochordal rest (GNR) is considered to be of notochordal derivation, but lacks radiologic evidence of bone destruction, and microscopically lacks a lobular pattern and pleomorphism. Giant notochordal rests infiltrate marrow spaces, but generally behave indolently.

Vascular lesions

The classification of vascular lesions, whether in bone, soft tissue, skin, or viscera, is confusing and often contradictory. In recent years an effort has been advanced by several international organizations to divide these lesions into two broad groups: tumors, characterized by endothelial proliferation, and malformations, representing structural abnormalities with normal endothelial turnover (46,47). Other recent classifications include malformations as benign hemangiomas and consider neoplasms together as benign, intermediate, and malignant tumors (48; see Chapter 1).

Benign neoplasms and malformations

Capillary hemangioma (CH)

Capillary hemangioma is a benign vascular neoplasm composed of capillary-sized blood vessels.

Clinical presentation: The patient may be asymptomatic or complain of solitary nodules. The lesions predominantly occur in vertebrae, but may be in the skull, facial bones, or flat and long bones. Osseous lesions are often associated with vascular lesions elsewhere. Vertebral radiological imaging shows an increase in trabeculations or sclerosis. Many lesions are lucent. Treatment consists of curettage, but for unresectable lesions, radiation therapy may be used. The prognosis is generally excellent.

Macroscopy: Capillary hemangioma appears cystic and dark red (Figure 12.53).

Histology: Capillary hemangioma is composed of capillary-sized vessels with larger feeder vessels, in a tree-like trunk and branch distribution. Some lesions have dilated vessels (Figure 12.54). The capillaries have pericytes around them that can be proliferative with increased normal mitoses. A solid appearance may be worrisome for malignancy. Smooth-muscle actin is positive in pericytes and confirms benignancy (intravascular process). Endothelial cells are positive for the vascular markers CD31, CD34, Fli1, and, particularly, Glut1.

Differential diagnosis: The lesions may appear similar to other vascular lesions and LCH may be considered on imaging. Granulation tissue in a fracture callus may be confused with CH, venous hemangiomas (VH), or venous malformations (VM). Hemangioendothelioma (HEA) and angiosarcoma (AS) can be distinguished from CH by their extravascular proliferation of atypical endothelial cells that lack normal surrounding smooth-muscle actin (SMA) positive pericytes.

Venous hemangioma (VH)/venous malformation (VM)

These are benign vascular proliferations of large venous channels, often dilated, with smooth muscle around the endothelium in VH/VM and thin-walled vessels in CH. They are also referred to as cavernous malformation (CAVM).

Clinical presentation: Venous hemangiomas and malformations occur in the first and second decades and commonly arise in craniofacial bones, vertebrae, and elsewhere, usually as localized lesions. Imaging appearances depend on site (49). Cranial lesions display bone expansion and new bone formation. In vertebral sites the bones are preserved with lysis. Long-bone lesions exhibit expansion and peripheral sclerosis. Thrombosis, reorganization, and phlebolith formation can be observed radiologically in these large spaces. Treatment for VH/VM includes excision and injection of sclerosing agents.

Genetics: A *T1E2* mutation has been described in some hereditary forms.

Macroscopy: Lesions are cystic and reddish-tan.

Histology: Venous hemangiomas and malformations are characterized by large venous channels with smooth muscle in the walls. Cavernous malformations are composed of dilated venous vessels without smooth muscle. Both can have thrombosis with dystrophic calcification and phlebolith formation. Within veins there can also be a specialized organization pattern of papillary endothelial hyperplasia (Masson). The endothelium is positive for CD31 and CD34, and negative for Glut1.

Differential diagnosis: Arteriovenous hemangioma/malformation (AVH/M), CH, and HEA should be considered.

Epithelioid hemangioma (EH)

Epithelioid hemangioma is a lobular proliferation of capillaries with plump epithelioid endothelial cells.

Clinical presentation: Epithelioid hemangioma occurs in the first and second decades, predominantly in the lower extremities and craniofacial bones. Skeletal lesions may be multiple. By imaging, single or multiple lesions display an osteolytic pattern with little sclerosis or expansive features.

Macroscopy: The tissue is bloody and dark red.

Histology: Epithelioid hemangioma resembles a lymph node with lymphocytes and germinal centers, with an entering feeder artery and central proliferating capillaries lined by plump hobnail epithelioid endothelial cells, with eosinophilic cytoplasm and cytoplasmic vacuoles that may represent primitive lumen formation, admixed with scattered eosinophils (Figure 12.55). Intraosseous EHs less frequently have lymphoid proliferation or an obvious feeder artery. Endothelial cells are positive for CD31, CD34, and factor VIIIRA, but Glut1, D2–40, and Prox1 are negative. Pericytes around each epithelioid capillary vessel are positive for SMA. Normally formed mitoses may

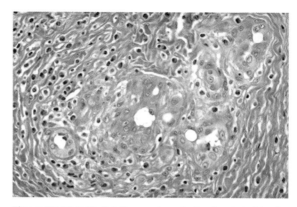

Figure 12.55 Epithelioid hemangioma. Lesional endothelial cells are plump with bland nuclei. Numerous infiltrating eosinophils are present (H&E × 20).

be present. CD31 assists in identifying vascular channels in bone when the endothelial lining abuts trabecular or cortical spicules; VEGFR3 is positive (50).

Differential diagnosis: Kimura disease of lymph nodes; CH or epithelial lesion within a lymph node should be considered.

Lymphangioma (LA)/lymphatic malformation (LM), and Gorham disease (GD)

The lesion is a benign malformation composed of lymphatic vessels.

Clinical presentation: Lymphangioma/lymphatic malformation occurs in craniofacial and appendicular bones throughout childhood, as well as in cervical soft tissue of Turner syndrome (XO). It can be florid, extensive, and multifocal. Bone formation is seen in the skull and resorption in vertebrae. Radiological imaging shows osteolysis and marginal sclerosis. When solitary or widespread bone loss is observed, the phenomenon is termed GD or Gorham–Stout (disappearing bone) disease.

Macroscopy: Lesions are pale tan and may be cystic.

Histology: Lymphangioma/lymphatic malformation is composed of anastomosing small thin-walled lymphatic vessels of variable caliber, lined by flat endothelium with valves, intraluminal proteinaceous material, and stromal lymphocytes. Bleeding may occur in lesional lymphatics. In GD, proliferation of blood capillaries or larger-caliber vessels may be present with bone loss and fibrosis. Bony involvement in these patients is accompanied by soft tissue and visceral lesions. Lymphatic endothelial cells are positive for D2–40, Prox1, and VEGFR3.

Arteriovenous hemangioma/malformation (AVHM)

Arteriovenous hemangioma/malformation is a benign mixed vascular process composed of arteries and veins, frequently with high-pressure phenomena.

Clinical presentation: Arteriovenous hemangioma/malformation occurs in the first and second decades, and involves the jaw or extremities. Radiologically, the lesions are osteolytic with minimal sclerosis. On angiograms rapid blood flow or arterial-to-venous shunting is observed, causing a clinical murmur. Radiologic-pathologic and clinicopathologic correlation is essential.

Macroscopy: The tissue is bloody and may be fibrous.

Histology: Large and small arteries, veins, indeterminate vessels, and loose fibrous stroma are seen. Thick muscular walls of vessels are often present. In soft tissue there is fatty replacement of skeletal muscle, and in bone there may be fatty marrow replacement. The endothelium is positive for CD31 and CD34.

Intermediate and malignant vascular lesions

Hemangioendothelioma (HEA) and epithelioid hemangioendothelioma (EHEA)

Hemangioendothelioma and EHEA are low-grade malignant lesions composed of extravascular endothelial cells, intermediate in behavior between HA and AS.

Clinical presentation: Hemangioendothelioma and EHEA are frequently multiple and occur in a variety of bones. The mean age is in the second decade. Radiological studies may show increased vascular flow or be non-specific. Metaphyseal lesions often display osteolysis.

Genetics: A t(1;3)(p36.3;q25) translocation has been identified in several cases (51).

Macroscopy: The tissue is soft, red, and bloody.

Histology: Hemangioendothelioma and EHEA are lobular with myxoid hyalinized stroma surrounding nests and cords of vaguely vascular tissue composed of plump cells with eosinophilic cytoplasm. Single cytoplasmic vacuoles characterize epithelioid endothelial cells (Figure 12.56). Higher-grade lesions display nuclear pleomorphism, necrosis, and mitoses, similar to angiosarcoma, but the hyalinized stroma of HEA/EHEA helps separate the two entities. Tumor cells are positive for endothelial markers and possibly for

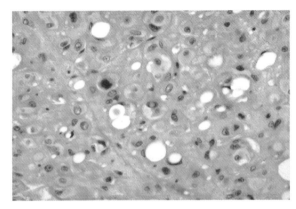

Figure 12.56 Epithelioid hemangioendothelioma. Hyaline matrix and embedded epithelioid endothelial cells characterize this low-grade malignancy. Mild to moderate nuclear atypia is seen. Vascular formation is vague, with cytoplasmic vacuolization (H&E × 40).

cytokeratins. There is loss of surrounding SMA-positive pericytes.

Differential diagnosis: Epithelioid hemangioma and AS are the main entities in the differential diagnosis. In adults, metastatic carcinoma is frequently considered. Other entities include CMF and adamantinoma (ADM).

Angiosarcoma (AS)

Angiosarcoma is an extravascular proliferation of atypical endothelial cells with mitotic activity.

Clinical presentation: Angiosarcoma is rare in both adults and children, occurring in the second decade in pediatric patients. Lesions occur in spine and pelvis but may involve any bone, and multifocal disease is common. Angiosarcoma is lytic on X-rays with no periosteal reaction. High-grade lesions demonstrate destruction and soft-tissue involvement. Treatment consists of surgery, with radiation therapy for incompletely resected or unresectable tumors. All ASs have a dismal prognosis.

Macroscopy: Lesions are soft, reddish, and bloody with no bony spicules. The borders are infiltrative.

Histology: Angiosarcoma is infiltrative, vasoformative, atypical, and mitotically active. Features include extravascular proliferation of atypical endothelial cells, with irregular tumor channels invading bone and accompanied by hemorrhage (Figures 12.57 and 12.58). Matrix is not seen. Criteria for grading include degree of mitotic activity, necrosis, nuclear pleomorphism and hyperchromasia, and intravascular budding. High-grade tumors display severe nuclear anaplasia, necrosis, sheet-like growth pattern, and

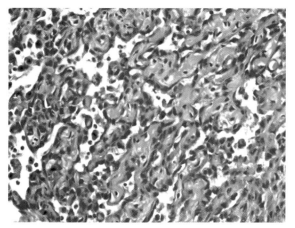

Figure 12.57 Angiosarcoma. The lesion is vasoformative with extravascular proliferation of atypical endothelial cells and mitotic activity, including atypical mitoses (H&E × 20).

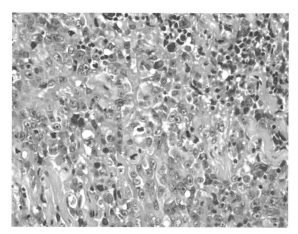

Figure 12.58 Epithelioid angiosarcoma. Leisonal cells are plump with vesicular nuclei containing prominent nucleoli. Vessels are difficult to discern (H&E × 40).

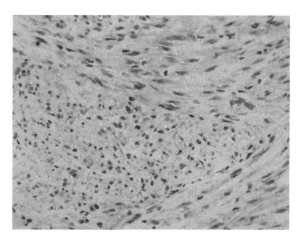

Figure 12.59 Myofibroma (myofibromatosis). These lesions have a bland biphasic appearance with myoid and pericytic components (H&E × 20).

atypical mitoses. Tumors are positive for CD31 and CD34, and cytokeratin reactivity may be observed (52,53).

Differential diagnosis: Papillary endothelial hyperplasia within vessels, CH, granulation tissue, and other soft-tissue sarcomas are in the differential diagnosis.

Myogenic, myopericytic, and epithelial tumors

Myofibroma (MF) and myofibromatosis (MFS)

Myofibroma and MFS are solitary and multiple benign myopericytic family tumors.

Clinical presentation: There is a wide age range, with multicentric forms more common in children and solitary lesions in adults. Any bone can be involved. Soft-tissue lesions may be superficial or deep, including organ involvement (see Chapter 11).

Genetics: An autosomal dominant inheritance pattern may be seen in MFS.

Macroscopy: Myofibroma can occur in the oral cavity submucosa or dermis or subcutis in other regions.

Histology: Myofibroma/MFS are biphasic with pink myoid and blue pericytoid regions (Figure 12.59). Vessels are veins surrounded by pericytes. An adult form suggests a reactive lesion of vessel wall. While cells may be mildly plump, mitoses are rare, and cytologic atypia and geographic necrosis are absent. SMA is positive, while desmin, CD34, S100 protein, and keratins are negative.

Differential diagnosis: Myofibroma and MFS should not be confused with solitary fibrous tumor or fibromatosis. Some myofibromas were previously termed infantile hemangiopericytoma. Smooth-muscle tumors are desmin-positive. The distinctive biphasic appearance, especially with multifocal lesions in children, should suggest the diagnosis. An aggressive growth pattern may be confused with spindle-cell malignancy. Myofibroma/MFS have overlapping features with nodular fasciitis in soft tissue and may be on a spectrum with one another.

Adamantinoma (ADM)

Adamantinoma is a low-grade malignant basaloid squamous-cell neoplasm that closely resembles

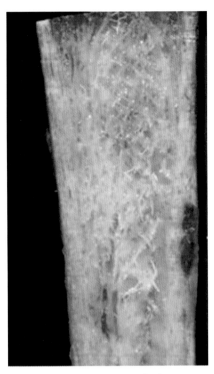

Figure 12.60 Adamantinoma. The lesion is eccentric, adjacent to cortex, well-circumscribed, and rubbery, with hemorrhage and necrosis. They are often adjacent to cortex and fleshy or yellow.

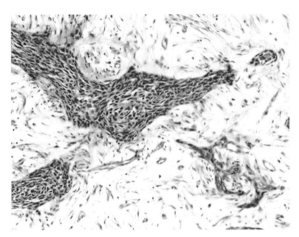

Figure 12.61 Adamantinoma. Islands of well-differentiated squamous cells lie in a fibrous stroma. The islands may have tubular, basaloid, spindle-cell, or osteofibrous dysplasia-like patterns (H&E × 20).

ameloblastoma of the jaw. It bears many similarities to osteofibrous dysplasia (OFD), and a relationship has been proposed consisting of a spectrum including OFD, differentiated (OFD-like) ADM, and conventional ADM. Genetic similarities between OFD and ADM support a relationship, but the association remains controversial (54).

Clinical presentation: Adamantinoma predominantly occurs along the anterior cortex of the tibia and occasionally fibula, and has a radiologic appearance similar to OFD with tibial bowing. It predominantly occurs in young adults in the second and third decades and is locally aggressive, requiring surgical excision. In 20–30% of cases pulmonary metastases develop.

Genetics: Lesions may display aneuploidy, particularly trisomies 7, 8, 12, 19, and 21 (54).

Macroscopy: If resected en bloc the lesions are well-circumscribed and rubbery, with hemorrhage and necrosis. They tend to be eccentric and adjacent to cortex with a fleshy or yellow appearance (Figure 12.60).

Histology: Adamantinoma displays various-sized islands of squamous cells in a fibrous stroma (Figure 12.61). The squamous cells may be arranged in a variety of patterns, including tubular, basaloid, with spindled nests lined by basal cells, squamous, with

prominent keratinization, and spindle-cell, which resembles monophasic synovial sarcoma (SS). An OFD-like pattern consists of desmoplastic stroma and spicules of woven bone lined by osteoblasts and osteoclasts, as seen in OFD, accompanied by clusters or strands of epithelial cells, rather than the single cytokeratin-positive cells seen in OFD. If the OFD-like pattern predominates, some authors refer to it as differentiated ADM. An adamantinomatous pattern has been described in association with the t(11;22) characteristic of ES/PNET; such a lesion is classified as a variant of ES/PNET rather than as ADM (55). The epithelial component is positive for pancytokeratin stains and cytokeratins 14, 19, 5/6, 17, and p63. CK5 and 17 suggest a resemblance to basaloid epithelial cells. The cells also may express Ki67, epidermal growth factor receptor (EGFR), fibroblast growth factor (FGF) 2, and p53.

Differential diagnosis: .019w?>The main consideration is OFD. Differentiated ADM occurs in younger patients; it is a fibro-osseous lesion with a paucity of epithelial cells. Aggressive tumors such as EHEA and SS are more commonly soft-tissue tumors or intraosseous (not intracortical), have much more atypia, and can be distinguished by applying appropriate immunostains and molecular studies.

Tumors of undefined neoplastic nature

Aneurysmal bone cyst (ABC)

Primary ABC is a multiloculated thin-walled cystic lesion with blood-filled spaces and walls composed of

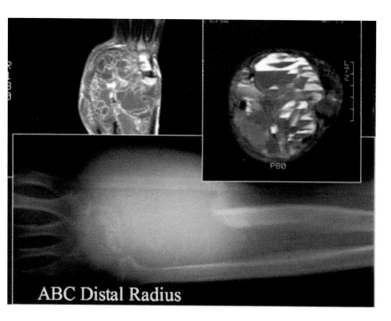

Figure 12.62 Aneurysmal bone cyst (imaging). Lesions are eccentric or intracortical, expansile, and multiloculated, fluid-fluid levels.

ABC Distal Radius

fibrous tissue, osteoclast-type giant cells, and reactive woven bone. Secondary ABC usually occurs as a cystic blood-filled component of other tumors such as GCTB, CBL, and CMF.

Clinical presentation: Primary ABC is an eccentric, sometimes intracortical solitary expansile multiloculated cystic lesion, with fluid-fluid levels seen on imaging (Figure 12.62). Although genetic abnormalities have been documented, ABC is probably a reactive organizing hematoma-like or MO-like lesion; in soft tissue it may have features of these entities. It is mainly found in long bones of young patients and less frequently in the spine. ABC is benign, but may recur locally.

Genetics: A balanced reciprocal translocation involving 17p is most characteristic (56). The partner is usually 16q, but other rearrangements have been observed.

Macroscopy: Primary ABC is entirely cystic with blood-filled spaces. Secondary ABC has a solid component that represents another tumor or thick walls that may represent telangiectatic OS.

Histology: Aneurysmal bone cyst cyst walls contain and may be lined by osteoclast-type giant cells, reactive woven bone rimmed by osteoblasts and fibrous walls with multiloculated blood-filled spaces (Figures 12.63 and 12.64). Bluish-tinged bony spicules may be present in the walls.

Differential diagnosis: Giant-cell reparative granuloma of long bone is synonymous with solid ABC, but GCTB should be excluded. Giant-cell tumor of bone may have secondary ABC; imaging is essential to

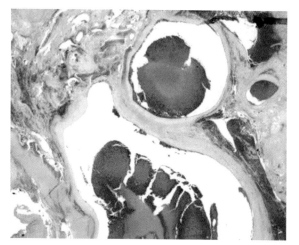

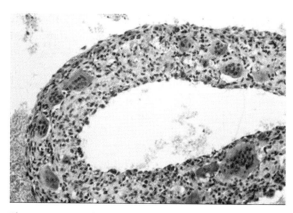

Figures 12.63 and 12.64 Aneurysmal bone cyst. Cystic spaces are filled with blood and lined by mesenchymal cells and osteoclast-like cells. Bony spicules are often present in the cyst walls (H&E × 10 and × 20).

421

document a solid component vs. an entirely cystic tumor. Telangiectatic OS has blood-filled cysts similar to those of ABC, but also displays thicker cyst walls, atypical cells, and rare osteoid production by malignant cells.

Simple bone cyst (SBC)

Simple bone cyst is a benign intramedullary commonly unilocular cyst filled with clear or straw-colored fluid; it is also called unicameral or solitary bone cyst.

Clinical presentation: Simple bone cyst most frequently occurs in the first two decades with a male predominance. The etiology is unknown, but has been attributed to a growth-plate disturbance or venous obstruction. The most common pediatric sites include proximal femur and humerus (ilial or calcaneal lesions in adults). Simple bone cyst first abuts the epiphysis and appears to move distally with bone growth. Bony expansion is usually limited to the width of the epiphyseal plate. The lesions may present with a pathologic fracture. Imaging demonstrates a unilocular smooth-walled cyst with condensation of surrounding bone, indicating indolence. At times a fragment may separate from the surrounding bone and migrate within the cyst cavity ("fallen fragment"). Cysts are often detected following fracture, as they are otherwise usually asymptomatic, or manifest mild swelling or local ache in older patients. Treatment by resection or curettage, previously used, is now often replaced by methylprednisolone injection. Removal largely precludes recurrence, while steroid injection may lead to recurrence in approximately 10–20% of patients. Sarcomas arising in SBC have been reported exceedingly rarely.

Genetics: Sporadic cases have been linked to t(7;12) (q21;q24.3) and other abnormalities (57).

Macroscopy: Simple bone cyst is rarely resected en bloc. On curettage the specimen demonstrates a thin white membrane attached to bony spicules.

Histology: The lining membrane is composed of fibrin and bland fibrous tissue without atypia. Rare septa may be seen (Figure 12.65). Reactive new bone, giant cells, chronic inflammation, cholesterol clefts, hemosiderin pigment, and following a fracture a callus may be seen; in those cases the lining and septa may be indistinguishable from ABC. Some cysts contain calcospherites, fibrinous deposits that resemble cementum in the wall.

Differential diagnosis: Aneurysmal bone cyst and GCTB must be excluded.

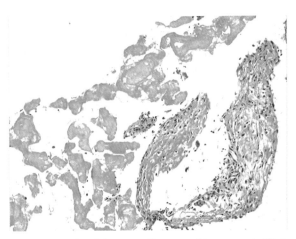

Figure 12.65 Simple bone cyst. The cyst wall is composed of fibrin and benign fibrous tissue, occasionally with calcospherites. Reactive features including new bone, giant cells, and inflammation; hemosiderin and callus may occur in fractured lesions and simulate aneurysmal bone cyst (H&E × 10).

Fibrous dysplasia (FD)

Fibrous dysplasia is a benign lesion composed of bone and fibrous tissue; it is generally regarded as a developmental defect (58).

Clinical presentation: Fibrous dysplasia may present in craniofacial bones, long bones of extremities, especially proximal femur and tibia, ribs, flat bones of the shoulder or pelvic girdle, or other bones. Male predominance occurs in rib and skull lesions, and female in jaws and long bones. Polyostotic FD occurs in about 30% of cases, and some of these may be associated with McCune–Albright syndrome, a genetic disorder with polyostotic FD accompanied by hyperfunctional endocrinopathies and pigmented skin lesions; in Mazabraud syndrome, FD is associated with soft-tissue myxomas, which often overlie the bony FD lesions. Osseous deformities may be caused by repeated fractures of FD. Sarcomas occur extremely rarely in FD cases. Imaging is extremely variable and presents a wide differential diagnosis, but lesions usually appear well-circumscribed and benign, with fusiform expansion of bone, sclerotic margins, and, on plain films, a classic ground-glass appearance. The lesion is limited to bone and may be covered only by periosteum. Central medullary lesions are surrounded by a dense bony shell. Secondary ABC may be present. The lesions are often followed without progression, but if necessary conservative excision by curettage is performed. Correction of deformities also requires surgery.

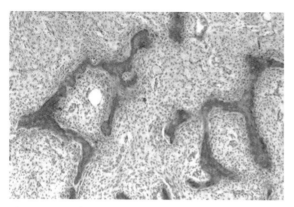

Figure 12.66 Fibrous dysplasia. Woven bone spicules with odd, sometimes cementomatous shapes, but no lining cells, lie in a fibrocollagenous stroma. Fractured lesions may have reactive osteoblasts and hemosiderin-laden macrophages (H&E × 20).

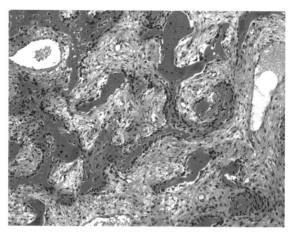

Figure 12.67 Osteofibrous dysplasia. Spicules of woven and lamellar bone are frequently lined by osteoclasts and osteoblasts. The stroma is composed of benign fibrocollagenous tissue with isolated cytokeratin-positive cells (H&E × 20).

Genetics: Trisomies 8 and 20 may be seen (34). Activating mutation in the *GNAS1* gene on 20q13.3, molecularly measured as the α-subunit of stimulatory G protein, is also found in McCune–Albright syndrome and solitary pituitary adenoma (59,60).

Macroscopy: The specimen commonly consists of bony fragments.

Histology: Spicules of woven bone with odd C or Y shapes comprise the osseous portion in a background of bland, plump, moderately cellular fibroblasts, probably preosteogenic, and collagenous tissue (Figure 12.66). No mitoses or nuclear atypia is seen. The woven bony spicules usually lack lining osteoblasts and blend imperceptibly with the surrounding stroma. If the lesion has fractured, osteoblasts may be accompanied by hemosiderin-laden macrophages. In some variants the spicules resemble those seen in cementomas, with rounded shapes. Xanthomatous or chondroid foci may be present.

Differential diagnosis: If atypia, permeative pattern, and mitoses are seen, an FD-like OS should be considered. Osteofibrous dysplasia is also in the differential diagnosis, particularly in the jaw; OFD is round and has prominent osteoblastic rimming, whereas FD is oval with few osteoblasts. Fibrocartilaginous mesenchymoma is a largely cartilaginous proliferation within FD.

Osteofibrous dysplasia (OFD)

Osteofibrous dysplasia is a benign lesion composed of bone and fibrous tissue. It was originally termed ossifying fibroma of long bones. "Ossifying fibroma" now refers to unrelated jaw lesions that have ossicles and resemble FD. It is controversial whether OFD is a precursor to ADM; not all cases progress, but sometimes OFD is found in the background of ADM (54).

Clinical presentation: Osteofibrous dysplasia most frequently occurs in anterior tibial cortex or rarely fibula in the first decade, with a slight male predominance. In younger patients, OFD is locally aggressive, but may regress spontaneously in the second decade. Radiography demonstrates a benign elongated lesion in the diaphyseal cortex, with lucent or cystic areas and a sclerotic margin. Anterior tibial bowing is common. Soft-tissue involvement may be seen. Osteofibrous dysplasia is benign, but may recur if incompletely excised, sometimes requiring partial bone resection rather than curettage.

Genetics: Genetic abnormalities include trisomies 7, 8, 12, 20, and 21, features also seen in ADM (34).

Macroscopy: Usually bony fragments are received. It is rarely excised en bloc.

Histology: On biopsy, OFD is composed of bland spindle cells in a collagenous matrix, with scattered woven and lamellar bone spicules frequently lined by osteoclasts and osteoblasts (Figure 12.67). Isolated cells in the soft-tissue portion are often immunoreactive for cytokeratins, including AE1/AE3 and cytokeratins 14, 19, 1, and 5.

Differential diagnosis: This includes FD and ADM.

Langerhans-cell histiocytosis (LCH)

Langerhans-cell histiocytosis consists of monostotic or polyostotic proliferations of clonal Langerhans-type

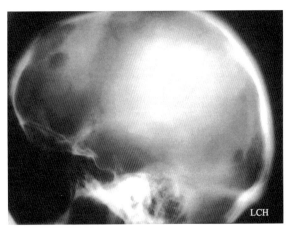

Figure 12.68 Langerhans-cell histiocytosis (imaging). Lesions have sharp borders and lytic centers. In the skull lesions have beveled edges and involve the tables unevenly.

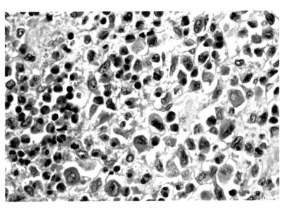

Figure 12.69 Langerhans-cell histiocytosis. Lesional cells have folded nuclei with bland chromatin and abundant pale eosinophilic cytoplasm. The lesional cells may be accompanied by eosinophils (H&E × 40).

dendritic cells, often accompanied by eosinophils and other inflammatory cells. It was formerly referred to variously as histiocytosis X, eosinophilic granuloma, Hand–Schüller–Christian disease, and Letterer–Siwe disease, depending on age, extent of disease, and related findings. Currently LCH is used, subdivided into monostotic, polyostotic, and/or soft-tissue or organ-involving forms, including lymph nodes, skin, or lung (61).

Clinical presentation: Most pediatric cases involve the skeleton, usually as a single lesion, or the skin in multisite disease. Single or multiple bone disease usually occurs between 5 and 15 years, while multisystem disease predominantly affects children < 5 years. Langerhans-cell histiocytosis is more common in males. Any bone may be involved, especially skull, vertebrae, ribs, pelvic bones, long bones, or facial bones. Patients present with pain, swelling, and tenderness; loose teeth may be observed. In multisystem disease, pituitary involvement may result in diabetes insipidus and orbital involvement with exophthalmos or proptosis. Langerhans-cell histiocytosis may occasionally be associated with hemophagocytic syndrome and some cases in early infancy may progress to a leukemia-like clinical picture with atypical Langerhans cells. On imaging, lesions have sharp borders and lytic centers initially, with ensuing chronic changes. Skull lesions characteristically have beveled edges and involve the tables unevenly (Figure 12.68). Monostotic lesions may resolve spontaneously or can be treated with curettage and corticosteroids. Multisystem disease is usually treated by chemotherapy regimens, including vinblastine and corticosteroids. Radiation therapy has been used for single lesions. COX2 expression has been observed, suggesting therapy using COX2 inhibitors such as celecoxib.

Genetics: Clonality has been demonstrated, but it is not clear whether the lesion is neoplastic or reactive, except in cases in infants with atypical Langerhans cells and a leukemic picture. 9p and 22q abnormalities and 1p loss have been observed (62).

Macroscopy: Curettage yields soft, tan, gray, or yellow tissue with hemorrhage.

Histology: Lesions are composed of loose clusters of plump LCH cells admixed with eosinophils, multinucleated osteoclast-like giant cells and sometimes other chronic inflammatory cells in varying proportions, with or without necrosis (Figure 12.69). Touch preparations often yield ideal specimens. On frozen section, eosinophils can resemble polymorphonuclear leukocytes and the lesion can be mistaken for acute infection. The diagnostic Langerhans cells are immunophenotypically dendritic cells, but lack dendritic processes. The cells have reniform nuclei with bland vesicular chromatin and frequent clefts or folds; multinucleation is common. The cytoplasm is abundant, plump, eccentric, and pale eosinophilic. Mitoses may be present, but are not atypical. Plasma cells may surround LCH lesions and suggest osteomyelitis (OML). CD1a and CD207 (Langerin), S100, CD68, and peanut lectin agglutinin are positive (Figure 12.70). The histiocytic markers fascin and factor XIIIa are negative. Specific membrane-associated structures known as Birbeck granules that resemble tennis racquets are diagnostic on ultrastructure, but EM is no longer required for diagnosis.

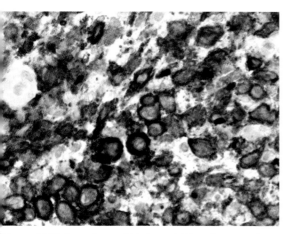

Figure 12.70 Langerhans cell histiocytosis. The cells are positive on CD1a immunostain (× 40).

Differential diagnosis: The differential diagnosis includes Rosai–Dorfman disease (RDD), juvenile xanthogranulomatosis, granulomatous disease, lymphoma, Erdheim–Chester disease (ECD) and fibro-osseous lesions. Early lesions may appear aggressive, prompting consideration of ES/PNET or OML. While LCH is typically metadiaphyseal, it can be present in the epiphysis and resemble CBL by imaging and histology, due to the giant cells and resemblance of Langerhans cells to chondroblasts. These other conditions lack CD1a or CD207 expression and eosinophils.

Erdheim–Chester disease (ECD)

Erdheim–Chester disease is a rare, benign histiocytosis with multiple bones involved by foamy histiocytes, fibrosis, and osteosclerosis. It is also termed polyostotic sclerosing histiocytosis.

Clinical presentation: More commonly an adult disease, there is a wide variety of patient ages, including the first decade, with a peak in the fifth through seventh decades. Systemic manifestations of mild bone pain, weight loss, fever, and weakness characterize ECD. Clinical features that overlap other benign and malignant histiocytoses include exophthalmos, diabetes insipidus, renal, cardiac, pulmonary or neurologic involvement, eyelid xanthomas, and hepatosplenomegaly. However, the lipid profile in ECD patients is normal. There is diffuse bilateral symmetrical osteosclerosis of the medullary cavity of long bones with relative epiphyseal sparing. Patients usually die within three years of renal, cardiopulmonary, or neurologic complications.

Genetics: One case with balanced chromosomal translocation t(12;15;20)(q11;q24;p13.3) has been identified. *BRAF (V600E)* mutations have been reported in multiple cases (63,64).

Macroscopy: Yellow, firm bony lesions.

Histology: Erdheim–Chester disease has diffuse marrow infiltration by foamy histiocytes associated with dense fibrosis, lymphocytes, plasma cells, and massive sclerosis of cortical and cancellous bone, with irregular cement lines. Histiocytic markers including CD68 and lysozyme are positive; S100 protein and CD1a are largely negative.

Differential diagnosis: This includes OML and other histiocytic processes, but these entities lack xanthomatous histiocytes.

Rosai–Dorfman disease (RDD)

Rosai–Dorfman disease is a rare solitary or multifocal histiocytic proliferative disease of possible viral etiology. It is also termed sinus histiocytosis with massive lymphadenopathy (SHML) (65; see Chapter 7).

Clinical presentation: Rosai–Dorfman disease or SHML usually presents with lymphadenopathy, but RDD may arise primarily in bone. Patients are usually young. Intraosseous locations include tibia, femur, clavicle, skull, maxilla, calcaneus, phalanx, metacarpal, and sacrum. Soft-tissue locations include subcutis in extremities, trunk, and head and neck. Simian virus 40 (SV40) has been identified in a few abdominal multicentric soft-tissue cases with persistent disease (66). Imaging demonstrates lytic lesions with well-defined, usually sclerotic margins. In general, RDD is solitary and follows a benign course with local excision.

Macroscopy: These are multilobulated, tan-yellow, and firm.

Histology: Rosai–Dorfman disease displays circumscribed nodules of large polygonal histiocytes with abundant pale eosinophilic cytoplasm demonstrating emperipolesis, and an aggregated and scattered background proliferation of lymphocytes and plasma cells, and sometimes pockets of numerous neutrophils (Figures 12.71 and 12.72). Rare spindling or mild cytologic atypia can be observed. Occasional pink cytoplasmic inclusions suggest viral etiology (66). The histiocytes are CD68- and S100-positive, and negative for CD1a and Langerin.

Differential diagnosis: This may include other histiocytic lesions, distinguished by morphology and immunophenotype.

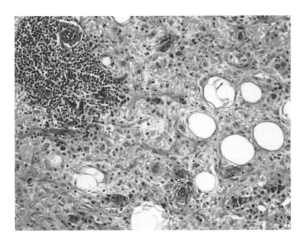

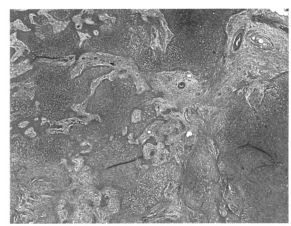

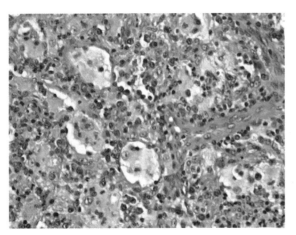

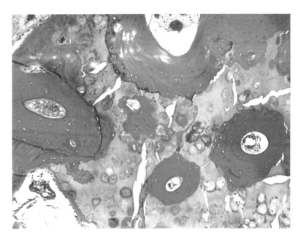

Figures 12.71 and 12.72 Rosai–Dorfman disease. Lesions are composed of lymphoid aggregates with plasma cells and polygonal histiocytes that display emperipolesis (H&E × 20 and × 40).

Figures 12.73 and 12.74 Fracture callus. An initial hematoma organizes with accompanying cellular cartilage and enchondral ossification (H&E × 20 and × 40).

Other bone lesions

Fracture callus (FC)

Fracture callus occurs as part of endochondral bony remodeling after fracture.

Clinical presentation: Microcallus can be observed in osteopenic osteoporotic bone and in healing fractures. In children, fractures often follow injury in long bones. Meningomyelocele can cause periarticular fractures resulting in Charcot joint. Avulsion fractures can be observed in the tibial tubercle in Osgood–Schlatter disease. Child abuse and osteogenesis imperfecta must be excluded in children with multiple fractures. Stress fracture (SF) with extensive periosteal new bone formation can be seen with repetitive trauma. Complications include fibrous non-union; pathologic fracture should not be missed. Imaging demonstrates linear cartilage.

Macroscopy: Approximation of fracture components can be observed.

Histology: Hematoma is present in recent fracture, followed by organization, linear cellular cartilage, and endochondral ossification (Figures 12.73 and 12.74).

Differential diagnosis: Fracture cartilage may be confused histologically with cartilaginous tumor; looking for linear cartilage and comparing with imaging studies is helpful.

Stress fracture (SF)

Definition and clinical presentation: Repetitive stress to bones in hikers, ballet dancers, and runners causes cumulative microfractures with reactive periosteal new bone formation, accompanied by chronic pain. Imaging demonstrates abundant periosteal new bone formation associated with a small fracture.

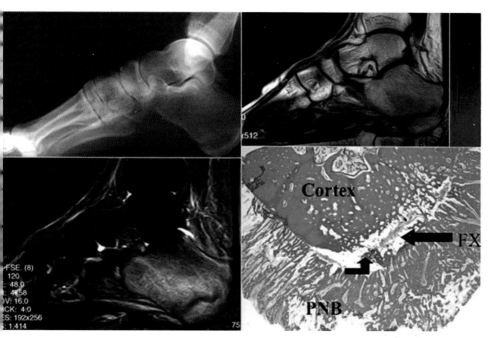

Figure 12.75 Stress fracture. The histology (bottom right) shows intramembranous (not endochondral) ossification (arrows) with a vigorous periosteal response.

Histology: The lesion demonstrates intramembranous rather than endochondral ossification, with a vigorous periosteal response (Figure 12.75).

Pseudarthrosis (PA)

Pseudarthrosis consists of fibrous tissue in place of normal bone development or FC, resulting in discontinuity of the bone.

Clinical presentation: Pseudarthrosis may arise in the context of healing fracture or congenitally. Congenital PA is seen at birth or in infancy, usually in the clavicle or mid-shaft of the tibia, radius, or ulna. The bone is discontinuous radiologically, with narrowing of bones on either side. Many cases in tibia arise in patients with neurofibromatosis type1. Pseudarthrosis may be difficult to treat, requiring amputation, and artificial limb placement.

Genetics: When associated with neurofibromatosis 1, double inactivation of the *NF1* gene has been proposed as an etiology (67).

Macroscopy: Following fracture, only dense fibrous tissue is observed instead of callus formation and reconstitution of intact bone. The specimen consists of white, rubbery, firm fibrous tissue.

Histology: The histologic lesion is composed of loose and dense fibrous connective tissue (Figure 12.76).

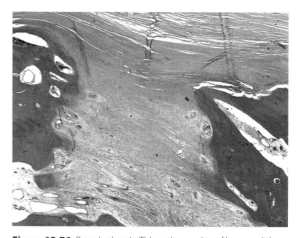

Figure 12.76 Pseudarthrosis. This entity consists of loose and dense fibrous connective tissue (H&E × 20).

Infectious osteomyelitis (IOML)

Infectious osteomyelitis may be acute or chronic, and caused by bacteria, fungi, mycobacteria, or other agents (68). Bacterial infection is the most common, usually *Staphylococcus aureus*. In many cases, no organisms are detected histologically or on culture. Proper diagnosis may then rest on response to surgery and antibiotic therapy.

Clinical presentation: Acute IOML may present with systemic signs and symptoms, including localized

427

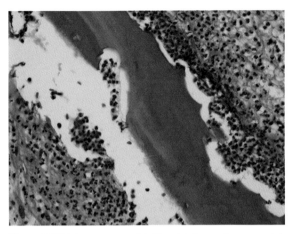

Figure 12.77 Acute osteomyelitis. There is inflammation appropriate to the infection; in this case we have purulent infiltrates in response to a bacterial infection, commonly *Staphylococcus*. The infection has obliterated marrow and dead bone is present (H&E × 40).

pain and swelling, fever, leukocytosis, and elevated C-reactive protein levels. Metaphyseal hematogenously spread IOML is more common in children, compared to IOML due to direct spread of organisms from injuries, or cellulitis due to poor wound healing in cases of diabetes, operative sites, or prostheses. Anatomic sites correlate with rapid bone growth, including proximal humerus, distal radius, distal femur, proximal tibia, calcaneus, and talus. Radiological changes appear after the first symptoms and are generally non diagnostic; positron emission tomography (PET), radionuclide and magnetic resonance (MRI) scans may assist in diagnosis and often demonstrate edema around the infection.

Macroscopy: Lesions may be biopsied or resected. Specimens are often loose or liquid, with sclerotic bony margins. Bacterial, fungal and mycobacterial cultures of the specimen are essential, but many specimens fail to yield positive cultures.

Histology: The acute lesion demonstrates inflammation appropriate to the infectious organisms: purulent infiltrates with bacterial infections, necrosis or granulomatous disease with fungi, and necrotizing granulomas with mycobacteria (Figure 12.77). Neonatal lesions are most commonly caused by *S. aureus*, *S. agalactiae*, or *E. coli*, probably acquired during delivery. The infection often obliterates hematogenous and fatty marrow, and abscesses with bone erosion may be seen. Chronic IOML is characterized by marrow fibrosis and reactive bony changes, with chronic inflammatory infiltrates that typically include plasma cells (Figure 12.78). Dead bone fragments, termed sequestra, often accompany inflammation

and may inhibit antibiotic penetration. When infection persists, reactive bone, the involucrum, may form a shell external to the normal cortex.

Genetics: Cases of mycobacterial IOML have been associated with interferon-γ receptor gene abnormalities. A *bax* gene nucleotide substitution is more frequent in patients with IOML, and *NOS3* polymorphism may be associated with IOML susceptibility (69–71).

Non-infectious osteomyelitis (NIOML)

This consists of bone and marrow inflammation without identifiable infectious cause; it is largely synonymous with chronic recurrent multifocal osteomyelitis (CRMO) (72).

Clinical presentation: This is similar to IOML, with multiple sites involved, one by one over time. No organisms are found, and CRMO is unresponsive to antibiotic therapy. It is often associated with Crohn's disease and purulent skin disorders. It is treated with steroids and non-steroidal antiinflammatory agents, and is often self-limited.

Genetics: Monogenic syndromic forms include Majeed syndrome due to *LPIN2* mutations, and interleukin-1 receptor antagonist deficiency due to *ILIRN* mutations. A susceptibility gene for this disorder at 18q21.3–18q22 has been linked to sporadic cases (73).

Microscopic: Chronic recurrent multifocal osteomyelitis resembles chronic IOML with reactive bony changes, loose myxoid fibrosis, and chronic inflammation, including plasma cells (Figure 12.79).

Differential diagnosis: Infection, benign or malignant neoplasms, and malformations are included. Langerhans-cell histiocytosis must be considered, as eosinophils can resemble polymorphonuclear leukocytes and Langerhans histiocytes can appear granulomatous.

Joint tumors and tumor-like lesions

Ganglion cyst (GC)

Ganglion cysts are benign cystic spaces in periarticular soft tissue, possibly related to synovial fluid leak with resultant mucoid cystic degeneration.

Clinical presentation: Ganglion cysts may be asymptomatic, but can be painful and palpable. The most common site is the wrist, especially with overuse.

Macroscopy: Gelatinous, cystic, whitish-tan soft tissue is seen.

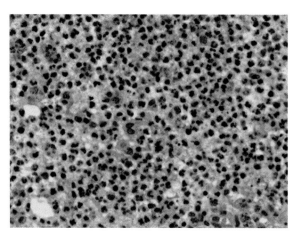

Figures 12.78 and 12.79 Chronic osteomyelitis. Chronic inflammatory infiltrates with plasma cells are accompanied by marrow fibrosis and necrotic bone lacking lacunar osteocytes. Micro-organisms are frequently absent. Chronic infectious osteomyelitis and chronic recurrent multifocal (non-infectious) osteomyelitis have similar appearances (H&E × 40 and × 20).

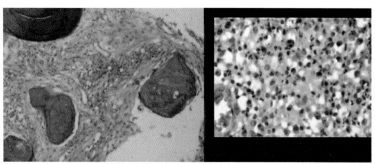

Histology: The lesion has fibromyxoid walls and sometimes interconnected cystic spaces that are filled with mucoid material and lack a synovial lining (Figure 12.80). Markers for vascular endothelium or epithelial cells are negative.

Differential diagnosis: A synovial cyst may be considered if synovial lining is present.

Synovial cyst (SCS)

Synovial cyst is a benign cystic outpouching of the synovial space caused by synovial fluid accumulation.

Clinical presentation: Synovial cyst most commonly occurs in the popliteal space, where it is known as Baker cyst, although it can occur in many locations. A palpable mass is cystic on sonography. Computed tomography demonstrates a homogenous mass with water density. Contrast may highlight septa in the cyst.

Macroscopy: The cysts have firm fibrotic walls.

Histology: Synovial cysts are lined by synovium, including an often attenuated dual cuboidal lining with underlying blood vessels.

Differential diagnosis: Ganglion cyst.

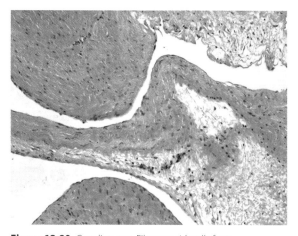

Figure 12.80 Ganglion cyst. Fibromyxoid walls form interconnected cystic spaces filled with mucoid material. No synovial lining is present (H&E × 20).

Pigmented villonodular synovitis (PVNS) and tenosynovial giant-cell tumor (TSGCT)

Tenosynovial giant-cell tumor and PVNS are benign histiocytoid synovial proliferations, termed PVNS if intra-articular and TSGCT if extra-articular. Either

429

can have a nodular or diffuse growth pattern (17,18,74).

Clinical presentation: Pigmented villonodular synovitis most commonly involves the knee, followed in frequency by the hip, ankle, shoulder, elbow, and spinal facet joints. It presents with monoarticular arthritic symptoms, such as pain, swelling, and joint dysfunction. Less commonly, a slow-growing palpable mass may have been present for years. Pigmented villonodular synovitis affects a wide age range, but tends to occur in young adults (< 40 years). Radiologically diffuse intra-articular PVNS shows subcapsular swelling with no lesional mineralization. Magnetic resonance imaging demonstrates low signal intensity on T1 and T2 weighted images due to hemosiderin deposits, sometimes thought to be diagnostic. Treatment for diffuse PVNS is total synovectomy; with complete excision the prognosis is good. With incomplete excision, 20–40% of patients may recur. However, the nodular or localized forms do not destroy the joint, and do well with complete excision. Tenosynovial giant-cell tumor is commonly found in the hand.

Genetics: Only a few cases have demonstrated molecular changes. Translocations involving the *CSF-1* gene on chromosome 1p11–3 are the most consistent rearrangements, although only found in a 2–16% of lesional cells (76).

Macroscopy: Diffuse intra-articular PVNS tends to be large (> 5.0 cm) with synovial thickening and a villonodular growth pattern. Depending on the number of hemosiderin- or lipid-laden macrophages, the tissue can vary in pigmentation, ranging from yellow to light brown.

Histology: The cells are histiocytoid with pale abundant eosinophilic cytoplasm, and small round to coffee-bean-shaped nuclei with small nucleoli, fine chromatin, and longitudinal grooves (Figure 12.81). While the cells may be plump and few mitoses may be present, marked mitotic activity, atypical mitoses, and marked cytologic atypia are absent. Scattered lymphocytes may be present. Lipid-laden macrophages (xanthoma cells) are almost always observed and osteoclast-type giant cells are often present, more frequently in extra-articular locations. The earliest lesion is a chronic proliferative synovitis with a vague villous growth pattern, and at least one osteoclast-type giant cell. Bone destruction and invasion do not indicate malignancy. Many cases cause degenerative joint disease. Synovial involvement by high-grade sarcoma with PVNS, or PVNS that recurs as high-grade

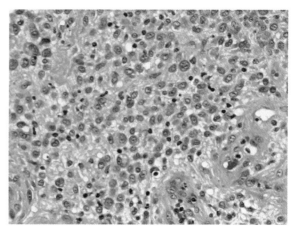

Figure 12.81 Pigmented villonodular synovitis. This is an intraarticular lesion with a diffuse (seen here) or nodular pattern (H&E × 40).

sarcoma, i.e. malignant TSGCT, is identified by marked pleomorphism, increased nuclear:cytoplasmic ratio, prominent nucleoli, sarcomatoid spindling, increased mitotic activity (> 20 per ten 40× fields) and necrosis. Malignant TSGCT/PVNS are controversial entities that are difficult to prove; they usually have a benign component in addition to a sarcoma. They should be separated from other sarcomas that involve joints by immunohistochemistry and morphology. The cells are CD68 positive in all subtypes including malignant. Dendritic-like desmin-positive cells can be observed in varying proportions (75).

Differential diagnosis: Diffuse PVNS can have plump rhabdoid cells and be worrisome for malignancy. The differential diagnosis may also include rheumatoid synovitis, hemosiderotic synovitis, or postarthroplasty changes. Villous hypertrophy may occur in rheumatoid synovitis or Lyme disease (LD); however, hemosiderin is usually not prominent and osteoclast-type giant cells are not found. Knee trauma (hemosiderotic synovitis (HS)), especially in those with a bleeding disorder such as hemophilia, can cause intra-articular chronic hemorrhage and surface hemosiderosis, but synovial hypertrophy, large nodules, villous fronds, and osteoclast-type giant cells are not identified. Foreign-body reaction as seen with arthroplasty or articular prosthesis can simulate PVNS. The history of joint replacement and use of methyl methacrylate bone cement or the presence of black metal particles within synoviocytes or subsynovial tissue favors a postarthroplasty reactive response vs. PVNS.

Synovial hemangioma (SH) and vascular malformation (VM)

These consist of benign CH, VM, or CAVM arising from the synovial lining (17,77).

Clinical presentation: Lesions generally arise in knees of children and young adults, predominantly in males, as masses with pain, swelling, or effusions; elbow or finger are also sites of occurrence. A mass over the joint can be palpated. Radiological findings are not specific, with joint-capsule thickening, soft-tissue mass, and occasionally bony erosion. Angiography and scans, particularly MRI, suggest a vascular lesion, either focal or diffuse, with occasional phleboliths. Treatment is limited to excision; diffuse lesions may present a surgical challenge. Recurrence after complete excision is rare.

Histology: Most commonly these lesions resemble VM (CAVM), with dilated thin-walled blood vessels in a loose myxoid matrix, at times accompanied by inflammation or hemosiderin-laden macrophages (78). Other patterns include CH, AVM, and VM, similar to their soft-tissue or osseous counterparts. Vascular spaces may develop papillary endothelial hyperplasia. The synovium may be villous. Recurrent hemorrhage may lead to HS.

Lipoma arborescens (LA)

Lipoma arborescens, also known as villous lipomatous proliferation of synovium, is a benign condition displaying fatty synovial soft tissue, possibly post-traumatic or related to synovitis. Lipoma arborescens related to post-traumatic enlargement of the fat pad flanking the patellar tendon is termed Hoffa syndrome (17,18).

Clinical presentation: Lipoma arborescens most commonly occurs in the knee, with painless swelling accompanied by effusion. On plain X-rays, the joint is full, and degenerative joint disease (DJD) may be seen. Computed tomography and MRI appearances are consistent with fat. The treatment is synovectomy.

Macroscopy: The synovium is bright yellow and usually papillary, but may be diffuse or nodular; DJD changes are often present.

Histology: The synovial lining is hyperplastic with replacement of underlying soft tissue by mature adipose tissue, with chronic inflammation and possibly myxoid change.

Differential diagnosis: Minimal fatty infiltration of synovium may be normal, and slight thickening is seen in DJD.

Other joint lesions

Rheumatoid arthritis (RA)

Rheumatoid arthritis consists of joint inflammation in patients with clinical and serologic evidence of rheumatoid disease (68).

Clinical presentation: Clinical, radiologic, and serologic features are necessary for diagnosis. Patients present with swelling and stiffness of several joints, and with radiologic evidence of joint inflammation, including articular erosion and osteopenia. Bilateral symmetric involvement is characteristic. Small joints and feet are involved initially, with any joint at risk. Serology for rheumatoid factor, anti-neutrophil antibodies, and cyclic citrullinated peptide (CCP) are diagnostic of RA. Rheumatoid factor consists of serum IgM that binds to the patient's IgG; it is associated with RA, but may be elevated in numerous disorders, particularly other collagen-vascular diseases.

Juvenile RA (juvenile idiopathic arthritis) generally begins in a large joint, in contrast to the small joints first affected in adults. Patients have distended joint capsules with fluid accumulation on radiologic imaging, especially on MRI and CT. Carpal bone damage often presents early. Bone ends may be enlarged. As in adult disease, rare late effects include joint and bone destruction. The disease is more proliferative than in adults. Spinal joints are often involved.

Genetics: Rheumatoid arthritis is associated with expression of HLA-DR4 associated with a gene on 6p; gene activity is involved in T-cell response to antigen-presenting cells.

Macroscopy: The synovium is red or reddish-brown, villous, and thickened with fibrin deposition. Cartilage is damaged and lost starting at the joint periphery, a form of secondary DJD. Meniscal destruction is common.

Histology: Neutrophils are found in synovial fluid. The synovium is hyperplastic with multinucleated giant cells; there is edema and expansion by infiltrates composed largely of plasma cells with Russell bodies, and lymphocytes with lymphoid follicles containing germinal centers. Synovial mesenchymal lining cells are prominent and enlarged. Vascular proliferation is seen. Fibrin may form rice bodies in the joint space. Pannus consists of synovial granulation tissue, inflammatory cells, and fibroblasts associated with cartilaginous destruction. The underlying bone may be chronically inflamed and display osteoporosis. As bone and cartilage are damaged, fragmentation further contributes to joint destruction.

431

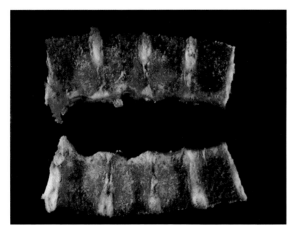

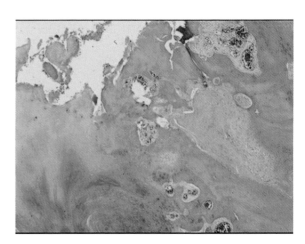

Figure 12.82 Degenerative joint disease (osteoarthritis).

Differential diagnosis: Similar clinicopathologic features may be seen in ankylosing spondylitis, psoriatic arthritis or other collagen-vascular disease-related arthritis, and Lyme disease. Lyme titers should be obtained at the time of RA serology.

Degenerative joint disease (DJD)

Degenerative joint disease consists of joint damage with cartilaginous destruction due to overuse, wear and tear, or malformations. Family genetics and inflammation play a role in later stages (68). Degenerative joint disease is often referred to as osteoarthritis.

Clinical presentation: In children, DJD is usually seen in congenitally malformed joints, such as in hip dysplasia.

Macroscopy: Initially the articular cartilage fibrillates or shreds, but over time cartilage disappears focally or diffusely, resulting in a polished or eburnated appearance of the exposed bone. Osteophytes form at the joint periphery (Figure 12.82).

Histology: The eburnated bone is sclerotic, with mucoid pseudocystic changes due to defects in subchondral bone with penetration of synovial fluid (Figure 12.83). Cartilage is often fibrillated (Figures 12.83 and 12.84). Osteophytes demonstrate peripheral endochondral ossification of cartilage and sclerosis. The synovial lining is hyperplastic, with variable stromal and perivascular chronic inflammation. Inflammation is significantly less impressive than that seen in RA.

Genetics: Patients with genetic disorders of collagen types or matrix proteins may develop DJD prematurely. Inborn errors of metabolism and Wilson disease may also manifest DJD (79).

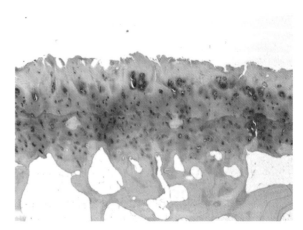

Figures 12.83 and 12.84 Degenerative joint disease. Articular cartilage is eroded, shredded, and ultimately lost or eburnated. Subchondral cysts may be present (H&E × 20).

Differential diagnosis: Generally the radiological, gross, and microscopic appearances are diagnostic.

Hemophilic arthropathy (HA), hemosiderotic synovitis (HS)

Hemophilic arthropathy consists of synovial inflammation and damage due to chronic intraarticular hemorrhage, often following minor trauma, in patients with hemophilia or, rarely, intra-articular vascular lesions (17,18).

Clinical presentation: Patients present with painful stiff joints due to DJD, usually involving the knee, elbow, or ankle, and less frequently in shoulders or hips. Radiological imaging of early lesions detects swelling due to effusion, epiphyseal overgrowth, and osteoporosis. Knee and elbow intercondylar notches may widen from synovial hypertrophy. In later stages, subchondral cysts are followed by cartilage damage and erosions, with subsequent joint-space narrowing. Magnetic resonance imaging is particularly helpful in defining early and late lesions. Treatment aims at management of joint degeneration. Hemophilic pseudotumors may lead to muscle and bone damage, infection, or neuropathy.

Genetics: Hemophilia A and B are X-linked disorders involving the genes for the coagulation factors VIII and IX.

Macroscopy: The synovium is brown or rust-colored with early villous projections. Nodules similar to PVNS are not observed. Later in the disease, synovium thickens and becomes opaque due to fibrotic scarring. Articular cartilage may display green-black discoloration. Hemophilic pseudotumors may occur in affected joints.

Histology: Synovial lining cells are plump, and contain hemosiderin granules, with perivascular hemosiderin-laden macrophages in soft tissue and cartilage, sometimes with chondrocyte necrosis. Lipidized and giant cells are not observed. Degenerative joint disease with cartilage destruction is often seen. Pseudotumors are composed of coagula of partially clotted blood and fibrotic membranes.

Differential diagnosis: Pigmented villonodular synovitis may manifest hemosiderin deposition and synovial hyperplasia, but displays more florid changes grossly, with microscopic clusters of synovial lining cells and multinucleated giant cells.

Lyme disease (LD)

Lyme disease is named for Lyme, Connecticut, where an epidemic of arthritis was associated with skin erythema. Lyme disease is caused by the spirochete *Borrelia burgdorferi*, an arthropod-borne infection transmitted by nymph-stage Ixodes deer ticks that affects joints, mostly as a secondary host response to the organism.

Clinical presentation: Patients are found in the north-eastern, eastern, and midwestern United States, Europe, and Japan. Patients present with fever, headache, and fatigue in endemic areas. The characteristic rash is erythema migrans, with an initial targetoid skin lesion followed by generalized arthralgias in the early disseminated stage; these stages can be treated with antibiotics. Arthritis is a late complication, as are encephalitis and cardiac disease; this phase is autoimmune and unresponsive to antibiotics. The diagnosis is made by serology, IgM and IgG testing, enzyme-linked immunosorbent assay (ELISA), and

confirmatory Western blotting. Polymerase chain reaction (PCR)-based detection of organisms from a skin lesion, synovial biopsy, or fluid is possible, but not routinely performed. IgM elevation for Lyme titer can be falsely positive with Epstein–Barr virus, cytomegalovirus, and rheumatoid arthritis.

Histology: With acute disease the synovium displays fibrin and polymorphonuclear leukocytes, as seen in infection, or pannus as seen in RA. Chronic changes include villous synovial proliferation with nodular aggregates of lymphoid cells and stromal fibrin, and microangiopathic lesions of small arterial occlusion with onion-skin-like myointimal proliferation. Warthin–Starry stain may demonstrate the spirochetes.

Differential diagnosis: The histology can mimic RA; plasma cells appear to be more numerous in RA. History and serology are helpful to separate RA and Lyme synovitis.

Tumoral calcinosis (TC)

Tumoral calcinosis consists of hydroxyapatite deposition with granulomatous response in patients with secondary hyperparathyroidism or hypercalcemia, idiopathic, or due to end-stage renal disease.

Clinical presentation: There are three types: (1) solitary without hyperphosphatemia; (2) multiple lesions with hyperphosphatemia, but not hypercalcemia (familial); and (3) those with hypercalcemia due to renal disease. Tumoral calcinosis occurs in all ages, including children, with a female predominance of mostly hands and feet, with mostly solitary to occasionally multiple lesions that may cause pain or limitation of joint mobility. Some patients report antecedent trauma, scleroderma (especially with acral lesions), long-standing osteoarthritis, or congenital bony deformities, including infants with congenital hand malformations, as well as chronic renal failure. Patients in type 1 can be from tropical or subtropical regions and these lesions can simulate parasite granulomas. Type 2 patients are often African-American adolescents with elevated serum 1,25-dihydroxyvitamin D levels, inherited as autosomal recessive or dominant. Type 3 is the most common, with end-stage renal disease and visceral involvement in older patients. Tumoral calcinosis is thought to arise from an error in phosphorus metabolism that leads to extracellular deposition of calcium hydroxyapatite crystals. Patients can also have dental abnormalities, periosteal thickening, and eye lesions. Shoulder, scapulae, hips, buttocks, and elbows are common locations, but not intra-articular sites. Radiologically, periarticular

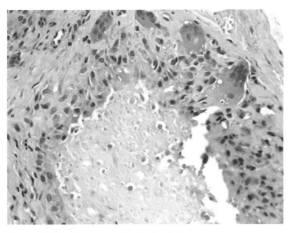

Figure 12.85 Tumoral calcinosis. The lesion demonstrates a histiocytic response to hydroxyapatite (H&E × 20).

mineralization is seen. A firm non-tender mass with signs of inflammation may be clinically present. Treatment, depending on type, includes surgery for types 1 and 2, and treatment of underlying renal disease for type 3 with phosphate binders, low-calcium dialysate, renal transplant, and parathyroidectomy. Sodium thiosulfate and vinpocetine are used to reduce mass size.

Genetics: The familial type 2 patients with multiple lesions have mutations in *GALNT3*, *FGF23*, and *KL*. *SMAD9* mutations have been detected in normophosphatemic familial patients of type 1.

Macroscopy: White, creamy material may be seen clinically. Sizes vary from smaller in distal lesions (0.3 cm) to large in proximal lesions, with multiloculated cystic, rubbery, gritty yellow to milky-white appearance. Subcutaneous lesions can cause superficial ulceration.

Histology: In tenosynovial, fascial, dermal, and, rarely, intra-articular sites, lesions are characterized by central pinkish calcification with calcospherites and surrounding mononuclear and multinucleated foreign-body and Langerhans histiocytes (Figure 12.85). Multiloculation and cystification can occur, with granulation tissue, fibrosis, and chronic inflammation, with progression to calcification, osseous metaplasia, and hyalinized fibrous tissue.

Differential diagnosis: Tophaceous pseudogout, granulomatous inflammatory disease, milk alkali syndrome, calcium deposits due to collagen vascular disease, such as dermatomyositis, and soft-tissue chondroma may be considered.

Acknowledgment

We are grateful to Steve Taylor, PA, for excellent assistance with illustrations.

Key references for further reading

1. Unni KK, Inwards C, Bridge JA, *et al. Tumors of the Bones and Joints. AFIP Atlas of Tumor Pathology*, fourth series, fascicle 2. Washington, DC: American Registry of Pathology in collaboration with the Armed Forces Institute of Pathology; 2005.

2. Vigorita, VJ. *Orthopaedic Pathology*, second edn. Philadelphia, PA: Wolters Kluwer; 2008.

3. Unni KK, Inwards CY. *Dahlin's Bone Tumors*, sixth edn. Philadelphia, PA: Wolters Kluwer; 2010.

4. Folpe AL, Inwards CY, editors. *Bone and Soft Tissue Pathology*. Philadelphia, PA: Saunders Elsevier; 2010.

5. Bullough PG. *Orthopaedic Pathology*, fifth edn. Edinburgh: Mosby; 2010.

6. Fletcher CDM, Bridge JA, Hogendoorn PCW, Mertens F, editors. *WHO Classification of Tumours of Soft Tissue and Bone*. Lyon: IARC Press; 2013.

References

7. Romeo S, Hogendoorn PC, Dei Tos AP. Benign cartilaginous tumors of bone: From morphology to somatic and germ-line genetics. Adv. Anat. Pathol. 2009;**16**:307–15.

8. Tallini G, Dorfman H, Brys P, *et al.* Correlation between clinicopathological features and karyotype in 100 cartilaginous and chordoid tumours. A report from the Chromosomes and Morphology (CHAMP) Collaborative Study Group. J. Pathol. 2002;**196**:194–203.

9. Fanburg JC, Meis-Kindblom JM, Rosenberg AE. Multiple enchondromas associated with spindle cell hemangioendotheliomas: An overlooked variant of Maffucci's syndrome. Am. J. Surg. Pathol. 1995;**19**:1029–38.

10. Pansuriya TC, van Eijk R, d'Adamo P, *et al.* Somatic mosaic IDH1 and IDH2 mutations are associated with enchondroma and spindle cell hemangioma in Ollier disease and Maffucci syndrome. Nat. Genet. 2011;**43**:1256–61.

11. Sjögren H, Orndal C, Tingby O, *et al.* Cytogenetic and spectral karyotype analyses of benign and malignant cartilage tumours. Int. J. Oncol. 2004;**24**:1385–91.

12. Mertens F, Möller E, Mandahl N, *et al.* The t(X;6) in subungual exostosis results in transcriptional deregulation of the gene for insulin receptor substrate 4. Int. J. Cancer 2011;**128**:487–91.

13. Nora FE, Dahlin DC, Beabout JW. Bizarre parosteal osteochondromatous proliferations of the hands and feet. Am. J. Surg. Pathol. 1983;**7**:245–50.

14. Moosavi CA, Al-Nahar LA, Murphey MD, *et al.* Fibroosseous pseudotumor of the digit: A

clinicopathologic study of 43 new cases. Ann. Diagn. Pathol. 2008;**12**:21–8.

15. Nilsson M, Domanski HA, Mertens F, *et al.* Molecular cytogenetic characterization of recurrent translocation breakpoints in bizarre parosteal osteochondromatous proliferation (Nora's lesion). Hum. Pathol. 2004;**35**:1063–9.

16. Murphey MD, Vidal JA, Fanburg-Smith JC, *et al.* From the archives of the AFIP. Imaging of synovial chondromatosis with radiologic-pathologic correlation. Radiologics 2007;**27**:1465–88.

17. Nielsen GP, Rosenberg AE, O'Connell JX, *et al.* Tumors and diseases of the joint. Semin. Diagn. Pathol. 2011;**28**:37–52.

18. O'Connell JX. Pathology of the synovium. Am. J. Clin. Pathol. 2000;**114**:773–84.

19. Davis RI, Hamilton A, Biggart JD. Primary synovial chondromatosis: A clinicopathologic review and assessment of malignant potential. Hum. Pathol. 1998;**29**:683–8.

20. Gadwal SR, Fanburg-Smith JC, Gannon FH, *et al.* Primary chondrosarcoma of the head and neck in pediatric patients: A clinicopathologic study of 14 cases with a review of the literature. Cancer 2000;**88**:2181–8.

21. Hameed M, Dorfman H. Primary malignant bone tumors–Recent developments. Semin. Diagn. Pathol. 2011;**28**:86–101.

22. Fanburg-Smith JC, Auerbach A, Marwaha JS, *et al.* Reappraisal of mesenchymal chondrosarcoma: Novel morphologic observations of the hyaline cartilage and endochondral ossification and beta-catenin, sox 9, and osteocalcin immunostaining. Hum. Pathol. 2010;**41**:653–62.

23. Fanburg-Smith JC, Auerbach A, Marwaha JS, *et al.* Immunoprofile of mesenchymal chondrosarcoma: Aberrant desmin and EMA expression, retention of INI1, and negative estrogen receptor in 22 female-predominant central nervous system and musculoskeletal cases. Ann. Diagn. Pathol. 2010;**14**:8–14.

24. Selesnick SH, Desloge RB, Bullough PG. Protuberant fibro-osseous lesions of the temporal bone: A unique clinicopathologic diagnosis. Am. J. Otol. 1999;**20**:394–6.

25. Sia SF, Davidson AS, Soper JR, *et al.* Protuberant fibro-osseous lesion of the temporal bone: "Bullough lesion". Am. J. Surg. Pathol. 2010;**34**:1217–23.

26. Gadwal SR, Gannon FH, Fanburg-Smith JC, *et al.* Primary osteosarcoma of the head and neck in pediatric patients: A clinicopathologic study of 22 cases with a review of the literature. Cancer 2001;**91**:598–605.

27. Bridge JA, Nelson M, McComb E, *et al.* Cytogenetic findings in 73 osteosarcoma specimens and a review of the literature. Cancer Genet. Cytogenet. 1997;**95**:74–87.

28. Bayani J, Zielenska M, Pandita A, *et al.* Spectral karyotyping identifies recurrent complex rearrangements of chromosomes 8, 17, and 20 in osteosarcomas. Genes Chromosomes Cancer 2003;**36**:7–16.

29. Fanburg JC, Rosenberg AE, Weaver DL, *et al.* Osteocalcin and osteonectin immunoreactivity in the diagnosis of osteosarcoma. Am. J. Clin. Pathol. 1997;**108**:464–73.

30. Dickman PS. Ewing's sarcoma/primitive neuroectodermal tumor. Pathol. Case Rev. 2000;**5**:60–70.

31. Tsokos M, Alaggio RD, Dehner LP, *et al.* Ewing sarcoma/peripheral primitive neuroectodermal tumor and related tumors. Pediatr. Dev. Pathol. 2012;**15**(1 Suppl):108–26.

32. Pinto A, Dickman P, Parham D. Pathobiologic markers of the Ewing sarcoma family of tumors: State of the art and prediction of behavior. Sarcoma 2011;**2011**:856190.

33. Moran CA, Vidal JA, Murphey MD, *et al.* Desmoplastic fibroma: More clearly defining this entity. A clinicopathologic and radiologic study of 58 cases. Mod. Patho.l 2007;**20**:67.

34. Bridge JA, Swarts SJ, Buresh C, *et al.* Trisomies 8 and 20 characterize a subgroup of benign fibrous lesions arising in both soft tissue and bone. Am. J. Pathol. 1999;**154**:729–33.

35. Ehrig T, Billings SD, Fanburg-Smith JC. Superficial primitive neuroectodermal tumor/Ewing sarcoma (PN/ES): Same tumor as deep PN/ES or new entity? Ann. Diagn. Pathol. 2007;**11**:153–9.

36. Lasota J, Fanburg-Smith JC. Genetics for the diagnosis and treatment of mesenchymal tumors. Semin. Musculoskelet. Radiol. 2007;**11**(3):215–30.

37. Folpe AL, Goldblum JR, Rubin BP, *et al.* Morphologic and immunophenotypic diversity in Ewing family tumors: A study of 66 genetically confirmed cases. Am. J. Surg. Pathol. 2005;**29**:1025–33.

38. Llombart-Bosch A, Machado I, Navarro S, *et al.* Histological heterogeneity of Ewing's sarcoma/PNET: An immunohistochemical analysis of 415 genetically confirmed cases with clinical support. Virchows Arch. 2009;**455**:397–411.

39. Ozdemirli M, Fanburg-Smith JC, Hartmann D-P, Azumi N, Miettinen M. Differentiating lymphoblastic lymphoma and Ewing's sarcoma: Lymphocyte markers and gene rearrangement. Mod. Pathol. 2001;**14**:1175–82.

40. Valent P, Horny HP, Escribano L, *et al.* Diagnostic criteria and classification of mastocytosis: A consensus proposal. Leuk. Res. 2001;**25**:603–25.

41. Amon U, Hartmann K, Horny HP, *et al.* Mastocytosis – an update. J. Dtsch. Dermatol. Ges. 2010;**8**:695–711.

42. Buresh CJ, Seemayer TA, Nelson M, *et al.* t(X;4)(q22; q31.3) in giant cell reparative granuloma. Cancer Genet. Cytogenet. 1999;**115**:80–1.

43. Ortiz-Cruz E, Quinn RH, Fanburg JC, *et al.* Late development of malignant fibrous histiocytoma at the site of a giant cell tumor. Clin. Orthop. 1995;**318**;199–204.

44. Gong L, Liu W, Sun X, *et al.* Histological and clinical characteristics of malignant giant cell tumor of bone. Virchows Arch. 2012;**460**:327–34.

45. Gorunova L, Vult von Steyern F, Storlazzi CT, *et al.* Cytogenetic analysis of 101 giant cell tumors of bone: Nonrandom patterns of telomeric associations and other structural aberrations. Genes Chromosomes Cancer 2009;**48**:583–602.

46. Bruder E, Perez-Atayde AR, Jundt G, *et al.* Vascular lesions of bone in children, adolescents, and young adults. A clinicopathologic reappraisal and application of the ISSVA classification. Virchows Arch. 2009;**454**:161–79.

47. Gupta A, Kozakewich H. Histopathology of vascular anomalies. Clin. Plastic Surg. 2011;**38**:31–44.

48. Kransdorf MJ, Murphey MD, Fanburg-Smith JC. Classification of benign vascular lesions: History, current nomenclature, and suggestions for imagers. Am. J. Roentgenol. 2011;**197**:8–11.

49. Cahill AM, Nijs EL. Pediatric vascular malformations: pathophysiology, diagnosis, and the role of interventional radiology. Cardiovasc. Intervent. Radiol. 2011;**34**:691–704.

50. Fanburg-Smith JC, Michal M, Partanen TA, *et al.* Papillary intralymphatic angioendothelioma (PILA). A report of twelve cases of a distinctive vascular tumor with phenotypic features of lymphatic vessels. Am. J. Surg. Pathol. 1999;**23** (9):1004–10.

51. Woelfel C, Liehr T, Weise A, *et al.* Molecular cytogenetic characterization of epithelioid hemangioendothelioma. Cancer Genet. 2011;**204**:671–6.

52. Abedalthagafi M, Rushing EJ, Auerbach A, *et al.* Sporadic cutaneous angiosarcomas generally lack hypoxia-inducible factor 1-α: A histologic and immunosthistochemical study of 45 cases. Ann. Diagn. Pathol. 2010;**14**:15–22.

53. Fanburg-Smith JC, Furlong MA, Childers ELB. Oral and salivary gland angiosarcoma. A clinicopathologic study of 29 cases. Mod. Pathol. 2003;**16**:263–71.

54. Gleason BC, Liegl-Atzwanger B, Kozakewich HP, *et al.* Osteofibrous dysplasia and adamantinoma in children and adolescents: A clinicopathologic reappraisal. Am. J. Surg. Pathol. 2008;**32**:363–76.

55. Bridge JA, Fidler ME, Neff JR, *et al.* Adamantinoma-like Ewing's sarcoma: Genomic confirmation, phenotypic drift. Am. J. Surg. Pathol. 1999;**23**:159–65.

56. Althof PA, Ohmori K, Zhou M, *et al.* Cytogenetic and molecular cytogenetic findings in 43 aneurysmal bone cysts: Aberrations of 17p mapped to 17p13.2 by fluorescence in situ hybridization. Mod. Pathol. 2004;**17**:518–25.

57. Sakai Junior N, Pereira MF, Kalil RK. A simple bone cyst of the distal humerus with a t(7;12)(q21;q24.3) in a patient with hypophosphatemic rickets. Cancer Genet. 2012;**205**:541–3.

58. Riddle ND, Bui MM. Fibrous dysplasia. Arch. Pathol. Lab. Med. 2013;**137**:134–8.

59. Lee SE, Lee EH, Park H, *et al.* The diagnostic utility of the GNAS mutation in patients with fibrous dysplasia: Meta-analysis of 168 sporadic cases. Hum. Pathol. 2012;**43**:1234–42.

60. Liang Q, Wei M, Hodge L, Fanburg-Smith, *et al.* Quantitative analysis of activating α subunit of the G protein (Gsα) mutation by pyrosequencing in fibrous dysplasia and other bone lesions. J. Mol. Diagn. 2011;**13**:137–42.

61. Kairouz S, Hashash J, Kabbara W, *et al.* Dendritic cell neoplasms: An overview. Am. J. Hematol. 2007;**82**:924–8.

62. Dacic S, Trusky C, Bakker A, *et al.* Genotypic analysis of pulmonary Langerhans cell histiocytosis. Hum. Pathol. 2003;**34**:1345–9.

63. Haroche J, Charlotte F, Arnaud L, *et al.* High prevalence of BRAF V600E mutations in Erdheim-Chester disease but not in other non-Langerhans cell histiocytoses. Blood 2012;**120**:2700–3.

64. Vencio EF, Jenkins RB, Schiller JL, *et al.* Clonal cytogenetic abnormalities in Erdheim-Chester disease. Am. J. Surg. Pathol. 2007;**31**:319–21.

65. Demicco EG, Rosenberg AE, Björnsson J, *et al.* Primary Rosai-Dorfman disease of bone: A clinicopathologic study of 15 cases. Am. J. Surg. Pathol. 2010;**34**:1324–33.

66. Al-Daraji W, Anandan V, Klassen-Fischer M, *et al.* Soft tissue Rosai Dorfman disease: 29 new lesions in 18 patients with detection of polyomavirus antigen in 3 abdominal cases. Ann. Diagn. Pathol. 2010;**14**:309–16.

67. Lee SM, Choi IH, Lee DY, *et al.* Is double inactivation of the NF1 gene responsible for the development of congenital pseudarthrosis of the tibia associated with NF1? J. Orthop. Res. 2012;**30**:1535–40.

68. DiCarlo EF, Kahn LB. Inflammatory diseases of the bones and joints. Semin. Diagn. Pathol. 2011;**28**:53–64.

69. Asensi V, Montes AH, Valle E, *et al.* The NOS3 (27-bp repeat, intron 4) polymorphism is associated with susceptibility to osteomyelitis. Nitric Oxide 2007;**16**:44–53.

70. Oca–a MG, Valle-Garay E, Montes AH, *et al.* Bax gene G(-248)A promoter polymorphism is associated with increased lifespan of the neutrophils of patients with osteomyelitis. Genet. Med. 2007;**9**:249–55.

71. Storgaard M, Varming K, Herlin T, *et al.* Novel mutation in the interferon-gamma-receptor gene and susceptibility to mycobacterial infections. Scand. J. Immunol. 2006;**64**:137–9.

72. Ferguson PJ, Sandu M. Current understanding of the pathogenesis and management of chronic recurrent multifocal osteomyelitis. Curr. Rheumatol. Rep. 2012;**14**:130–41.

73. Golla A, Jansson A, Ramser J, *et al.* Chronic recurrent multifocal osteomyelitis (CRMO): Evidence for a susceptibility gene located on chromosome 18q21.3–18q22. Eur. J. Hum. Genet. 2002;**10**:217–21.

74. Murphey MD, Rhee JH, Lewis RB, *et al.* Pigmented villonodular synovitis: Radiologic-pathologic correlation. Radiologics 2008;**28**:1493–518.

75. O'Connell JX, Fanburg JC, Rosenberg AE. Giant cell tumor of tendon sheath and pigmented villonodular synovitis: Immunophenotype suggests a synovial cell origin. Hum. Pathol. 1995;**26**:771–5.

76. Cupp JS, Miller MA, Montgomery KD, *et al.* Translocation and expression of CSF1 in pigmented villonodular synovitis, tenosynovial giant cell tumor, rheumatoid arthritis and other reactive synovitides. Am. J. Surg. Pathol. 2007;**31**:970–6.

77. Greenspan A, Azouz EM, Matthews J 2nd, *et al.* Synovial hemangioma: Imaging features in eight histologically proven cases, review of the literature, and differential diagnosis. Skeletal. Radiol. 1995;**24**:583–90.

78. Devaney K, Vinh TN, Sweet DE. Synovial hemangioma: A report of 20 cases with differential diagnostic considerations. Hum. Pathol. 1993;**24**:737–45.

79. Bálint G, Szebenyi B. Hereditary disorders mimicking and/or causing premature osteoarthritis. Bailliercs Best. Pract. Res. Clin. Rheumatol. 2000;**14**:219–50.

Chapter 13

Neuropathology

David A. Ramsay and Fabiana Lubieniecki

Introduction

Surgical pediatric neuropathology is a specialized branch of pathology that is usually carried out by neuropathologists. Accordingly, a comprehensive account of surgical neuropathology lies beyond the "essentials" of surgical pediatric pathology. However, a surgical pediatric pathologist should be able to recognize common lesions and be capable of ensuring the optimal preservation of biopsies from patients with other unusual, rare, or complex disorders so that the material can be referred to regional neuropathologists.

The majority of pediatric surgical neuropathology biopsies are from tumors and skeletal muscle; less frequently specimens are received from "epilepsy neurosurgery," brain biopsies are carried out in cases of progressive atypical neurological disorders (which are usually rare inflammatory disorders or infections in immune-suppressed patients), and peripheral nerves may be sampled to attempt to delineate the cause of a neuropathy.

As a general principle, pathologists should be aware of the clinical history, neuroimaging findings, and the results of relevant ancillary investigations before they formulate their diagnoses. Molecular biological findings are also playing an increasing role in diagnostic formulations (1,2).

Tumors of the central nervous system (CNS)

In this section, many of the more common CNS tumors are described; standard texts should be consulted for further information on and comprehensive illustrations of these lesions (3,4). There are also numerous rare pediatric brain tumors that represent, as a group, a significant part of a pediatric surgical

pathology practice; for this reason, these tumors are briefly mentioned here, and appropriate citations in the medical literature are provided.

General comments

Classification, grading, and incidence

Pediatric intracranial tumors can be roughly categorized as gliomas and glioneuronal tumors, undifferentiated or embryonal neoplasms, germ-cell tumors, tumors of the meninges, and miscellaneous other tumors. The incidence of primary brain tumors in the 0 to 14 years age group is 4.61/100 000 patient years; the commonest tumors are various astrocytomas (40%), medulloblastomas, and other primitive or embryonal neoplasms (21%), ependymomas and anaplastic ependymomas (8%), and "unclassified" primary brain tumors (6%) (5). Of the astrocytomas, the pilocytic astrocytoma is the commonest (56%), the others being "not otherwise classified" (NOS; 17%), glioblastomas (9%), and "unique variants," such as the pleomorphic xanthoastrocytoma (7%), anaplastic astrocytomas (7%), and diffuse astrocytomas (4%). Other significant tumors include germ-cell tumors, nerve-sheath tumors, craniopharyngiomas, oligodendrogliomas, and anaplastic oligodendrogliomas, meningiomas, choroid plexus tumors, and pituitary-region tumors.

The relatively numerous "unclassified" primary brain tumors and "astrocytomas NOS" reflect the difficulty in accurately categorizing a significant proportion of pediatric brain tumors, either because the biopsy is small and non-representative or the appearances of the tumor do not fit recognized categories.

All CNS tumors are graded on a scale of I to IV, depending on their expected prognosis (3); accordingly,

Essentials of Surgical Pediatric Pathology, ed. Marta C. Cohen and Irene Scheimberg. Published by Cambridge University Press.
© Cambridge University Press 2014.

at the extremes, a "benign" meningioma is a WHO grade I "brain tumor" whereas the "malignant" medulloblastoma or glioblastoma is a WHO grade IV "brain tumor."

The completeness of resection is also an important prognostic feature; for example, the histologically "benign" hypothalamic pilocytic astrocytoma (WHO Grade I) and the diffuse astrocytoma (WHO Grade II) cannot be completely resected, owing to their critical location and capacity for widespread infiltration respectively, and they may accordingly exhibit a "malignant" course – similarly, the completeness of resection of a meningioma (the "Simpson grade") is a better prognostic indicator than the tumor grade.

Clinical presentation and the diagnostic significance of patient age and tumor location

The signs and symptoms caused by brain tumors are legion, but fall into one or more broad categories: seizures (especially temporal and frontal lesions); loss of function (when "sensitive" or "eloquent" regions of the brain are involved, such as the motor cortex, visual axis, and brain stem); symptoms of raised intracranial pressure (i.e., headache, nausea, vomiting, obtundation or coma, and third and fourth cranial nerve palsies) – this category of signs and symptoms is particularly characteristic of lesions that cause hydrocephalus by interfering with the flow of colony stimulating factor through the cerebral aqueduct (e.g., tumors of the pineal region and fourth ventricle) or in cases where the tumor and its associated brain swelling are extensive.

The age of the patient, the pace of evolution of the clinical signs and symptoms, and the location and neuroimaging appearance of the neoplasm provide useful clues to the identity of the tumor:

- The age of presentation varies somewhat for different types of tumors; for example, atypical teratoid/rhabdoid tumors occur in the first three years of life, medulloblastomas and pilocytic astrocytomas appear from around three years of age onwards, and diffuse astrocytic tumors (including the glioblastomas) and germ-cell tumors generally occur at the end of the first and in the second decade of life (6,7).
- A long history favors a lower-grade tumor and a short history an aggressive tumor; e.g., an uncomfortable child with a several- month-long history of worsening nocturnal headaches, may have a cerebellar pilocytic astrocytoma, whereas a fractious, miserable, headache-ridden child with a short history may have a medulloblastoma.

Table 13.1 CNS location and tumor type

Site	Common tumor type
Cerebral hemispheres (solid tumors)	Diffuse astrocytoma Desmoplastic (infantile) astrocytoma/ganglioglioma Primitive neuroectodermal tumor Atypical teratoid/malignant rhabdoid tumors
Cerebral hemispheres ('cystic' tumors)	High-grade glioma with cyst-like central necrosis Pilocytic astrocytoma Pleomorphic xanthoastrocytoma
Pineal region	Pineoblastoma Germ-cell tumor
Suprasellar region/ hypothalamus	Craniopharyngioma Germ-cell tumor
Other midline tumor and tumor-like lesions	Dermoid and epidermoid cysts
Intraventricular and juxtaventricular region	Choroid plexus papilloma and carcinoma Ependymoma Subependymal giant-cell astrocytoma Meningioma (intraventricular)
Brain stem	Brain stem glioma
Cerebellum	Medulloblastoma Pilocytic astrocytoma
Spinal cord	Diffuse astrocytoma Ependymoma Pilocytic astrocytoma
	Myxopapillary ependymoma (filum terminal) Paraganglioma (filum terminal)

- The site of occurrence of the tumor is also diagnostically useful. Intracranial tumors that are outside the brain (i.e., extra-axial tumors) are likely to be meningiomas or schwannomas. Table 13.1 provides a list of sites and their frequently associated "intraparenchymal" tumors.
- A "ring-enhancing" intracranial lesion has a broad differential diagnosis, including a necrotic neoplasm with perinecrosis enhancement, enhancement around the margins of a pleomorphic xanthoastrocytoma or pilocytic astrocytoma, or perilesional enhancement related to a bacterial abscess, an acute demyelinating plaque or an organizing intracerebral hematoma.
- There are several familial tumor syndromes that may involve the nervous system. The most common is neurofibromatosis (NF) 1 and 2 in which there is

439

increased risk of meningiomas, intracranial schwannomas, optic-nerve gliomas, and various intra-axial glioma-like hamartomas (3).

Technical considerations and comments on the frozen section

Brain tumors may be difficult to access surgically or they may be in functionally critical parts of the brain. For this reason it is common to receive tiny samples of tissue. In such circumstances, the possibility of a "non-representative" biopsy should always be taken into account and, even more so than usual, the histological findings should be interpreted in the clinical and neuroimaging context.

Intraoperative diagnoses from smear (squash) preparations or frozen sections are commonly requested by the neurosurgeons on biopsies of intracranial tumors, whether to ensure that the tissue is "lesional," as a matter of routine, or out of curiosity. The frozen-section diagnosis may be of doubtful use for intraoperative management, but the opportunity should not be missed for sampling fresh tissue for molecular studies, flow cytometry (in suspected lymphoproliferative disorders), and electron microscope examination (especially when an unusual or bizarre lesion is encountered, or there is a discrepancy between the neuroimaging and provisional frozen-section diagnoses).

Since brain tumors are often biopsied or removed piecemeal, their gross appearances are seldom of diagnostic use. An exception is the meningioma, in which a careful search for brain tissue attached to the tumor surface and the sampling of these areas for microscopic examination are essential to determine whether or not prognostically important brain invasion is apparent.

Some useful immunohistochemical antibodies for oncologic surgical neuropathology are listed in Table 13.2.

Astrocytic neoplasms

Pilocytic astrocytoma (WHO Grade I)

A well-differentiated, circumscribed, slow-growing, often cystic astrocytic neoplasm.

Clinical and neuroimaging comments: Pilocytic astrocytomas (PAs) usually occur in the cerebellum ("juvenile cerebellar astrocytoma"). Less commonly, they develop in the thalamus or hypothalamus, cerebral hemispheres (usually in older patients), optic nerve ("optic glioma"), and spinal cord. The classic

Table 13.2 Commonly used neuro-oncologic immunohistochemical markers

Significance	Antibody
Astrocytic differentiation	Glial fibrillary acidic protein (GFAP), p53 (nuclear labelling)
Ependymal differentiation	Epithelial membrane antigen (EMA) – granular or dot-like pattern
Mesenchymal differentiation	Vimentin (gliosarcomas, meningiomas), EMA (meningioma), CD34 (solitary fibrous tumors/ hemangioperiytoma)
Neural differentiation	Chromgranin, neu N (nuclear labelling), neurofilaments (neuronal and glioneuronal tumors, cortical dysplasias); S100 (nerve sheath tumors)
Infiltrative activity	Neurofilaments, synaptophysin (tumor cells between labelled axons)
Primitive neuroectodermal tumors (PNETs) vs. atypical teratoid/malignant rhabdoid tumor (AT/RT)	AT/RT nuclei are immunonegative for INI1
Proliferative activity, prognostic information	MIB 1 (Ki 67), IDH1 (positivity in gliomas may indicate a better prognosis)

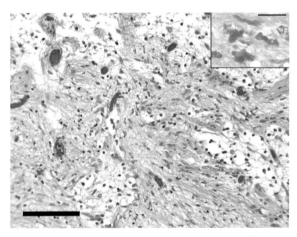

Figure 13.1 Pilocytic astrocytoma showing compact and loosely arranged areas (H&E; scale bar 100 µm). Inset: brightly eosinophilic Rosenthal fibers (H&E; scale bar 20 µm).

neuroimaging finding is a cystic, ring-enhancing neoplasm with an enhancing "mural nodule," although the tumor may be solid.

Histology (Figure 13.1): The classic PA exhibits a biphasic pattern that includes areas of compactly arranged astrocytes with elongated hair-like "piloid" processes alternating with loosely arranged microcystic areas that contain multipolar cells. Eosinophilic granular cytoplasmic bodies and Rosenthal fibers are also common. Pilocytic astrocytomas may exhibit a complex array of other histological findings, including endothelial proliferation and glomeruloid structures, necrosis, vascular mural hyalinosis (to the extent that in some cases the tumor may appear as a fibrous mass of tissue), siderophages, areas indistinguishable from oligodendrogliomas, large multinucleated cells, and extracellular myxoid material. Mitoses may also be observed. Inconsequential invasion of the subarachnoid space occurs.

Immunohistochemistry: The spindled cells are strongly glial fibrillary acidic protein (GFAP)-immunopositive. There is minimal nuclear MIB-1 immunolabelling of the tumor cells, and often extensive MIB-1 immunopositivity of the proliferating endothelium.

Molecular pathology: Many sporadic PAs have focal duplication of chromosome 7q34, associated with the expression of a novel fusion transcript between KIAA1549 locus and the BRAF gene, which activates the MAPK/ERK pathway (1). Although this mutation is characteristic of PAs, it is occasionally found in "diffuse astrocytoma" in which it indicates a better than usual prognosis. Pilocytic astrocytomas lack the genetic changes commonly seen in "diffuse astrocytomas," such as alterations of p53, p16, epidermal growth factor receptor (EGFR), RB, and PTEN. Some PAs, particularly those of the optic nerve, occur in patients with NF1 in which a germline mutation at 17q11.2 leads to a defect in neurofibromin, a tumor-suppressor gene; the KIAA1549-BRAF fusion mutation is not observed in NF1-associated PAs.

Prognosis: Cerebellar PAs, being surgically accessible, have a better prognosis than do similar tumors in the hypothalamus and other inaccessible parts of the brain. Pilocytic astrocytomas associated with NF1 seem to behave in a less aggressive manner than the sporadic forms. The presence of marked necrosis, endothelial proliferation, hypercellularity, mitosis, and spinal drop metastases may, but does not invariably, indicate a more aggressive tumor.

Differential diagnosis: The diagnosis of the PA is usually straightforward when adequate amounts of tissue are provided. The main differential diagnosis is a pilomyxoid astrocytoma, as discussed in the next section. Rosenthal fibers, although characteristic of PAs, are non-specific and in general indicate a slow-growing neoplasm (such as a PA, pleomorphic xanthoastrocytoma, or ganglioglioma) or chronic "irritation" of the nervous system at the margins of a tumor (e.g., a craniopharyngioma).

Pilomyxoid astrocytoma (WHO Grade II)

A pilomyxoid astrocytoma resembles a PA histologically, but it has a more aggressive course. It typically occurs in the suprasellar and hypothalamic region in very young children. The criteria for distinguishing between PAs and pilomyxoid astrocytomas are uncertain, but "unusual" amounts of myxoid material, and a lack of Rosenthal fibers and eosinophilic granular bodies in a PA-like tumor from the suprasellar or hypothalamic region in a very young child is highly suggestive of a pilomyxoid astrocytoma.

Diffuse astrocytoma (WHO grade II)

A glioma with astrocytic morphology whose cells infiltrate normal brain tissue and have a predisposition to undergo malignant transformation.

Clinical and neuroimaging comments: Diffuse astrocytomas occur in the cerebral hemispheres and brainstem in older children. They do not enhance and they may be associated with marked brain swelling.

Histology: The key features are mild-to-moderate glial hypercellularity in the absence of necrosis and endothelial proliferation or hyperplasia. The white-matter hypercellularity is haphazard, whereas the tumor cells that infiltrate the cortex tend to collect around neurons, blood vessels, and under the pia. The tumor-cell cytoplasm is often indistinct and the nuclei are, in comparison to normal glial-cell nuclei, more variable in size and shape, and are hyperchromatic; mitoses are rare. Most tumor cells have "fibrillary" morphology, but gemistocytic (8) and "protoplasmic" forms also occur.

Immunohistochemistry: The tumor-cell cytoplasm is strongly GFAP-immunopositive. Scant nuclear MIB1 immunolabelling is usual.

Molecular pathology: Pediatric diffuse astrocytomas are less likely than their adult counterparts to exhibit mutations of the TP53 and IDH1/2 genes.

Prognosis: Diffuse astrocytomas are difficult to resect completely because of their infiltrative behavior, and their treatment usually requires adjuvant chemo- and radiotherapy.

Differential diagnosis: The main diagnostic difficulties are in distinguishing between a diffuse astrocytoma and an oligodendroglioma (chromosome 1 and 19 loss of heterozygosity may occur in the latter, though is less common in children than in adults), a pilocytic astrocytoma (the neuroimaging features, the presence of infiltration, and the BRAF status are helpful distinguishing features), and reactive gliosis. The distinction between reactive glial cells and neoplastic astrocytes in diffuse gliomas of low cellularity can be extremely difficult, particularly in small biopsies; helpful clues include the tendency for the nuclei of neoplastic astrocytes to be more hyperchromatic and pleomorphic than those of normal glial cells and for scattered neoplastic nuclei to be MIB1 immunopositive (but rare "normal" glial nuclei may be MIB1 immunopositive).

Anaplastic astrocytoma (WHO Grade III)

Anaplastic astrocytomas are essentially diffuse astrocytomas with "increased" cellularity, nuclear pleomorphism, and unequivocal mitotic activity. There may also be a subtle or uncertain impression of hypertrophy of endothelial cells. Anaplastic astrocytomas develop *de novo* or they may evolve from diffuse astrocytomas.

Glioblastoma (WHO Grade IV)

Diffusely infiltrative, high-grade gliomas.

Clinical and neuroimaging comments: No part of the CNS is spared, although glioblastomas commonly occur in the cerebral hemispheres. Extensive enhancement, particularly "ring enhancement," and perilesional edema are the characteristic neuroimaging findings, the tumor exhibiting a tendency to invade and expand the corpus callosum and to spread under the ependyma.

*Histology (*Figure 13.2*)*: The original name of this neoplasm, "glioblastoma *multiforme*," is a reminder of the highly varied histological features that characterize this neoplasm. Many glioblastomas exhibit a range of cytological features, including small undifferentiated cells with minimal cytoplasm, spindled cells with long GFAP-immunopositive processes, large epithelioid cells, and multinucleated giant cells with voluminous eosinophilic cytoplasm, while other glioblastomas may be composed of cells with uniform morphology.

Depending on the dominant histological features, some glioblastomas can be subclassified as small-cell type, giant-cell type, and epithelioid-, lipidized-, or granular-cell type. Gliosarcomas contain discrete

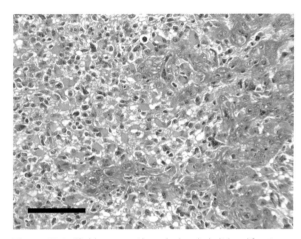

Figure 13.2 Glioblastoma with marked endothelial proliferation, pleomorphic nuclei and gemistocytes (H&E; scale bar 100 μm).

GFAP-immunopositive "glial" areas (identical to glioblastomas) interspersed with reticulin-rich vimentin-immunopositive "sarcomatoid" areas (with or without other mesenchymal metaplasia, including bone, cartilage, and skeletal muscle).

Immunohistochemistry: Cytoplasmic GFAP-immunopositivity of the tumor cells is usual, although it may be inconspicuous and focal. The tumor cells may also be immunopositive for S100 and vimentin. MIB1 nuclear immunopositivity is usually obvious (i.e., > 10% of nuclei are immunolabelled) and sometimes conspicuous (e.g., > 25% of nuclei are labelled). The tumor cells may also exhibit focal non-specific chromogranin-, EMA-, synaptophysin- and/or neurofilament-immunopositivity. Some of the nuclei may be INI1-immunonegative.

Molecular pathology: Methylation of the MGMT (6-methylguanine-DNA methyltransferase) promoter region, which indicates a better prognosis and response to alkylating agents, is present in approximately 50% of pediatric glioblastoma patients.

Prognosis: The prognosis for a glioblastoma is poor, irrespective of its subtype.

Differential diagnosis: Although the histological features of the classic glioblastoma are distinctive, diagnostic problems may arise in glioblastomas with monomorphic histological patterns, and in small biopsies. The "small-cell" glioblastoma may be confused with an anaplastic oligodendroglioma (chromosome 1 and 19 LOH may distinguish the latter). A predominant population of large cells raises the differential diagnosis of a ganglioglioma (in which case the large cells exhibit strong neurofilament and chromogranin immunopositivity), or a pleomorphic xanthoastrocytoma (a cystic neoplasm with extensive intervascular/pericellular reticulin and lacking evidence of significant proliferative activity). The presence of marked endothelial proliferation and foci of necrosis in a pilocytic astrocytoma should not be confused with a glioblastoma, which rarely occurs in the cerebellum.

Diffuse astrocytoma, anaplastic astrocytoma, and glioblastoma: additional comments

Histological spectrum: Rather than being in discrete and readily recognizable grade categories, the diffuse astrocytomas, anaplastic astrocytomas, and glioblastomas represent a spectrum of progressively increasing cellularity, nuclear pleomorphism, and proliferative activity. The distinction between the three categories may therefore be difficult and a matter of opinion, especially when the diagnosis is based on a small biopsy, but endothelial proliferation and necrosis is the *sine qua non* of a glioblastoma.

Brain-stem gliomas

Most brain-stem gliomas are diffuse astrocytomas (WHO Grade II), but some may be glioblastomas, and others, particularly those with exophytic growth, are pilocytic astrocytomas.

Gliomatosis cerebri

In a few cases neuroimaging may reveal a multicentric, often enhancing neoplasm that, on biopsy, has the histological features of a well-differentiated or anaplastic glioma; this combination of findings indicates "gliomatosis cerebri," for which the prognosis is poor irrespective of the tumor grade; these tumors are extreme examples of the infiltrative capacities of this group of brain tumors.

Primary leptomeningeal gliomas

On rare occasions, extensive leptomeningeal growth of a well-differentiated glioma, usually an astrocytoma, but sometimes an oligodendroglioma, suggests a primary leptomeningeal glioma (9). Whether these tumors represent primary neoplastic transformation of meningeal glial heterotopias or are neoplasms in which a small primary intraparenchymal primary focus has not been detected remains uncertain.

Pleomorphic xanthoastrocytoma (PXA) (WHO Grade II)

A circumscribed, superficially located, reticulin-rich, glial neoplasm with distinctive large-cell morphology.

Clinical and neuroimaging comments: The clinical symptoms are usually seizures (both acute and

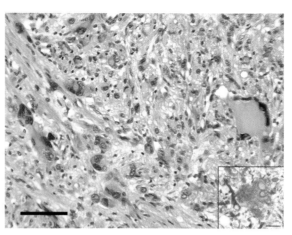

Figure 13.3 Pleomorphic xanthoastrocytoma with large cells characterized by marked nuclear pleomorphism and inconspicuous cytoplasmic xanthomatous change (H&E; scale bar 50 μm). Inset: GFAP-immunolabelled cells (GFAP; scale bar 20 μm).

chronic) and/or those of slowly evolving intracranial hypertension. The neuroimaging appearances are of a cystic or a cystic-solid, superficially located neoplasm, with enhancement of the cyst margins and the solid components. The tumor is usually, but not always well demarcated. Cerebral edema is inconspicuous, reflecting the neoplasm's minimal infiltrative properties.

Microscopic findings (Figure 13.3): The characteristic histological findings are large, pleomorphic, multinucleated giant cells, cells with xanthomatous cytoplasm, and pericellular reticulin. Various other cell types are found, including spindled cells and epithelioid cells. Mitoses are rare. Eosinophilic granular bodies are common. Infiltration of the adjacent brain tissue is unusual, and necrosis and endothelial proliferation is lacking. Perivascular inflammation may be found and mineralization is common.

Immunohistochemistry: Strong GFAP immunolabelling is characteristic. Many examples are CD34 immunopositive. In some cases neu-N-, neurofilament-, and chromogranin-immunolabelling indicates neuronal differentiation and therefore a variant of a glioneuronal tumor ("PXA with neuronal differentiation").

Molecular biology: BRAF v600E mutations are found in the majority of PXA (10).

Prognosis: Complete resection and long-term survival is to be expected, but up to 40% recur. The recurrences may exhibit more aggressive histological features, including necrosis, endothelial proliferation, and marked proliferative activity, with a corresponding poor prognosis.

Differential diagnosis: The differential diagnosis includes any primary brain tumor in which large and/or multinucleated cells are found, particularly gangliogliomas and giant-cell glioblastomas.

Oligodendroglial tumors

Oligodendroglioma and anaplastic oligodendroglioma (WHO Grades II and III) (11)

Diffusely infiltrating glioma composed of cells that resemble oligodendroglia.

Clinical and neuroimaging comments: Oligodendrogliomas are rare in childhood. The median age of presentation is 11 years (with a range of from 10 months to 18 years). Oligodendrogliomas are characterized radiologically by discrete, non-enhancing masses with minimal cerebral edema.

Histology (Figure 13.4): Oligodendrogliomas are sparsely to moderately cellular infiltrative neoplasms composed of sheets of monomorphic, round cells with perinuclear cytoplasmic vacuolation ("halos" – an artefact of fixation) and round monomorphic nuclei. The infiltrating cells form striking perineuronal, perivascular, and subpial clusters, and in some instances, as they pass through the cortex, their nuclei become elongated. Small monomorphic cells with eccentrically placed nuclei and small amounts of discrete eosinophilic cytoplasm (micro- or mini-gemistocytes) are common. A fine network of narrow capillaries forms a "chicken wire" or "curlicue-like" pattern, and mineralization and calcospherites are frequent. There may be sheets

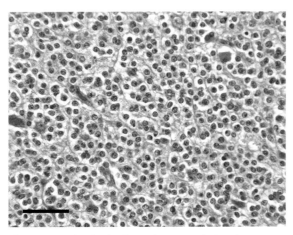

Figure 13.4 Oligodendroglioma showing marked nuclear uniformity and perinuclear cytoplasmic vacuolation (H&E; scale bar 50 µm).

of bland fibrillary material embedded in and adjacent to the cellular areas.

Anaplastic oligodendrogliomas are recognized by their endothelial proliferation (which is rarely conspicuous), hypercellularity, angular or "tented" cytological morphology, and focal necrosis; minigemistocytes tend to be more numerous and the prevalence of mitosis also increases (but scattered mitoses are acceptable in WHO Grade II oligodendrogliomas).

Immunohistochemistry: There is no reliable, specific immunohistochemical method for identifying oligodendroglioma cells. They are, however, frequently microtubule-associated protein 2-immunopositive. The microgemistocytes exhibit weak GFAP immunopositivity; otherwise, this immunohistochemical method reveals a background plexus of the supporting glial-cell processes and the stellate bodies of embedded reactive astrocytes. Many oligodendrogliomas are synaptophysin-immunopositive, but this hint of neuronal differentiation is not supported by chromogranin-, neu N- and neurofilament-immunopositivity.

Molecular pathology: Unlike their adult counterparts, 1p and 19q co-deletion is unusual in pediatric oligodendrogliomas, and when present does not appear to indicate a better prognosis (12).

Prognosis: The five-year progression-free survival and overall survival intervals for ordinary oligodendrogliomas are 66.4% and 93.4%, respectively, the prognosis being better for children over three years of age and after a gross total resection (11). A correspondingly worse prognosis is associated with the anaplastic form and, irrespective of grade, when there is enhancement by neuroimaging.

Differential diagnosis: An adequately sampled oligodendroglioma or anaplastic oligodendroglioma is readily recognizable. The principal differential diagnosis in pediatric patients is the dysembryoplastic neuroepithelial tumor. Other possibilities include the clear cell ependymoma (in which there is likely to be at least a hint of perivascular or ependymal rosettes and focal granular epithelial membrane antigen immunolabeling) or a central neurocytoma (usually an intraventricular or periventricular tumor, and chromogranin- and neu N-immunopositive). Glioblastomas may also exhibit focal oligodendroglioma differentiation.

Mixed oligo-astrocytomas and anaplastic oligo-astrocytomas (WHO Grades II and III)

These tumors, which are rare in childhood (13), contain well-defined oligodendrogliomatous and diffuse astrocytomatous areas. The prognosis is intermediate between an oligodendroglioma and a diffuse astrocytoma.

Ependymal tumors

Ependymoma and anaplastic ependymoma (WHO Grades II and III)

Circumscribed glial neoplasms that tend to occur in or adjacent to the ventricles and which exhibit ependymal rosettes and/or perivascular pseudorosettes.

Clinical and neuroimaging comments: Ependymomas can arise throughout the neuroaxis, but most of them are intracranial, two-thirds of these being in the posterior fossa, associated with the fourth ventricle. They are solid, well-circumscribed enhancing masses. On rare occasions they occur at a distance from a ventricular surface.

Histology (Figure 13.5): An ependymoma exhibits areas of relative hypercellularity interrupted by perivascular eosinophilic, fibrillary, nuclear-free zones ("perivascular pseudorosettes"). The tumors may also contain "ependymal rosettes," characterized by rings of cuboidal, sometimes ciliated ependymal cells around a clear lumen; small intensely eosinophilic, dPAS-positive foci similarly surrounded by ependymoma cells are the more common "microrosettes," whose central ultrastructure is of tangled, closely opposed microvillus processes. Ependymomas may also be surrounded by or contain areas of bland fibrillary hypocellularity. The ependymoma cell nuclei may have distinctive crisp granular or speckled chromatin.

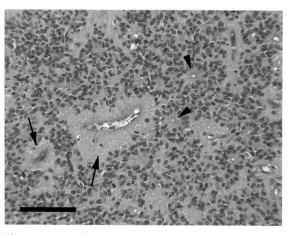

Figure 13.5 Ependymoma showing perivascular pseudorosettes (arrows) and ependymal rosettes (arrowheads) (H&E; scale bar 100 μm).

The presence of necrosis, endothelial proliferation, significant mitotic activity, and/or marked hypercellularity indicates anaplastic ependymoma.

There are several rare ependymoma variants, including clear-cell, giant-cell and papillary forms (14–16).

Immunohistochemistry: Most ependymomas exhibit GFAP immunopositivity, which tends to be most prominent in the nuclear free zones of the perivascular pseudorosettes. Granular or dot-like cytoplasmic epithelial membrane antigen (EMA) immunolabelling is a useful distinguishing feature.

Molecular pathology (17,18): Ependymomas contain numerous cytogenetic abnormalities, but their diagnostic and therapeutic utility is unproven.

Prognosis: The ependymoma is often well-circumscribed and may be completely excised; nevertheless, even with apparent complete excision, there is a significant risk of local recurrence. In general, pediatric ependymomas have a poorer prognosis than in adults and their five-year survival rate is from 39% to 64%. The WHO grade is only poorly correlated with prognosis and is therefore somewhat inadequate for prognostication purposes (19).

Differential diagnosis: Although there may be some difficulty deciding on their WHO grade, the histological appearance of most ependymomas is distinctive. However, depending on location, various papillary neoplasms of the CNS should be considered in the differential diagnosis, including angiocentric gliomas, astroblastomas, chordoid gliomas, papillary pineal region tumors, and papillary glioneuronal tumors. The clear-cell ependymomas may be difficult to distinguish from oligodendrogliomas, although the presence of rosettes, whether perivascular pseudorosettes, ependymal rosettes, or microrosettes, usually allows the correct diagnoses to be reached. Many glioblastomas contain focal ependymal differentiation.

Unusual and rare gliomas

Although these tumors are rare, consideration of them frequently plays a role in the differential diagnosis applied to the commoner gliomas, especially when the latter have unusual clinical, neuroimaging, and histological features (Table 13.3).

Neuronal and mixed glioneuronal tumors

These include a disparate group of tumors that exhibit various forms and degrees of glial and neuronal differentiation.

445

Table 13.3 Unusual and rare gliomas

Tumor	WHO grade	Key clinical and imaging features	Key histological features	Differential diagnosis
Angiocentric glioma (20,21)	I	Intractable seizures Non-enhancing (resembling diffuse astrocytomas) May be cystic Periphery of cerebral hemispheres	Infiltrative and cellular Perivascular accumulation of tumor cells (various patterns) Schwannoma-like fascicles of spindled astrocytes Adjacent cortical dysplasia	Diffuse astrocytoma Ependymoma Pilomyxoid astrocytoma
Astroblastoma (22,23)	II (some III or IV)	Seizures, effects of space-occupancy Long history Periphery of cerebral hemispheres Some periventricular Circumscribed, enhancing, often cystic Curative resection possible, but significant risk of long-term recurrence	Papillary architecture Poor intervascular cohesion Fibrosis of blood vessels GFAP+ radially arranged unipolar spindle cells	Ependymoma Choroid plexus tumors Metastatic papillary neoplasms
Chordoid glioma (24)	II	Rare in children Third ventricular tumor Solid, contrast-enhancing Resectable subject to anatomical limitations	Clusters and cords of GFAP+ epithelioid cells Mucinous, vacuolated stroma Lymphoplasmacytic infiltrate	Chordoid meningioma
Desmoplastic infantile astrocytoma and ganglioglioma (25–27)	I (some II or III?)	First two years of life; "non-infantile" forms occur Cystic and heterogeneously enhancing Attached to convexity meninges Curative resection possible	Abundant pericellular reticulin GFAP+ spindle cells Ganglion cells in some cases Some cases have malignant histology	Meningioma Hemangiopericytoma Diffuse astrocytoma Ganglioglioma
Myxopapillary ependymoma (28)	I	Second decade Usually cauda equina/filum terminale region Curative resection possible, but significant risk of recurrence	Papillary morphology GFAP+/EMA+ ("dot-like") Mucinous papillary and intervascular degeneration	Distinctive histology Other cauda equina tumors (astrocytomas, ependymomas, paragangliomas)
Subependymoma (29,30)	I	Rare in children Slow growing, often an incidental finding Peri- or intra-ventricular	Paucicellular fibrillary background Small nests of ependymal cells	Ependymoma May contain elements of other gliomas, especially ependymomas (i.e., "mixed gliomatous pattern") (30)

Dysembryoplastic neuroepithelial tumor (DNET) (WHO Grade I)

Well-differentiated, well-circumscribed, usually supratentorial glioneuronal neoplasm that forms discrete cortical nodules and which presents with refractory epilepsy.

Clinical and neuroimaging comments: Dysembryoplastic neuroepithelial tumors may present throughout childhood and they show a predilection for the temporal lobe. Neuroimaging reveals a characteristic multicystic nodular cortical pattern, which may resemble macrogyri, and a lack of peritumoral edema. Enhancement is not usually present, although it may appear in response to intratumoral hemorrhage or ischemia. The overlying calvarium may be hypoplastic.

Histology (Figure 13.6): The tumor is a nodular or multinodular, sharply demarcated lesion composed of a network of fine strands of neuroglial tissue that demarcate a honeycomb arrangement of cysts in which mature neurons may appear to be "floating" ("specific glioneuronal" pattern). The morphology of many of the glial cells is identical to oligodendroglia. In some tumors, the "specific glioneuronal" pattern ("simple" DNET) may be complicated by areas that resemble conventional gliomas and/or by a more diffuse growth of the glioneuronal elements ("complex"

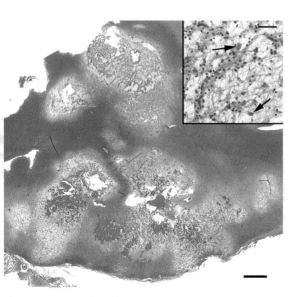

Figure 13.6 Dysembryoplastic neuroepithelial tumor. Note the nodular growth pattern and focal hemorrhage (H&E; scale bar 1 mm). Inset: characteristic strands of neuroglial tissue and "floating neurones" (arrows) (H&E; scale bar 50 μm).

DNET). Other not uncommon findings include various vascular abnormalities (that may lead to intratumoral hemorrhage), mineralization, ischemic necrosis, and perilesional neuronal dysplasia.

Prognosis: Excision of the tumor is usually curative and abolishes the seizures. In unresectable cases there is characteristically minimal evidence of growth in the residual tumor; new neuroimaging features are more likely to be related to secondary bleeding and ischemic injury. Malignant transformation is exceptionally rare.

Differential diagnosis: It may be difficult to distinguish DNETs and oligodendrogliomas, particularly in small biopsies and when the "specific glioneuronal pattern" is inconspicuous. The demonstration of chromosome 1 and 19 loss of heterozygosity in oligodendrogliomas may help in the distinction. Gangliogliomas, unlike DNETS, may be grossly cystic and often contain lymphocytes and intratumoral reticulin.

Ganglioglioma and gangliocytoma (mostly WHO Grade I)

Rare, well-differentiated, slowly growing neoplasms composed of neoplastic mature ganglion cells (gangliocytoma) or a mixture of these cells and neoplastic glial cells (ganglioglioma).

Clinical and neuroimaging comments: Gangliogliomas occur throughout childhood and into adulthood, typically causing seizures. The majority are found in the temporal and frontal lobes. Neuroimaging studies generally reveal a circumscribed solid mass or a cyst with a mural nodule; the degree and pattern of enhancement varies from case to case.

Histology: The gangliocytoma, which is rare, is composed of irregular groups of dysplastic, otherwise mature neurons embedded in a non-neoplastic glial stroma. Reticulin is commonly found.

The ganglioglioma contains similar neurons, but, in addition, there is an obvious well-differentiated gliomatous component that may resemble pilocytic astrocytomas, oligodendrogliomas, and/or diffuse astrocytomas (Figure 13.7). Rosenthal fibers and eosinophilic granular bodies are often present, in line with the indolent nature of the neoplasm. Intravascular reticulin is frequent, and mineralization and extensive lymphoid infiltrates (particularly in the perivascular spaces) are common. In rare cases, anaplastic transformation of the glial elements of the tumor may occur.

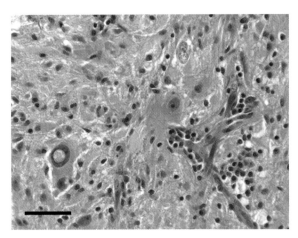

Figure 13.7 Ganglioglioma showing scant perivascular lymphocytes, large atypical neurones and a fibrillary glial background (H&E; scale bar 50 μm).

Prognosis: The prognosis is usually good. The outlook for gangliogliomas with anaplastic change reflects that of the anaplastic gliomatous component.

Differential diagnosis: The principal differential diagnosis is a diffuse glioma with normal neurones trapped by the infiltrative growth of the tumor. If the neurones in question have normal morphology they are likely to be "trapped," whereas those of a ganglioglioma have atypical features, including irregularly shaped nuclei, multiple nuclei, and chromatolysis.

Other neuronal and glioneuronal tumors and tumor-like lesions: Table 13.4

Embryonal tumors

The histological classification of these tumors is controversial. Some schools of thought, arguing a common progenitor, favor classifying them under the single rubric of primitive neuroectodermal tumor ("PNET"). Others prefer classifying these tumors as medulloblastomas (when they occur in the cerebellum) or, in other regions of the CNS, as PNETs with astrocytic, neural (i.e., cerebral neuroblastomas), ependymal (i.e., ependymoblastoma), or mixed differentiation (the differentiation does not materially affect the prognosis), based on their appearance in sections stained with hematoxylin and eosin, and the immunohistochemical findings. It is highly probable that, in the near future, specific molecular criteria will supplement or even replace the histological classification of these tumors.

Medulloblastoma (WHO Grade IV)

An embryonal neuroepithelial tumor of the cerebellum and the most common malignant brain tumor of childhood.

Clinical and neuroimaging comments: The incidence of medulloblastomas shows a bimodal peak, at 3–4 years of age and at 8–9 years of age; medulloblastomas also occur in adults. Seventy percent to 90% of medulloblastomas occur in the midline, mostly arising in the inferior vermis, whereas the remainder arise in the cerebellar hemispheres (usually in older children and adults). The medulloblastoma is typically a well-defined, diffusely enhancing, homogeneous mass, with mild to moderate peritumoral vasogenic edema; a minority of cases are calcified and cysts or necrotic, non-enhancing regions are commonly observed.

Histology: Medulloblastomas are characterized by sheets of poorly differentiated cells with minimal cytoplasm and round or slightly elongated hyperchromatic nuclei (Figure 13.8). There may be foci of necrosis, inconspicuous endothelial proliferation and, in a minority of cases, neural (Homer–Wright) rosettes, characterized by a circular arrangement of tumor-cell nuclei around a central tangle of fine cytoplasmic processes. Mitoses are usually found and often abundant. The tumor cells invade the adjacent brain parenchyma and the subarachnoid space.

Various other configurations may be observed, including ill-defined streaming fascicles of tumor cells, neural differentiation (characterized by small groups of neurocytic or ganglion cells in a neuropil background) and, rarely, ependymal differentiation, melanotic epithelioid cells ("melanotic medulloblastoma") and rhabdomyoblasts ("medullomyoblastoma").

Four distinct histological patterns are recognizable (3):

- Classic medulloblastoma (75%) – predominantly sheet-like or ill-defined fascicular morphology.
- Desmoplastic medulloblastoma (7%) – fields of poorly differentiated tumor cells interspersed by hypocellular, reticulin-rich regions with a neurofibrillary background matrix and scattered neurocytes.
- Medulloblastoma with extensive nodularity (MDEN) (3%) – resembles the desmoplastic medulloblastoma, but the paucicellular regions do not contain reticulin (usually in infants).

Table 13.4 Other neuronal and glioneuronal tumors and tumor-like lesions

Tumor	WHO grade	Key clinical and imaging features	Key histological features	Differential diagnosis
Central (3) and extraventricular neurocytoma (31)	II	Rare, second decade Usually intraventricular, close to the foramen of Munro Symptoms of intermittent intracranial hypertension Sharply demarcated, calcified (extraventricular forms may be cystic +/− mural nodule) Dissemination possible (32)	Sheets of monomorphic round cells embedded in fibrillary neuropil Synaptophysin and neu N immunopositive	Oligodendroglioma
Dysplastic cerebellar gangliocytoma (Lhermitte–Duclos disease) (33)	I	Part of the "PTEN hamartoma tumor syndrome" Pathognomonic of Cowden's syndrome Associated with megalocephaly and seizures Isolated cerebellar mass–neoplasm or hamartoma?	Expansion and disruption of cerebellar folia by dysplastic ganglion cells and scattered granule cells Aberrant myelin bundles in outer molecular layer Calcification common	Distinctive lesion – basic cerebellar cortical morphology retained
Papillary glioneuronal tumor (34)	I	Seizures Temporal lobe Enhancing, solid or cystic (with or without mural nodule)	Pseudopapillary with interpapillary gangliocytoid cells (synaptophysin +, neu N +) Hyalinized papillary blood vessels Simple or pseudostratified GFAP+ cuboidal epithelium	Ependymoma Choroid plexus tumor Astroblastoma
Rosette-forming glioneuronal tumor (35)	Undetermined, indolent	Usually in fourth ventricle Inconsistent imaging characteristics (solid/cystic with or without enhancement and calcium)	Two cell populations. GFAP+ pilocytic astrocytes Neu N+/synaptophysin+ neurocytes forming Homer–Wright or perivascular pseudorosettes	Pilocytic astrocytoma Ganglioglioma Central neurocytoma
Tuberous sclerosis	Not applicable	A phakomatosis characterized by cortical tubers and periventricular glioneuronal hamartomas ('candle gutterings') or tumors (subependymal giant-cell astrocytoma)	Hypocellular region with ballooned neurones or neuron-like cells with a background stroma of spindled glial cells in the periventricular lesions. Mixed pattern of GFAP+ and neural marker + immunohistochemistry for neuron-like cells. Strong GFAP+ in stromal glia	Cortical dysplasia Various astrocytomas

Table 13.5 Molecular pathology of medulloblastomas (2,36–38)

Group	Fraction of cases	Molecular abnormalities	Morphology	Age	Five-year survival
WNT	10%	β-Catenin (CTNNB1) mutation (WNT signaling effector)	Classic	>3 years	95%
SHH	30%	Inhibition of sonic hedgehog (SHH) gene by somatic mutation of patched 1 (PTCH1) and suppressor of fused homologue (SFU) genes	Usually classic Other patterns rarely	<3 years, adults	75%
Group 3	25%	Marked genomic instability High levels of MYC proto-oncogene amplification. Aberrant MYC expression. Gains in chromosomes 1q, 7, 17q Deletions of chromosome 10q, 11, 16q, 17p	Classic Large cell/anaplastic	>3 years	50%
Group 4	35%	Amplification of the MYC proto-oncogene and cyclin-dependent kinase 6 (CDK6), the latter rare in Group 3	Usually classic. Rarely large cell/ anaplastic	>3 years	75%

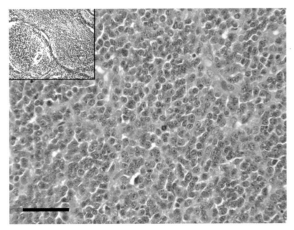

Figure 13.8 Medulloblastoma with sheets of poorly differentiated "small blue cells" and a solitary mitosis. (H&E; scale bar 50 μm). Inset: low-power view of a "medulloblastoma with extensive nodularity."

- Large cell/anaplastic medulloblastoma (10–22%) – there are extensive areas of densely packed, molded, pleomorphic polyhedral cells with very high mitotic and apoptotic rates (i.e., "anaplastic" morphology), supplemented in some cases with a significant population of large cells whose nuclei are two or three times larger than those of the classic medulloblastoma and which have prominent nucleoli (i.e., "large-cell" morphology).

Immunohistochemistry: The immunophenotype of a medulloblastoma is varied. Many of these tumors exhibit diffuse or patchy synaptophysin labelling. There may be focal GFAP immunolabelling of reactive astrocytes and their processes and/or in the cytoplasm of tumor-cell groups. Strong synaptophysin and neurofilament immunolabelling may be present in the neuropil in regions exhibiting ganglion-cell differentiation.

Molecular findings: The molecular classification and subclassification of medulloblastomas is developing rapidly, and will soon be in widespread use for prognostic purposes and to tailor the treatment of medulloblastomas for individual cases (Table 13.5).

Prognosis: The overall five-year survival rate for patients with medulloblastomas is between 70% and 80% when complex treatment protocols are used, including surgery, craniospinal radiotherapy, and chemotherapy. The survival is, however, at the cost of considerable disability, related partly to the effects of the tumor and partly to its treatment. In clinical terms, infants three years of age and under, patients with residual tumor after surgery, and/or those exhibiting leptomeningeal dissemination at the time of diagnosis are considered to be "high risk"; all other patients are deemed to be "average risk." In terms of histology, the nodular medulloblastomas (both the desmoplastic and MDEN variants) have a better prognosis and the anaplastic/large-cell variants have a worse prognosis (Table 13.5).

Differential diagnosis: The principal differential diagnosis is an atypical teratoid/malignant rhabdoid tumor. Extensive reticulin may be found in any of the medulloblastoma variants that are growing close to or into the leptomeninges and should not be interpreted as evidence of a desmoplastic medulloblastoma.

Primitive neuroectodermal tumor (39–42) (WHO Grade 4)

Rare, extracerebellar, poorly differentiated neuroepithelial embryonal neoplasm of the brain.

Clinical and neuroimaging comments: The mean age of presentation of PNETs is from 3–5 years. They usually arise in the cerebral hemispheres, although they may occur in the spinal cord. They are well-circumscribed heterogeneous masses, with both solid and cystic components. They are frequently mineralized and heterogeneous enhancement is the rule. Leptomeningeal dissemination, including in the spinal subarachnoid space, is common.

Histology: The tumor is formed by highly cellular monotonous sheets of "small round" cells that have inconspicuous cytoplasm, round, angulated, or cleaved nuclei, and coarse chromatin. A few tumors may also exhibit larger cells with more prominent eosinophilic cytoplasm and/or spindle cells. A fine fibrillary neuropil may be observed around the tumor cells and adjacent to blood vessels. Homer–Wright and ependymal rosettes are unusual findings. Mitoses are often numerous. Foci of coagulative necrosis and endothelial hyperplasia are usually apparent. Fibrous septa or stroma may also be observed.

Immunohistochemistry: The tumor cells are NSE-, neu N-, and synaptophysin-immunopositive. Chromogranin immunolabelling is not observed, although a minority of cells exhibit irregularly distributed neurofilament immunopositivity. Glial fibrillary acidic protein (GFAP) immunopositivity is also found, usually in groups of cells, some of which are perivascular. Epithelial membrane antigen immunolabeling is common in various patterns (including diffuse cytoplasmic, membranous, and/or paranuclear dot labeling). The MIB1 nuclear immunolabelling index is usually high. There may also be evidence of muscle and melanocytic differentiation.

Molecular pathology: There is evidence that the WNT/β-catenin pathway is activated in cerebral PNETs, but that the responsible genes are different from those implicated in the WNT group of medulloblastomas (43). A subset of cerebral hemispheric PNETs contain t(11;22) translocation (EWSR1/FLI1 fusion gene) and exhibit the corresponding MIC2/CD99 membrane immunolabelling, which is characteristic of a peripheral PNET/Ewing's sarcoma. There is some evidence that the prognosis for these tumors is better than for the "ordinary" PNETs and, as a result, their treatment is different (44).

Prognosis: The five-year survival is approximately 40% to 50%.

Differential diagnosis: The differential diagnosis includes atypical teratoid/malignant rhabdoid tumor (AT/RT), small-cell glioblastoma (which tends not to be immunopositive for neural markers), medulloepithelioma (see Table 14.9) and metastatic "small blue-cell" or "malignant monomorphic" tumors.

Atypical teratoid/malignant rhabdoid (AT/RT) tumor (7,45,46) (WHO Grade IV)

A highly malignant embryonal tumor of the CNS that resembles PNETs and medulloblastomas.

Clinical and neuroimaging comments: The median age of diagnosis of AT/RTs is 1.4 years; these tumors are rare in children older than two years, although they may present at any time in childhood from the neonatal period to adolescence (7). Approximately 50% of AT/RTs arise in the posterior fossa, and the majority will have disseminated through the spinal subarachnoid space at the time of presentation. By neuroimaging, the tumor is a heterogeneous and hyperdense mass, and exhibits variable enhancement. The heterogeneity is related to abundant foci of intratumoral necrosis, cysts, and hemorrhages. Perilesional edema is usually mild.

Histology (Figure 13.9): The histological appearance is varied. There is usually necrosis, sometimes with dystrophic calcification, and broad fibrous septa may be apparent. The cytological features include various combinations of small, poorly differentiated cells and larger epithelioid cells (sometimes deceptively bland, cells that resemble rhabdoid cells and which have eccentric nuclei and abundant, inclusion-like, hyaline, or eosinophilic cytoplasm). In rare cases the

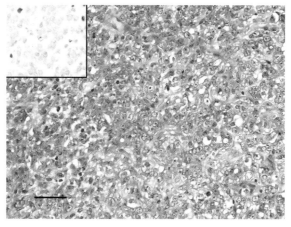

Figure 13.9 Atypical teratoid/rhabdoid tumor formed by pleomorphic, poorly differentiated cells (H&E; scale bar 50 μm); Inset: characteristic lack of nuclear INI1 nuclear immunolabelling (rare inflammatory cells are immunopositive) (INI1 immunohistochemistry; same magnification). (Courtesy of Dr. C. Hawkins, Toronto Hospital for Sick Children.)

tumors exhibit mesenchymal differentiation (reminiscent of a chordoma or characterized by fascicles of spindle cells) or epithelial differentiation (characterized by ill-defined glands and papillae). Although the histological appearance is characteristically pleomorphic, monomorphic forms may be observed in which the primitive neuroectodermal or the epithelioid cell pattern predominate. Abundant reticulin is common, particularly in the perivascular regions.

Immunohistochemistry: In general, these tumors show striking polyimmunophenotypic immunoreactivity. Diffuse vimentin immunopositivity is seen in all tumors. Glial fibrillary acidic protein immunolabelling in single cells and small clusters of cells is also characteristic; a similar pattern of cytokeratin immunolabelling is also frequently present. The epithelioid (including rhabdoid) cells and the glandular epithelium are EMA-immunopositive. Smooth-muscle actin immunolabelling may be present in both the spindled and rhabdoid cells. α-Fetoprotein immunolabelling may also be seen in the large cells, but there is no evidence of placental alkaline phosphatase and β-hCG immunolabelling. There is inconsistent immunolabelling for chromogranin (in neuron-like elements), HMB-45 (rare isolated cells), neurofilament, S100, and synaptophysin.

Molecular pathology: Atypical teratoid/malignant rhabdoid tumor exhibit biallellic inactivation of the tumor-suppressor gene SMARCB1 (hSNF5/INI1) at chromosome locus 22q.11.23. The histological substrate of this abnormality is absence of nuclear INI1 immunolabelling, an important microscopic feature that allows AT/RTs to be distinguished from other embryonal neoplasms.

Prognosis: The prognosis is generally poor (five-year survival 39.5%), but the chance of survival is improved if gross total resection is possible.

Differential diagnosis: The varied primitive, mesenchymal, and epithelial morphology of the AT/RT may resemble many types of malignant CNS tumors, including PNETs/medulloblastomas, choroid plexus carcinomas, germ-cell tumors, and malignant gliomas. Awareness of the possibility of an AT/RT as a relatively common malignant brain tumor in infants, the clinical and neuroimaging findings, and the lack of INI1 nuclear immunolabelling will generally resolve this differential diagnosis.

Pineal region tumors

Pineal region tumors account for 2.8% of CNS tumors in children. They include pineal parenchymal tumors (47) (i.e., pineocytomas, pineal parenchymal tumors of intermediate differentiation, pineoblastomas), germ-cell tumors, and papillary tumors of the pineal region. Pineoblastomas and germ-cell tumors are the most common pineal region tumors in childhood.

Pinealoblastoma (WHO Grade IV)

A poorly differentiated malignant tumor of the pineal region that resembles a PNET.

Clinical and neuroimaging comments: These tumors usually present at the beginning of the second decade of life with rapidly progressive symptoms of local compression, including hydrocephalus and Parinaud's syndrome. Spinal leptomeningeal metastases are common and pineoblastomas tend to be locally invasive. These neoplasms may also occur with bilateral retinoblastomas ("trilateral retinoblastoma").

Histology: Pineoblastomas are made up of sheets, nodular arrays, or haphazardly distributed, poorly differentiated cells with minimal cytoplasm and irregularly shaped, round to oval hyperchromatic nuclei. The nucleus–cytoplasm ratio is high, molding of nuclei is frequent, and mitoses are numerous. Homer–Wright rosettes may be observed and there may also be retinoblastoma-like features, including Flexner–Wintersteiner rosettes (which resemble ependymal rosettes) and "fleurettes" (characterized by slightly bulbous, radially arranged, club like process surrounded by a ring of tumor-cell nuclei); however, the tumors do not contain pineocytomatous rosettes. Necrosis is frequent and of variable extent, and there may be desmoplastic foci. The tumor may also exhibit anaplastic features, similar to anaplastic medulloblastomas. Melanin, cartilage, and skeletal muscle ("ectomesenchymal") differentiation may be observed in otherwise typical pineoblastomas, usually in infants, indicating the diagnosis of a "pineal anlage tumor" (48).

Immunochemistry: There is usually at least focal immunopositivity for neuronal and neuroendocrine markers. Glial fibrillary acidic protein immunolabelling is focal and variable. Extensive nuclear MIB1 nuclear immunopositivity is typical.

Molecular pathology: Approximately 50% of pineoblastomas are hereditary. Numerous genes (UBEC2, TERT, TEP1, PRAME, CD24) and transcription factors (POU4F2, SOX4, HOXD13) are highly expressed in pineoblastomas. A germline mutation of the RB gene is found in cases of "trilateral retinoblastoma".

Table 13.6 Other non-germ-cell pineal region tumors

Tumor	WHO grade	Key clinical and imaging features	Key histological features	Differential diagnosis
Pineocytoma	I	Extremely rare in childhood	Pineocytomatous (pineocytic) rosette (resembles Homer–Wright rosette) Ganglion cell differentiation	Normal pineal gland
Pineal parenchymal tumor of intermediate differentiation (49–51)	I, II	Unusual in children	Transitional (resembling pineocytomas), lobulated (resembling neuroendocrine cells) and diffuse patterns (similar to oligodendrogliomas and neurocytomas) WHO Grade 2 = any pattern and < 6 mitoses/HPF. WHO Grade 3 = lobulated/diffuse pattern and > 5 mitoses/HPF	Pineoblastoma Oligodendroglioma Neurocytoma
Papillary tumor of the pineal region (52)	II, III	Commoner in adults Well-circumscribed, solid or cystic, enhancing pineal mass Local recurrence is common	Papillae (fibrovascular cores lined by cytokeratin+ columnar or cuboidal epithelium) Solid areas of epithelioid cells + immunopositive for EMA ("dot-like"), GFAP (focal), MAP2, S100, vimentin	Papillary tumors (choroid plexus tumors, papillary ependymoma, papillary meningioma)

Differential diagnosis: The differential diagnosis includes a PNET/medulloblastoma (which has a better prognosis) and an AT/RT.

Prognosis: Like most CNS tumors composed of poorly differentiated cells, the prognosis is poor, and there is a high risk of CSF and systemic metastasis. The five-year survival is approximately 10%.

Other non-germ-cell pineal tumors: Table 13.6

Tumors of cranial, spinal, and peripheral nerves (53)

These tumors include Schwannomas, neurofibromas, perineuromas, malignant peripheral nerve-sheet tumors, and benign hybrid nerve-sheath tumors. Generally speaking, their appearances are distinctive and the diagnosis is usually straightforward.

Schwannoma (WHO Grade I)

A benign nerve-sheath tumor composed of Schwann cells.

Clinical and neuroimaging comments: Most schwannomas are sporadic, but bilateral eighth cranial nerve schwannomas are virtually pathognomomic of neurofibromatosis type 2, whereas multiple peripheral Schwannomas are characteristic of schwannomatosis (a usually sporadic disorder without other manifestations of neurofibromatosis and associated with non-germline inactivation of the NF2 gene). The sporadic

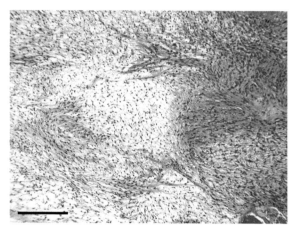

Figure 13.10 Schwannoma with biphasic cellular (Antoni A) and hypocellular (Antonia B) regions (H&E; scale bar 200 μm).

schwannomas typically involve the fifth and eighth cranial nerves, the dorsal spinal nerve roots, and various peripheral nerves. Intracerebral schwannomas have also been described. Neuroimaging reveals a heterogeneously enhancing, well-demarcated, sometimes cystic mass, which may be associated with bone erosion.

Histology (Figure 13.10): The tumor grows to one side of and displaces the nerve (unlike the neurofibroma, which diffusely expands the nerve and encompasses the axons); accordingly, nerve bundles are often found in the capsule of the neoplasm. The microscopic features are highly variable and include many degenerative changes, such as large hyperchromatic nuclei, vascular mural hyalinosis, acute and organizing microhemorrhages, and various degrees of fibrosis. The classic schwannoma has areas of compactly arranged, elongated cells whose nuclei at times form ill-defined palisades (Antoni A pattern) interspersed with more loosely arranged process-bearing cells that often have small, hyperchromatic nuclei (Antoni B pattern). Cellular, plexiform, and melanotic variants are described.

Immunohistochemistry: The tumor-cell cytoplasm and nuclei are generally S100 immunoreactive; focal GFAP immunolabelling is common.

Prognosis: Schwannomas are benign tumors that rarely recur or undergo malignant change. An increased risk of recurrence is associated with cellular schwannomas.

Neurofibroma (WHO Grade I)

A well-demarcated or diffusely infiltrating neoplasm composed of Schwann cells, fibroblasts, and perineurial cells.

Clinical and neuroimaging comments: The tumor is sporadic or, when multiple and/or plexiform, is associated with neurofibromatosis type I. Neurofibromas usually develop in the peripheral nervous system, although involvement of the spinal nerve roots also regularly occurs in NF2.

Histology: The solitary neurofibroma is a fusiform, well-circumscribed swelling of the nerve, whereas a plexiform neurofibroma is characterized by a tangled multinodular expansion of the nerve. The tumors are formed by haphazardly and loosely arranged small fibroblasts and small Schwann cells (which may be scant), and variable numbers of collagen bundles.

Immunohistochemistry: The Schwann cells are S100-immunopositive. Neurofilament immunolabelling will identify scattered axons wandering through the tumor.

Prognosis: The isolated solitary fusiform neurofibroma carries a good prognosis, but plexiform neurofibromas and neurofibromas of major nerves have a significant risk of malignant transformation.

Nerve-sheath tumors: differential diagnosis

Difficulties may be encountered in distinguishing schwannomas from meningiomas at the time of frozen sections (tight whorls and nuclear pseudoinclusions favor the former, whereas very loose or no whorls suggest the latter), in determining whether a neurofibroma with increased cellularity and nuclear pleomorphism is a low-grade peripheral nerve-sheath tumor (which is favored by the presence of mitoses),

identifying the rare intraparenchymal schwannoma (which, being a GFAP- and S100-immunopositive spindle-cell neoplasm, may resemble an astrocytoma – the presence of pericellular reticulin and the ultrastructural demonstration of a basal lamina indicates a schwannoma), and remembering that tumors with mixed Schwannian and neurofibroma morphology occur.

Other nerve-sheath tumors: Table 13.7

Sellar and suprasellar neoplasms (57,58) (see also Chapter 6)

Tumors of the midline in the hypothalamic and pituitary region (sellar and suprasellar neoplasms) are common in childhood and account for 15% to 20% of all pediatric brain tumors. The tumors include craniopharyngiomas and pituitary adenomas, as well as other rarer lesions, including optic gliomas (usually pilocytic astrocytomas in the context of neurofibromatosis type 1), dermoid/epidermal cysts, hamartomas, germ-cell tumors, and various astrocytomas. These lesions present with endocrine dysfunction, visual disturbance, and/or signs and symptoms of intracranial space-occupancy. Endocrine dysfunction tends to be the earliest and most subtle indicator of a lesion in this region. More than 90% of purely intrasellar tumors are pituitary adenomas and the others are developmental lesions, such as Rathke cleft cysts or craniopharyngiomas.

Craniopharyngioma (WHO Grade 1)

A common pediatric brain tumor that is derived from the residual epithelium between the neurohypophysis and adenohypophysis (Rathke's cleft).

Clinical and neuroimaging characteristics: Craniopharyngiomas develop in the second decade of life, most involve the pituitary fossa, and many extend into the suprasellar region. They cause headaches (due to raised intracranial pressure), visual-field defects (because of compression on the optic apparatus), and, by interfering with the pituitary axis, various endocrine signs and symptoms, including growth retardation (due to growth-hormone deficiency), and delayed puberty (related to hyposecretion of the gonadotrophic hormones); the pituitary stalk is infrequently involved, which accounts for the relative infrequency of secondary ("stalk compression") hyperprolactinemia. Neuroimaging reveals a cystic or solid, enhancing neoplasm with areas of mineralization.

Table 13.7 Other nerve-sheath tumors

Tumor	WHO grade	Key clinical and imaging features	Key histological features	Differential diagnosis
Perineuroma (54)	I	Rare in children Peripheral nerve sheath tumor Most associated with neurofibromatosis Tumor has chromosome 22 monsomy	Innumerable small whorls EMA+, S100–	Traumatic neuroma (extraneural Schwann cells, S100+, hemosiderin present) Demyelinating neuropathy (history of symmetrical neuropathy)
Benign hybrid nerve-sheath tumor (55,56)	I	Some are associated with NF2 and schwannosis	Mixed histological features of a schwannoma and neurofibroma or neurofibroma and perineuroma	Other 'pure' nerve sheath tumors
Malignant peripheral nerve-sheath tumor (3)	II, III, IV	Rare in children Arises in soft tissues or a peripheral nerve Associated with NF1 Infiltrating mass Five- and ten-year survival rates are 34% and 23%, respectively	Approximates, in various degrees, to a sarcoma WHO Grade II – cellular neurofibroma with rare mitoses WHO Grade III – "significant" numbers of mitoses WHO Grade IV – necrosis May exhibit mesenchymal (usually rhabdomyosarcomatous = malignant Triton tumor) and glandular differentiation	Other sarcomas

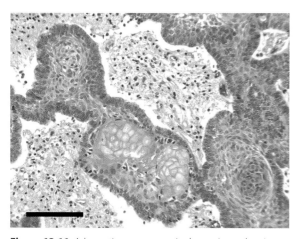

Figure 13.11 Adamantinomatous craniopharyngioma showing a nodule of "wet" keratinization (H&E; scale bar 100 µm).

Histology (Figure 13.11): Adamantinomatous craniopharyngiomas are typically cystic and calcified. The tumor is characterized by epithelial-lined cysts (filled with dark, cholesterol and hemosiderin-rich fluid resembling crank-case oil) with loosely arranged stellate and spindled cells or brain parenchyma between the cysts. Characteristic of this tumor are islands of plump squamous cells with clear or watery cytoplasm ("wet keratin") that undergo calcification.

Prognosis: Although these tumors are histologically low grade they exhibit locally infiltrative behavior and a tendency to engulf vital structures of the sellar and suprasellar region, rendering them difficult to resect. Escape of cyst contents into the ventricles or subarachnoid space can induce an intense clinical ventriculitis or meningitis. On rare occassions the Rosenthal fiber-bearing perilesional astrocytosis may be so intense as to obscure the cranipharyngioma and masquerade as a pilocyctic astrocytoma.

Pituitary adenomas (59–61) (WHO Grade I)

Pituitary adenomas are histologically benign neoplasms of the adenohypophysis.

Clinical and neuroimaging comments: Pituitary adenomas form approximately 3% of all intracranial pediatric neoplasms:

- Prolactinomas are the most common adenoma in adolescence.
- ACTH-secreting adenomas arc the most common adenoma in prepubescent children.
- The third most common adenoma, usually appearing in adolescence, is the growth-hormone-secreting adenoma.

The presenting symptoms include those of endocrine dysfunction (such as growth delay, primary amenorrhea, Cushing's disease, and gigantism) or, less

455

frequently, headache and visual loss related to the space-occupying effects of the neoplasm.

A pituitary macroadenoma is a non-enhancing neoplasm that is readily identified using standard MRI techniques. However, many pediatric pituitary adenomas are difficult to detect because they are microadenomas; such neoplasms, suspected because of their symptoms, may require specialized neuroimaging and other techniques for their identification (57).

Histology: Adenomas are characterized cytologically by bland, monomorphic neuroendocrine morphology, the tumor cells forming sheets or ill-defined papillary structures. The concentration of secretory vesicles determines whether the tumor-cell cytoplasm will be lightly stained ("chromophobic"), strongly eosinophilic (prolactinomas, somatotroph adenomas), or basophilic (corticotropic, gonadotropic, and thyrotropic adenomas).

Immunohistochemistry: The type of adenoma is defined by its immunohistochemical profile, antibodies for all the pituitary hormones being readily available. Immunopositivity for a given pituitary hormone does not always mean that the hormone is being secreted, and many pituitary adenomas may show plurihormonal immunolabelling.

Molecular pathology: Early childhood pituitary adenomas are apt to occur in a familial setting or in association with multiple endocrine neoplasia type 1 (prolactinomas) or various genetic defects, including GNAS, menin, PRKAR1A, AIP, and p27 (CDKN1B) mutations (somatotroph and corticotroph adenomas).

Prognosis: Pediatric pituitary adenomas may be more aggressive than the adult forms, but the prognosis is usually excellent if gross total resection of the neoplasm can be achieved and the somatic effects of hormone hypersecretion are not too advanced.

Mesenchymal neoplasms

Meningiomas (62) (WHO Grade I, II, or III)

Meningiomas are phenotypically highly pleomorphic "extra-axial" neoplasms that arise from the arachnoid cap cells.

Clinical and neuroimaging comments: In childhood, meningiomas are unusual, accounting for less than 3% of all primary CNS tumors. In comparison to their adult counterparts, they have a greater predilection for uncommon sites, such as the cerebral ventricles and the infratentorial compartment.

The average age presentation is 13–14 years and there is a slight male predominance. Predisposing factors include neurofibromatosis types 1 and 2,

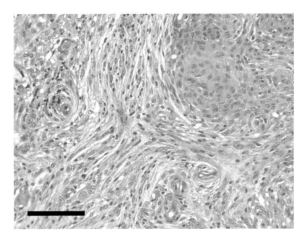

Figure 13.12 Transitional meningioma with fibrous and syncytial areas, and small whorls (H&E; scale bar 100 μm).

Gorlin syndrome, and previous therapeutic craniospinal radiation (e.g., after treatment of a medulloblastoma or acute lymphocytic leukemia). The percentages of supratentorial, infratentorial, intraventricular, and spinal tumors are 72%, 11%, 11%, and 6% respectively.

Neuroimaging studies reveal discrete, enhancing, dural-based masses, often with a "tail" of enhancement extending away from the body of the tumor into the adjacent dura, that indent the brain or spinal cord, and are associated with various degrees of brain swelling (particularly in the microcystic, angiomatous, and lymphoplasmacytoid-rich variants); cystic change is common.

Histology (Figure 13.12): Meningiomas are graded as WHO Grade I (80%), Grade II (10%), or Grade III (10%) tumors. Although the histological findings are highly varied, to the extent that meningiomas may be considered as the great mimics of intracranial neoplasms, the basic histological features of a meningioma are small meningothelial whorls, elongated fibrocytic or fibroblastic cells, and psammoma bodies. Table 13.8 summarizes the varied histological features of these neoplasms.

Immunohistochemistry: All meningiomas are vimentin-immunopositive. Many exhibit focal S100 immunolabelling. Focal or diffuse membranous EMA immunopositivity is characteristic of most meningiomas, but may be inconspicuous in the higher-grade tumor. The lack of nuclear progesterone receptor immunopositivity is a poor prognostic finding in high-grade meningiomas, but not in the WHO grade I tumors.

Molecular pathology: The meningiomas are associated with numerous genetic alterations, which become more prominent with increasing grade. None appear to carry special prognostic value.

Table 13.8 Meningioma summary

WHO grade (proportion)	Type	Key histological features	10-Year relapse-free (survival) rates
I (80%)	Syncytial	Many whorls, epithelioid cells with indistinct borders arranged in lobules	74% (83%)
	Fibrous (fibroblastic)	Spindle cells arranged in ill-defined, haphazardly arranged fascicles, many strands of collagen	
	Transitional	Mixed features of syncytial and fibrous	
	Angiomatous	Abundant thin-walled blood vessels	
	Lymphoplasmacytoid	Abundant lymphocytes and plasma cells. May resemble an inflammatory pseudotumor	
	Metaplastic	Prominent metaplastic bone, cartilage, and/or lipid	
	Microcystic	Marked microcystic change	
	Psammomatous	Abundant psammoma bodies. Commoner in spinal meningiomas	
	Secretory	Numerous epithelioid cells with discrete dPAS+ /CEA+ cytoplasmic inclusions	
II (10%)	Chordoid	Cords or trabeculae of eosinophilic cells, prominent mucoid background	58% (75%)
	Clear cell	Abundant cells with glycogen-rich, clear cytoplasm and small, round hyperchromatic nuclei	
	Atypical	Grade I characteristics, plus four or more mitoses/10 HPFs OR three or more of: monotonous growth pattern ("sheeting"); foci of small, poorly differentiated, lymphocyte-like cells; large ("macro") nucleoli; and geographic necrosis	
	"Brain-invasive"	Brain invasion beyond the Virchow–Robin spaces (GFAP useful to demonstrate)	
III (10%)	Papillary	Prominent perivascular pseudopapillary pattern	30% (72%)
	Rhabdoid	Plump, epithelioid cells with eccentric nuclei, prominent nucleolus, and inclusion-like, strongly vimentin+ eosinophilic cytoplasm	
	Anaplastic/malignant	Frank malignant microscopic morphology, reminiscent of a carcinoma or a high-grade sarcoma, usually 20 or more mitoses per 10 HPFs	

Prognosis: The extent of resection is the strongest independent prognostic factor for pediatric meningiomas. Irrespective of grade, the 15-year relapse-free survival rate is 78%, and 11% for grossly or subtotally resected tumors, respectively. The WHO grade is somewhat unreliable and well-differentiated meningiomas may behave in an aggressive fashion. Children aged 3–11 years appear to have a better prognosis than those younger than 3 years, or 12 years or older (also see Table 13.8).

Differential diagnosis: In frozen sections some meningothelial meningiomas may resemble well-differentiated adenocarcinoma (although the prominent nucleoli in the latter are distinctive) and it may also be difficult to distinguish between infratentorial meningiomas (with inconspicuous whorls) and schwannomas (with loosely arranged whorl-like structures). The fibroblastic meningiomas may be confused with a schwannoma, but the extensive S100 immunopositivity of the latter and the EMA immunolabelling of the former usually resolve the difficulty. The presence of bone in a meningioma may be taken as evidence of skull invasion, but it may also be a metaplastic change. The distinction between an inflammatory pseudotumor and a lymphoplasmacytoid meningioma may be problematic if inflammation is the dominant feature. Some difficulty may be encountered in distinguishing anaplastic meningiomas from intracranial fibrosarcomas and, if there is extensive brain invasion, from gliosarcomas. Other peripherally located, reticulin-rich gliomas (desmoplastic ganglioglioma, pleomorphic astrocytoma) may present radiologically as "meningiomas."

Other subdural lesions

Most subdural masses are meningiomas. However, on rare occasions they may be non-meningiomatous mesenchymal tumors of various sorts (Table 14.9) or, exceptionally rare in children, inflammatory pseudotumors (63) (which may also be intraparenchymal (64).

Germ-cell neoplasms

Germ-cell tumors of the CNS form approximately 3% of all childhood CNS tumors. They resemble germ-cell tumors found elsewhere in the body (see Chapter 9) and include teratomas, germinomas, and non-germinomatous germ-cell tumors (NGGCT).

Clinical and neuroimaging comments: Germinomas account for the majority of intracranial germ-cell tumors. Non-germinomatous germ-cell tumors include choriocarcinomas, endodermal sinus tumors (yolk-sac tumors), embryonal carcinomas, and tumors with mixed morphology. Intracranial germ-cell tumors usually arise in the pineal gland or, approximately half as frequently, in the suprasellar region; simultaneous suprasellar and pineal region tumors occur in approximately 10% of cases. Germinomas most often present between 10–12 years of age, but NGGCTs tend to occur in younger patients. The commonest CNS site for teratomas is the sacrococcygeal region, the patients usually presenting in infancy. By neuroimaging, non-teratomatous tumors are solid and enhancing, whereas teratomas are usually cystic, often calcified, and rarely enhance. Intratumoral hemorrhage is common in the choriocarcinomas.

Histology: The histological appearances are very similar to extraneural germ-cell tumors. In summary, teratomas contain mature ectodermal (skin, brain, choroid plexus), mesenchymal (cartilage, bone, fat, and striated and smooth muscle), and endodermal elements (cysts lined by respiratory or enteric epithelia). The presence of immature mitotically active primitive mesenchymal and/ or neuroectodermal elements, no matter how minor, indicates an immature teratoma; such tumors are exceptionally rare in the CNS. Teratomas with malignant transformation contain malignant components such as rhabdomyosarcoma, undifferentiated sarcoma, and, less commonly, various carcinomas.

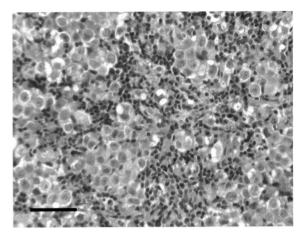

Figure 13.13 Germinoma showing seams of lymphocytes among the large pale epithelioid tumor cells (H&E; scale bar 50 μm).

Germinomas are characterized by large epithelioid cells with abundant cytoplasm that are arranged in nests and small lobules separated by bands of connective tissue – lymphocytic inflammation is common and at times marked (Figure 13.13). Embryonal carcinomas contain focally necrotic sheets of highly mitotically active large cells. Hyperchromatic, multinucleated, syncytiotrophoblast characterize the choriocarcinoma, and primitive epithelial cells with a sinusoidal growth pattern, occasionally investing a papillary core (Schiller–Duval body), indicate a yolk-sac tumor.

Immunohistochemistry: A panel of immunohistochemical methods may be used to distinguish between the various types of germ-cell tumors. Germinomas are typically immunopositive for placental alkaline phosphatase and CD 117 (c-kit); a few examples may be focally cytokeratin-immunopositive (CAM 5.2, AE1/3). Yolk-sac tumors and embryonal carcinomas are immunopositive for α-fetoprotein and CD30, respectively, and both are cytokeratin-immunopositive; they may also be PLAP-immunopositive. The syncytiotrophoblast in choriocarcinomas is hCG-immunopositive.

Molecular pathology: The molecular characteristics of the CNS germ-cell tumors have not been extensively studied, but they appear to be similar to those of extramural germ-cell neoplasms.

Differential diagnosis: The principal problem is determining which and how many of the various malignant germ-cell elements are present in a germinoma and, with reference to the teratoma, where in the axis of maturity, immaturity, and malignancy a given teratoma should be classified. An intracerebral hematoma may belie a choriocarcinoma, and intense lymphocytic inflammation can obscure a germinoma. More generally, there are a host of other CNS tumors that may superficially resemble various germ-cell neoplasms, but the basic hematoxylin and eosin appearances, clinical context and neuroimaging findings, and the judicious use of immunohistochemical methods will usually allow the correct diagnosis to be reached.

Prognosis: Pure germinomas and mature teratomas have a good prognosis, whereas a poor prognosis is expected for choriocarcinomas, yolk-sac tumors, embryonal carcinomas, and mixed tumors composed predominantly of these elements. The prognosis for the remainder, including mixed tumors composed mainly of germinomatous or teratomatous elements, is intermediate.

Choroid plexus tumors

Choroid plexus tumors are neoplasms of the cerebral ventricular system, which include choroid plexus papillomas (CPPs) and choroid plexus carcinomas (CPCs).

Clinical and neuroimaging comments: Although choroid plexus tumors occur throughout life and in all cerebral ventricles, they are most common in the first year of life and show a predisposition for the lateral ventricles in the pediatric population. Choroid plexus papillomas are more common than CPCs. Choroid plexus tumors typically present with hydrocephalus and, in infants, with increasing head circumference. By neuroimaging, they exhibit irregular contrast enhancement and they are usually well-delineated unless there is brain invasion. Dissemination through the CSF pathways may occur.

Histology: Choroid plexus papillomas resemble normal choroid plexus, although their papillae are more crowded and their epithelial cells are more elongated. They are characterized by delicate fibrovascular cores lined by a single layer of cuboidal or columnar epithelium (Figure 13.14). Brain invasion and mitoses may be observed; however, two or more mitoses per 10 HPF indicate an atypical CPP. Choroid plexus carcinomas are distinguished by loss of papillary morphology, areas of necrosis, frank cytological evidence of malignancy, mitoses (> 5/10 HPF), and brain invasion.

Immunochemistry: There is no specific immunohistochemical marker for choroid plexus neoplasms. Most of them are cytokeratin- and vimentin-immunopositive (less so with the CPCs), many are

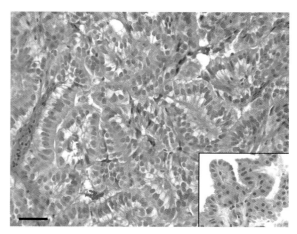

Figure 13.14 Choroid plexus papilloma. Note the tightly packed papillae and more columnar epithelium in comparison to the normal choroid plexus shown in the inset (both H&E; scale bar 50 μm).

transthyretin (prealbumin)-immunopositive, and a few may be GFAP-immunopositive.

Differential diagnosis: The principal differential diagnosis for the CPP is normal choroid plexus or, unlikely to be a problem in children, a metastatic papillary carcinoma. The presence of INI1 nuclear immunolabelling distinguishes the CPC from an AT/RT, which it may closely resemble.

Prognosis: Surgical excision of a choroid plexus tumor may be curative. There is a low risk of recurrence for CPPs and a higher risk for the CPCs. Dissemination of the tumor through the CSF pathways is a poor prognostic sign.

Miscellaneous other tumors and tumor-like conditions: Table 13.9

Metastases to and from the CNS and "second" tumors

With the increasingly effective management and long survival of children with malignant tumors, "second malignancies," whether as a complication of the immune-suppression associated with the management of the first tumor, or due to an underlying genetic predisposition, and metastases (both from and to the CNS) are being increasingly encountered (Table 13.10).

The surgical pathology of refractory epilepsy

The neuroimaging and electrophysiological investigation of children with refractory (drug-resistant)

Table 13.9 Miscellaneous other primary CNS tumors

Tumor	WHO grade	Key clinical and imaging features	Key histological features	Differential diagnosis
Non-meningiomatous subdural, intradural and/or epidural neoplasms (3)	I to IV	Appear to arise from inner face of cranium, dura or arachnoid. Rarely occur elsewhere in brain. Resemble their extracranial counterparts	Rhabdomyosarcoma. Fibroma and fibrosarcoma. Ewing's sarcoma. Leiomyoma and leiomyosarcoma. Lipoma and angiolipoma. Solitary fibrous hist ocytoma. Pigmented hamartomas and neoplasms, e.g., diffuse meningeal melanocytosis, meningeal melanocytomas and melanomas (rare in children)	Desmoplastic astrocytoma/ganglioglioma. Other sarcomas
Hemangioblastoma (3)	I	Associated with and frequently multiple in von Hippel–Lindau disease. Typically occur in cerebellum, brainstem, and rostral spinal cord. Enhancing, cystic mass with mural nodule	Large vacuolated stroma cells (predominate in cellular variant). Plexus of thin-walled sinusoidal vessels (predominate in reticular variant). Inhibin +, cytokeratin –	Metastatic clear-cell carcinoma
Various epithelial-lined cysts (65–67)	N/A	Extra-axial (and sometimes intra-axial) epithelial-lined cysts can rarely occur throughout the neuroaxis, particularly in the midline	Dermoid/epidermal morphology ("pearly" tumor). Neuroenteric (enterogenous) cysts. Ependymal cysts	Cystic neoplasms. Teratomas (dermoid cysts). Cyst contents may cause chemical meningitis
Primary CNS lymphomas (68)	N/A	Rare in children (more common in immune-suppression)	Poorly differentiated, non-cohesive cells. Perivascular reticulin networks. Various types (standard lymphoma IHC work-up)	Other neoplasms composed of malignant monomorphic (small blue) cells
Langerhans-cell histiocytosis (69)	N/A	Rare. Solitary eosinophilic granuloma of skull commonest	Histiocytic lesion (+/– erythrophagocytic histiocytosis). Apparent mixed inflammatory infiltrate including abundant eosinophils CD1a-immunopositive. Birbeck granules by electron microscopy	Vasculitis, various histiocytic lesions, inflammatory pseudotumors, histiocytoid neoplasms
Medulloepithelioma	IV	Most occur in the first five years of life. Often periventricular. May be associated with peripheral nerves. Circumscribed, solid or cystic, non-enhancing at presentation	Papillary non-ciliated tubular or trabecular neoplastic neuroepithelium buried in sheets of poorly or partly differentiated neuroepithelial cells. Resembles embryonic neural tube. Epithelium is nestin + and vimentin +. The remaining cells show various degrees of astrocytic, ependymal, and oligodendroglial differentiation	Various embryonal neoplasms (medulloblastoma, PNET). Choroid plexus carcinoma
Malignant ectomesenchymoma (70)	Undetermined	Possible good prognosis after gross total resection and adjuvant craniospinal radiotherapy	Neuroectodermal elements (poorly differentiated neuroepithelial cells, atypical ganglion cells). Rhabdomyoblasts, cells reminiscent of rhabdomyosarcoma	Various polyphenotypic tumors
Primitive polar spongioblastoma (71)	Variable	Prognosis is of principal tumor	Closely packed GFAP+ spindled cells arranged in striking parallel palisades. Pattern resembles primitive spongioblasts	Probably not a specific neoplasm. Pattern found focally or diffusely in ependymomas, hemispheric and cerebellar pilocytic astrocytomas, oligodendrogliomas, glioblastomas, PNETs and medulloblastomas

Table 13.10 Metastases from CNS tumors; cerebral metastases; second malignancies

Process	Tumor type and findings	Comments
Extracranial metastasis from primary CNS tumors (72–74) (Note: *Intracranial and intraspinal* leptomeningeal and, to a lesser extent, ventricular metastases are a significant and prognostically important problem, especially with the embryonal tumors)	Medulloblastoma to bone marrow and lymph nodes Gliomas (oligodendrogliomas, glioblastomas) to lung, liver and lymph nodes	Associated with extensive surgical resection, especially if cerebral sinuses and veins are involved
Cerebral metastases from extracranial tumors (75,76)	Malignant meningitis and perivascular intracerebral spread in hematopoietic malignancies Especially from clear-cell sarcoma and pleuropulmonary blastoma Sometimes from choriocarcinoma (hemorrhagic), Ewing's sarcoma, osteogenic sarcoma, alveolar rhabdomyosarcoma	May be present at time of diagnosis (especially leukemic meningitis) but usually develop after diagnosis and treatment of primary tumor (median 20 months) Concurrent pulmonary metastases are frequent Develop clinically in 2% of cases Present in 6–13% of fatal cases
"Second" neoplasms (77–79)	*After treatment of primary CNS tumor* (usually with a several years-long latency): leukaemia, carcinoma, bone tumors, *de novo* second CNS neoplasms *CNS tumors after treatment of extracranial tumors*: usually meningiomas (after craniospinal irradiation) and high-grade gliomas	Cumulative risk for all "second" neoplasms is 3.2% after 20 years Etiology uncertain, but likely to be related to direct effects of irradiation on exposed tissue, systemic effects of chemotherapy and genetic tumor predisposition

epilepsy may reveal focal, resectable, structural lesions of the brain, or cases in which, despite negative neuro-imaging, there is a seizure focus that may prove amenable to resection and consequently to improved control or abolition of seizures. Such epileptogenic lesions are often in the temporal lobe, but they may also occur elsewhere, particularly the frontal lobes.

The commonest pathological samples received from these cases include part or all of the affected temporal lobe and the medial temporal structures or a small sample of cortex and white matter containing an electrophysiologically identified seizure focus (a "lesionectomy"). Specimens from epilepsy cases should be cut into multiple thin slices, perpendicular to the cortical surface, and a generous sampling submitted for microscopic examination. As well as routine stains, immunohistochemistry for GFAP, neu N, neurofilaments, and synaptophysin should be used in cases in which focal cortical dysplasia is suspected.

A detailed account of epilepsy pathology is beyond the scope of this chapter, but in summary, epileptogenic pathological abnormalities include:

- Malformations, which are usually areas of focal cortical dysplasia, characterized by microscopic

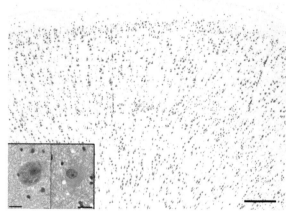

Figure 13.15 Cortical dysplasia. There are cortical architectural abnormalities in the form of spaces between and short columns of neurones (cortical dysplasia type Ia; Neu N immunohistochemistry; scale bar 500 μm); Inset: a dysplastic neuron (left) and "balloon" cell (right), typical of cortical dysplasia type IIb (H&E; scale bar 20 μm).

focal disruption of the cortical neuronal laminae, dysplastic neurons, and ballooned neurons (Figure 13.15; 80). Other malformations are only rarely encountered in surgical pathology but may include hemimegalencephaly, polymicrogyria, and cerebral heterotopias (81).

- Low-grade tumors (particularly DNETs and other glioneuronal tumors) (82).

461

- Organizing destructive lesions, such as old infarcts and contusions.
- Other focal structural defects, including vascular malformations.
- Rasmussen's encephalitis (a progressive disorder that usually affects one hemisphere and whose histological features of perivascular lymphocytic inflammation, neuronal loss, and gliosis resemble chronic autoimmune encephalitis) (83).
- Non-specific findings are common in epilepsy specimens, including subpial (Chaslin's) gliosis, perivascular clustering of white matter oligodendroglia, and leptomeningeal inflammation (usually in children who have had surface electroencephalographic monitoring of the brain prior to surgery).

Mesial temporal sclerosis is commonly associated with seizures of various etiologies. It is a striking, but non-specific finding whose precise etiology remains uncertain and is characterized by loss of neurons from Ammon's horn and the amygdala, associated with gliosis and variable degrees of loss of and dispersal of the dentate gyrus neurons.

Light and electron microscopic examination of skin biopsies and muscle biopsies may be requested in patients with myoclonic seizures and/or progressive neurological diseases. A specific diagnoses is possible from these biopsies in some cases, particularly Lafora body disease (Lafora bodies are PAS-positive inclusions and glycogen-like material in the apocrine sweat glands), neuronal ceroid lipofuscinoses, and mitochondrial cytopathies (especially the syndrome of "myoclonic epilepsy with ragged red fibers") (84).

Cerbrovascular disorders

The incidence of pediatric vascular disease is similar to that of brain tumors (85), but it is unusual to receive a surgical sample from such cases. These unusual specimens may include:

- Arteriovenous malformation: A tangle of large veins, thick-walled "arterialized" veins and a "feeder" artery, the vascular profiles being separated by gliotic brain tissue.
- Cavernous angioma: A nodule composed of back-to-back, thin-walled vascular profiles, and abundant perilesional hemosiderin – the lesion may be familial (86).
- Vasculitis: In such cases a brain biopsy will have been carried out to resolve an unexplained encephalopathy or when primary "small-vessel" angiitis of the nervous system was suspected. The histological features are of mononuclear intramural and perivascular infiltrates composed of lymphocytes and histiocytes, associated with leptomeningeal inflammation (87).
- Epilepsy "lesionectomy" specimen: Usually old infarcts, dating from infancy, that are localized, chaotic areas of gliosis, cavitation, mineralized neurons, aberrant myelination, and bundles of coarse astrocytes resembling wheat sheaves.

Neuromuscular disorders

The study of these disorders is a specialized activity that is usually carried out by neuropathologists. Pediatric pathologists may be asked to advise on the optimal method for sampling skeletal muscle and peripheral nerve, and to provide a provisional diagnosis, pending an opinion from a neuropathologist. Detailed information on various disorders is available in standard specialized texts (88–90).

Technical considerations

Muscle biopsies should be carried out on muscle that is only moderately involved by the disease process (severely involved muscle may display non-specific end-stage findings), and at sites that have not been used for needle electromyography. Skeletal muscle biopsies must be handled gently to avoid causing handling artefacts. A core of tissue 1 cm in diameter and 3–4 cm long should be removed surgically. (Some centers routinely carry out needle biopsies, saving the open biopsies for complex cases and cases in which the findings in the needle biopsy have not resolved the diagnosis.)

Samples from the biopsy are prepared for frozen sectioning and electron microscopy; there are various methods for freezing skeletal muscle, and advice should be sought from the appropriate neuropathology referral laboratory. When metabolic disease is suspected, additional samples should be stored in liquid nitrogen and in cases of possible mitochondrial dysfunction, fresh tissue may be needed for the isolation and testing of mitochondrial function. Surplus tissue may be fixed in formalin although the microscopic examination of this tissue rarely adds much diagnostic information; however, examination of serial paraffin sections provides an efficient method of searching for inflammation when an inflammatory myopathy is suspected. A battery of stains, histochemical methods, and immunohistochemical methods are usually carried out on skeletal muscle biopsies (89).

Peripheral nerve biopsies are rarely carried out and therefore will not be further considered here; technical details and a summary of the principal current practical use of this procedure are provided in the medical literature (91,92).

Inflammatory myopathy

The most likely muscle disorder to be encountered in general pediatric surgical practice is an inflammatory myopathy. Inflammation in skeletal muscle usually indicates an idiopathic inflammatory myopathy (although it may also be found in the dystrophies or infectious myopathies). The pediatric idiopathic inflammatory myopathies include juvenile dermatomyositis, polymyositis, and myositis associated with connective tissue disorders ("myositis plus"). Juvenile dermatomyositis is by far the commonest pediatric myositis; polymyositis (which tends to be a more aggressive illness) and "myositis plus" each make up about 10% of cases of idiopathic inflammatory myopathy (93). The heliotrope rash and other clinical manifestations may be so distinctive in dermatomyositis that a muscle biopsy is not needed; juvenile dermatomyositis, unlike the adult form, is rarely paraneoplastic.

The histological features of an inflammatory myopathy include muscle-fiber necrosis (which is often inconspicuous or absent in dermatomyositis), regenerating fibers, focal mild perimysial and endomysial fibrosis, mild myocyte hypertrophy, and inflammatory endomysial, perimysial, and perivascular infiltrates composed of various combinations of lymphocytes, histiocytes, and plasma cells. The perivascular lymphocytes tend to be B-cells (which are more numerous in dermatomyositis), whereas those elsewhere are T-cells; CD8 lymphocytes predominate in polymyositis and CD4 lymphocytes in dermatomyositis.

Although it may not be possible to distinguish between the various idiopathic inflammatory myopathies from the biopsy findings, selective involvement and atrophy of muscle fibers around the edges of the fascicles (perifascicular atrophy – Figure 13.16), perimysial inflammation, and loss of capillaries with mural thickening and hyalinosis of the surviving capillaries suggest dermatomyositis; invasion of necrotic fibers by lymphocytes is more characteristic of polymyositis.

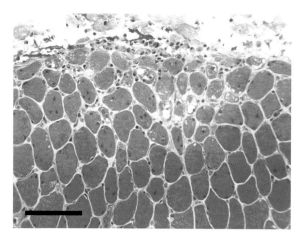

Figure 13.16 Dermatomyositis with perifascicular histiocytic infiltrates and muscle fiber changes (H&E; scale bar 100 μm).

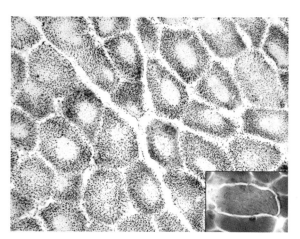

Figure 13.17 Many pediatric muscle diseases show distinctive histological features, including the central areas lacking succinic dehydrogenase activity in central core disease in the main frame and, in the inset, the ragged red fibers of a mitochondrial myopathy (Gomori's modified trichrome).

The inflammation in the idiopathic inflammatory myopathies is patchy, so a "negative" biopsy does not exclude the diagnosis. However, the immunohistochemical demonstration of sarcolemmal MHC class 1 antigens, which are normally only expressed in the blood vessels, is suggestive of an inflammatory myopathy (but also occurs in some dystrophinopathies and dysferlinopathies).

Other muscle disorders

A general overview of various pediatric disorders of skeletal muscle is provided in Table 13.11. For a more

463

Table 13.11 Examples of some muscle diseases and their key features

Class of disorder	Subclasses and examples of specific diagnoses		Immunohistochemical findings and other key features
DYSTROPHIES	Congenital muscular dystrophy (CMD)	Dystroglycanopathies, including muscle-eye- brain disease, Fukuyama and Walker–Warburg syndromes	Abnormal glycosylation of α-dystroglycan (DG) causes defective sarcolemmal α-DG IHL
		"Merosin deficiency" CMD (MDC1A)	Defective sarcolemmal laminin α2 IHL
		Ullrich CMD	Defective sarcolemmal and/or perimysial collagen VI IHL
	Classic muscular dystrophy	Duchenne dystrophy	Widespread defects in sarcolemmal dystrophin IHL
		Becker dystrophy	Focal defects in sarcolemmal dystrophin IHL
	Limb girdle muscular dystrophy (LGMD)	Dysferlinopathy (LGMD2B, Miyoshi myopathy)	Defective sarcolemmal dysferlin IHL and positive sarcoplasmic dysferlin IHL
		Sarcoglycanopathy; LGMD2-C is the commonest of these rare disorders	Defective sarcolemmal sarcoglycan IHL There are four sarcoglycan subunits, each associated with its own LGMD, e.g., α (LGMD2D), β (LGMD2E), γ (LGMD2C – Duchenne-like presentation) or δ (LGMD2F)
CONGENITAL MYOPATHIES	Nemaline rod disease		Nemaline rods (GMT, EM)
	Central core disease (see Figure 13.17) multi-mini core disease		Central or patchy (multi-mini cores) loss of oxidative enzyme activity (e.g., NADH), various sarcomeric and myofilamentous abnormalities (EM)
	Centronuclear and myotubular X-linked myopathy		Central nuclei (H&E)
	Congenital fiber type disproportion		Predominance and hypoplasia of Type 1 fibers (ATPase methods)
INFLAMMATORY MYOPATHY AND MUSCLE INFLAMMATION	Dermatomyositis (see Figure 13.16)		Perifascicular atrophy (H&E).
	Muscle inflammation in vasculitis		Intramuscular small vessel vasculitis, neurogenic changes (H&E, ATPase methods).
	"Secondary inflammation" in various dystrophies		e.g., LGMD2B (see above)
METABOLIC MYOPATHIES	Glycogen storage disorders (Pompe, Andersen, Tarui, Macardle)		Excessive sarcoplasmic membrane-bound glycogen (PAS, EM)
	Mitochondrial myopathies (see Figure 13.17)		Ragged red fibers (GMT), altered mitochondrial enzyme activity (increased SDH in fibers with diminished COX activity), abnormalities of mitochondrial ultrastructure.
NEUROGENIC CHANGES	Werdnig–Hoffman disease (spinal muscular atrophy Type 1). Neuropathy-associated muscle changes.		Acute changes – central cores Chronic changes – large groups of atrophic muscle fibers ("group atrophy"), large groups of type 1 and type 2 fibers ("type grouping")

(Abbreviations: COX = cytochrome C oxidase histochemistry (HC); GMT = Gomori's modified trichrome stain; IHL = immunohistochemical labelling; NADH = Nicotinamide adenine dinucleotide-tetrazolium reductase HC; SDH = succinic dehydrogenase HC

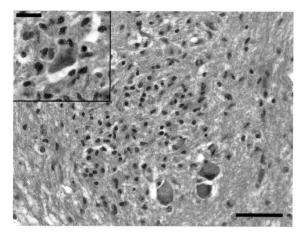

Figure 13.18 Arbovirus (West Nile) encephalitis showing focally prominent microglial activation (H&E; bar; scale bar scale bar 50 μm). Inset: a dying eosinophilic neuron (H&E; scale bar 20 μm). (Courtesy of Dr. R. Hammond, London Health Sciences Centre, London, Ontario.)

detailed and complete description of the various pediatric disorders of skeletal muscle other sources should be consulted (89,90). In general terms, muscle disorders can be classified as congenital myopathies (Figure 13.17), muscular dystrophies, metabolic myopathies, miscellaneous muscle diseases (including myofibrillary myopathies), inflammatory myopathies, and muscle with neurogenic changes. Genetic defects lead to deficiencies in: sarcolemmal proteins (causing the dystrophies); intermediate filaments and sarcoplasmic proteins (causing the myofibrillary myopathies); mitochondrial proteins and enzymes (causing mitochondrial cytopathies or myopathies); and cytosolic enzymes (causing various metabolic and storage disorders). In many instances the effects of these genetic disorders may be limited to the skeletal muscle, but extramuscular involvement is frequent.

Other surgical neuropathological disorders

General comments

It is unusual to receive neurosurgical specimens from other than tumor, epilepsy, and muscle disease cases. However, a discrete lesion may be biopsied to distinguish between a neoplasm and an infection, such as an abscess or a tuberculoma. A diagnostic biopsy may also be performed when the clinical features, neuroimaging, and other laboratory investigations have failed to elucidate the cause of a multifocal or diffuse brain disease,

typical examples being viral encephalitis, opportunistic infections in the setting of immune-deficiency, vasculitis, sarcoidosis, and various metabolic disorders.

The key in these situations is an intraoperative assessment of the tissue so that the presence of lesional tissue in the biopsy is confirmed and samples can be properly processed for appropriate investigations. Depending on the circumstances, these tests include cultures for bacterial, viral, and fungal infections, molecular studies on frozen tissue in cases of suspected metabolic disease, chromosomal and other analysis of cells in tissue culture in cases of suspected storage disorders, and electron microscopic examination of thin sections from tissue preserved in glutaraldehyde, also in cases of suspected storage disorders.

Infectious and inflammatory diseases of the CNS

The various organisms that cause CNS infections vary from region to region and country to country, and are dependent on the immune-competency of the individual. It is invariably worthwhile to discuss likely endemic causes of a suspected CNS infection with a microbiologist or infectious disease expert. With a few exceptions, the histological features of CNS infections are similar to the same infections elsewhere in the body.

Abscesses and abscess-like lesions

"Ring enhancement" on neuroimaging is characteristic of these lesions. Malignant gliomas, metastases, acute multiple sclerosis, and a capsule around an organizing hematoma may also be associated with ring enhancement.

Abscesses are characterized by polymorphonuclear infiltrates and, depending on the chronicity of the infection, various degrees of lymphohistiocytosis of, and connective tissue (reticulin and collagen) in, the wall of the abscess. Perilesional reactive astrocytosis may be marked and in a small non-representative biopsy may resemble a glioma.

Tuberculomas are characterized by caseating necrosis and inflammation, of which multinucleated histiocytes are typical; in some cases the latter may be absent or inconspicuous, and a reactive T-cell lymphocytosis may dominate the lesion; acid-fast bacilli may be found only after reviewing multiple levels from the biopsy. Toxoplasmosis may also cause an abscess-like lesion (see below).

Fungal infections

Fungal infections are commonly vasotropic or vasocentric and, to a variable degree, hemorrhagic, depending on the extent of vascular destruction. The causal organism is usually readily demonstrated with special stains such as dPAS, Gomori's methenamine silver, and mucicarmine although the precise identification of the fungus depends on its characteristics in culture.

Viral infections

The classic features of viral infections are perivascular and, to a lesser extent, parenchymal lymphocytic inflammation, viral inclusions (which are usually intranuclear, the exception being the cytoplasmic Negri bodies of rabies), or viral-induced nuclear dysmorphism (i.e., a blurring and faint dusky eosinophilia of the neuronal and/or glial nuclei), and microglial collections and "neuronophagia" (the engulfment and eventual phagocytosis of the infected neuron by microglia/histiocytes) (Figure 13.18). In addition, in some infections, the dominant histological findings may be of necrosis and petechial hemorrhages, which may mask the inflammatory reaction.

Viral infections may predominantly affect the gray matter (i.e., polioencephalitis caused by, for example, enteroviruses and arboviruses – including the West Nile virus) or result in necrosis of gray matter and white matter (i.e., panencephalitis, caused for example by herpes simplex 1 (HSV), varicella zoster (VCV), cytomegalovirus (CMV), and some arboviruses). Different regions of the brain and spinal cord are also preferentially affected by different viruses (e.g., temporal lobe by HSV, periventricular areas by CMV, brain stem by West Nile virus and VZV, spinal cord by poliovirus and VZV), and the effects of a given virus may be compounded by those of a secondary small vessel vasculitis (e.g., VZV).

'Atypical' viral (including HIV) infections

Progressive multifocal leucoencephalopathy (widely referred to by its abbreviation, PHL) is a demyelinating white matter infection caused by reactivation of the polyoma virus, usually in immune-suppressed patients. The lesions are multifocal and characterized by demyelination (i.e., a myelin stain shows loss of myelin in which preserved axons can be visualized using Bielschowsky's method or neurofilament immunohistochemistry), ground-glass viral nuclear inclusions in the oligodendroglia and bizarre, pleomorphic, hypertrophic astrocytes (which may be misinterpreted as a glioma in inadequately sampled lesions) (Figure 13.19).

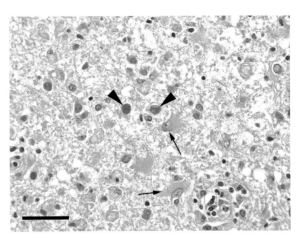

Figure 13.19 Progressive multifocal leucoencephalopathy showing large, "muddy" glial nuclear viral inclusions (arrow-heads) and atypical astrocytes (arrows) (H&E; scale bar 50 μm).

Measles may rarely cause a chronic, progressive, non-necrotising panencephalitis in which gliosis and neuronal loss predominate, inflammation is scant or inconspicuous, and viral inclusions few (subacute sclerosing panencephalitis).

Human immuno-deficiency virus (HIV)-associated lesions of the CNS include a leucoencephalitis characterized by scattered microglia nodules, giant cells with circumferentially and peripherally arranged nuclei (reminiscent of lipid-free "Touton" giant cells), a non-specific leucoencephalopathy (recognized by the presence of diffuse pallor of the white matter), and a vacuolar myelopathy (with extensive microvacuolation of the spinal cord white matter, whose histology is vaguely reminiscent of, but much more extensive than, that of subacute combined degeneration).

Opportunistic CNS infections

Common opportunistic CNS infections in immune-suppressed patients include those caused by cryptococcosis (lymphocytic meningitis, "soap bubble" abscesses), toxoplasma (abscesses/encephalitis – characterized by irregularly shaped areas of histiocyte-rich necrosis surrounded by an ill-defined pseudocapsule of neutrophils, histiocytes, and scattered tachyzoites), PML, mycobacterial infections, and CMV and VZV encephalitis.

Other infectious and inflammatory disorders (Figure 13.20)

There are also a legion of other infections and inflammatory disorders of the child's nervous system, which may be rare in some regions and common in others,

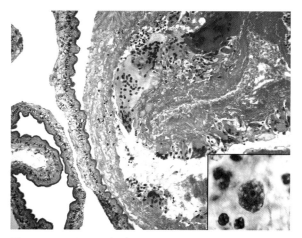

Figure 13.20 Protozoal infections may have distinctive features. Main figure: a foreign-body giant cell to the membrane of a cysticercosis cyst (H&E). Inset: trophozoite with its relatively small nucleus (compared to histiocytes) in a case of Balamuthia granulomatous amoebic encephalitis (Giemsa stain).

whose detailed analysis is beyond the scope of this chapter. However, attention to basic tissue reactions in the context of an odd clinical and neuroimaging picture may provide important clues:

- Eosinophils should prompt the consideration of a protozoal infection (of which cysticercosis is common; the lesion can be solitary, "burnt-out," and neoplasm-like, or active and multiple).
- Multinucleated giant cells suggest sarcoidosis and fungal infections.
- Abundant macrophages raise numerous possibilities: acute multiple sclerosis, toxoplasmosis, an unexpected infarct; and, when predominantly perivascular, cerebral Whipple's disease (with dPAS-, Gram- and Grocott-positive histiocytic granular inclusions).
- A predominantly perivascular distribution of lymphocytes, particularly when intramural, suggests small-vessel vasculitis, if viral infections can be ruled out.

References

1. Rodriguez FJ, Lim KS, Bowers D, et al. Pathological and molecular advances in pediatric low-grade astrocytoma. Annu. Rev. Pathol. 2013;**8**:361–79.

2. Taylor MD, Northcott PA, Korshunov A, *et al.* Molecular subgroups of medulloblastoma: the current consensus. Acta Neuropathol. 2012;**123**:465–72.

3. Louis DN, Ohgaki H, Wiestler OD, *et al. WHO Classification of Tumors of the Central Nervous System.* Lyon: IARC; 2007.

4. Ironside JW, Moss TH, Louis DN, *et al. Diagnostic Pathology of Nervous System Tumors.* London: Churchill Livingstone; 2002.

5. CBTRUS. Statistical Report: Primary Brain Tumors in the United States, 2000–2004. 2008. Central Brain Tumor Registry of the United States.

6. Rosemberg S, Fujiwara D. Epidemiology of pediatric tumors of the nervous system according to the WHO 2000 classification: A report of 1,195 cases from a single institution. Childs Nerv. Syst. 2005;**21**:940–4.

7. Woehrer A, Slavc I, Waldhoer T, *et al.* Incidence of atypical teratoid/rhabdoid tumors in children: A population-based study by the Austrian Brain Tumor Registry, 1996–2006. Cancer 2010;**116**:5725–32.

8. Tihan T, Vohra P, Berger MS, *et al.* Definition and diagnostic implications of gemistocytic astrocytomas: A pathological perspective. J. NeuroOncol. 2006;**76**:175–83.

9. Dorner L, Fritsch MJ, Hugo HH, *et al.* Primary diffuse leptomeningeal gliomatosis in a 2-year-old girl. Surg. Neurol. 2009;**71**:713–9.

10. Dias-Santagata D, Lam Q, Vernovsky K, *et al.* BRAF V600E mutations are common in pleomorphic xanthoastrocytoma: diagnostic and therapeutic implications. PLoS One 2011;**6**:e17948.

11. Creach KM, Rubin JB, Leonard JR, *et al.* Oligodendrogliomas in children. J. Neuro-Oncol. 2012;**106**:377–82.

12. Kreiger PA, Okada Y, Simon S, *et al.* Losses of chromosomes 1p and 19q are rare in pediatric oligodendrogliomas. Acta Neuropathol. 2005;**109**:387–92.

13. Hyder DJ, Sung L, Pollack IF, *et al.* Anaplastic mixed gliomas and anaplastic oligodendroglioma in children: results from the CCG 945 experience. J. Neuro-Oncol. 2007;**83**:1–8.

14. Seyithanoglu H, Guzey FK, Emel E, *et al.* Clear cell ependymoma of the temporal lobe in a child: A case report. Pediatr. Neurosurg. 2008;**44**:79–84.

15. Li JY, Lopez JI, Powell SZ, *et al.* Giant cell ependymoma-report of three cases and review of the literature. Int. J. Clin. Exp. Pathol. 2012;**5**:458–62.

16. Kleinman GM, Zagzag D, Miller DC. Epithelioid ependymoma: A new variant of ependymoma: report of three cases. Neurosurgery 2003;**53**:743–7.

17. Grill J, Bergthold G, Ferreira C. Pediatric ependymomas: Will molecular biology change patient management? Curr. Opin. Oncol. 2011;**23**:638–42.

18. Kilday JP, Rahman R, Dyer S, *et al.* Pediatric ependymoma: Biological perspectives. Mol. Cancer Res. 2009;7:765–86.

19. Raghunathan A, Wani K, Armstrong TS, *et al.* Histological predictors of outcome in ependymoma are dependent on anatomic site within the central nervous system. Brain Pathol. 2013;23:584–94.

20. Shakur SF, McGirt MJ, Johnson MW, *et al.* Angiocentric glioma: A case series. J. Neurosurg. Pediatr. 2009;3:197–202.

21. Marburger T, Prayson R. Angiocentric glioma: A clinicopathologic review of 5 tumors with identification of associated cortical dysplasia. Arch. Pathol. Lab. Med. 2011;135:1037–41.

22. Navarro R, Reitman AJ, de Leon GA, *et al.* Astroblastoma in childhood: pathological and clinical analysis. Childs Nerv. Syst. 2005;21:211–20.

23. Kantar M, Ertan Y, Turhan T, *et al.* Anaplastic astroblastoma of childhood: Aggressive behavior. Childs Nerv. Syst. 2009;25:1125–9.

24. Castellano-Sanchez AA, Schemankewitz E, Mazewski, *et al.* Pediatric chordoid glioma with chondroid metaplasia. Pediatr. Dev. Pathol. 2001;4:564–7.

25. Phi JH, Koh EJ, Kim SK, *et al.* Desmoplastic infantile astrocytoma: recurrence with malignant transformation into glioblastoma: A case report. Childs Nerv. Syst. 2011;27:2177–81.

26. Hummel TR, Miles L, Mangano FT, *et al.* Clinical heterogeneity of desmoplastic infantile ganglioglioma: A case series and literature review. J. Pediatr. Hematol. Oncol. 2012;34:e232–e236.

27. Gelabert-Gonzalez M, Serramito-Garcia R, Arcos-Algaba A. Desmoplastic infantile and non-infantile ganglioglioma. Review of the literature. Neurosurg. Rev. 2010;34:151–8.

28. Stephen JH, Sievert AJ, Madsen PJ, *et al.* Spinal cord ependymomas and myxopapillary ependymomas in the first 2 decades of life: A clinicopathological and immunohistochemical characterization of 19 cases. J. Neurosurg. Pediatr. 2012;9:646–53.

29. Hou Z, Wu Z, Zhang J, *et al.* Clinical features and management of intracranial subependymomas in children. J. Clin. Neurosci. 2013;20:84–8.

30. Rushing EJ, Cooper PB, Quezado M, *et al.* Subependymoma revisited: clinicopathological evaluation of 83 cases. J. Neuro-Oncol. 2007;85:297–305.

31. Garber ST, Brockmeyer DL. A rare case of a pediatric extraventricular neurocytoma: case report and review of the literature. Childs Nerv. Syst. 2012;28:321–6.

32. Stapleton CJ, Walcott BP, Kahle KT, *et al.* Diffuse central neurocytoma with craniospinal dissemination. J. Clin. Neurosci. 2012;19:163–6.

33. Hobert JA, Eng C. PTEN hamartoma tumor syndrome: An overview. Genet. Med. 2009;11:687–94.

34. Demetriades AK, Al Hyassat S, Al-Sarraj S, *et al.* Papillary glioneuronal tumor: A review of the literature with two illustrative cases. Br. J. Neurosurg. 2012;27:401–4.

35. Thurston B, Gunny R, Anderson G, *et al.* Fourth ventricle rosette-forming glioneuronal tumor in children: An unusual presentation in an 8-year-old patient, discussion and review of the literature. Childs Nerv. Syst. 2012;29:839–47.

36. Northcott PA, Jones DT, Kool M, *et al.* Medulloblastomics: the end of the beginning. Nat. Rev. Cancer 2012;12: 818–34.

37. Northcott PA, Korshunov A, Witt H, *et al.* Medulloblastoma comprises four distinct molecular variants. J. Clin. Oncol. 2011;29: 1408–14.

38. Kool M, Korshunov A, Remke M, *et al.* Molecular subgroups of medulloblastoma: An international meta-analysis of transcriptome, genetic aberrations, and clinical data of WNT, SHH, Group 3, and Group 4 medulloblastomas. Acta Neuropathol. 2012;123:473–84.

39. Dirks PB, Harris L, Hoffman HJ, *et al.* Supratentorial primitive neuroectodermal tumors in children. J. NeuroOncol. 1996;29:75–84.

40. Rorke LB, Trojanowski JQ, Lee VM, *et al.* Primitive neuroectodermal tumors of the central nervous system. Brain Pathol. 1997;7:765–84.

41. Visee S, Soltner C, Rialland X, *et al.* Supratentorial primitive neuroectodermal tumors of the brain: multidirectional differentiation does not influence prognosis. A clinicopathological report of 18 patients. Histopathology 2005;46:403–12.

42. Vogel H, Fuller GN. Primitive neuroectodermal tumors, embryonal tumors, and other small cell and poorly differentiated malignant neoplasms of the central and peripheral nervous systems. Ann. Diagn. Pathol. 2003;7:387–98.

43. Rogers HA, Miller S, Lowe J, *et al.* An investigation of WNT pathway activation and association with survival in central nervous system primitive neuroectodermal tumors (CNS PNET). Br. J. Cancer 2009;100:1292–302.

44. Kazmi SA, Perry A, Pressey JG, *et al.* Primary Ewing sarcoma of the brain: A case report and literature review. Diagn. Mol. Pathol. 2007;16:108–11.

45. Burger PC, Yu IT, Tihan T, *et al.* Atypical teratoid/rhabdoid tumor of the central nervous system: A highly malignant tumor of infancy and childhood frequently mistaken for medulloblastoma: A Paediatric Oncology Group study. Am. J. Surg. Pathol. 1998;22:1083–92.

46. Poretti A, Meoded A, Huisman TA. Neuroimaging of pediatric posterior fossa tumors including review of the literature. J. Magn. Reson. Imaging 2012;**35**:32–47.

47. Dahiya S, Perry A. Pineal tumors. Adv. Anat. Pathol. 2010;**17**:419–27.

48. Olaya JE, Raghavan R, Totaro L, et al. Pineal anlage tumor in a 5-month-old boy. J. Neurosurg. Pediatr. 2010;**5**:636–40.

49. Li G, Mitra S, Karamchandani J, et al. Pineal parenchymal tumor of intermediate differentiation: clinicopathological report and analysis of epidermal growth factor receptor variant III expression. Neurosurgery 2010;**66**:963–8.

50. Komakula S, Warmuth-Metz M, Hildenbrand P, et al. Pineal parenchymal tumor of intermediate differentiation: imaging spectrum of an unusual tumor in 11 cases. Neuroradiology 2011;**53**:577–84.

51. Fukuoka K, Sasaki A, Yanagisawa T, et al. Pineal parenchymal tumor of intermediate differentiation with marked elevation of MIB-1 labeling index. Brain Tumor Pathol. 2012;**29**:229–34.

52. Fevre MM, Vasiljevic A, Bergemer Fouquet AM, et al. Histopathologic and ultrastructural features and claudin expression in papillary tumors of the pineal region: A multicenter analysis. Am. J. Surg. Pathol. 2012;**36**:916–28.

53. Rodriguez FJ, Folpe AL, Giannini C, et al. Pathology of peripheral nerve sheath tumors: diagnostic overview and update on selected diagnostic problems. Acta Neuropathol. 2012;**123**:295–319.

54. Merlini L, Viallon M, De CG, et al. MRI neurography and diffusion tensor imaging of a sciatic perineuroma in a child. Pediatr. Radiol. 2008;**38**:1009–12.

55. Feany MB, Anthony DC, Fletcher CD. Nerve sheath tumors with hybrid features of neurofibroma and schwannoma: A conceptual challenge. Histopathology 1998;**32**:405–10.

56. Hornick JL, Bundock EA, Fletcher CD. Hybrid schwannoma/perineurioma: clinicopathologic analysis of 42 distinctive benign nerve sheath tumors. Am. J. Surg. Pathol. 2009;**33**:1554–61.

57. Keil MF, Stratakis CA. Pituitary tumors in childhood: update of diagnosis, treatment and molecular genetics. Expert Rev. Neurother. 2008;**8**:563–74.

58. Taylor M, Couto-Silva AC, Adan L, et al. Hypothalamic-pituitary lesions in pediatric patients: endocrine symptoms often precede neuro-ophthalmic presenting symptoms. J. Pediatr. 2012;**161**:855–63.

59. Kunwar S, Wilson CB. Pediatric pituitary adenomas. J. Clin. Endocrinol. Metab. 1999;**84**:4385–9.

60. Partington MD, Davis DH, Laws ER, et al. Pituitary adenomas in childhood and adolescence. Results of transsphenoidal surgery. J. Neurosurg. 1994;**80**:209–16.

61. Webb C, Prayson RA. Pediatric pituitary adenomas. Arch. Pathol. Lab. Med. 2008;**132**:77–80.

62. Kotecha RS, Pascoe EM, Rushing EJ, et al. Meningiomas in children and adolescents: A meta-analysis of individual patient data. Lancet Oncol. 2011;**12**:1229–39.

63. Suri V, Shukla B, Garg A, et al. Intracranial inflammatory pseudotumor: report of a rare case. Neuropathology 2008;**28**:444–7.

64. Radi-Bencteux S, Proust F, Vannier JP, et al. Intracerebral inflammatory pseudotumor in a 16-month-old boy. Neuropediatrics 2003;**34**:330–3.

65. Preece MT, Osborn AG, Chin SS, et al. Intracranial neurenteric cysts: imaging and pathology spectrum. AJNR Am. J. Neuroradiol. 2006;**27**:1211–16.

66. Hirano A, Hirano M. Benign cysts in the central nervous system: neuropathological observations of the cyst walls. Neuropathology 2004;**24**:1–7.

67. Caldarelli M, Massimi L, Kondageski C, et al. Intracranial midline dermoid and epidermoid cysts in children. J. Neurosurg. 2004;**100**:473–80.

68. Abla O, Weitzman S. Primary central nervous system lymphoma in children. Neurosurg. Focus 2006;**21**:E8.

69. Grois N, Prayer D, Prosch H, et al. Neuropathology of CNS disease in Langerhans cell histiocytosis. Brain 2005;**128**:829–38.

70. Weiss E, Albrecht CF, Herms J, et al. Malignant ectomesenchymoma of the cerebrum. Case report and discussion of therapeutic options. Eur. J. Pediatr. 2005;**164**:345–9.

71. Schiffer D, Cravioto H, Giordana MT, et al. Is polar spongioblastoma a tumor entity? J. Neurosurg. 1993;**78**:587–91.

72. Campbell AN, Chan HS, Becker LE, et al. Extracranial metastases in childhood primary intracranial tumors. A report of 21 cases and review of the literature. Cancer 1984;**53**:974–81.

73. Berger MS, Baumeister B, Geyer JR, et al. The risks of metastases from shunting in children with primary central nervous system tumors. J. Neurosurg. 1991;**74**:872–7.

74. Kochbati L, Bouaouina N, Hentati D, et al. (Medulloblastoma with extracentral nervous system metastases: clinical presentation and risk factors). Cancer Radiother. 2006;**10**:107–11.

75. Kebudi R, Ayan I, Gorgun O, et al. Brain metastasis in pediatric extracranial solid tumors: survey and literature review. J. NeuroOncol. 2005;**71**:43–8.

76. Stefanowicz J, Izycka-Swieszewska E, Szurowska E, et al. Brain metastases in paediatric patients: characteristics of a patient series and review of the literature. Folia Neuropathol. 2011;**49**:271–81.

77. Smith MB, Xue H, Strong L, *et al.* Forty-year experience with second malignancies after treatment of childhood cancer: Analysis of outcome following the development of the second malignancy. J. Pediatr. Surg. 1993;**28**:1342–8.

78. Vasudevan V, Cheung MC, Yang R, *et al.* Pediatric solid tumors and second malignancies: characteristics and survival outcomes. J. Surg. Res. 2010;**160**:184–9.

79. Elbabaa SK, Gokden M, Crawford JR, *et al.* Radiation-associated meningiomas in children: clinical, pathological, and cytogenetic characteristics with a critical review of the literature. J. Neurosurg. Pediatr. 2012;**10**:281–90.

80. Al Sufian F, Ang LC. Neuropathology of temporal lobe epilepsy. Epilepsy Res. Treat. 2012; article ID 624519.

81. Barkovich AJ, Guerrini R, Kuzniecky RI, *et al.* A developmental and genetic classification for malformations of cortical development: update 2012. Brain 2012;**135**:1348–69.

82. Prayson RA. Tumors arising in the setting of paediatric chronic epilepsy. Pathology 2010;**42**:426–31.

83. Pardo CA, Vining EP, Guo L, *et al.* The pathology of Rasmussen syndrome: stages of cortical involvement and neuropathological studies in 45 hemispherectomies. Epilepsia 2004;**45**:516–26.

84. Abramovich CM, Prayson RA, McMahon JT, *et al.* Ultrastructural examination of the axillary skin biopsy in the diagnosis of metabolic diseases. Hum. Pathol. 2001;**32**:649–55.

85. Beslow LA, Jordan LC. Pediatric stroke: the importance of cerebral arteriopathy and vascular malformations. Childs Nerv. Syst. 2010;**26**:1263–73.

86. Acciarri N, Galassi E, Giulioni M, *et al.* Cavernous malformations of the central nervous system in the pediatric age group. Pediatr. Neurosurg. 2009;**45**:81–104.

87. Twilt M, Benseler SM. The spectrum of CNS vasculitis in children and adults. Nat. Rev. Rheumatol. 2012;**8**:97–107.

88. Midroni G, Bilbao JM. *Biopsy Diagnosis of Peripheral Neuropathy*. Newton, MA: Butterworth-Heinemann, 1995.

89. Dubowitz V, Sewry CA, Oldfors A. *Muscle Biopsy: A Practical Approach*, Fourth edn. Elsevier, 2013.

90. Karpati G. *Structural and Molecular Basis of Skeletal Muscle Diseases*. Basel: ISN Neuropath Press; 2002.

91. Vallat JM, Vital A, Magy L, *et al.* An update on nerve biopsy. J. Neuropathol. Exp. Neurol. 2009;**68**:833–44.

92. Mellgren SI, Lindal S. Nerve biopsy: Some comments on procedures and indications. Acta Neurol. Scand. Suppl. 2011;64–70.

93. Shah M, Mamyrova G, Targoff IN, *et al.* The clinical phenotypes of the juvenile idiopathic inflammatory myopathies. Medicine (Baltimore) 2013;**92**:25–41.

Chapter 14

Introduction to small round-cell tumors

Erin R. Rudzinski

Small round-cell tumors present a common, yet challenging, diagnostic category in pediatric pathology. Characterized by high nuclear:cytoplasmic ratios, the histologic features of these tumors may be remarkably similar (Table 14.1). Correct identification of the specific tumor type is important as the various types have very different treatments. Thankfully, modern ancillary tests, including immunohistochemical, cytogenetic, and molecular techniques, aid in diagnostic confirmation. Since these biopsies are often small, knowledge of the general clinical and histologic features of these tumors is helpful in appropriately triaging limited tissue. The purpose of this chapter is to provide a general overview of small round-cell tumors in childhood, including specimen handling and an approach to the differential diagnosis and work-up of these common pediatric neoplasms.

Initial specimen handling

Typically, pediatric tumors first come to the attention of the pathologist when the surgeon requests a frozen-section diagnosis. Although sometimes amenable to simple histologic diagnosis, more often intraoperative consultation provides an opportunity to ensure the receipt of adequate diagnostic material. This is particularly important in small round-cell tumors in which the need for well-fixed tissue for histology and immunohistochemistry competes with the need for fresh tissue for cytogenetics and/or flow cytometry, as well as frozen tissue for research and biologic tests (Table 14.2).

Although each case is different, developing a routine for handling tissue ensures appropriate diagnosis and treatment later. If the specimen is a primary resection, it should also be sampled adequately for both staging and diagnostic purposes.

Our knowledge of the molecular features of pediatric small round-cell tumors has advanced tremendously; however, light microscopy remains a powerful tool for diagnosing these pediatric malignancies. With adequate sampling, many tumors are readily diagnosed by histopathological features and a panel of immunohistochemical stains; thus, obtaining well-fixed tissue for routine processing is critical.

Unique to small round-cell tumors is the fact than many are characterized by recurrent cytogenetic abnormalities, which may aid or confirm the histopathological impression (Table 14.3). Although several techniques (including fluorescence *in situ* hybridization (FISH) and Reverse transcriptase, Polymerase chain reaction (RT-PCR) can use formalin-fixed paraffin-embedded tissue, small specimens requiring an extensive immunohistochemical panel may be exhausted prior to completing all the desired ancillary studies. Therefore, for small specimens such as needle biopsies, touch preparations may not only aid in diagnosis, but air-dried slides may also be used for ancillary tests such as FISH. Touch preparations offer the advantage of requiring no additional sacrifice of tissue and may be made from fresh or previously frozen tissue.

If tissue is sufficient, reserving fresh tissue for routine cytogenetics (e.g., karyotyping) may reveal unexpected abnormalities or help characterize variant translocations detected on FISH (see Chapter 15). If leukemia/lymphoma remains in the differential diagnosis, then fresh tissue should also be obtained for flow cytometry studies. Additionally, many pediatric patients with small round-cell malignancies are enrolled on clinical trials requiring frozen tissue as part of the eligibility requirements. Regardless of whether this tissue is required for study or research purposes, freezing tissue allows the opportunity for additional biologic and prognostic testing (such as

Table 14.1 Small round-cell tumors in childhood

Common
Non-Hodgkin's lymphoma
Extramedullary leukemia
Neuroblastoma
Rhabdomyosarcoma
Ewing's sarcoma/peripheral neuroectodermal tumor (PNET)
Wilms' tumor (nephroblastoma)
Desmoplastic small round-cell tumor

Less common
Synovial sarcoma (poorly differentiated)
Malignant peripheral nerve-sheath tumor (poorly differentiated)
Undifferentiated sarcoma
Mesenchymal chondrosarcoma
Osteosarcoma (small-cell variant)
Melanotic neuroectodermal tumor of infancy
Hepatoblastoma (small-cell variant)
Pleuropulmonary blastoma

Table 14.2 Handling of pediatric small round-cell tumors

Fresh
– Cytogenetics and/or flow cytometry

Frozen
– Research protocols or other prognostic/biologic studies (ie. loss of heterozygosity, DNA-ploidy)
– Snap frozen or preserved in frozen-section media

Touch preparations
– Cytologic features aid in diagnosis
– Conserves tissue when handling limited specimens
– Air-dried slides may be used for FISH

Formalin fixation
– Routine light microscopy and immunohistochemistry
– Molecular genetic techniques (FISH, RT-PCR)

Electron microscopy
– May be useful in cases without histologic or immunohistochemical differentiation
– Requires miniscule amounts of tissue in appropriate fixative (i.e., glutaraldehyde)

Table 14.3 Recurrent chromosomal translocations in pediatric small round-cell tumors

Ewing's/peripheral neuroectodermal tumor (PNET)	t(11;22)(q24;q12)	*FLI1-EWSR1*	90%
	t(12;22)(q22;q12)	*ERG-EWSR1*	5–10%
	t(7;22)(p22;q12)	*ETV1-EWSR1*	<1%
	t(17;22)(q12;q12)	*E1AF-EWSR1*	<1%
	t(2;22)(q23;q12)	*FEV-EWSR1*	<1%
Alveolar rhabdomyosarcoma	t(2;13)(q35;q14)	*PAX3-FOXO1*	~75%
	t(1;13)(p36;q14)	*PAX7-FOXO1*	~10%
	t(X;2)(q13;q35)	*AFX-PAX3*	<1%
Desmoplastic small round-cell tumor	t(11;22)(p13;q12)	*WT1-EWSR1*	~95%
Synovial sarcoma	t(X;18)(p11;q11)	*SS18-SSX1, SSX2, SSX4*	~95%
Mesenchymal chondrosarcoma	t(8;8)(q13;q21)	*HEY1-NCOA2*	
	der(13;21)(q10;q10)		
Undifferentiated sarcoma	t(4;19)(q35;q13)	*CIC-DUX4*	
	t(10;19)(q26;q13)		
	t(x;x)(11.4; 11.22) BCOR – CCNB3		

loss of heterozygosity in Wilms' tumor or neuroblastoma). Snap freezing tissue in liquid nitrogen is recommended, but if material is scant then cryoembedded tissue used for frozen-section diagnosis provides an alternative means of preserving frozen tissue.

Finally, saving tissue for electron microscopy may be useful in difficult cases that fail to show histological, immunohistochemical, or molecular evidence of differentiation. The tissue required for this test is miniscule (1 mm^3 is recommended for optimal fixation).

The sample can also be stored in glutaraldehyde for a short period of time, or embedded in resin and held indefinitely should the primary work-up fail to provide a definitive diagnosis.

Differential diagnosis

After describing the specimen and allocating tissue, the next task for the pathologist is to decide on the most effective panel of ancillary tests to make a diagnosis. In

Table 14.4 Differential diagnosis of pediatric small round-cell tumors by site

Head and Neck
Rhabdomyosarcoma, Ewing's/PNET, melanotic neuroectodermal tumor of infancy, metastatic neuroblastoma, non-Hodgkin's lymphoma

Soft Tissue
Rhabdomyosarcoma, extraosseous Ewing's/PNET, extramedullary leukemia, non-Hodgkin's lymphoma, synovial sarcoma, MPNST, undifferentiated sarcoma

Bone
Ewing's sarcoma, leukemia/lymphoma, small cell variant of osteosarcoma, mesenchymal chondrosarcoma, metastatic rhabdomyosarcoma or neuroblastoma

Abdominal mass
Neuroblastoma, rhabdomyosarcoma, Wilms' tumor, desmoplastic small round-cell tumor, germ-cell tumor

Kidney
Wilms' tumor, PNET, rhabdoid tumor

Adrenal/paravertebral sympathetic ganglia
Neuroblastoma

Liver
Hepatoblastoma (small-cell variant), undifferentiated embryonal sarcoma, rhabdomyosarcoma, rhabdoid tumor, metastatic neuroblastoma

Genitourinary
Rhabdomyosarcoma, germ-cell tumors

Chest – midline
Lymphoma, germ-cell tumor, NUT-midline carcinoma

Chest – lateral
Ewing's sarcoma, osteosarcoma

Lung
Pleuropulmonary blastoma, metastatic disease

PNET: primitive neuroectodermal tumor; MPNST: malignant peripheral nerve-sheath tumor

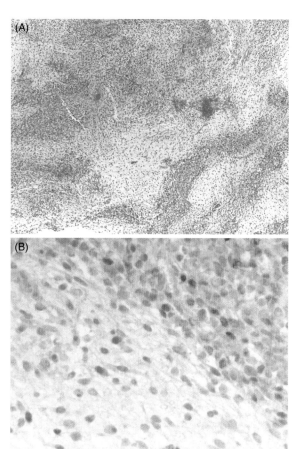

Figure 14.1 (A) Embryonal rhabdomyosarcoma (H&E × 100), showing alternating regions of dense and loose cellularity with a myxoid background. (B) Myogenin immunohistochemistry shows nuclear expression in malignant cells, strongest in regions of dense cellularity (× 400).

many instances, these tumors recapitulate the histology of the developing fetal organ or cell type, and recognizing these features ensures accurate diagnosis. Making the best choices based on the clinical and histological characteristics hastens the time to diagnosis and allows maximum preservation of tissue for diagnostic studies. The following sections provide a short discussion of the differential diagnosis of various pediatric malignancies based on common clinical presentations (Table 14.4). More information on the common tumor types can be found in the corresponding chapters.

Head and neck

Several types of small round-cell tumors arise in the head and neck region. Rhabdomyosarcomas

commonly occur in the soft tissues of the orbit, sinonasal, or parameningeal regions. The embryonal subtype predominates in the head and neck, although the alveolar subtype is often seen in parameningeal or paranasal sinus masses. Embryonal rhabdomyosarcoma typically shows spindled to ovoid nuclei, and rhabdomyoblastic differentiation may be seen as cells with abundant eosinophilic cytoplasm or even cross-striations (see Chapter 11). Typical embryonal rhabdomyosarcoma histology includes regions of dense cellularity alternating with hypocellular areas in a myxoid background resembling primitive mesenchyme (Figure 14.1A; 1). Some tumors may have uniformly dense cellularity with little differentiation and may be difficult to distinguish from the alveolar subtype or other small round-cell tumors. Alveolar rhabdomyosarcoma is characterized by discohesive,

473

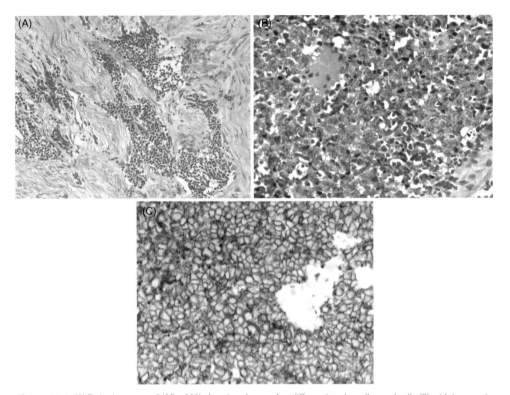

Figure 14.2 (A) Ewing's sarcoma (H&E × 200), showing sheets of undifferentiated small round cells, (B) with inconspicuous nucleoli (H&E × 400). (C) Immunohistochemistry for CD99 shows strong, diffuse membrane expression (× 400).

monomorphous round-cell cytology, and can resemble leukemia/lymphoma. Classic alveolar architecture is a helpful diagnostic clue if present, but this is absent in the solid variant of alveolar rhabdomyosarcoma (1).

For all histologic patterns of rhabdomyosarcoma, myogenin and desmin immunohistochemistry confirm the diagnosis. Notably, embryonal rhabdomyosarcoma typically has weak expression of myogenin, often expressed in 50% of tumor nuclei or less (Figure 14.1B). This may be helpful in distinguishing embryonal from alveolar rhabdomyosarcoma, which typically shows strong, uniform myogenin expression in nearly all tumor nuclei. For alveolar rhabdomyosarcoma diagnoses, or in cases where the subtype is uncertain, material should also be sent to test for presence of the *PAX/FOXO1* fusion transcript, which not only confirms alveolar histology, but may also play a role in determining risk stratification and treatment (2). Rhabdomyosarcoma is further discussed in Chapter 11.

Some small round-cell tumors may also involve the bones of the skull. Ewing family tumors (EFTs) arise in the skull in rare cases (3). As at other sites, EFTs are characterized by undifferentiated small round cells with a deceptively low mitotic index. Nuclei are uniform, with fine

chromatin and inconspicuous nucleoli (Figure 14.2A–C). Cytoplasm is scant and pale, and typically contains glycogen, which can be demonstrated with PAS staining. Strong membranous staining for CD99 is the hallmark immunohistochemical finding of EFT, although care should be taken to exclude leukemia/lymphoma, which may also show membranous expression of CD99. Lack of hematopoietic markers such as TdT or CD43 and presence of an *EWS* fusion transcript support the diagnosis of EFT. Chapter 11 provides additional discussion on EFT.

Melanotic neuroectodermal tumor of infancy (MNTI) is an uncommon neoplasm that affects infants less than one year of age (4). This tumor often arises from the mandible or maxilla, but may also involve the calvarium or other regions of the head and neck. Radiographic imaging may suggest an aggressive tumor with bony erosion, but MNTI typically behaves in a benign fashion, and patients do well after complete resection. Knowledge of MNTI and its histologic appearance are essential, as there are no specific immunohistochemical features. Melanotic neuroectodermal tumor of infancy demonstrate nests of small, undifferentiated round cells in a densely fibrotic stroma. Scattered pigmented,

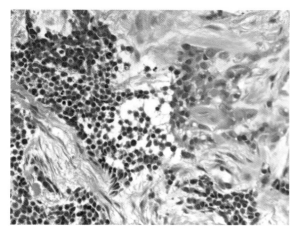

Figure 14.3 Melanotic neuroectodermal tumor of infancy showing nests of undifferentiated round cells in a dense, fibrotic stroma (H&E × 200). Higher-power examination shows clusters of epithelioid cells at the periphery of the nests, some with fine pigment (× 400).

melanin-containing, epithelioid cells are present, at least focally, around the periphery of the primitive nests (Figure 14.3). The small, undifferentiated cells may express neural markers such as synaptophysin or glial fibrillary acidic protein (GFAP), while the larger epithelioid cells may express melanocytic markers, including S100 and HMB-45, although the expression patterns are inconsistent.

Hematopoietic neoplasms may present with cervical lymphadenopathy and a neck mass, although there is usually a clinical suspicion of lymphoma in this setting. Finally, although it is an uncommon presentation, metastatic small-cell malignancies, such as neuroblastoma, may present as primary head and neck tumors. In the absence of CD99 expression, close attention to the presence of neuropil, Homer–Wright rosettes, or occasional cells with neuronal differentiation may provide clues to this unusual presentation.

Soft tissue and bone

Many of the same tumors that occur in the head and neck also enter the differential diagnosis for pediatric soft tissue tumors. Rhabdomyosarcomas often present as soft-tissue masses, and in the extremities and perineum these tumors are more often alveolar than embryonal. Ewing family tumors classically present as primary bone lesions centered in the metaphysis with an onion-skin appearance on X-ray (5). They may also present as a primary soft tissue mass, however. The histologic features of each of these tumor types are described above.

Soft-tissue tumors common in adolescents and young adults, such as synovial sarcoma and malignant peripheral nerve-sheath tumors (MPNST), have poorly differentiated round-cell variants that must be included in the differential diagnosis as well. Malignant peripheral nerve-sheath tumors should be considered if there is a clinical history of neurofibromatosis, or if spindled regions more typical of a nerve-sheath tumor with S100 expression are seen elsewhere in the tumor. Poorly differentiated synovial sarcoma may be difficult to distinguish from EFT (6). Synovial sarcomas may show CD99 expression, although not typically in the strong and diffuse, membranous pattern seen with EFT. Nuclear TLE1 (transducin-like enhancer of split 1) expression, a highly specific marker for synovial sarcoma, is present in approximately 80% of cases and may be useful (7). Molecular and/or cytogenetic analysis for the *SS18-SSX* fusion transcript should be considered for undifferentiated small round-cell tumors lacking an *EWS* translocation. These soft-tissue tumors are discussed in more detail in the corresponding chapter (Chapter 11).

Some undifferentiated round-cell tumors continue to show no evidence of differentiation, despite immunohistochemistry and molecular genetic tests, and one may be left with the diagnosis of undifferentiated sarcoma. While this group is heterogeneous, recurrent mutations have been recently identified in a subset of these tumors. A recurrent t(4:19) resulting in a CIC–DUX4 fusion has been identified in nearly two-thirds os soft-tissue tumors with undifferentiated round-cell morphology (8). Similarly, a recurrent BCOR-CCNB3 fusion has been identified in a subset of round-cell sarcomas arising in bone (9). These tumors may demonstrate patchy membranous staining for CD99, suggesting a diagnosis of EFT, although molecular genetic analysis will show no evidence of an EWS translocation. Current studies suggest these tumors with variant translocations behave aggressively and should be treated with intensive chemotherapy similar to EFT.

Hematopoietic neoplasms may present as soft-tissue masses if enlarged axillary or groin lymph nodes are not recognized. Non-Hodgkin's lymphoma or extramedullary leukemias may also present as subcutaneous or soft-tissue nodules (Figure 14.4). As mentioned in the previous sections, lymphoblastic leukemia/lymphoma may show membranous CD99 expression, and this diagnosis should be excluded with CD43 and/or TdT immunohistochemistry. Finally, metastatic neuroblastoma may occasionally present with subcutaneous nodules or a bone lesion, although a primary mass is usually identified.

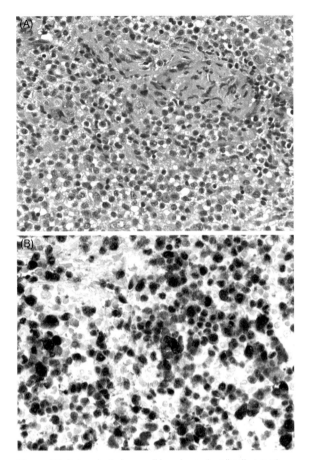

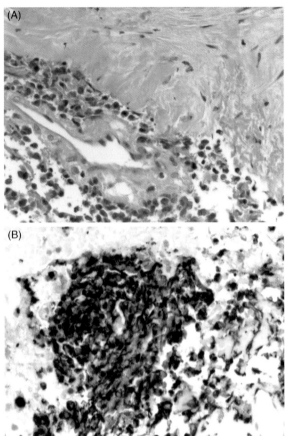

Figure 14.4 Anaplastic large-cell lymphoma (small-cell variant): (A) sheets of monomorphic small round cells with clear to eosinophilic cytoplasm (H&E × 400); (B) the tumor cells show strong nuclear and cytoplasmic expression of ALK protein (× 400).

Figure 14.5 (A) Desmoplastic small round-cell tumor demonstrated nests of undifferentiated small round blue cells in a densely fibrotic background (H&E × 400). (B) Characteristic cytoplasmic expression of desmin, with dot-like accentuation (× 400).

Mesenchymal chondrosarcoma and the small-cell variant of osteosarcoma are rare primary bone malignancies in children. Mesenchymal chondrosarcoma may be histologically indistinguishable from EFT, except for scattered nodules of well-differentiated hyaline cartilage within the tumor (6). Similarly, the small-cell variant of osteosarcoma may mimic EFT, but one should be able to identify at least focal osteoid production (6). Both of these tumors lack the t(11;22) translocation characteristic of EFT. Although a few recurrent genetic abnormalities have been found in mesenchymal chondrosarcoma, the frequency of these changes is unknown and many tumors show complex cytogenetics (10,11).

Intra-abdominal/pelvic mass

Abdominal and pelvic masses may be large, displacing normal structures and making a point of origin difficult to determine radiographically. In these cases, the differential diagnosis may be broad. Organ-based tumors (i.e., neuroblastoma, Wilms' tumor, germ-cell tumors) should be considered, and these entities are discussed later. Soft-tissue tumors involving the retroperitoneum, such as rhabdomyosarcoma, should be included in the differential diagnosis as well.

Desmoplastic small round-cell tumors (DSRCTs) are unique to this location, however, and show no evidence of arising from a particular organ. These tumors often present as multiple peritoneal nodules or masses at the time of diagnosis. Histologically, DSRCTs have a fibrotic to myxoid stroma, with nests of undifferentiated small round cells (Figure 14.5A). The immunophenotype of the undifferentiated cells is characteristic, with co-expression of cytokeratin, vimentin, and some neural markers. Desmin-expression is also present, typically in a dot pattern

(Figure 14.5B). These tumors also show nuclear expression of WT-1 protein, although some tumors may express variant transcripts of this protein, resulting in loss of the protein terminus antibody target and false-negative staining. This occurs because the characteristic translocation of DSRCT, *WT1-EWSR1*, creates a chimeric fusion protein between the N-terminal end of EWSR1 and the C-terminal end of WT-1. The N-terminus of WT-1 is often truncated in the resulting fusion product, and immunohistochemical antibodies targeting the N-terminus may be negative (12). Fusion studies should also be interpreted with caution, as an EWSR1 break-apart probe will be positive in both EFT and DSRCT. Correlation of cytogenetic results and immunophenotype with the clinical setting and histopathologic features are necessary for this diagnosis.

Adrenal/extra-adrenal paraganglia

Neuroblastoma is the most common solid tumor of childhood, and is further discussed in Chapter 6. It typically arises from the adrenal gland or from paraganglia in the paraspinal soft tissues (13). The diagnosis may be suspected based on location, and elevated serum tumor markers vanillylmandelic acid (VMA) and homovanillic acid (HVA) may be known at the time of surgery. At paravertebral sites, the tumor may extend into neural foramen, causing spinal-cord compression, in which case rapid diagnosis is essential to early treatment. Bone, skin, and liver are common sites of metastasis and these metastatic foci may occasionally be the presenting lesion,

as discussed in the above sections. The histologic features of neuroblastoma remain the same regardless of location. Neuroblastomas are characterized by small neuroblasts in a background of fibrillary neuropil. Homer–Wright rosettes may be present, and there are varying degrees of ganglion-cell differentiation (Figure 14.6). Undifferentiated neuroblastomas show none of the above features, and immunohistochemistry is required to distinguish this histologic subtype from EFT, rhabdomyosarcoma, or the blastemal component of Wilms' tumor. Neuroblastomas show expression of neural markers including synaptophysin, chromogranin, NB84, and PGP9.5. In contrast to EFT, however, neuroblastomas lack CD99 expression. Biologic studies are particularly important for risk categorization and determining treatment in neuroblastoma, and obtaining adequate tissue for these tests is critical. Fresh and frozen tissue should be collected for analysis of *MYCN* amplification, loss of heterozygosity, and DNA ploidy in all cases.

Kidney

Wilms' tumor (nephroblastoma) is the most common primary renal malignancy in children (see Chapter 8). The classic histologic appearance is of a triphasic neoplasm, including blastemal, epithelial, and stromal components (Figure 14.7). When all three components are present the diagnosis is relatively simple, but this may become more difficult when one component predominates. With regard to small round-cell tumors in children, the diagnosis may be particularly

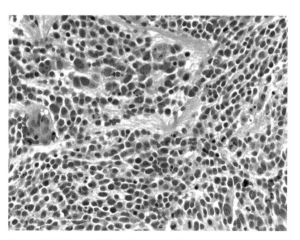

Figure 14.6 Poorly differentiated neuroblastoma demonstrating small neuroblasts in a background of fibrillary neuropil with rare ganglion cell differentiation (H&E × 400).

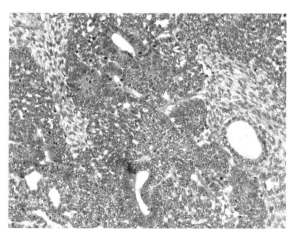

Figure 14.7 Wilms' tumor with primitive tubules surrounded by undifferentiated blastemal elements and spindled stroma (H&E × 400).

challenging when there is a predominantly blastemal pattern of Wilms' tumor. In this setting, one may consider the possibility of a primary renal PNET, or less likely, a neuroblastoma with invasion into the kidney. The imaging appearance is helpful in evaluating the latter possibility, and immunohistochemistry for WT-1 will show diffuse nuclear expression in Wilms' tumors. In contrast, primary renal PNET lack WT-1 expression and show membranous CD99 expression.

At times, the stromal component of a Wilms' tumor may predominate and show extensive rhabdomyoblastic differentiation. In these cases, Wilms' tumor should always be excluded before a diagnosis of a primary renal rhabdomyosarcoma is considered. Wilms' tumors may also rarely be extrarenal in origin. In these cases, the presence of epithelial elements amongst the stroma and blastema is the key histologic feature for making this diagnosis.

Genitourinary

Rhabdomyosarcoma is the classic small round-cell tumor of the genitourinary tract in children. When associated with mucosal surfaces of the bladder, vagina, or prostate, a botryoid pattern is typically observed. The classic histologic feature of this variant is the presence of a cambium layer, or densely aggregating tumor cells just beneath the mucosal surface. The overall cellularity may be sparse, and one should look closely to rule out the presence of malignant cells in inflamed mucosal biopsies in young patients.

In the scrotum, the spindle-cell (leiomyomatoid) variant is most common and typically presents as a paratesticular mass (see Chapter 9). As the name suggests, these tumors do not have the typical small round-cell appearance, and instead resemble smooth-muscle tumors with fascicles of spindled cells. Immunohistochemistry for desmin and myogenin confirms the diagnosis, as discussed above.

Liver

Hepatoblastoma is the most common primary hepatic malignancy in children. An elevated α-fetoprotein (AFP) level may suggest this diagnosis, although care should be taken to interpret these values with consideration of the normal ranges in young infants. Most hepatoblastomas show epithelial differentiation, and the fetal and embryonal patterns resemble well- or moderately differentiated fetal liver, respectively

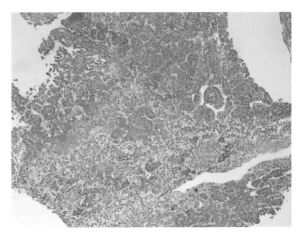

Figure 14.8 Hepatoblastoma, epithelial type with fetal and embryonal patterns. The fetal component shows an alternating light and dark pattern, with glycogenated cells with clear cytoplasm alternating with deeply eosinophilic cells arranged in cords and acini. Occasional nests of smaller, less differentiated cells with scant cytoplasm representing the embryonal pattern are interspersed throughout the biopsy (H&E × 200).

(Figure 14.8). Mesenchymal elements may also be encountered, particularly as islands of osteoid formation. Occasionally, teratoid features with melanin or neuroectodermal differentiation may also be seen. More information can be found in Chapter 3.

Hepatoblastomas may have focal or diffuse, poorly differentiated or small-cell areas. These areas appear as sheets of undifferentiated cells resembling neuroblasts. If this component alone is sampled, the diagnosis may be challenging, particularly as these undifferentiated tumors often have low AFP levels (14). Identification of focal fetal or embryonal patterns may be the only clue to diagnosis, and one should exclude metastatic small round-cell tumors in these cases. Hepatoblastomas may express AFP, but otherwise are not immunoreactive for other typical small round-cell tumor markers such as desmin, myogenin, CD99, WT-1, or synaptophysin. Additionally, a subset of small-cell hepatoblastomas appears to lack INI-1 expression (15). There is some controversy about whether loss of INI-1 indicates a diagnosis of a primary rhabdoid tumor or whether loss of INI-1 is also seen in the small-cell variant of hepatoblastoma. In general, tumors with focal fetal or embryonal patterns are thought to represent small-cell undifferentiated hepatoblastoma, and may show variable INI-1 expression. When the tumor is composed entirely of otherwise undifferentiated small cells that lack INI-1 expression, the diagnosis of malignant rhabdoid tumor should be rendered. In both cases, prognosis is poor, and patients require aggressive chemotherapy.

Although the name sounds similar to other small round-cell malignancies, embryonal (undifferentiated) sarcoma is a unique liver tumor in children. The cells in this tumor are spindled, and classically show PAS-positive, diastase-resistant hyaline globules. The morphologic features are the main clue to diagnosis, as again – immunohistochemistry is mainly useful to exclude other small round-cell tumors (16). Embryonal sarcomas may show vimentin expression with patchy, focal cytokeratin and α-1 antitrypsin expression. They are negative for myogenin, caldesmon, S100, hepatocyte antigen, AFP, and CD34. Importantly in this differential, embryonal rhabdomyosarcomas may present as primary hepatic masses arising from the biliary tree. Presence or absence of myogenin expression helps resolve this dilemma, however.

Chest

The location within the chest is important for approaching the differential diagnosis of tumors in this region. For tumors involving the mediastinum, lymphoma is the primary diagnostic consideration, and material should always be obtained fresh for flow cytometry and cytogenetics. As children generally get blastic, intermediate, or large cell-type lymphomas, preliminary immunohistochemical panels should include CD43 and TdT to evaluate for lymphoblastic lymphoma, as well as B- and T-cell markers, CD30, and anaplastic lymphoma kinase (ALK) to evaluate for Burkitt's, large B-cell lymphomas or anaplastic large-cell lymphoma (see Chapter 7).

Other types of tumors encountered in the mediastinum include germ-cell tumors, particularly in adolescent males. Seminomas/germinomas may resemble small round-cell tumors, and immunohistochemistry for placental alkaline phosphatase (PLAP), OCT 3/4, or c-kit (CD117) will help resolve this differential diagnosis. Uncommonly, children may get poorly differentiated carcinomas, often associated with *NUT* (nuclear protein in testis) gene rearrangements, which may be detected by immunohistochemistry using a monoclonal antibody to NUT or by confirmation of a *BRD-NUT* or *NUT*-variant fusion by FISH or RT-PCR (17).

The lateral chest wall raises a separate list of diagnostic considerations, including primary bone tumors. Ewing's sarcoma of the chest wall is referred to as

Askin's tumor, and shows typical features of EFT. Osteosarcomas may arise from the axial skeleton as well.

Finally, primary lung masses are rare in the pediatric population. Some tumors, such as Ewing's sarcoma and osteosarcoma, frequently metastasize to the lung, but these usually manifest as small, subcentimeter nodules. Pleuropulmonary blastoma (PPB) should be considered for large primary lung-based masses, particularly if there is a cystic component. These tumors may have markedly varied histology with well-differentiated cystic-type 1 PPB being clinically and radiographically indistinguishable from benign lung cysts (18). In contrast, type 3 PPB is a solid lesion containing blastemal and sarcomatous elements, often with nodules of primitive cartilage. Similar to Wilms' tumor, there is often prominent rhabdomyoblastic differentiation, and this finding in a primary lung lesion should raise the possibility of pleuropulmonary blastoma. Familial PPB is associated with loss of DICER1 expression in the epithelium of the lung (19). Some patients with PPB may have other cysts or tumor growths, including renal cysts, benign nasal tumors, rhabdomyosarcomas, thyroid nodules, ovarian Sertoli–Leydig cell tumors, dysgerminomas/seminomas, and some leukemias (20,21).

References

1. Newton WA, Gehan EA, Webber BL, *et al.* Classification of rhabdomyosarcomas: pathologic aspects and proposal for a new classification – an Intergroup Rhabdomyosarcoma Study. Cancer 1995;**76**:1073–85.

2. Missiaglia E, Williamson D, Chisholm J, *et al. PAX3/ FOXO1* fusion gene status is the key prognostic molecular marker in rhabdomyosarcoma and significantly improves current risk stratification. J. Clin. Oncol. 2012;**30**:1670–7.

3. Khoury JD. Ewing sarcoma family of tumors (review). Adv. Anat. Pathol. 2005;**12**:212–20.

4. Stocker JT, Dehner LP, editors. *Pediatric Pathology*, second edn. Philadephia, PA: Lippincott Williams and Wilkins;2002:1372–3.

5. Hameed M. Small round-cell tumors of bone. Arch. Pathol. Lab. Med. 2007;**131**:192–204.

6. Fletcher C, Bridge JA, Hogendoorn P, Mertens F, editors. *Pathology and Genetics: Tumors of Soft Tissue and Bone. World Health Organization Classification of Tumours.* Lyon, France: IARC, 4th Edition; 2013.

7. Foo, WC, Cruise MW, Wick MR, Hornick JL. Immunohistochemical staining for TLE1 distinguishes

479

synovial sarcoma from histologic mimics. Am. J. Clin. Pathol. 2011;**135**:839–44.

8. Italiano A, Sung YS, Zhang L, *et al.* High prevalence of CIC fusion with double-homeobox (DUX4) transcription factors in EWSR1-negative undifferentiated small round blue cell sarcomas. Genes Chromosomes Cancer 2012;**51**:207–18.

9. Pierron G, Thirode, F, Lucchesi C, *et al.* A new subtype of bone sarcoma defined by BCOR-CCNB3 gene fusion. Nature Genetics 2012;**44**:461–468.

10. Naumann S, Krallman PA, Unni K, *et al.* Translocation der(13;21)(q10;q10) in skeletal and extraskeletal mesenchymal chondrosarcoma. Mod. Pathol. 2002;**15**:572–6.

11. Wang L, Motoi T, Khanin R, *et al.* Identification of a novel, recurrent HEY1-NCOA2 fusion in mesenchymal chondrosarcoma based on genome-wide screen of exon-level expression data. Genes Chromosomes Cancer 2012;**51**:127–39.

12. Murphy AJ, Bishop K, Pereira, C *et al.* A new molecular variant of desmoplastic small round-cell tumor: significant of WT1 immunostaining in this entity. Hum. Pathol. 2008;**39**:1763–70.

13. Shimada H, Ambros IM, Dehner, LP *et al.* Terminology and morphologic criteria of neuroblastic tumors: recommendations by the International Neuroblastoma Pathology Committee. Cancer 1999;**86**:349–63.

14. De Ioris M, Brugieres L, Zimermann A, *et al.* Hepatoblastoma with a low serum α-fetoprotein level at diagnosis: the SIOPEL group experience. Eur. J. Cancer 2008;**44**:545–50.

15. Trobaugh-Lotrario AD, Tomlinson GE, Finegold MJ, *et al.* Small cell undifferentiated variant of hepatoblastoma: Adverse clinical and molecular features similar to rhabdoid tumors. Pediatr. Blood Cancer 2009;**52**:328–34.

16. Kiani B, Ferrell LD, Qualman S and Frankel WL. Immunohistochemical analysis of embryonal sarcoma of the liver. Appl. Immunohistochem. Mol. Morphol. 2006;**14**:193–7.

17. French CA. NUT midline carcinoma (review). Cancer Genet. Cytogenet. 2010;**203**:16–20.

18. Priest JR, Williams GM, Hill DA, *et al.* Pulmonary cysts in early childhood and the risk of malignancy. Pediatr. Pulmonol. 2009;**44**:14–30.

19. Hill DA, Ivanovich J, Priest JR, *et al.* Germline DICER1 mutations in familial pleuropulmonary blastoma. Science 2009;**325**:965–8.

20. Priest JR, Watterson J, Strong L, *et al.* Pleuropulmonary blastoma: A marker for familial disease. J. Pediatr. 1996;**128**:220–4.

21. Priest JR, Williams GM, Hill DA, *et al.* Pulmonary cyst in early childhood and the risk of malignancy. Pediatr. Pulmonol. 2009;**44**:14–30.

Chapter 15

Molecular genetics and diagnostic techniques

Luc Laurier Oligny

Introduction

Molecular biology is taking an ever-increasing role in diagnostic medicine. As such, many "old" diagnostic tests have been replaced by molecular tests. Hence, an understanding of molecular diagnostic techniques is now essential to the practice of pathology. Molecular diagnostic techniques are evolving at an astounding rate. This chapter lays foundations to allow understanding of old and new techniques, and of their applications.

This chapter aims to provide an illustrated overview of the many different techniques used in the molecular diagnostic field, and to highlight their clinical use. It covers basic molecular diagnostic techniques: Polymerase chain reaction (PCR), quantitative PCR (Q-PCR), and reverse transcriptase PCR (RT-PCR), *Southern blotting, Dot-blotting*, allele-specific oligonucleotides (*ASOs*), restriction-fragment length polymorphisms (*RFLPs*), *sequencing* and *Northern* and *Western blotting*. Cytogenetic techniques and their molecular offshoots are also reviewed: Fluorescent *in situ* hybridization with *break-apart and fusion probes, DNA and RNA microarrays*, including single nucleotide polymorphisms (*SNPs*) and comparative genomic hybridization (*CGH*). Techniques that allow *sequencing* of the *whole genome*, the *exome*, the *transcriptome*, and the *epigenome* conclude the technical portion of this chapter, along with their impact on *personalized gene-targeted therapy*.

This chapter is designed for practicing pathologists, and provides an introduction to the current tests used in molecular diagnosis. Most techniques are illustrated, to facilitate understanding. It is designed to allow the reader to gain a working knowledge of all these techniques and their applications, and to understand which technique is best suited to answer molecular diagnostic-related questions. An overview of molecular genetics in embryogenesis and paediatrics, and of chromosomal abnormalities is beyond the scope of this chapter (1,2). For more details regarding molecular diagnostic techniques, the reader is referred to either Wikipedia or textbooks (3–5).

The Human Genome Organization (HUGO) sequenced the entire human genome; the project was initiated in 1990, and was completed in 2003 (two years ahead of schedule):

– 3.5 billion nucleotides in the haploid genome (i.e., 7 billion base pairs per diploid nucleus)
– 20–25 000 genes (but alternative splicing allows the synthesis of much more than 25 000 proteins).

This sequencing effort has had an extremely significant impact on all spheres of medicine.

PCR (polymerase chain reaction) and variants

In 1993, Kary Mullis received a Nobel Prize for his elaboration of the PCR technique. Polymerase chain reaction is an ingenious method to reveal the presence or absence of short sequences of DNA. A pair of primers (very short segments of DNA) is used to flank the region of interest, and with a DNA polymerase, the region included between these primers is synthesized. The polymerase functions only in the 5' to 3' direction: each DNA strand is thus synthesized during a cycle, which doubles the number of strands during each cycle. Thus, the DNA of a single cell can be amplified a million-fold (10 cycles = 2^{10} ~ 1000 amplicons; 20 cycles = 2^{20} ~ one million amplicons).

The PCR technique is simple: DNA from as few as one cell is suspended in a solution containing the

Essentials of Surgical Pediatric Pathology, ed. Marta C. Cohen and Irene Scheimberg. Published by Cambridge University Press. © Cambridge University Press 2014.

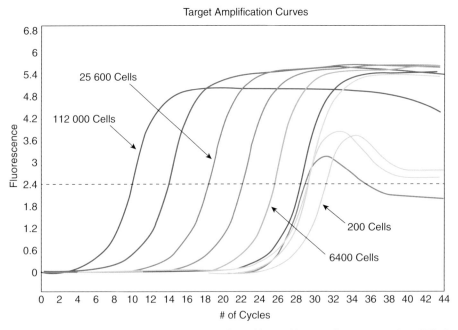

Figure 15.1 Quantitative PCR (Q-PCR): The test is calibrated by amplifying single-copy genes (e.g., *CFTR* of cystic fibrosis), to determine the number of cycles required to yield a given number of fluorescence units (2.4 in this case) with respect to the number of copies of the gene in the sample (two copies per cell)

primers in excess, nucleotides (A, T, G, and C), and DNA polymerase (Taq polymerase, which is stable at 100 °C). In one cycle, the solution is heated to 95 °C in order to denature the DNA (i.e., to render it in a single-stranded form – ssDNA), cooled to 60 °C to allow annealing of the primers, and then brought to 72 °C to enable the polymerase to synthesize the new strands of DNA. Multiple cycles are performed, with an exponential rise in the number of fragments produced.

Once the cycling is done, the solution is subject to electrophoresis, to determine if amplification occurred. As one generally knows the length of the amplified fragment, finding a band of the correct length confirms that the sequence of DNA sought is present in the sample. Hybridization after blotting onto a membrane can be performed to prove that the fragment found is indeed the sequence sought.

Quantitative PCR (Q-PCR or real-time PCR)

Amplification of DNA with the PCR technique can be performed using nucleotides labelled with a fluorochrome; the intensity of fluorescence emitted is proportional to the number of labelled nucleotides bound in DNA. This amount of fluorescence is quantified in real time throughout the PCR cycles. Quantitative PCR can be divided in three phases: the first phase, or lag phase, is an exponential amplification, but the fluorescent signal is too low to be detected, as it is below the background fluorescence; the second phase is also exponential, but the signal is strong enough to be detected; the third phase is a plateau, where amplification is no longer exponential (Figure 15.1).

The amount of DNA in a sample can be assessed through Q-PCR, using the properties of these three phases: the smaller the number of DNA copies to be amplified, the longer the lag phase. The number of copies present within the sample is determined by the number of amplification cycles required to yield 2.4 units of fluorescence. This can be used to assess the number of copies of MYCN in a neuroblastoma, or the Epstein–Barr virus load in patients at risk for a post-transplant lymphoproliferative disorder.

Reverse transcriptase PCR (RT-PCR)

Reverse transcriptase PCR allows one to determine if a gene of interest is transcribed: the cell extract is digested with DNAse to remove all traces of DNA; then, the remaining mRNA is converted into cDNA with a reverse transcriptase – note that the cDNA thus

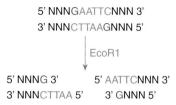

5' NNNGAATTCNNN 3'
3' NNNCTTAAGNNN 5'

|
EcoR1

5' NNNG 3'   5' AATTCNNN 3'
3' NNNCTTAA 5'   3' GNNN 5'

Figure 15.2 Restriction enzymes such as EcoR1 cut double-stranded DNA palindromes, to produce "sticky ends." N indicates non-specific nucleotides.

(A)

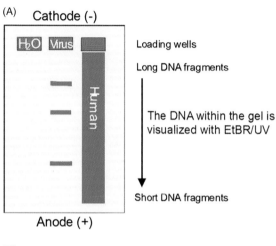

Cathode (-)

H₂O   Virus

Human

Loading wells

Long DNA fragments

The DNA within the gel is visualized with EtBR/UV

Short DNA fragments

Anode (+)

(B)

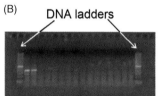

DNA ladders

Figure 15.4 (A) Southern blotting. An agarose gel is prepared containing wells. Purified and cut DNA is added to the wells and the restriction fragments are separated by electrophoresis: the anode attracts negatively charged DNA, causing these fragments to migrate in the direction of the arrow according to their length; longer fragments are less mobile and encounter more resistance from the agarose molecules than shorter fragments. Note that the viral genome (Figure 15.3) contains only three restriction sites, and thus shows only three bands on the gel. The human genome, being orders of magnitude longer, appears as a single band, but this band is composed of millions of bands overlying one another, from the longest (on top) to the shortest (at the bottom). This diagram shows only three wells; however, in routine usage, gels contain up to 36 wells to study multiple samples at once. The well into which no DNA has been added (water) is the negative control, and should show no band; should a band be seen, contamination must be considered. (B) Gel visualized under fluorescent light, after the DNA is stained with ethidium bromide. The length of the fragments can be evaluated by comparison with standardized fragments (DNA ladders).

produced is composed exclusively of exons devoid of introns. This cDNA can then be amplified by PCR or Q-PCR, in a routine fashion.

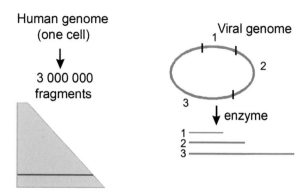

Human genome (one cell)

↓

3 000 000 fragments

Viral genome

↓ enzyme

1 ————
2 ————
3 ————

Figure 15.3 Digestion of human and viral DNA with a restriction enzyme to generate restriction fragments. The human genome generates thousands to millions of restriction fragments, from very short to very long; one such fragment is highlighted in red. The viral genome is much less complex, and generates only three restriction fragments. These segments can be separated by size, using electrophoresis.

Southern blotting

Dr Edwin Southern described this technique in 1975. Note that the Northern and Western blots have been so-named in humoristic honor of Dr Southern. No technique has yet been found to merit the appellation Eastern blotting.

Southern blots require "large" quantities of purified DNA, compared to PCR. The DNA from thousands to millions of cells is then digested by one (or more) restriction enzyme, in order to obtain thousands to millions of each restriction fragment. Furthermore, each of these fragments has a molecular weight and an electrical charge that differs from all the other fragments. These physical properties are exploited in the Southern technique.

Southern blotting involves cutting the purified DNA into restriction fragments (Figure 15.2 and 15.3). Each sample is placed in a well within an agarose gel (Figure 15.4A). The agarose concentration determines the speed of migration of the restriction fragments within the gel, when subjected to electrophoresis (Figure 15.4B and 15.5). The restriction fragments can thus be separated according to length. The DNA is then transferred onto a membrane (Figure 15.6), where it can be hybridized with specific probes.

Purification of DNA

Many molecular techniques require purified DNA. Cells are lysed, DNA is extracted and purified (many commercial kits are available, yielding "genomic DNA," containing the introns and exons of genes, in

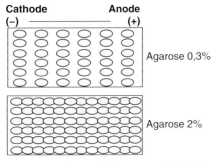

Figure 15.5 The speed of migration of the DNA within the agarose gel depends on the intensity of the electrophoresis current and the density of the agarose. A low concentration of agarose separates long fragments, whereas a denser agarose gel is better to separate short DNA fragments (dense agarose has a greater discrimination power for short fragments of similar lengths, but requires longer migration times).

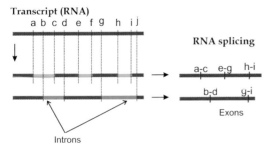

Figure 15.7 DNA is transcribed into RNA, which is spliced to remove the introns, generating the RNA segment composed of the coding exons. Some RNA segments can be spliced differently, and this alternative splicing can generate two or more different mRNAs, each generating one protein. Some genes can be spliced to generate more than 1000 different proteins.

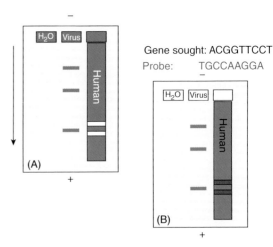

Figure 15.6 (A) DNA is transferred from the agarose gel onto a membrane. The left-hand well is a negative control (water) into which no DNA is added. The central well contains DNA from a digested virus, and the right-hand well contains the digested human DNA. Prior to hybridization, the alleles of the gene of interest cannot be visualized (albeit shown here in white). (B) After hybridizing the membrane with the probe, the membrane is washed and exposed to a radiographic film to reveal the presence and location of the alleles recognized by the probe (shown in red).

Restriction enzymes

These enzymes recognize and cut DNA sequences with great specificity, such that a difference of a single nucleotide prevents their action. This allows the identification of a point mutation, which suppresses or induces a restriction site.

For example, EcoR1 is a restriction enzyme that cuts DNA and generates sticky ends.

In Figure 15.2, the enzyme has cut the DNA segment between G and A. Note that the two extremities are single-stranded, with the 5′ segment (on either strand) being longer than the 3′; furthermore, each extremity

read in the 5′ to 3′ direction is identical to its homologous strand, as the sequence recognized by EcoR1 is a palindrome (i.e., a word which reads identically from left to right and from right to left, e.g., WOW).

Such cuts are said to generate "sticky ends," as two different DNA fragments cut by EcoR1 will hybridize, and can be joined.

Restriction enzymes can recognize and cut sequences ranging from 4 to 12 nucleotides (nt = bp, base pairs):

- recognition of a 4 bp sequence yields one cut every 256 bp $(4)^4$ on average
- recognition of a 6 bp sequence yields one cut every 4096 bp $(4)^6$ on average
- recognition of an 8 bp sequence yields one cut every 655356 bp $(4)^8$ on average.

Viral genomes range from 10^3 bp (1 Kb: kilobase) to 2×10^6 bp (2 Mb: megabases), whereas the human genome is composed of $3.5 \ 10^9$ bp – it is thus 10^3 to 10^6 times larger than viral genomes. Hence, depending on the restriction enzyme used to cut the human genome, we can generate between 3×10^3 and 3×10^6 restriction fragments, some very short, others very long (Figure 15.3).

If the sample contains 10^6 cells, then there will be 10^6 identical copies of each restriction fragment after

addition to non-coding DNA; genomic DNA must be distinguished from complementary DNA (cDNA), which is composed of coding DNA (i.e., DNA exons, whose introns have been spliced out; Figure 15.7).

digestion. These segments can then be separated, from longest to shortest, through electrophoresis on an agarose gel: digested DNA is placed in wells within the gel, and migrates towards the anode. Shorter segments migrate faster, which allows size-based separation. Fragments of similar sizes can be better discriminated by using higher-density gels.

Transfer of the DNA onto a membrane

Once the DNA fragments are separated by electrophoresis, the DNA is transferred (i.e., blotted) from the agarose gel onto a membrane (generally nylon or nitrocellulose) which has a great affinity for DNA. The DNA is thus fixed onto this membrane, which can be manipulated with much greater ease than the gel (Figure 15.6). After the transfer, the position which each band occupies on the membrane is identical to that which it occupied on the gel. Membranes can be hybridized with probes, to determine the presence or absence of DNA sequences of interest.

To reveal the presence or absence of a gene or of a segment of DNA, probes complementary to the sequence of interest are used: in DNA, adenine pairs with thymidine (**AT**), through two hydrogen bonds, and guanine pairs with cytosine (**GC**) through three hydrogen bonds; GC bonds are thus more difficult to dissociate than AT bonds. In RNA, thymidine is replaced by uracil. Probes are segments of DNA or RNA that are either radioactive, or linked with an enzyme or a fluorochrome, enabling their visualization; probes are then hybridized to the denatured DNA (i.e., the DNA that has been rendered single stranded – ssDNA).

Allele-specific oligonucleotides (ASOs)

A difference of a single nucleotide within a probe of 15–50 nt is sufficient to prevent its hybridization with the DNA under study; one can change the hybridization conditions to favor stringency (conditions allowing hybridization only if the probe is perfectly complementary with the DNA segment), or to allow a more permissive hybridization.

Stringency vs. permissivity

The more a solution of DNA is heated, the more the strands have a tendency to dissociate (i.e., to denature). On the other hand, the greater the homology between the two strands of DNA, the greater their affinity for one another and the tendency to remain together. This property is exploited in the ASO technique (allele-specific oligonucleotide): first, one must determine the temperature which separates ASO probes that are perfectly matched with the genomic sequence under study. Once this "melting" temperature is known, the ASO probe can be used clinically: after hybridization, the probe–genomic-DNA mixture is heated to temperatures just below the melting point – a perfect match will not dissociate, enabling the probe to yield a signal; dissociation of the probe from the genomic DNA will not yield a signal, which indicates that the genomic sequence differs from the probe by at least one nucleotide.

A reaction is said to be stringent when the hybridization conditions (temperature and ionic concentration of the solution) prevent a non-perfect match, whereas the reaction is permissive when the probe can hybridize with the genomic DNA even when the match is not perfect. Depending on what is sought, hybridization conditions will be stringent (e.g., in ASO probes) or permissive.

Dot blot

Dot blotting is a variation of the Southern blot that does not require digesting the DNA or electrophoresis: a drop of the DNA solution is placed onto a membrane and directly hybridized with a probe. This technique is much faster than Southern, as the sample is not digested (which requires 6 to 24 hours, depending on the enzyme used), there is no electrophoresis (2 to 12 hours), and there is no transfer from gel to membrane (up to 12 hours). However, as in Southern blotting, the membrane must be hybridized, washed, and placed to expose the signal onto a film (12 hours to several days) before the signal is revealed. Up to 10 000 samples can be blotted onto the membrane – dot blotting is thus ideal for evaluating the presence or absence of a gene in large numbers of samples, or when the length of the fragment is not important (Figure 15.8).

Dot blotting was once used to detect blood samples contaminated by HIV, hepatitis B, CMV, and other viruses. The membrane is simultaneously hybridized with various probes jointly recognizing all of these viruses – a positive signal renders the blood unusable, regardless of the infectious agent. Hence, identification of the infectious agent is irrelevant for this purpose.

ASO–dot blot

Dot-blotted membranes can be hybridized using the ASO technique – one probe recognizes the normal allele, the other recognizes the mutated allele. The

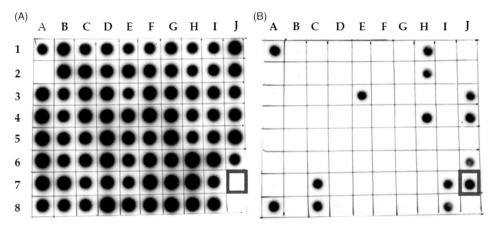

Figure 15.8 Dot blot, using the ASO technique. Dot blot allows testing multiple samples at once – it is limited only by the size of the membrane. Membrane (A) is hybridized with a probe recognizing the normal Factor-V allele, and membrane (B) with a probe recognizing the allele with a Factor-V-Leiden mutation. A1 is a heterozygous control, B1 is a homozygous normal control. A2 and J8 are controls devoid of DNA, and J7 is a patient with a homozygous mutation. Heterozygous carriers are frequent. (Courtesy of Françoise Couture and Dr Georges-Étienne Rivard, CHU Sainte-Justine.)

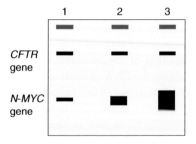

Figure 15.9 Semi-quantitative Southern: *N-MYC* is amplified in the tumors of patients 2 and 3 (well 1 is a normal control). The intensity of the signal vs. that of the CFTR gene (normally present in two copies per cell) allows the estimation of the number of copies of *N-MYC* per tumor cell.

membrane is then hybridized sequentially with the probes recognizing the normal *and* the mutant alleles. A carrier will give a positive signal with both probes (Figure 15.8).

Summary

Southern blotting requires the extraction of DNA, its purification, digestion, electrophoresis in an agarose gel, its transfer onto a membrane, which is then hybridized with a probe, and revelation of the radioactive probe using a radiographic film. This technique is widely used in molecular diagnostic laboratories. It allows:

1. Detection of a mutated allele whose molecular weight differs from that of the normal allele (see RFLPs, below).

2. Evaluation of the quantity of DNA within a sample, such as the amplification of *N-MYC* in neuroblastomas. The membrane is hybridized with two probes, one recognizing *N-MYC*, the other recognizing a single-copy gene (e.g., *CFTR*, the gene involved in cystic fibrosis). The intensity of the *N-MYC* signal is then compared with that of the control gene (Figure 15.9).

3. Detection of mutated alleles when this mutation induces or suppresses a restriction site (Figure 15.10).

The drawbacks of Southern blotting are:

1. Expensive, requiring numerous manipulations and considerable technician time.

2. Procedure is long, preventing Southern blotting from yielding a diagnosis in less than a few days, regardless of the clinical urgency.

3. Southern blotting cannot be achieved on microsamples, as relatively large quantities of DNA are required to bind the labelled probe in order to generate a detectable signal.

RFLP (Restriction fragment length polymorphism)

Everyone possesses two different chromosomes for each pair of autosomes: their exact molecular DNA sequence always differs. With the exception of identical twins, there are no two individuals on earth who

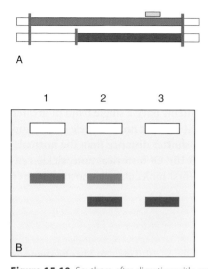

Figure 15.10 Southern after digestion with enzymes recognizing a point mutation, in the diagnosis of sickle-cell anaemia (SCA). (A) Genomic DNA (light blue) is cut by the restriction enzyme (green lines). In this heterozygous patient, the enzyme recognizes the point mutation in the abnormal allele (bottom), creating a shorter restriction fragment (red). Both the normal and abnormal segments are recognized by the probe (orange bar). (B) The digested DNA is assayed by Southern blot. Patient 1 has only one normal-sized signal, ruling out the presence of the SCA mutation. Patient 2 has an additional signal (red), and this second fragment is shorter than the normal fragment, indicating a heterozygous state (sickle cell trait). Patient 3 has only the abnormal allele, and is thus homozygous for the SCA mutation.

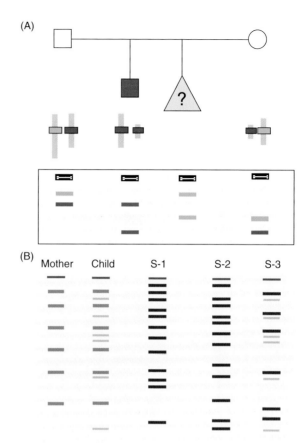

Figure 15.11 (A) Southern blotting, prenatal screening. Pedigree of a couple with one child suffering from an autosomal recessive disease. The DNA of the parents, affected child and fetus is cut using a restriction enzyme chosen to generate restriction fragments of different lengths. This allows the identification of four different parental alleles (polymorphisms). As the affected child must possess both mutated alleles, the normal alleles can easily be identified. In this pedigree, using a chorionic villous biopsy sample, the fetus can be diagnosed to be homozygous normal, with certainty. (B) Restriction fragment length polymorphisms: multiple probes are used to identify multiple polymorphic alleles. RFLPs can be used for medicolegal purposes, as they allow discrimination between individuals with near certainty when a sufficient number of probes recognizing highly polymorphic alleles are used. This allows the determination of a father in paternity testing: all the bands shared between mother and child are of maternal origin; the father must have each and every one of the child's other bands. Note that in these diagrams, the bands are shown in color for didactic purposes, but they are black on real films.

have molecularly identical chromosomes. These variations (i.e., polymorphisms) are generally devoid of any pathological effect, and are said to be silent polymorphisms as they do not impact gene transcription or function.

In the context of RFLPs, the term "allele" is used to designate the DNA fragments on which the genes of interest are localized. These restriction fragments may be of variable lengths, even if the segment of DNA containing the gene of interest (i.e., the portion included between the TATA box and the Stop codon) is of identical length on both chromosomes.

The RFLP technique is used to distinguish both alleles of a gene of interest; hence, in Figure 15.11A, the ability to distinguish all four parental alleles allows the determination of the carrier status of the fetal alleles. If a greater number of probes is used, this technique also allows the incrimination or the exoneration of a suspect by comparing his/her DNA with DNA found at the crime scene. Using 15 to 60 probes, one can discriminate between two individuals with a risk of error of less than one in a million (Figure 15.11B).

There are two reasons for differences in the lengths of the restriction fragments:

1. The segment included between the restriction sites may contain repeated sequences (e.g., CA dinucleotides, ALU or LINE sequences, and microsatellites), all of which may be extremely variably repeated from one allele to the next (Figure 15.12 and 15.13). Hence, by choosing a restriction enzyme which includes a repeated sequence within the allele (i.e., restriction fragment), one can generate polymorphisms in the

487

lengths of these fragments, as evidenced with a Southern blot (Figure 15.12).

2. Single nucleotide variability may generate restriction sites, thus truncating or expanding the restriction fragment. These variations may be found within coding or non-coding DNA, and may be silent (polymorphisms) or pathogenic (point mutations). For example, sickle-cell anemia

results from a point mutation that converts the codon GAG to GTG in a coding segment of the hemoglobin gene, which leads to an abnormal function of this molecule; this substitution of an adenine by a thymine abolishes the restriction site recognized by the restriction enzyme MSTII, and homozygous patients have a single band of greater molecular weight than the normal allele – this band thus migrates a shorter distance than the normal allele (Figure 15.10). Of historical note, sickle-cell anemia was the first molecular diagnostic test ever to be reported.

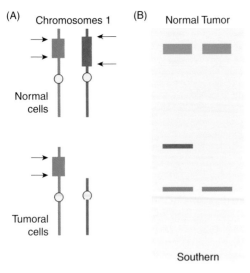

Figure 15.12 Loss of heterozygosity (LOH). The pair of chromosomes 1 has one copy of paternal origin (blue), and one of maternal (red). (A) In normal cells, these two chromosomes yield different restriction fragments (cleavage sites shown by arrows), defined as heterozygosity. All the restriction fragments originating from the same allele are identical. (B). In a Southern blot, a probe identifying these two fragments would generate two signals, a "light" and "heavy" band, respectively of paternal and maternal origin. In tumoral cells, chromosomal segments are often lost (often containing anti-oncogenes) therefore the probe can only hybridize to the non-deleted segment of the paternal chromosome, the deleted maternal segment being lost.

RFLP and PCR

Fragment-length polymorphisms can also be demonstrated through PCR: the segment is amplified with primers flanking the polymorphic sequence; the amplification product is then migrated on an electrophoresis gel to separate the alleles according to their length. There is no need to cut the amplification product. The fragments studied by PCR must be much shorter than those that can be studied by Southern, but the PCR-based technique is much faster than Southern, much cheaper, and can be used on minute amounts of DNA, which makes it useful for medicolegal applications.

Northern blot

This technique is similar to Southern blotting, but studies mRNA rather than DNA. mRNA is extracted from the cells, but does not require cutting by restricting enzymes as all mRNAs from the same allele have identical molecular weight (when they are spliced similarly). The mRNA fragments are separated by

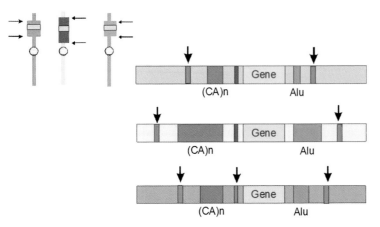

Figure 15.13 Polymorphisms in the lengths of restriction fragments (RFLPs, generated by recognition of specific sequences recognized by the restriction enzymes (arrows)) result from variations in the numbers of repeats in the (CA) dinucleotides, in the Alu sequences, in the SINE and LINE segments (not shown), and in polymorphisms in sequences recognized by the restriction enzymes. These polymorphisms often involve non-coding DNA, rather than the sequence of the gene itself.

electrophoresis, and transferred onto a membrane to be hybridized with labelled probes. Contrary to Southern, Northern does not assess the presence of the gene in the tissue, but rather whether the gene is transcribed or not. Northern blotting thus studies which genes are transcribed (i.e., active) in a tissue, at any given time. This has been particularly useful to determine gene expression, e.g., the chronological expression of *HOX* genes in the development of the upper limb, gene expression profiling, etc.

Southern blot, PCR, Northern blot, and RT-PCR: Summary

In summary, there are two general types of diagnostic modalities: those that assess DNA, and those that assess RNA. The distinction is fundamental, as DNA-based tests yield no information on transcription, i.e., whether a gene is active or not in the tissue studied. It is crucial to remember that *Southern blotting and PCR are DNA based*, and as such, they both assess the presence of a gene in a sample.

On the other hand, *Northern blots and RT-PCR assess the presence of RNA, which tells us if a gene is active (transcribed)* or not, and quantitative methods allow us to determine the degree to which it is active.

Blots vs. PCR: Southern and Northern are time-consuming techniques (days vs. hours), they require larger amounts of DNA (milligrams of tissue vs. a single cell), but PCR requires knowledge of the sequence sought to generate primers, and can only analyze relatively small segments (few thousands of base pairs, vs. megabases).

Hence, *PCR and RT-PCR are preferred over the blotting techniques when they can solve the clinical question.*

Western blot

Western blotting studies cellular protein expression through gel electrophoresis. Different proteins have different molecular weights and electrical charges, and thus migrate at different speeds. The proteins in the gel are then transferred onto a membrane which is subsequently exposed to labelled antibodies to identify the protein of interest. Western blotting identifies polymorphisms and mutations affecting the size, tertiary structure, and charge of the proteins of interest, as well as post-translational errors which prevent synthesis of the protein or which alter their half-life. It is more sensitive than immunohistochemical studies, as the protein of interest from all the cells within the sample is concentrated in a single band, but the ability to localize this protein within the tissue is lost.

Oligonucleotide synthesis

When oligonucleotides are required, for example to serve as probes or primers, one only needs to write out the desired sequence and send it by internet to the provider of choice, and the oligonucleotide is delivered within days. No further detail shall be provided.

Fluorescent *in situ* hybridization (FISH)

Fluorescent *in situ* hybridization is a technique used to identify the presence of segments of chromosomes spread onto a slide using probes. The chromosomes can be either in metaphase or in interphase, depending on the technique used and on the specificity of the probe. It can also be used quantitatively, to determine the number of genes in a cell (e.g., to assess N-MYC amplification in neuroblastoma; Figure 15.14). Several types of probes can be used, including fusion and break-apart probes, whole chromosome painting, spectral karyotyping (SKY), and chromosome-based comparative genomic hybridization (CGH).

Break-apart probes consist of a series of two probes, each labelled in a different color (generally red and green fluorochromes), which hybridize to one segment immediately above the breakpoint of an oncogenic translocation, and the other hybridizing immediately below that locus (Figure 15.15A1–A2). Normal cells will yield two yellow signals from the merged red and yellow spots. A translocation involving the gene of interest will separate these signals: such cells show a yellow signal, corresponding to the normal chromosome, and both a red and a green signal corresponding to the translocation breakpoints (Figure 15.15B1–B2).

Fusion probes detect balanced translocations when the two translocation partners are anticipated (Figure 15.15C). One probe labelled in red hybridizes to one of the genes (*EWSR1* in this case), the other probe is labelled in green and hybridizes to the other gene (*FLI1*). Normal cells (Figure 15.15C1) show four signals, two red and two green. Cells with a t(11;22)(q24.3;q12.2) show one normal green and red signal, and the combined yellow signal of the EWSR1-FLI1 translocation (Figure 15.5C2).

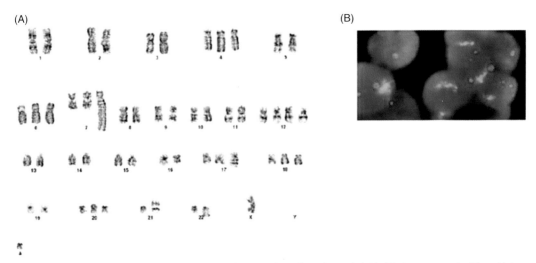

(A)

(B)

Figure 15.14 (A) Karyotype from a neuroblastoma. This metaphase shows hyperdiploidy (54 chromosomes) with multiple rearrangements. One chromosome 7 is noteworthy, with a large homogeneously staining region (HSR). (B) FISH confirmed that this HSR corresponds to *MYCN* amplification (*MYCN* shows an intense signal, green probe, intimately associated with chromosome 7, identified with an orange centromeric probe). (Courtesy of Diane Lachance, Lysanne Le Brock and Dr Amanda Fortier, CHU Sainte-Justine.)

There are three major types of oncogenic translocations: (1) those that disrupt a tumor-suppressor gene, or cause its deletion; (2) those that join a physiologically active promoter to a normally inactive oncogene (Figure 15.16A); and (3) those that form a chimeric protein (Figure 15.16B1–B2). These translocations can be documented by either FISH or Southern. However, the large quantity of non-coding DNA between potential primer sites prevents the identification of the latter two types of translocations by PCR, but chimeric RNA can be diagnosed by RT-PCR.

Whole chromosome painting (WCP) uses multiple same-color probes that all hybridize to different portions of one pair of chromosomes, to cover its whole length. Chromosomes spread in metaphases will thus be visualized, and translocations involving small segments of these chromosomes will be readily identified (2).

Spectral karyotyping (SKY) is a variation of whole chromosome painting, where every chromosome is painted with a different-colored probe (24 colors, 22 for the autosomes, plus one for the X and one for the Y). It allows characterization of complex translocations that cannot be resolved by conventional cytogenetic techniques (2). Spectral karyotyping can only be used on metaphases; this can be problematic as malignant cells do not always grow in culture. It is a very powerful technology, but is extremely expensive and is now generally replaced by newer techniques.

Single nucleotide polymorphisms (SNP) micro-arrays

The sequencing of the human genome has revealed polymorphisms that are frequent and span all regions of each chromosome. Single nucleotide polymorphisms study the differences involving only one nucleotide in a specific sequence, with probes specifically recognizing these variations. This technique is similar to ASOs, but allows the study of the whole genome through microarrays, rather than studying a single gene on a membrane. Microarrays can contain probes spanning upwards of 1 million loci (i.e., 2 million probes). The signals are analyzed by computer.

A normal person possesses 46 different chromosomes, with such polymorphisms uniformly distributed throughout the genome. If a sufficient number of loci are studied with two probes for each of these loci, each chromosomal region (i.e., a segment containing several thousands of loci) should reveal polymorphisms (i.e., heterozygous alleles); each locus can thus express the polymorphism A or B, and thus, the genotype of each locus can be AA, AB, or BB (Figure 15.17A–C).

Cells trisomic for a chromosome (e.g., trisomy 8 in tumoral cells) will have three chromosomes 8 rather than two. As such, each locus studied can be either AAA, AAB, ABB, or BBB (Figure 15.17D), rather than AA, AB, and BB in normal disomic cells.

Chapter 15: Molecular genetics and diagnostic techniques

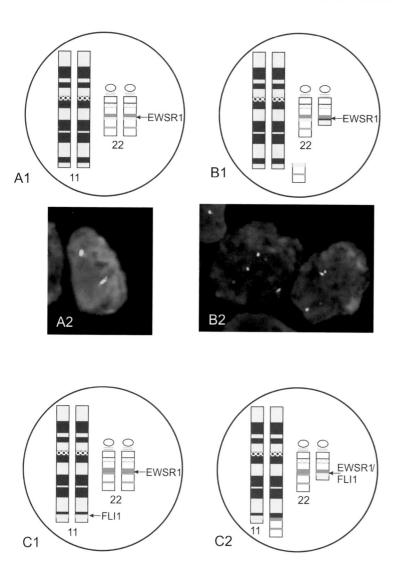

Figure 15.15 (A) Break apart probes. A red probe hybridizes above the *EWSR1* gene (and includes *EWSR1*), and a green probe hybridizes below the *EWSR1* gene on 22q12.2. In normal cells (A1 in metaphase, A2 in interphase), two yellow signals (or contiguous red-green signals) are seen (red + green photons = yellow). (B) Translocations involving the *EWSR1* gene (B1-B2) separate the two signals, the red remaining on chromosome 22 and the green being translocated on the derivative chromosome 11; this yields one red and one green signal, in addition to the normal signal. Break-apart probes are useful to study oncogenic genes that have multiple translocation partners, as in this case of Ewing's sarcoma, where the two most common translocations involve EWSR1, either with *FLI1* on 11q24.3 or *ERG* on 22q22.2. (C) Fusion probes. A red probe hybridizes to the *EWSR1* gene, and a green probe to *FLI1*. In normal cells, four independent signals are seen: two green and two red. When a translocation involves the EWSR1 and FLI1 genes, their red and green signals unite, yielding three signals: the normal red and green signals, and the translocated red-green signal. Fusion probes allow the translocation partners to be ascertained, e.g., in a desmoplastic small round blue-cell tumor, a break-apart EWSR1 probe would show the rearrangement, but would not allow a molecular distinction between a t(11q24.3;22q12.2) of Ewing sarcoma and a t(11p13; 22q12.2) of DSRCT, which involves *WT1* rather than *FLI1*. (A2 and B2 courtesy of Diane Lachance, Lysanne Le Brock and Dr Amanda Fortier, CHU Sainte-Justine.)

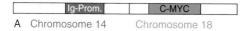

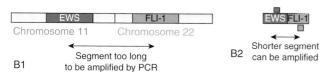

Figure 15.16 Translocations can be of two types: (A) The promoter of a normally active gene becomes adjacent to a normally silenced proto-oncogene, resulting in its abnormal activation, e.g., the t(8;14) of Burkitt's lymphoma places *C-MYC* under the control of the highly active immunoglobulin promoter, producing excessive quantities of the normal C-MYC protein. Note that the distance separating the promoter from the gene which it activates can be substantial, preventing their identification with PCR using probes hybridizing to the promoter and *C-MYC*. These translocations can be diagnosed by FISH and by Southern blotting. (B1) Translocations can fuse two genes, causing a segment of one protein to become continuous with the segment of another protein, as in the t(11;22) merging *EWS* and *FLI-1* to create the chimeric protein of Ewing's sarcoma. On the translocated chromosome, *EWS* and *FLI-1* are too distant to allow detection by PCR. (B2) Once the introns are removed, the resulting mRNA can be easily and specifically identified through RT-PCR using primers specific for EWS and FLI-1 (red and green squares).

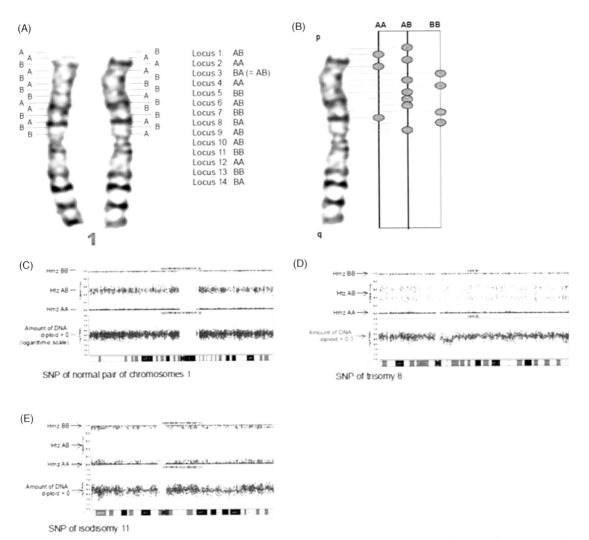

(A)

Locus 1:	AB
Locus 2:	AA
Locus 3:	BA (= AB)
Locus 4:	AA
Locus 5:	BB
Locus 6:	AB
Locus 7:	BB
Locus 8:	BA
Locus 9:	AB
Locus 10:	AB
Locus 11:	BB
Locus 12:	AA
Locus 13:	BB
Locus 14:	BA

(B)

(C) SNP of normal pair of chromosomes 1

(D) SNP of trisomy 8

(E) SNP of isodisomy 11

Figure 15.17 (A) SNPs spanning the short arm of chromosome 1. Note that only 14 loci (28 probes) are shown; a microarray would comprise hundreds of thousands of loci in a chromosomal segment of this length. On average, for each locus, ¼ are homozygous AA, ¼ are BB and ½ are heterozygous AB. (B) Same information, in diagrammatic view. (C) Printout of a SNP array of a normal pair of chromosomes 1. Each dot corresponds to a probe hybridized with its homologous chromosomal segment. On average, for each locus, ¼ are AA, ¼ are BB and ½ are AB. The amount of DNA from chromosome 1, per cell, is shown as a logarithmic scale (red line); 0 = diploidy. (D) SNP array of a tumor with trisomy 8. The result would be similar in cases of fetal trisomy 13, 18, or 21. This methodology also allows easy diagnosis of monosomy X in Turner syndrome (the amount of chromosome X DNA per cell would be less than normal, every chromosome X locus would be homozygous, and there would be no signal for chromosome Y). (E) SNP array of a tumor with an isodisomy of chromosome 11. As cells are diploid, the amount of chromosome 11 DNA is normal; since both copies of chromosome 11 are identical, there are no heterozygous loci. (SNP assay printouts from Illumina chips, courtesy of Drs Anne-Laure Rougemont, Dorothée Dal Soglio and Jean-Christophe Fournet, CHU Sainte-Justine.)

Single nucleotide polymorphisms also allow the detection of a loss of heterozygosity (LOH) in tumors: the chromosome or a chromosomal segment shows exclusively AA and BB alleles, with the AB alleles being absent; in these cases, the quantity of DNA is reduced to the haploid state. When the quantity of DNA is normal in such segments, a diagnosis of isodisomy is made (i.e., the quantity of DNA is diploid, but both chromosomal segments are identical; Figure 15.17E).

DNA microarrays (DNA chips)

The human genome has been sequenced, and it has been cloned in millions of small segments in its entirety. Each one of these clones has been characterized with respect to its location on chromosomal bands, and to its location compared to other adjacent clones. Furthermore, each of these clones is characterized with respect to the genes from which it arises, and its location within this gene – these segments are sufficiently small that tens to hundreds span the length of each gene, including their introns.

Thousands to millions of these DNA segments are individually spotted onto chips. These chips are then hybridized to the DNA to be tested. The signals are analyzed by software programs.

Comparative genomic hybridization microarrays

The patient's DNA is labelled in green, and this DNA is mixed with the same quantity of a same-sex control DNA which has been labelled in red. This mixture is hybridized onto the microarray; if the control and the test DNA are present in equimolar quantities, as much red DNA will hybridize onto the probe as green DNA, resulting in a yellow signal (red + green photons = yellow light). If the test DNA is in excess, the signal will be green (e.g., trisomy 21, N-MYC amplification, etc.). If the test DNA is present in lesser quantities, the signal will be red (e.g., deletion of P53, del 5p syndrome, etc.) (Figure 15.18).

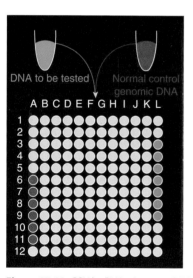

Figure 15.18 CGH by DNA-microarray. DNA to be tested (patient's genomic or tumoral DNA) and from a sex-matched control are mixed in equimolar quantities and hybridized to a DNA chip spotted with up to several million probes, spanning the whole genome (144 probes shown). Diploid genes from the test sample bind equally to the probes as the control DNA, yielding yellow signals. Genes that are over-represented (e.g., MYCN when amplified in neuroblastoma, or all the probes corresponding to chromosome 21 in a patient with Down syndrome) will yield a predominantly green signal, the intensity of which is proportional to its copy number. Genes that are deleted (e.g., P53, genes in the 11p15.5mat region, etc.) will yield a red signal, and the intensity of this red signal will be stronger when both alleles are lost.

Comparative genomic hybridization chips may contain more than 2 million probes that span all chromosomes (2 million probes spanning ~ 25 000 genes yields an extremely high sensitivity).

RNA microarrays (gene-expression microarrays)

Gene-expression microarrays can determine the degree of expression of genes of interest; DNA is digested with DNAses, and the residual RNA (i.e., the RNA from every gene expressed by all the cells within the sample) is converted into cDNA using reverse transcriptase; after labelling this cDNA in green, it is hybridized onto a microarray. The intensity of the signal correlates with the degree of expression of the genes of interest (i.e., of the genes recognized by the probes spotted onto the microarray).

CGH–SNP microarrays

Newer generation chips combine standard CGH and SNP probes. These combined chips are extremely powerful. They allow high-resolution detection of numerical anomalies (whole chromosome or segmental trisomies and monosomies, polyploidy), LOH and isodisomies, thus yielding useful information on imprinted genes. Furthermore, the newer generation chips are designed to evaluate clinically relevant regions (syndromes, cancer genes, telomeres), as the probes are selected to target these hot spots.

Chips have replaced karyotyping as the gold standard for the evaluation of malformations and developmental disabilities (7). It is anticipated that chips will also change our diagnostic approach in the study of oncological specimens, as they are much more sensitive than karyotypes (450 band vs. 2.7 million band resolution), they do not require live cells (as few as 100 ng of purified DNA suffices), and provide results in 48 hours. Furthermore, considering that karyotypes cost US \$300–500 and that FISH studies cost US \$250–400, the chip technology is cost-efficient. Chips are presently being developed to identify oncogenic translocations. However, it must be pointed out that at this time, chip technology does not detect balanced translocations, which is a major caveat for constitutional genetics.

DNA chips are also developed to assess the status of *all* the genes known to play a role in a certain disease. Such *clinical chips* will undoubtedly play a very major role in genetic counselling, once a proband has been identified. For example, 11 different genes can lead to hypertrophic cardiomyopathy. In families at risk, disease-specific chips can be used to assess the status of each and every one of these genes, including the search for all known mutations for each of these genes. These chips use an ASO methodology, with thousands of ASO probes spotted onto the chip. Family screening can thus be performed with great sensitivity, at great speeds (approximately two days), and at a much cheaper cost than using conventional methodologies (e.g., Southern blotting, sequencing, etc., which must be performed for each one of these genes).

Such chips are now either on the market or being developed for a variety of diseases: mitochondriopathies, dilated cardiomyopathies, Noonan's disease, pediatric hearing loss, neonatal jaundice-inducing liver diseases, retinitis pigmentosa, polycystic kidney disease, congenital glycosylation disorders, Duchenne muscular dystrophy, SCIDs, amyotrophic lateral sclerosis, cystic fibrosis, familial cancer genes, diabetic uremia, X-linked mental retardation, neurofibromatosis, pharmacogenomic testing, and others. This technology will certainly revolutionize clinical genetics, oncology, pharmacology, and pathology.

Summary

DNA-based tests include Southern, PCR, FISH, CGH, and SNP. These tests yield information on the number of copies of a gene present in a cell, and whether their alleles are normal or not. On the other hand, the tests assessing gene expression are Northern, RT-PCR, RNA-based microarrays, and Western blotting.

Sequencing

Sequencing consists in determining the nucleotide sequence of a segment of DNA. Real-time PCR allows effortless sequencing (Figure 15.19) of short segments of DNA. Over the last five years, the sequencing technology has evolved extremely rapidly. Many companies using different technologies have sprouted, allowing sequencing of the whole genome at ever-increasing speeds and decreasing costs. It will soon be cheaper to study patients through whole genome sequencing than to sequence a few genes

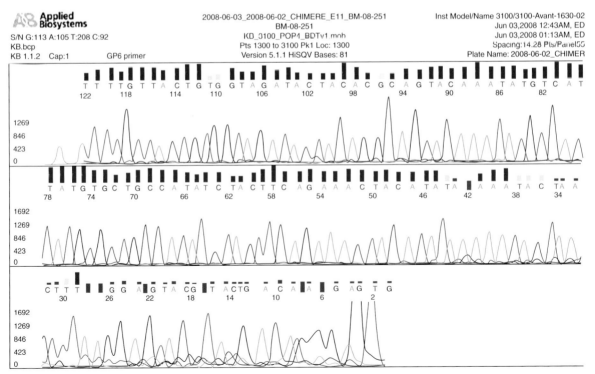

Figure 15.19 HPV genome present in all HPVs, such as the GP6 sequence, is amplified using primers. Sequencing is automated, and allows specific typing (HPV 16 in this case). Sequencing is also used to identify point mutations.

raised by the differential diagnosis. The caveat is that the amount of information obtained from a single patient is enormous – ~1 Tb; considering the extent of neutral polymorphisms in our genome (i.e., differences in genetic sequences that have no clinical impact), obtaining useful practical information from this data requires massive bioinformatics resources (7). The ethical problems raised by this technology are beyond the scope of this review (8).

The American College of Medical Genetics and Genomics has put out guidelines (March 2013) regarding the reporting of genome sequencing. They advocate mandatory reporting of mutations affecting any one of 57 genes (e.g., cancer genes such as *BRCA1*, *TP53*, *MLH1*, *APC*, *RET*, and *RB*, as well as for non-cancer mutations such as those causing Marfan syndrome, hypertrophic cardiomyopathy, arrhythmogenic right ventricular cardiomyopathy, etc.) (9).

Sequencing of tumors will certainly prove to be a major challenge: clonal evolution generates tremendous genetic heterogeneity within tumors, and more so within their metastases. Furthermore, this "evolution" is an ongoing process that progresses with every round of mitoses. The sequencing of a single tumoral region will yield only partial information regarding a whole tumor's biology, and for most tumor types much further research and studies will be needed before sequencing data translates directly to personalized therapy.

Whole genome sequencing (WGS)

It is expected that these improvements, referred to as *next-generation sequencing (NGS)*, will allow WGS to become routine in the clinical setting in the very near future. This will impact all of medicine: genes involved in familial cancers, in neurodegenerative diseases, and in cardiovascular health will all be assessed in a single test, along with all other genes of medical and social impact. We are facing a medical revolution.

As its name implies, WGS sequences the whole genome: all 24 chromosomes (i.e., the 22 autosomes, and the X and Y chromosomes), introns, exons, and "junk DNA," which is now realized to play a much more important function than previously estimated (10,11). Whole genome sequencing will thus be used to assess patients' constitutional DNA as well as their tumors' mutated genomes. Furthermore, WGS can identify balanced and unbalanced translocations.

Whole genome sequencing will also play a major role in assessing fetuses. Pilot studies are underway to perform prenatal diagnosis using WGS on circulating fetal DNA to avoid the complications of amniocentesis and chorionic villous sampling (Dr Guy Rouleau, personal communication).

Whole exome sequencing (WExS)

The *exome* is the part of the genome formed by exons, that is, the coding portion of mRNA. It consists of all DNA that is transcribed into mature RNA in cells of any type. The exome of the human genome consists of roughly 180 000 exons corresponding to about 1% of the total genome, or about 30 megabases of DNA. Though comprising a very small fraction of the genome, mutations in the exome are thought to harbor 85% of disease-causing mutations. By sheer virtue of this size difference, WExS is easier to analyze than WGS. Whole exome sequencing has proved to be an efficient strategy to determine the genetic basis of several mendelian or single gene disorders (12) and to investigate children and families with cancer predisposition syndromes (13). One can focus the information obtained with WGS and WExS by using software panels that highlight the regions/genes of interest with respect to the differential diagnosis. This methodology has proven particularly useful in syndromes with a heterogeneous clinical presentation; the fact that ethically sensitive genes are hidden by these panels is an added advantage (14).

Whole exome sequencing has obvious applications both in medical diseases (15) and in surgical pathology (16–18). It can even be performed on a single cancer cell (19), or on a single embryonic cell for preimplantation genetic diagnosis or screening (20,21).

Transcriptome sequencing

The *transcriptome* is the set of all RNA molecules, including mRNA, rRNA, tRNA, and other non-coding RNAs produced in one or a population of cells. It differs from the exome in that it includes only those RNA molecules found in a specified cell population (all of the coding and non-coding RNAs), and usually includes the amount or concentration of each RNA molecule. The transcriptome includes long non-coding RNAs that play an important role in the epigenetic control of gene transcription (10).

Epigenome sequencing (WEpS)

The *epigenome* consists of the record of the chemical changes to the DNA (e.g., cytosine methylation) and histone proteins of an organism; these changes can be passed down from one cell to its descendants, and to an organism's offspring. Changes to the epigenome can result in changes to the structure of chromatin and control the transcription of the genome. Tumor cells do not need to mutate to become malignant, they only need to reactivate embryonic dormant genes. Cells reactivating proto-oncogenes, telomerase, angiogenic factors, and enzymes digesting the extracellular matrix become more aggressive; changing the cell-adhesion molecules (CAMs) on their cytoplasmic membrane promotes metastasis, and the specific CAM determines where metastases implant. Epigenetic alterations can also silence genes that should normally be active; silencing tumor-suppressor genes, inhibitors of angiogenesis, and CAMs that glue cells to their neighbors and thus prevent their migration away from their normal site also promote aggressivity during clonal evolution. During the development of neoplasia and of clonal evolution, such epigenetic alterations are more common than mutations.

Studying the epigenome of a cancer allows the determination of the genes that are reactivated and those that are abnormally silenced. New therapeutic agents can make epigenetic modifications, but these cannot yet be targeted to specific genes, for activation or inactivation (22–25). Epigenetic therapy of solid tumors has met with limited success, but such regimens hold greater promise for hematologic malignancies (26).

Thousands of human cancers have been subjected to WEpS. It should not come as a surprise that in cancers, many genes that control the epigenome are mutated, leading to a synergy between conventional mutations and epigenetic alterations: genetic and epigenetic mechanisms are intertwined and synergize during tumorigenesis. Epigenetic mechanisms can lead to genetic mutations, and genetic mutations in epigenetic regulators lead to an altered epigenome. This collusion between epigenetics and genetics in cancer has been reviewed (27).

Future perspectives

The pathologist's role is to give the most accurate diagnosis possible, in order to allow clinicians to give the treatment that is best suited for that child–tumor pair. We are entering an era of personalized medicine, where a patient's characteristics can be assessed to maximize treatment. *MYCN* amplification was found to correlate with an aggressive course,

and this status directs which chemotherapeutic course is given to neuroblastoma patients. The KIT cascade is inhibited by imatinib in gastrointestinal stromal tumors, with a dramatically increased survival. Breast cancers shown to overexpress *HER2* by FISH respond to Herceptin. The new sequencing techniques hold the promise of detecting *all* the genes that can be specifically targeted in a patient's cancer, with a single test. Furthermore, this test will yield other lines of important information, such as regarding the enzymes involved in the metabolic pathway of the drugs used, which impact on their half-life and thus on their dosage regimen. These techniques are at our doorstep (28).

In summary, there are two general types of diagnostic modalities: those that assess DNA, and those that assess RNA. The distinction is fundamental, as DNA-based tests yield no information on transcription, i.e., whether a gene is active or not in the tissue studied.

Acknowledgements

Dr Oligny is grateful to Drs Anne-Laure Rougemont, Dorothée Dal Soglio and Jean-Christophe Fournet of CHU Sainte-Justine, Université de Montréal, for allowing inclusion of their data (Figure 15.17C-E). Drs Isabelle Thiffault and Roland Auer are thanked for their insightful criticism of this manuscript.

References

1. Wilson GN, Oligny LL. Mechanisms of development and growth: molecular genetics. In Gilbert-Barness E, editor, *Potter's Pathology of the Fetus, Infant and Child*. Philadelphia, PA: Elsevier; 2007:3–64.

2. Gilbert-Barnes E, Oligny LL. Chromosomal abnormalities. In Gilbert-Barness E, editor, *Potter's Pathology of the Fetus, Infant and Child*. Philadelphia, PA: Elsevier; 2007:213–75.

3. www.wikipedia.com provides more in depth information on most of these techniques.

4. Patrinos G, Ansorge W. *Molecular Diagnostics*, first edn. Philadelphia, PA: Elsevier; 2009.

5. Coleman WB, Tsongalis GJ. *Molecular Pathology: The Molecular Basis of Human Disease*, first edn. Philadelphia, PA: Elsevier; 2009.

6. Miller DT, Adam MP, Aradhya S, *et al.* Consensus statement: chromosomal microarray is a first-tier clinical diagnostic test for individuals with developmental disabilities or congenital anomalies. Am. J. Hum. Genet. 2010;**86**:749–64.

7. Gullapalli RR, Desai KV, Santana-Santos L, Kant JA, Becich MJ. Next generation sequencing in clinical medicine: Challenges and lessons for pathology and biomedical informatics. J. Pathol. Inform. 2012;**3**:40.

8. May T, Zusevics KL, Strong KA. On the ethics of clinical whole genome sequencing of children. Pediatrics 2013;**132**(2):207–9.

9. Green RC, Berg JS, Grody WW, *et al.* ACMG recommendations for reporting of incidental findings in clinical exome and genome sequencing. http://www.acmg.net/docs/ACMG_Releases_Highly-Anticipated_Recommendations_on_Incidental_Findings_in_Clinical_Exome_and_Genome_Sequencing.pdf (accessed November 2013).

10. Derrien T, Guigo R, Johnson R. The long non-coding RNAs: A new (p)layer in the "dark matter". Front Genet. 2011;**2**:107.

11. Meyerson M, Gabriel S, Getz G. Advances in understanding cancer genomes through second-generation sequencing. Nat. Rev. Genet. 2010;**11**:685–96.

12. Majewski J, Schwartzentruber J, Lalonde E, Montpetit A, Jabado N. What can exome sequencing do for you? J. Med. Genet. 2011;**48**:580–9.

13. Schiffman JD, Geller JI, Mundt E, *et al.* Update on pediatric cancer predisposition syndromes. Pediatr. Blood Cancer 2013;**60**:1247–52.

14. Bell CJ, Dinwiddie DL, Miller NA, *et al.* Carrier testing for severe childhood recessive diseases by next-generation sequencing. Sci. Transl. Med. 2011;**3**:65ra4.

15. Foo JN, Liu JJ, Tan EK. Whole-genome and whole-exome sequencing in neurological diseases. Nat. Rev. Neurol. 2012;**8**:508–17.

16. Meldrum C, Doyle MA, Tothill RW. Next-generation sequencing for cancer diagnostics: A practical perspective. Clin. Biochem. Rev. 2011;**32**:177–95.

17. Ku CS, Cooper DN, Ziogas DE, *et al.* Research and clinical applications of cancer genome sequencing. Curr. Opin. Obstet. Gynecol. 2013;**25**:3–10.

18. Shyr D, Liu Q. Next generation sequencing in cancer research and clinical application. Biol. Proced Online. 2013;**15**:4.

19. Navin N, Hicks J. Future medical applications of single-cell sequencing in cancer. Genome Med. 2011;**3**:31.

20. Martín J, Cervero A, Mir P, *et al.* The impact of next-generation sequencing technology on preimplantation genetic diagnosis and screening. Fertil. Steril. 2013;**99**:1054–61.

21. Handyside AH. 24-chromosome copy number analysis: A comparison of available technologies. Fertil. Steril. 2013;**100**:595–602.

22. Baylin SB, Jones PA. A decade of exploring the cancer epigenome: biological and translational implications. Nat. Rev Cancer 2011;**11**:726–34.

23. Karpathakis A, Dibra H, Thirlwell C. Neuroendocrine tumours: cracking the epigenetic code. Endocr. Relat. Cancer 2013;**20**:R65–82.

24. Batora NV, Sturm D, Jones DT, *et al.* Transitioning from genotypes to epigenotypes: Why the time has come for medulloblastoma epigenomics. Neuroscience. 2014;**264**:171–85.

25. Clarke J, Penas C, Pastori C, *et al.* Epigenetic pathways and glioblastoma treatment. Epigenetics 2013;**8**:785–95.

26. Azad N, Zahnow CA, Rudin CM, Baylin SB. The future of epigenetic therapy in solid tumours: Lessons from the past. Nat. Rev. Clin. Oncol. 2013;**10**:256–66.

27. You JS, Jones PA. Cancer genetics and epigenetics: two sides of the same coin? Cancer Cell. 2012;**22**:9–20.

28. Roychowdhury S, Iyer MK, Robinson DR, *et al.* Personalized oncology through integrative high-throughput sequencing: A pilot study. Sci. Transl. Med. 2011;**3**:111ra121.

Index

498

Terms and Conditions of Use

1. License

a) Cambridge University Press grants the customer a non-exclusive license to use this DVD-ROM **either** (i) on a single computer for use by one or more people at different times **or** (ii) by a single user on one or more computers (provided the DVD-ROM is used only on one computer at one time and is always used by the same user).

b) The customer must not: (i) copy or authorize the copying of the DVD-ROM, except that library customers may make one copy for archiving purposes only, (ii) translate the DVD-ROM, (iii) reverse-engineer, disassemble, or decompile the DVD-ROM, (iv) transfer, sell, assign, or otherwise convey any portion of the DVD-ROM from a network or mainframe system.

c) The customer may use the DVD-ROM for educational and research purposes as follows: Material contained on a simple screen may be printed out and used within a fair use/fair dealing context; the images may be downloaded for bona fide teaching purposes but may not be further distributed in any form or made available for sale. An archive copy of the product may be made where libraries have this facility, on condition that the copy is for archiving purposes only and is not used or circulated within or beyond the library where the copy is made.

2. Copyright

All material within the DVD-ROM is protected by copyright. All rights are reserved except those expressly licensed.

3. Liability

To the extent permitted by applicable law, Cambridge University Press accepts no liability for consequential loss or damage of any kind resulting from use of the DVD-ROM or from errors or faults contained in it.

Every effort has been made in preparing this content to provide accurate and up-to-date information which is in accord with accepted standards and practice at the time of publication. Nevertheless, the authors, editors and publishers can make no warranties that the information contained herein is totally free from error, not least because clinical standards are constantly changing through research and regulation. The authors, editors and publishers therefore disclaim all liability for direct or consequential damages resulting from the use of this content. Users are strongly advised to pay careful attention to information provided by the manufacturer of any drugs or equipment that they plan to use.

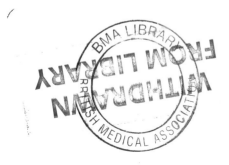